ACUTE CARE HANDBOOK FOR PHYSICAL THERAPISTS

FOURTH EDITION

ACUTE CARE HANDBOOK FOR PHYSICAL THERAPISTS

Jaime C. Paz, PT, DPT, MS
Associate Chair
Clinical Professor
Division of Physical Therapy
Walsh University
North Canton, Ohio

Michele P. West, MS, PT
Physical Therapist
St. Joseph Hospital
Nashua, New Hampshire

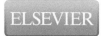

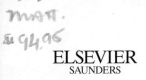

(handwritten notes) 12/13 matt. $94.95

ELSEVIER
SAUNDERS

3251 Riverport Lane
St. Louis, Missouri 63043

Notices

Knowledge and best practice in this field are constantly changing. As new research and experience broaden our understanding, changes in research methods, professional practices, or medical treatment may become necessary.

Practitioners and researchers must always rely on their own experience and knowledge in evaluating and using any information, methods, compounds, or experiments described herein. In using such information or methods they should be mindful of their own safety and the safety of others, including parties for whom they have a professional responsibility.

With respect to any drug or pharmaceutical products identified, readers are advised to check the most current information provided (i) on procedures featured or (ii) by the manufacturer of each product to be administered, to verify the recommended dose or formula, the method and duration of administration, and contraindications. It is the responsibility of practitioners, relying on their own experience and knowledge of their patients, to make diagnoses, to determine dosages and the best treatment for each individual patient, and to take all appropriate safety precautions.

To the fullest extent of the law, neither the Publisher nor the authors, contributors, or editors, assume any liability for any injury and/or damage to persons or property as a matter of products liability, negligence or otherwise, or from any use or operation of any methods, products, instructions, or ideas contained in the material herein.

Vice President and Publisher: Linda Duncan
Content Strategist: Jolynn Gower
Content Development Specialist: Megan Fennell
Publishing Services Manager: Catherine Jackson
Senior Project Manager: David Stein
Design Direction: Paula Catalano

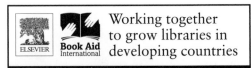

Working together to grow libraries in developing countries

www.elsevier.com • www.bookaid.org

Printed in the United States

Last digit is the print number: 9 8 7 6 5 4 3 2 1

Contributors to the Fourth Edition

Sean M. Collins, PT, ScD
Associate Professor of Physical Therapy
    and Biomedical Engineering
Director, Human Assessment Lab
College of Health Sciences
University of Massachusetts–Lowell
Lowell, Massachusetts

Konrad J. Dias, PT, DPT, CCS
Associate Professor
Physical Therapy Program
Maryville University of St. Louis
St. Louis, Missouri

Margarita V. DiVall, PharmD
Associate Clinical Professor
Director of Assessment
School of Pharmacy
Northeastern University
Boston, Massachusetts

Cathy S. Elrod, PhD, PT
Chair and Associate Professor
Department of Physical Therapy
Marymount University
Arlington, Virginia

Harold Merriman, PT, PhD, CLT
Associate Professor
General Medicine Coordinator
Doctor of Physical Therapy Program
Department of Health & Sport Science
University of Dayton
Dayton, Ohio

Kathryn Panasci, PT, DPT, CBIS, CWS
Assistant Professor
Doctor of Physical Therapy Program
Department of Rehabilitation Sciences
Texas Tech University Health Sciences Center
Lubbock, Texas

Danika Quinlan, PT, DPT
Staff Physical Therapist
Dayton VAMC
Dayton, Ohio

Hillary A. Reinhold, DPT, CBIS
Senior Physical Therapist
Inpatient Complex Medical
Spaulding Hospital–Cambridge
Cambridge, Massachusetts

Paul E.H. Ricard, PT, DPT, CCS
Clinical Specialist
Rehabilitation Services
Brigham and Women's Hospital
Boston, Massachusetts;
Adjunct Faculty
Physical Therapy
University of Massachusetts–Lowell
Lowell, Massachusetts;
Part-Time Lecturer
Physical Therapy
Northeastern University
Boston, Massachusetts

Falguni Vashi, PT, DPT
Physical Therapist
Rehabilitation Services
St. Joseph Hospital
Nashua, New Hampshire

Karen Vitak, PT, DPT
Clinical Assistant Professor
Director of Clinical Education
School of Health Sciences
Cleveland State University
Cleveland, Ohio

Jessika Vizmeg, PT, DPT
Staff Physical Therapist
St. Vincent Charity Medical Center
Cleveland, Ohio

Kelsea A. Ziegler
Bouvé College of Health Sciences
School of Pharmacy
Northeastern University
Boston, Massachusetts

Contributors to Previous Editions

James J. Gaydos, MS, PT
Senior Physical Therapist
Department of Inpatient Acute Care
New England Baptist Hospital
Boston, Massachusetts
Musculoskeletal System

Marka Gehrig, MPT
Department of Rehabilitation Medicine
The Cleveland Clinic Foundation
Cleveland, Ohio;
Therapy Partners
Cleveland, Ohio
Musculoskeletal System

Jennifer Lee Hunt, MS, PT
Physical Therapist
Rehabilitation Services
Lahey Clinic
Burlington, Massachusetts
Organ Transplantation

Marie Jarell-Gracious, PT
Owner
Specialty Care
Mokena, Illinois
Burns and Wounds

Kimberly Knowlton, PT
Clinical Lead Physical Therapist
Rehabilitation Services
University of Massachusetts Memorial Medical Center
Worcester, Massachusetts
Burns and Wounds

Eileen F. Lang, PT, DPT
Senior Physical Therapist
Rehabilitation Services
Lahey Clinic North Shore
Peabody, Massachusetts
Medical-Surgical Equipment in the Acute Care Setting

V. Nicole Lombard, MS, PT
Staff Physical Therapist
Department of Physical Therapy
New England Baptist Hospital
Boston, Massachusetts
Infectious Diseases

Rachael Maiocco, MSPT
Physical Therapist
Brigham and Women's Hospital
Boston, Massachusetts
Infectious Diseases

Cheryl L. Maurer, PT
Senior Physical Therapist
Outpatient Physical Therapy Services
Massachusetts General Hospital
Boston, Massachusetts
Musculoskeletal System

Leah Moinzadeh, PT
Physical Therapist
Inpatient Rehabilitation
Rehabilitation Services
Lahey Clinic
Burlington, Massachusetts
Organ Transplantation

Jackie A. Mulgrew, PT, CCS
Clinical Specialist
Physical Therapy Services
Massachusetts General Hospital
Boston, Massachusetts
Circulatory Assist Devices

David Nicoloro, PT, MS
In-Patient Physical Therapy Coordinator
Department of Rehabilitation Services
Newton-Wellesley Hospital
Newton, Massachusetts;
Clinical Instructor
Northeastern University
Department of Physical Therapy
Boston, Massachusetts
Gastrointestinal System

Kara O'Leary, MS, PT, CCS
Senior Physical Therapist
Inpatient Physical Therapy and Outpatient
   Pulmonary Rehabilitation
Rehabilitation Services
Lahey Clinic
Burlington, Massachusetts
Pulmonary System

Susan Polich, PT, MA (ASCP), MEd
Assistant Clinical Specialist
Department of Physical Therapy
Northeastern University
Boston, Massachusetts;
Adjunct Instructor
Physical Therapy Assistant Program
Community College of Rhode Island
Newport, Rhode Island
Oncology
Fluid and Electrolyte Imbalances

Jason D. Rand, PT
Physical Therapist
Inpatient Physical Therapy Services
Winthrop University Hospital
Mineola, New York
Amputation

Marie R. Reardon, PT
Clinical Specialist
Inpatient Physical Therapy Services
Massachusetts General Hospital
Boston, Massachusetts
Musculoskeletal System

Jennifer A. Silva, MS, PT
Physical Therapist
Outpatient Rehabilitation Center
South Shore Hospital
South Weymouth, Massachusetts
Functional Tests

Timothy J. Troiano, PT
Senior Physical Therapist
Outpatient Physical Therapy Services
Massachusetts General Hospital
Boston, Massachusetts
Oncology

For my loving wife, Tallie, and my spirited boys,
Will and Henry—thanks for bringing life to me.

To Nay and Tay, thank you for the gift of promise
and hope.

J.C.P.

For my husband, Jim, the reader...
and the many new chapters in our life.

For my daughters, Isabelle and Genevieve,
you make motherhood an honor and a true pleasure.

For my sister, Marie, an author in her own right.

M.P.W.

Preface

Acute Care Handbook for Physical Therapists was originally developed to provide clinicians with a handy reference for patient care in the hospital setting. It was created primarily for physical therapy students and clinicians unfamiliar with entry-level acute care practice. This handbook was never intended to be a formal comprehensive textbook; however, over the past three editions, many students and physical therapy programs have adopted this reference as part of their curricula. Given the recent advances in acute care literature and practice, we are thankful to be able to contribute to this area of clinical practice.

For this edition, we have retained past contributors and again have added new contributors from around the country, providing this edition with a broader perspective. Four of these new contributors are faculty members, which helps this edition be more commensurate with the advancement of the profession toward an entry-level clinical doctorate degree. The overall mix of clinicians and faculty as contributors provides a good balance of clinically applicable information that is current with evidence.

Thus the fourth edition was revised to serve its original purpose and includes a revision of all chapters with updated literature, available at the time of revision, to assist with implementing evidence-based practice in this setting, such as:
- A review of anticoagulation and international normalized ratio (INR) parameters.
- Information on minimally invasive surgery for cardiac patients.
- Updates on bariatric surgery and physical therapy management.
- Burn and wound care management by a certified wound care specialist.
- A more streamlined orthopedic chapter aimed at facilitating clinically applicable information.
- Information on multimodal neuromonitoring.
- An updated pharmacology chapter written by a pharmacology expert that includes pharmacologic implications for physical therapists concerning medication side effects and the use of combination drugs.
- Expanded sections on standardized outcome measures that are appropriate to clinical practice in the acute care setting.
- Pertinent issues related to the acute care setting including documentation, patient confidentiality, electronic health records, latex allergy, fall risk prevention, and medication reconciliation.
- Unique considerations including intensive care unit (ICU) psychosis, alcohol withdrawal syndrome, and end-of-life issues.

- An improved design that includes a new order of chapters, with each chapter formatted to highlight informative tables and clinical tips.

As a member of the health care team, the physical therapist is often expected to understand hospital protocol, safety, medical-surgical "lingo," and the many aspects of patient care from the emergency room setting to the ICU to the general ward. This handbook is therefore intended to be a resource to aid in the interpretation and understanding of the medical-surgical aspects of acute care.

Each chapter about a major body system or diagnosis in this edition of *Acute Care Handbook for Physical Therapists* includes:
- A review of body structure and function.
- An overview of the medical-surgical evaluation of a patient admitted to the hospital, including pertinent diagnostic procedures and laboratory tests.
- A review of health conditions that emphasizes information pertinent to physical therapy management.
- Guidelines for physical therapy examination and intervention.

Clinical Tips appear throughout each chapter. These helpful hints are intended to maximize safety, quality, and efficiency of care. These clinical tips are suggestions from the editors and contributors that, from clinical experience, have proved to be valuable in acclimating therapists to the acute care setting. With advances in literature pertaining to acute care, more of these tips have become validated and thus are referenced accordingly in this new edition.

It is important to remember that all the information presented in this book is intended to serve as a guide to stimulate independent critical thinking within the scope of practice of physical therapy and the spectrum of medical-surgical techniques and trends. As health care practice continues to evolve with either shortened lengths of stay or the creation of new types of settings, clinicians will need to adapt information to the best of their ability. As is the case with evidence-based practice, this reference should serve as one of the many resources involved with clinical decision making. Developing and maintaining a rapport with the medical-surgical team are highly recommended because the open exchange of information among professionals is invaluable. We believe this new edition of *Acute Care Handbook for Physical Therapists* can enhance the clinical experience by providing readers with valuable information while they are reviewing charts, preparing for therapy intervention, and making clinical decisions in the acute care setting.

J.C.P.
M.P.W.

Acknowledgments

We offer sincere gratitude to the following people:
- Kathy Falk, Jolynn Gower, and Elsevier for their confidence in creating a fourth edition of this book.
- Megan Fennell for her vision and creativity in helping redesign the format of the textbook along with her endless supply of patience, support, guidance, and resourcefulness during the editorial process.
- David Stein and his colleagues for their high level of professionalism and dedication toward producing a high-quality text.
- The contributors—both past and present—we sincerely appreciate your expertise and the time taken out of your lives to enhance this textbook.
- The many patients and students, who continually challenge yet enrich our lives, both professionally and personally.

Personal thanks from Jaime to the following:
- Tallie, for all her support and positive encouragement during this revision.
- Michele West, for her ongoing editorial contributions, insights, and ideas, which continually add value to this text.
- Katherine Valek for her work in providing research assistance to the Oncology chapter.
- Maggie Zronek and Susan Shultz for their help in gathering articles for the Genitourinary and Endocrine chapters.

- The community at Walsh University for providing an atmosphere of collegiality and professional development.
- The many clinicians from around the country who have spoken to me and offered positive feedback and suggestions for this textbook to help make it a true resource for them.
- My faith and church community who has helped me to see beyond the scope of everyday life.

Personal thanks from Michele to the following:
- My husband, Jim, for your patience and understanding during the writing of this manuscript, especially during the summertime.
- My daughters Isabelle and Genevieve, for motivating me in many ways.
- My family and friends, who offered encouragement throughout the publishing process.
- My co-workers and patients, who inspire me to become a better clinician.
- Erin Monahan, for your assistance with articles on telemetry.
- Beth Derego, for your insight on current post-anesthesia nursing care.
- Cindy Sloan, Medical Librarian at St. Joseph Hospital, for your assistance with literature searches.

Contents

CHAPTER 1

Acute Care Setting

Michele P. West

CHAPTER OBJECTIVES

The objectives of this chapter are the following:

1. Review the basic safety guidelines and principles in the hospital setting for the physical therapist and the patient
2. Discuss the multisystem effects of prolonged bed rest that can occur with hospitalization and the relevant physical therapy considerations
3. Review the unique characteristics of and patient response(s) to the intensive care unit
4. Review briefly alcohol abuse and alcohol withdrawal syndrome
5. Discuss end-of-life issues and palliative care concepts

PREFERRED PRACTICE PATTERNS

The acute care setting is multifactorial and applies to many body systems. For this reason, specific practice patterns are not delineated in this chapter. Please refer to Appendix A for a complete list of the preferred practice patterns to identify the most applicable practice pattern for a given diagnosis.

The physical therapist must have an appreciation for the distinct aspects of inpatient acute care. The purpose of this chapter is to present briefly information about the acute care environment, including safety and the use of physical restraints; the effects of prolonged bed rest; end-of-life issues; and some of the unique circumstances, conditions, and patient responses encountered in the hospital setting.

The acute care or hospital setting is a unique environment with protocols and standards of practice and safety that may not be applicable to other areas of health care delivery, such as an outpatient clinic or school system. Hospitals are designed to accommodate a wide variety of routine, urgent, or emergent patient care needs. The clinical expertise of the staff and the medical-surgical equipment used in the acute care setting (see Chapter 18) reflect these needs. The nature of the hospital setting is to provide 24-hour care; thus the patient, family, and caregivers are faced with the physical, psychologic, and emotional sequelae of illness and hospitalization. This can include the response(s) to a change in daily routine; a lack of privacy and independence; or perhaps a response to a potential lifestyle change, medical crisis, critical illness, or long-term illness.

Safe Caregiver and Patient Environment

Patient safety is a top priority. The physical therapist should strive to keep the patient safe at all times, comply with hospital initiatives that maximize patient safety, and understand the

Joint Commission's (TJC) annual National Patient Safety Goals. Basic guidelines for providing a safe caregiver and patient environment include the following:

- Always follow Standard Precautions, including thorough hand washing. Refer to Table 13-3 for a summary of infection-prevention precautions, including airborne, droplet, and contact precautions.
- Be familiar with the different alarm systems, including how and when to use such equipment as code call buttons, staff assist buttons, and bathroom call lights.
- Know the facility's policy for accidental chemical, waste, or sharps exposure, as well as emergency procedures for evacuation, fire, internal situation, and natural disaster. Know how to contact the employee health service and hospital security.
- Confirm that you are with the correct patient before initiating physical therapy intervention according to the facility's policy. Most acute care hospitals require two patient identifiers (by patient report or on an identification bracelet), such as name and hospital identification (ID) number or another patient-specific number. A patient's room number or physical location may not be used as an identifier.[1] Notify the nurse if a patient is missing an ID bracelet.
- Elevate the height of the bed as needed to ensure your use of proper body mechanics when performing a bedside intervention (e.g., stretching or bed mobility training).
- Leave the bed or chair (e.g., stretcher chair) in the lowest position with wheels locked after physical therapy intervention is complete. Leave the top bed rails up for all patients.
- Use only equipment (e.g., assistive devices, recliner chairs, wheelchairs) that is in good working condition. If equipment is unsafe, then label it as such and contact the appropriate personnel to repair or discard it.
- Keep the patient's room as neat and clutter free as possible to minimize the risk of trips and falls. Pick up objects that have fallen on the floor. Secure electrical cords (i.e., for the bed or intravenous pumps) out of the way. Keep small equipment used for physical therapy intervention (e.g., cuff weights) in a drawer or closet. Do not block the doorway or pathway to and from the patient's bed.
- Store assistive devices at the perimeter of the room when not in use. However, when patients are allowed to ambulate independently in their rooms with an assistive device, the device should be in safe proximity to the patient.
- Provide enough light for the patient to move about the room or read educational materials.
- Reorient a patient who is confused or disoriented. In general, patients who are confused are assigned rooms closer to the nursing station.
- Always leave the patient with the call bell or other communication devices within close reach. These include eyeglasses and hearing aids.
- Make recommendations to nursing staff members for the use of bathroom equipment (e.g., tub bench or raised toilet seat) if the patient has functional limitations that may pose a safety risk.
- Dispose of linens, dressings, sharps, and garbage according to the policies of the facility.

Fall Risk

A fall is defined as "an event which results in a person coming to rest inadvertently on the ground or floor or other lower level."[2] A fall by this definition applies to the conscious or unconscious patient. For hospitalized patients, a fall is one of the most common adverse events and accounts for increased hospital personnel needs, length of stay, cost, and morbidity and mortality, especially among older adults.[3] Fall prevention during hospitalization includes a fall risk assessment performed on admission by the nurse. Further prevention of falls involves a multitude of strategies and safety initiatives to prevent falls, including personal alarms, proper footwear, medication review, frequent toileting, adequate room lighting, and routine mobilization. The standardized fall risk assessment performed on admission varies from hospital to hospital; however, common components include prior falls, age, polypharmacy, the use of diuretics or antihypertensive agents, bowel and bladder incontinence, visual acuity, presence of lines and tubes, medical conditions associated with falls, and a history of dementia or impaired short-term memory.[4] Depending on the fall risk score and the subsequent designation of increased fall risk, a patient is identified as such (depending on hospital policy) by a specialized wristband, on a sign at the doorway to the room, and in the medical record.

Use of Restraints

The use of a restraint may be indicated for the patient who is at risk of self-harm or harm to others, including health care providers, or is so active or agitated that essential medical-surgical care cannot be completed.[5] A restraint is defined as "any manual method, physical or mechanical device, material or equipment that immobilizes or reduces the ability of a patient to move his or her arms, legs, body or head freely; or a drug or medication when it is used as a restriction to manage the patient's behavior or restrict the patient's freedom of movement and is not a standard treatment or dosage for the patient's condition."[6]

The most common types of physical restraints in the acute care setting are wrist or ankle restraints, mitt restraints, or a vest restraint. Side rails on a bed are considered a restraint when all four are raised.[7] The use of restraint requires an order from a licensed independent practitioner that must be updated approximately every 24 hours.[8] A patient must be monitored on a frequent basis, either continuously, hourly, or every 4 to 8 hours, depending on the type of restraint used or according to facility policy and procedure.[8]

Although restraints are used with the intent to prevent injury, morbidity and mortality risks are associated with physical restraint use.[7] Most notably, the presence of the restraint and the resultant limitation of patient mobility can increase agitation. New-onset pressure ulcers or alterations in skin integrity, urinary incontinence, constipation, pneumonia, and physical deconditioning also can occur.[9] Musculoskeletal or nerve injury from prolonged positioning or from pushing or pulling on the restraint or strangulation/asphyxiation from the restraint as a result of entrapment can occur if the patient is not monitored closely.[9] Many hospital care plans and policies reflect the trend of minimizing restraint use and using alternatives to restraints, including scheduled toileting, food and fluids, sleep, and walking; diversions such as reading material or activity kits; recruitment of help from family or other patient care companions; relaxation techniques; camouflaging medical devices; and adequate pain management.[9] Nonrestraint strategies for minimizing fall risk include bed and chair alarms that alert staff when a patient has moved from a bed or chair unassisted.

General guidelines most applicable to the physical therapist for the use of restraints include the following:

- Use a slipknot to secure a restraint rather than a square knot if the restraint does not have a quick-release connector. This ensures that the restraint can be untied rapidly in an emergency.
- Do not secure the restraint to a moveable object (e.g., the bed rail), to an object that the patient is not lying or sitting on, or where the patient can easily remove it.
- Ensure the restraint is secure but not too tight. Place two fingers between the restraint and the patient to be sure circulation and skin integrity are not impaired.
- Always replace the restraint after a physical therapy session.
- Be sure the patient does not trip on the ties or "tails" of the restraint during functional mobility training.
- Consult with the health care team to determine whether a patient needs to have continued restraint use, especially if you feel the patient's behavior and safety have improved.
- Remember that the side effects of a chemical restraint may make a patient drowsy or alter his or her mental status; thus participation in a physical therapy session may be limited.

Medication Reconciliation

Medication reconciliation is the process of comparing a list of the medication(s) a patient is taking to that which is ordered on admission, on transfer between areas of the hospital, and on discharge for the purpose of ensuring an up-to-date medication list.[10] Medication reconciliation has become an important safety initiative in hospitals to prevent medication errors such as inadvertent omission or duplication of a medication, incorrect dosing, and drug interactions and to ensure that all health care providers can access a similar and complete medication list.[11]

Latex Allergy

A latex allergy is a hypersensitivity to the proteins in natural rubber latex. If the reaction is immediate, then it is IgE-mediated with systemic symptoms resulting from histamine release.[12] If the reaction is delayed, typically 48 to 96 hours after exposure, then it is T cell–mediated with symptoms at the area of contact and related to the processing chemicals used in the production of natural rubber latex.[12] Signs and symptoms of an allergic reaction to latex may include urticaria, contact dermatitis, rhinitis, asthma, or even anaphylaxis.[13]

Natural rubber latex can be found in a multitude of products and equipment found in the acute care setting. The products most commonly used in the hospital setting include gloves, stethoscopes, blood pressure cuffs, Ambu bags, adhesive tape, electrode pads, catheters, tubes, and hand grips on assistive devices. Many hospitals have minimized or eliminated latex products, particularly powdered latex gloves; they have been replaced with vinyl products for the benefit of the patient and health care provider.

Between 5% and 10% of the general population has a sensitization to latex; health care workers have a greater incidence.[13] Persons with spina bifida, congenital or urogenital defects, indwelling urinary catheters or condom catheters, multiple childhood surgeries, occupational exposures to latex, or food allergies are at increased risk for latex allergy.[14] An association exists between latex sensitivity and food allergy, in which a person can have a cross-reactive protein allergy to a food (often a fruit) that is linked allergenically to natural rubber latex.[15] This cross-reactivity is known as latex-fruit syndrome; those fruits most strongly identified with a reaction include banana, kiwi, avocado, and chestnuts.[15] Although not all people with latex sensitivity will also be allergic to certain foods, awareness of the possibility is important.

If a patient has an allergy or hypersensitivity to latex, then it is documented in the medical record and at the patient's bedside. Hospitals will provide a special "latex-free kit," which consists of latex-free products for use with the patient. Health care providers may be at risk for developing latex allergy from increased exposure to latex in the work setting primarily from repeated latex glove use. The allergen is leached directly from the glove by skin moisture or from the powder in the glove or is inhaled when the allergen becomes airborne with glove use.[13] If you suspect a latex hypersensitivity or allergy, seek assistance from the employee health office or a primary care physician.

Effects of Prolonged Bed Rest

The effects of short-term (days to weeks) or long-term (weeks to months) bed rest can be deleterious and affect every organ system in the body. For the purposes of this discussion, bed rest incorporates immobilization, disuse, and recumbence. The physical therapist must recognize that a patient in the acute care setting is likely to have an alteration in physiology (i.e., a traumatic or medical-surgical disease or dysfunction) superimposed on bed rest, a second abnormal physiologic state.[16] In general, the physiologic consequences of bed rest include fluid volume redistribution, altered distribution of body weight and pressure, muscular inactivity, and aerobic deconditioning.[17]

The degree of impaired aerobic capacity is directly related to the duration of bed rest.[18] Most patients on bed rest have been in the intensive care unit (ICU) for many weeks with multisystem organ failure or hemodynamic instability requiring sedation and mechanical ventilation. Other clinical situations classically associated with long-term bed rest include severe burns and multitrauma, spinal cord injury, acute respiratory distress syndrome (ARDS), or grade IV nonhealing wounds of the lower extremity or sacrum. The decline of cardiac and pulmonary function occurs at a faster rate than musculoskeletal changes, especially in older adults, and the rate of recovery is generally slower than the initial decline.[17] It is beyond the scope of this book to discuss in detail the physiologic and cellular mechanisms of the sequelae of prolonged bed rest; however, Table 1-1 lists major systemic changes.

Physical Therapy Considerations

- Monitor vital signs carefully, especially during mobilization out of bed for the first few times.
- Progressively raise the head of the bed before or during a physical therapy session to allow blood pressure to regulate.
- Consider the use of lower extremity antiembolism stockings with or without elastic wrapping for the patient performing initial static sitting activities to minimize pooling of blood in the lower extremities if hypotension persists more than a few sessions.
- Use stretcher chairs (chairs that can position the patient from supine to different degrees of reclined or upright sitting) if

orthostatic hypotension or activity intolerance prevents standing activity or if the patient may need to quickly return to a supine position.
- Time frames for physical therapy goals will likely be longer for the patient who has been on prolonged bed rest.
- Supplement formal physical therapy sessions with independent or family-assisted therapeutic exercise for a more timely recovery.
- Be aware of the psychosocial aspects of prolonged bed rest. Sensory deprivation, boredom, depression, and a sense of loss of control can occur.[19] These feelings may manifest as emotional lability or irritability, and caregivers may incorrectly perceive the patient to be uncooperative.
- As much as the patient wants to be off bed rest, the patient will likely be fearful the first time out of bed, especially if

TABLE 1-1 Systemic Effects of Prolonged Bed Rest

Body System	Effects
Cardiac	Increased heart rate at rest and with submaximal exercise Decreased stroke volume and left ventricular end-diastolic volume at rest Decreased cardiac output, $\dot{V}O_{2max}$ with submaximal and maximal exercise Orthostatic hypotension
Hematologic	Decreased total blood volume, red blood cell mass, and plasma volume Increased hematocrit Venous stasis, hypercoagulability, and blood vessel damage (Virchow triad), causing increased risk of venous thromboembolism
Respiratory	Increased respiratory rate Decreased lung volumes and capacities, especially FRC, FVC, and FEV_1 Decreased mucociliary clearance Increased risk of pneumonia and pulmonary embolism Ventilation-perfusion mismatch
Gastrointestinal	Decreased appetite, fluid intake, bowel motility, and gastric bicarbonate secretion Gastroesophageal reflux Difficulty swallowing
Genitourinary	Increased mineral excretion, kidney stones, difficulty voiding, urinary retention, and overflow incontinence Decreased glomerular filtration rate Increased risk of urinary tract infection
Endocrine	Altered temperature and sweating responses, circadian rhythm, regulation of hormones, increased cortisol secretion, and glucose intolerance Decreased overall metabolism
Musculoskeletal	Muscle: increased muscle weakness (especially in antigravity muscles), atrophy, risk of contracture, weakened myotendinous junction, and altered muscle excitation Bone: disuse osteoporosis Joints: degeneration of cartilage, synovial atrophy, and ankylosis
Neurologic	Sensory and sleep deprivation Decreased dopamine, noradrenaline, and serotonin levels Depression, restlessness, insomnia Decreased balance, coordination, and visual acuity Increased risk of compression neuropathy Reduced pain threshold
Integumentary	Increased risk of pressure ulcer formation and skin infection
Body composition	Increased sodium, calcium, potassium, phosphorus, sulfur, and nitrogen loss Increased body fat and decreased lean body mass Fluid shift from the legs to the abdomen/thorax/head, diuresis, natriuresis, dehydration

Data from Buschbacher RM, Porter CD: Deconditioning, conditioning, and the benefits of exercise. In Braddom RL, editor: Physical medicine and rehabilitation, ed 2, Philadelphia, 2000, Saunders; Knight J, Nigam Y, Jones A: Effects of bedrest 1: cardiovascular, respiratory, and haemotological systems. Effects of bedrest 2: Gastrointestinal, endocrine, renal, reproductive, and nervous systems. Effects of bedrest 3: musculoskeletal and immune systems, skin and self-perception (website): http://www.nursingtimes.net. Accessed July 11, 2012.

FRC, Functional residual capacity; *FVC,* forced vital capacity; *FEV₁,* forced expiratory volume in 1 second; $\dot{V}O_{2max}$, maximum oxygen uptake.

the patient has insight into his or her muscular weakness and impaired aerobic capacity.

- Leave the patient with necessities or commonly used objects (e.g., the call bell, telephone, reading material, beverages, tissues) within reach to minimize feelings of confinement.

Intensive Care Unit Setting

The intensive care unit (ICU), as its name suggests, is a place of intensive medical-surgical care for patients who require continuous monitoring, usually in conjunction with therapies such as vasoactive medications, sedation, circulatory assist devices, and mechanical ventilation. ICUs may be named according to the specialized care that they provide, such as the coronary care unit (CCU) or surgical ICU (SICU). The patient in the ICU requires a high level of care; thus the nurse-to-patient ratio is 1:1 or 1:2.

Common Patient and Family Responses to the Intensive Care Unit

Psychosocial alterations and behavioral changes or disturbances can occur in the patient who is critically ill as a result of distress caused by physically or psychologically invasive, communication-impairing, or movement-restricting procedures.[20] When combined with the environmental and psychologic reactions to the ICU, mental status and personality can be altered. Environmental stressors can include crowding, bright overhead lighting, strong odors, noise, and touch associated with procedures or from those the patient cannot see.[18] Psychologic stressors can include diminished dignity and self-esteem, powerlessness, vulnerability, fear, anxiety, isolation, and spiritual distress.[21]

The patient's family usually is overwhelmed by the ICU. Family members may experience fear, shock, anxiety, helplessness, anger, and denial.[18,22] Like the patient, the family may be overwhelmed by the stimuli and technology of the ICU, in addition to the stress of a loved one's critical or life-threatening illness.

An acute state of delirium, often termed ICU delirium or psychosis, is a state of delirium that can occur during admission to the ICU. Delirium is a "disturbance in consciousness with inattention accompanied by a change in cognition or perceptual disturbance that develops over a short period of time (hours to days) and fluctuates over time."[19,23]

ICU delirium may be hyperactive (characterized by agitation and restlessness); hypoactive (characterized by withdrawal and flat affect or by decreased responsiveness); or mixed (a fluctuation between the two).[24]

Delirium in the ICU, which is reversible, is associated with many precipitating factors, including mechanical ventilation, opioid and benzodiazepine use, presence of restraints and lines, sleep deprivation, polypharmacy, pain, and the ICU environment.[19,25] Risk factors associated with delirium in the ICU include male gender, advanced age, malnutrition, and a history of dementia.[26] Conditions associated with delirium in the ICU include trauma, sepsis, hypoxia, metabolic disorders, dehydration, central nervous system (CNS) pathology such as stroke, and hip fracture.[26] ICU delirium can be assessed by standardized

tests. The most common is the Confusion Assessment Method for the Intensive Care Unit (CAM-ICU). It is a four-part assessment used in tandem with the Richmond Agitation-Sedation Scale (RASS) and has been validated for use with a verbal patient or a patient on mechanical ventilation.[25] Treatment for delirium consists of elimination or reduction of precipitating factors, antipsychotic medications (e.g., haloperidol), the discontinuation of nonessential medications, proper oxygenation, hydration, pain management, early mobilization, maximization of a normal sleep pattern, and the company of family or others.[23]

The transfer of a patient from the ICU to a general floor also can be a stress to the patient and family. Referred to as transfer anxiety, the patient and family may voice concerns of leaving staff members whom they have come to recognize and know by name; they may have to learn to trust new staff or fear that the level of care is inferior to that in the ICU.[22] To minimize this anxiety, the physical therapist may continue to treat the patient (if staffing allows), slowly transition care to another therapist, or assure the patient and family that the general goals of physical therapy are unchanged.

Critical Illness Polyneuropathy

Critical illness polyneuropathy (CIP), otherwise known as ICU neuropathy or the neuropathy of critical illness, is the acute or subacute onset of widespread symmetric weakness in the patient with critical illness, most commonly with sepsis, respiratory failure, multisystem organ failure, or septic inflammatory response syndrome (SIRS).[27] The patient presents with distal extremity weakness, wasting, and sensory loss, as well as paresthesia and decreased or absent deep tendon reflexes.[28,29] Frequently, CIP is discovered when the mechanically ventilated patient fails to wean from the ventilator; it is possibly the most common neuromuscular cause of prolonged ventilator dependence.[28] The clinical features that distinguish CIP from other neuromuscular disorders (e.g., Guillain-Barré syndrome) are a lack of ophthalmoplegia, dysautonomia, cranial nerve involvement, and normal cerebrospinal fluid analysis.[30] Nerve conduction studies show decreased motor and sensory action potentials.[30] The specific pathophysiology of critical illness polyneuropathy is unknown; however, it is hypothesized to be related to drug, nutritional, metabolic, and toxic factors; prolonged ICU stay; the number of invasive procedures; increased glucose level; decreased albumin level; and the severity of multisystem organ failure.[28] Medical management of CIP includes supportive and symptomatic care, treatment of the causative factor, and physical therapy. No proven cure exists for CIP; however, an intensive insulin regimen has been associated with a lower incidence of CIP.[31]

Critical Illness Myopathy

Critical illness myopathy (CIM), otherwise known as acute quadriplegic myopathy or acute steroid myopathy, is the acute or subacute onset of diffuse quadriparesis, respiratory muscle weakness, and decreased deep tendon reflexes[27] with exposure to short-term or long-term high-dose corticosteroids and simultaneous neuromuscular blockade.[32] Researchers suggest that neuromuscular blockade causes a functional denervation that renders muscle fibers vulnerable to the catabolic effects of steroids.[28] Muscle weakness appears to affect large proximal muscles, and sensation typically remains intact.[29] Diagnostic tests demonstrate elevated serum creatine kinase (CK) levels at the onset of the myopathy.

Three types of CIM exist:

- Thick filament myopathy,[32] which is highly associated with asthma requiring ventilator support, mildly increased CK levels, and muscle biopsy, does not show thick myosin filaments.
- Acute necrotizing myopathy, which is highly associated with myoglobulinuria, significantly increased CK levels, and muscle biopsy, shows widespread necrosis.
- Disuse (cachectic) myopathy, a diagnosis of exclusion associated with significant muscle wasting with muscle biopsy, shows Type II fiber atrophy.

Sleep Pattern Disturbance

The interruption or deprivation of the quality or hours of sleep or rest can interfere with a patient's energy level, personality, and ability to heal and perform tasks. The defining characteristics of sleep pattern disturbance are difficulty falling or remaining asleep with or without fatigue on awakening, drowsiness during the day, decreased overall functioning, inability to concentrate, and mood alterations.[33]

In the acute care setting, sleep disturbance may be related to frequent awakenings associated with a medical procedure or the need for nursing intervention (e.g., vital sign monitoring); pain; an inability to assume normal sleeping position; loss of routine or privacy; elevated noise level; and excessive daytime sleeping resulting from medication side effects, stress, or environmental changes.[34] Sleep pattern disturbance is often more prevalent in the older adult population because of changes in circadian rhythms, coexisting health conditions, and dementia.[35]

The physical therapist should be aware of the patient who has altered sleep patterns or difficulty sleeping because lack of sleep can affect a patient's ability to participate during a therapy session. The patient may have trouble concentrating and performing higher-level cognitive tasks. The pain threshold may be decreased, and the patient also may exhibit decreased emotional control.[36]

Substance Abuse and Withdrawal

The casual or habitual abuse of alcohol, drugs (e.g., cocaine), or medications (e.g., opioids) is a known contributor of acute and chronic illness, traumatic accidents, drowning, burn injury, and suicide.[37] The patient in the acute care setting may present with acute intoxication or drug overdose or with a known (i.e., documented) or unknown substance abuse problem.

The physical therapist is not involved in the care of the patient with acute intoxication or overdose until the patient is medically stable. However, the physical therapist may become involved secondarily when the patient presents with impaired strength, balance, coordination, and functional mobility as a result of chemical toxicity or prolonged bed rest.

The patient with unknown substance abuse who is hospitalized for days to weeks is a challenge to the hospital staff when substance withdrawal occurs. In this text, alcohol withdrawal is discussed because of its relatively high occurrence. Alcohol use disorders include alcohol abuse and alcohol dependence (alcoholism).

Data suggest that one in five patients admitted to a hospital or one in four medical-surgical patients has an alcohol use disorder.[38] An estimated 18 million persons in the United States have an alcohol use disorder.[39] Alcohol withdrawal syndrome (AWS) is an acute toxic state resulting from the sudden cessation of alcohol intake after prolonged alcohol consumption.[40] The signs and symptoms of AWS are the result of a hyperadrenergic state from increased CNS neuronal activity that attempts to compensate for the inhibition of neurotransmitters with chronic alcohol use.[41] The signs and symptoms of AWS begin 6 to 12 hours after alcohol use is discontinued; they may be mild, moderate, or severe and can continue to emerge 48 to 72 hours after admission[42]:

- Mild signs/symptoms of AWS include hypertension, tachycardia, fine tremor, diaphoresis, headache, nausea and vomiting, anxiety, and insomnia.
- Moderate signs/symptoms of AWS include persistent or worsened hypertension, tachycardia, and nausea and vomiting, in addition to moderate anxiety, agitation, and transient confusion.
- Severe AWS symptoms (formerly known as delirium tremens [DTs]) can include uncontrollable shaking, hallucinations, hypothermia, and seizure.

Interventions to prevent or minimize AWS include hydration, electrolyte replacement, adequate nutrition, thiamine, glucose, reality orientation, and the use of benzodiazepines. Optimally, an objective scale is used by the nursing staff to grade AWS symptoms and dose medication or other interventions accordingly. The Clinical Institute Withdrawal Assessment for Alcohol (CIWA-Ar) is the gold standard for grading withdrawal severity and guiding medical treatment.[38]

End-of-Life Issues

End-of-life issues are often complex moral, ethical, or legal dilemmas, or a combination of these, regarding a patient's vital physiologic functions, medical-surgical prognosis, quality of life, and personal values and beliefs.[43] End-of-life issues facing patients, family, and caregivers include the following:

- Resuscitation status
- Withholding and withdrawing medical therapies
- Palliative care
- Coma, vegetative state, and brain death

Resuscitation Status

Each patient has a "code" status. The designation *full code* means all appropriate efforts will be made to revive a patient after cardiopulmonary arrest. Another code status *do not resuscitate*

(DNR) is the predetermined decision to decline cardiopulmonary resuscitation, including defibrillation and pharmacologic cardioversion in case of cardiorespiratory arrest. The code status *do not intubate* (DNI) is the predetermined decision to decline intubation for the purpose of subsequent mechanical ventilation in case of respiratory arrest. Either full code or DNR and/or DNI status is documented officially in the medical record by the attending physician. If a patient has a DNR or DNI status, he or she will wear a wristband with that designation. The physical therapist must be aware of each patient's resuscitation or "code" status. DNR/DNI orders do not directly affect the physical therapy plan of care.

Withholding and Withdrawing Medical Therapies

Withholding support is not initiating a treatment because it is not beneficial for the patient, whereas withdrawing support is the discontinuation of a treatment (but not a discontinuation of care).[44] Forgoing treatment is the combination of withholding and withdrawing support, in which disease progression is allowed to take its course.[44] In the case of forgoing medical-surgical therapies, an order for "comfort measures only" (CMO) is written by the physician. The patient with CMO status receives medications for pain control or sedation or to otherwise eliminate distress. The patient on CMO status does not receive physical therapy.

Palliative Care

Over the past few years, the concept of palliative care has become an important component of acute care; many hospitals have created palliative care teams. The goal of palliative care is to "prevent and relieve suffering, and to support the best possible quality of life for patients and their families, regardless of their stage of disease or the need for other therapies, in accordance with their values and preferences."[45] Palliative care is not synonymous with hospice care: the patient does not have to forgo curative treatment, and the prognosis is not necessarily less than 6 months.[46] Palliative care affirms life and supports the dying process throughout the course of illness.[45] Palliative care is often interdisciplinary, including physical therapy, with an emphasis on pain and fatigue management or the relief of other symptoms. Key components of palliative care are spirituality, family involvement, and nontraditional therapies.

Physical therapy intervention in this patient population focuses on functional training, endurance training, energy conservation techniques, lymphedema management, the use of modalities/therapeutic exercise, and family/caregiver training to improve the quality of life during hospitalization or in preparation for home.[47] Physical therapists are uniquely equipped to meet the needs of this population because of the ability to provide a continuum of care, to provide services when a patient has a change in medical status, and to use a knowledge base encompassing movement dysfunction, ergonomics, and pain management.[48] The role of physical therapy in hospital-based palliative care may be consultative or ongoing.

Coma, Vegetative State, and Brain Death

The diagnosis of coma, vegetative state, or brain death can be devastating. These conditions involve unconsciousness and absent self-awareness but are distinct in terms of neurologic function and recovery. Coma is a state of unconsciousness without arousal or awareness characterized by a lack of eye opening and sleep/wake cycles with intact brain stem reflex responses; however, no meaningful interaction with the environment occurs.[49,50] Coma is a symptom of another condition such as neurologic disease (e.g., stroke), a mass (e.g., brain tumor), trauma (e.g., traumatic brain injury), or a metabolic derangement (e.g., encephalopathy); or it may be due to drug and alcohol overdose, poisoning, or infection; or it may be psychogenic.[49] A vegetative state (VS) is a transient state of wakefulness without awareness characterized by cyclic sleep patterns, spontaneous eye opening and movement, and normal body temperature yet a lack of purposeful responsiveness to stimuli, cognitive function, and speech. VS is considered persistent if it lasts longer than 1 month after an acute trauma; it is considered permanent 3 months after nontraumatic brain injury or 12 months after a traumatic brain injury.[50] The clinical criteria for brain death include the absence of brain stem reflexes or cerebral motor responses in addition to apnea, in the setting of a known irreversible cause typically with radiographic evidence of an acute catastrophic event.[51] Brain death usually is confirmed by cerebral angiography, somatosensory-evoked potential testing, electroencephalography, transcranial Doppler echography, or (^{99m}Tc-HMPAO) single-photon emission computed tomography.[52] Refer to Chapter 6 for more information on these neurologic diagnostic tests.

References

1. The Joint Commission: 2012 National Patient Safety Goals. NPSG01.01.01 Element of Performance (website): http://www.joint commission.org. Accessed July 11, 2012.
2. World Health Organization: Falls fact sheet no. 344. August 2010 (website): http://www.who.int/mediacentre/factsheets/fs344/en/index/html. Accessed July 22, 2012.
3. Ferrari M, Harrison B, Rawashdeh O et al: Clinical feasibility trial of a motion detection system for fall prevention in hospitalized older adult patients, Geriatr Nurs 33(3):177-183, 2012.
4. Day JR, Ramos LC, Hendrix CC: Fall prevention through patient partnerships, Nurse Pract 37(7):14-20, 2012.
5. Smith SF, Duell DJ, Martin BC, editors: Restraints. In Clinical nursing skills: basic to advanced skills, ed 5, Upper Saddle River, NJ, 2000, Prentice Hall, pp 139-146.
6. Department of Health and Human Services: Medicare and Medicaid programs: hospital conditions of participation: patients rights, CMS 42 CFR Part 482, Fed Regist 71(236):71383, 2006.
7. Craven R, Hirnle C, Jensen S: Safety. In Craven R, Hirnle C, Jensen S, editors: Fundamentals of nursing human health and function, ed 7, Philadelphia, 2013, Wolters Kluwer Health.

8. The Joint Commission: Provision of care, treatment, and services, CAMH Update 2, March 2012. Standard PC.03.05.05.

9. Radziewicz, RM, Amato S, Bradas C et al: Use of physical restraints with elderly patients. Hartford Institute for Geriatric Nursing (website): http://consultgerirn.org. Accessed July 11, 2012.

10. Agency for Healthcare Research and Quality, U.S. Department of Health & Human Services: Medication reconciliation (website): http://psnet.ahrq.gov/primer. Accessed July 21, 2012.

11. The Joint Commission: Sentinel event alert issue 35—January 25, 2006 (website): http://www.jointcommission.org/SentinelEvents. Accessed July 21, 2012.

12. American Latex Allergy Association: About latex allergy: definition (website): http://www.latexallergyresources.org. Accessed July 11, 2012.

13. Yunginger JW: Natural rubber latex allergy. In Adkinson NF et al, editors: Middleton's allergy: principles and practice, ed 7, St Louis, 2009, Mosby, pp 1019-1026.

14. Infection prevention and control. In Potter PA, Perry AG, Stockert PA et al, editors: Basic nursing, ed 7, St Louis, 2011, Mosby, pp 248-249.

15. Grier T: Latex allergy: latex cross-reactive foods fact sheet (website): http://www.latexallergyresource.org. Accessed July 11, 2012.

16. Downey RJ, Weissman C: Physiological changes associated with bed rest and major body injury. In Gonzalez EG, Myers SJ, Edelstein JE et al, editors: Downey and Darling's physiological basis of rehabilitation medicine, ed 3, Boston, 2001, Butterworth-Heinemann, p 449.

17. Dean E, Butcher S: Mobilization and exercises: physiological basis for assessment, evaluation, and training. In Frownfelter D, Dean E, editors: Cardiovascular and pulmonary physical therapy evidence to practice, ed 5, St Louis, 2013, Elsevier, pp 244-272.

18. Malone DJ: Bed rest, deconditioning, and hospital-acquired neuromuscular disorders. In Malone DJ, Bishop-Lindsay KL, editors: Physical therapy in acute care: a clinician's guide, Thorofare, NJ, 2006, Slack.

19. Knight J, Nigam Y, Jones A: Effects of bedrest 3: musculoskeletal and immune systems, skin and self-perception (website): http://www.nursingtimes.net. Accessed July 11, 2012.

20. Urban N: Patient and family responses to the critical care environment. In Kinney MR, Dunbar SB, Brooks-Brunn J et al, editors: AACN's clinical reference for critical care nursing, ed 4, St Louis, 1998, Mosby, pp 145-162.

21. Urden LD: Psychosocial alterations. In Urden LD, Stacy KM, Lough ME, editors: Critical care nursing diagnosis and management, ed 6, St Louis, 2010, Mosby, pp 75-91.

22. Urden LD: Patient and family education. In Urden LD, Stacy KM, Lough ME, editors: Critical care nursing diagnosis and management, ed 6, St Louis, 2010, Mosby, pp 58-74.

23. Vanderbilt University Medical Center, Center for Health Sciences Research: Delirium overview (website): http://www.mc.vanderbilt.edu/icudelirium/overview.html. Accessed July 20, 2012.

24. Vanderbilt University Medical Center: Confusion Assessment Method for the ICU (CAM-ICU), the complete training manual, revised edition, October 2010 (website): http://www.mc.vanderbilt.edu/icudelirium/docs/CAM_ICU_training.pdf. Accessed July 22, 2012.

25. Lough ME: Sedation, agitation, delirium: assessment and management. In Urden LD, Stacy KM, Lough ME, editors: Critical care nursing diagnosis and management, ed 6, St Louis, 2010, Mosby, pp 160-174.

26. Moldonado JR: Delirium in the acute care setting: characteristics, diagnosis and treatment, Crit Care Clin 24:657-702, 2008.

27. Centers for Disease Control and Prevention: Critical illness polyneuropathy critical illness myopathy (website): http://www.cdc.gov/nchs/data/icd9/icd501a.pdf. Accessed July 20, 2012.

28. Juel VC, Bleck TP: Neuromuscular disorders in the ICU. In Vincent JL et al, editors: Textbook of critical care, ed 6, Philadelphia, 2011, Saunders, pp 212-219.

29. Robinson E: Weakness after critical illness—just deconditioning? Or something more? Acute Care Perspect 15:7-9, 2006.

30. Latronico N, Bolton CF: Critical illness polyneuropathy and myopathy: a major cause of muscle weakness and paralysis, Lancet Neurol 10(10):931-941, 2011.

31. Lorin S, Nierman DM: Critical illness neuromuscular abnormalities, Crit Care Clin 18:553-568, 2002.

32. Chawla J, Gruener G: Management of critical illness polyneuropathy and myopathy, Neurol Clin 28:961-977, 2010.

33. Landis CA: Sleep and rest. In Craven R, Hirnle C, Jensen S, editors: Fundamentals of nursing human health and function, ed 7, Philadelphia, 2013, Wolters Kluwer Health, pp 1118-1143.

34. Sullivan SC: Sleep alterations and management. In Urden LD, Stacy KM, Lough ME, editors: Critical care nursing: diagnosis and management, ed 6, St Louis, 2010, Mosby, pp 92-107.

35. Cole C, Richards K: Sleep disruption in older adults, Am J Nurs 107:40-49, 2007.

36. Carpenito LJ: Sleep pattern disturbance. In Nursing diagnosis: application to clinical practice, ed 8, Philadelphia, 2000, Lippincott, pp 858-865.

37. Shaffer J: Substance abuse and withdrawal: alcohol, cocaine, and opioids. In Civetta JM, Taylor RW, Kirby RR, editors: Critical care, Philadelphia, 1997, Lippincott-Raven, pp 1511-1514.

38. Elliott DY, Geyer C, Lionetti T et al: Managing alcohol withdrawal in hospitalized patients, Nursing, April 22-30, 2012.

39. National Institute on Alcohol Abuse and Alcoholism: Alcohol use disorders (website): http://www.niaaa.nih.gov. Accessed July 20, 2012.

40. Meltzer SC, Bare BG, Hinkle JL et al, editors: Emergency nursing. In Brunner & Suddarth's textbook of medical-surgical nursing, ed 11, Philadelphia, 2007, Lippincott Williams & Wilkins, p 2549.

41. Jennings-Ingle S: The sobering facts about alcohol withdrawal syndrome, Nursing Made Incredibly Easy, January/February 2007.

42. Lussier-Cushing M et al, editors: Is your medical/surgical patient withdrawing from alcohol? Nursing 37(10):50-55, 2007.

43. Tidswell M, Jodka PG, Steingrub JS: Medical ethics and end-of-life care. In Irwin RS, Rippe JM, editors: Irwin and Rippe's intensive care medicine, ed 6, Philadelphia, 2008, Lippincott Williams & Wilkins, pp 239-249.

44. Levin PD, Sprung CL: Beyond technology: caring for the critically ill. In Vincent JL et al, editors: Textbook of critical care, ed 6, Philadelphia, 2011, Saunders, pp 1559-1562.

45. American Academy of Hospice and Palliative Medicine: Statement on clinical practice guidelines for quality palliative care (website): http://www.aahpm.org. Accessed July 12, 2012.

46. National Hospice and Palliative Care Organization: Living with illness: palliative care (website): http://www.caringinfo.org. Accessed July 12, 2012.

47. Ries E: A special place: physical therapy in hospice and palliative care, PT in Motion, March 2007 (serial online): http://www.apta.org. Accessed July 12, 2012.

48. The role of physical therapy in hospice and palliative care HOD P06-11-14-11(position paper) (website): http://www.apta.org. Accessed July 12, 2012.

49. Baumann JJ: Neurologic disorders and therapeutic management. In Urden LD, Stacy KM, Lough ME, editors: Critical care nursing diagnosis and management, ed 6, St Louis, 2010, Mosby, pp 724-763.

50. Stubgen JP, Plum F, Kochanek P: Coma. In Vincent JL et al, editors: Textbook of critical care, ed 6, Philadelphia, 2011, Saunders, pp 153-165.

51. Blazek JD, Burton MJ, Clark D et al: Organ donation and transplantation. In Urden LD, Stacy KM, Lough ME, editors: Critical care nursing diagnosis and management, ed 6, St Louis, 2010, Mosby, pp 1043-1090.

52. Jacobs T, Bleck TP: Determination of brain death. In Vincent JL et al, editors: Textbook of critical care, ed 6, Philadelphia, 2011, Saunders, pp 1585-1586.

The Medical Record

Michele P. West

CHAPTER OBJECTIVES

The objectives for this chapter are the following:

1. Briefly describe the medical record in paper and electronic forms, including medical record confidentiality and security
2. Review documentation standards for the physical therapist and physical therapist assistant
3. Describe the different components of the medical record, including a detailed outline of the admission history and physical

PREFERRED PRACTICE PATTERNS

The medical record is multifactorial and applies to many body systems. For this reason, specific practice patterns are not delineated in this chapter. Please refer to Appendix A for a complete list of the preferred practice patterns to identify the most applicable practice pattern for a given diagnosis.

The medical record, whether paper or electronic, is a legal document that chronicles a patient's clinical course during hospitalization and is the primary means of communication between the various clinicians caring for a single patient. More specifically, the medical record contains information about past or present symptoms and disease(s), test and examination results, interventions, and the medical-surgical outcome.[1] Additionally, the medical record may be used for educational purposes and for performing quality improvement studies, conducting research, and resolving legal issues such as competency or disability.[2]

The widespread use of electronic health records (EHR) has been promoted by the Health Information Technology for Economic and Clinical Health (HITECH) Act, which consists of three-stage criteria, including financial incentives for hospitals to comply with an EHR. Stage 1 calls for EHR compliance by the end of 2014, with penalties for those institutions or providers not in compliance.[3] Stages 2 and 3 are yet to be specifically defined. In conjunction with the transition to EHR, an initiative known as "meaningful use" has been developed to ensure providers are able to enhance the quality of patient care with the implementation of EHR.[4]

Specific advantages of an EHR compared with a paper record include complete and accurate patient health data that is readily available and shared with multiple providers to improve care coordination, the convenience of electronic prescriptions, the ability to track quality data, patient empowerment (by giving them access to their own records), and the potential for improved automatic patient follow-up.[5]

Confidentiality

According to the Health Insurance Portability and Accountability Act (HIPAA) *Privacy Rule,* any information in the medical record that contains "protected health information (PHI)" should be kept confidential, and all health care providers should safeguard the availability and integrity of health care information in oral, written, or electronic forms.[6] PHI includes any information that pertains to the past, present, or future physical or mental health conditions of an individual, including provision of care, payment of care, and demographics.[7] A subset of the *Privacy Rule* is the *Security Rule,* which specifically addresses the confidentiality of electronic PHI (e-PHI). The *Security Rule* states that a covered entity must ensure the integrity and availability of e-PHI that it creates, maintains, or transmits.[8] The goal of the *Security Rule* is to protect e-PHI as institutions such as hospitals adopt new and efficient technologies.[8] Specific topics, such as human immunodeficiency virus status, substance abuse, domestic abuse, or psychiatric history, are privileged information, and discussion of them is subject to additional ethical and regulatory guidelines.[9]

The physical therapist must be compliant with HIPAA,[10] the American Physical Therapy Association's *Guide for Professional Conduct* and *Code of Ethics for Physical Therapists*,[11,11a] and any policies and procedures of the facility or state in regard to sharing medical record information with the patient, family, caretakers, visitors, or third parties.

✎ CLINICAL TIP

To ensure confidentiality of PHI in the acute care setting, the physical therapist should log off the computer when not in use, keep the written medical chart and flow books closed when not in use, cover any paperwork kept on clipboards when traveling in the facility, and use discretion when discussing patient information in shared rooms, hallways, and/or elevators.

Physical Therapist Documentation

The physical therapist should comply with the documentation standards including, but not limited to, the policies/procedures of the organization, the state, and the American Physical Therapy Association's *Guidelines for Physical Therapy Documentation of Patient/Client Management*.[12]

In general, documentation must be:

- Dated and timed with an authenticated signature, including therapist credentials
- Legible and in black ink (in a paper chart)
- Clearly labeled with the appropriate patient identification
- Complete, accurate, and objective
- Cosigned for a physical therapist assistant or student therapist

Documentation should be free of ambiguous acronyms or abbreviations to minimize misinterpretation and prevent errors that could result in patient safety issues (Table 2-1).[13]

These standards apply to the examination, evaluation, and plan of care portions of physical therapist documentation, including flow sheets. A documentation entry is required for every physical therapist visit and should include the following, if applicable[14]:

- Phone calls or conversations with other health care providers
- Handouts provided to the patient, including exercise programs or educational materials
- The use of interpreter services
- Therapist response and assessment of an adverse event or situation

Ideally, documentation of physical therapy intervention should occur at point of service or as close to the time of intervention as possible. If a documentation error is noted, correct the error as soon as possible. Be familiar with your institution's policy for correcting chart errors in written or electronic formats.

Physical Therapy Considerations

- Be sure to document when a patient/family member declines or refuses therapy intervention or requests a specific time of day for therapy, including a rationale for such.
- Documentation of deferring or "holding" therapy should include a rationale and the source of the deferral, whether it is from the physician, nursing, or other providers. Deferring physical therapy when originated from the therapist's perspective should be succinctly described.
- Documentation of patient unavailability (e.g., off the floor at a test) is also suggested.

Components of the Medical Record

The organization of the medical record can vary from institution to institution; however, the medical record typically is composed of the following basic sections.

TABLE 2-1   Prohibitive Abbreviations*

Do Not Use	Potential Problem	Use Instead
U, u (unit)	Mistaken for "0" (zero), the number "4" (four) or "cc"	Write "unit"
IU (International Unit)	Mistaken for IV (intravenous) or the number 10 (ten)	Write "International Unit"
Q.D, QD, q.d., qd (daily)	Mistaken for each other	Write "daily"
QOD., QOD, q.o.d., qod (every other day)	Period after Q mistaken for "I" and the "O" mistaken for the "I"	Write "every other day"
Trailing zero (X.0 mg)†	Decimal point is missed	Write X mg
Lack of trailing zero (.X mg)		Write 0.X mg
MS	Can mean morphine sulfate or magnesium sulfate	Write "morphine sulfate"
MSO$_4$ and MgSO$_4$	Confused for one another	Write "magnesium sulfate"

*Applies to all orders and all medication-related documentation that is handwritten (including free-text computer entry) or on preprinted forms.

†Exception: A "trailing zero" may be used only where required to demonstrate the level of precision of the value being reported, such as for laboratory results, imaging studies that report size of lesions, or catheter/tube sizes. It may not be used in medication orders or other medication-related documentation. Data from The Joint Commission Official "Do Not Use " List. www.jointcommission.org. Last accessed June 9, 2012.

Orders

The order section is a log of all instructions of the plan of care for the patient, including medications, diagnostic or therapeutic tests and procedures, vital sign parameters, activity level, diet, the need for consultation services, and resuscitation status. Orders may be written by a physician, physician assistant, or nurse practitioner. An order may be taken by a nurse or other health care provider, including a physical therapist, according to departmental, facility, and state policies. In the interest of patient safety and error prevention, the process of taking a verbal order, especially for medications, has been minimized in many hospitals.[15] All (telephone) orders must be dated, timed, and signed or cosigned by the appropriate personnel. In addition, a telephone order should be read back to the person giving the order for the purpose of verification.[16]

Physical Therapy Considerations

- The order section of the patient's medical record should be reviewed before the initial and any subsequent physical therapy intervention(s) for the following: the order for physical therapy, patient activity level, weight-bearing status (if applicable), vital sign parameters, and positioning restrictions (if applicable). On subsequent physical therapy sessions, the review of the order section offers a "snapshot" of change(s) in a patient. Look for new or discontinued medications, changes in PO status, and new laboratory or diagnostic testing orders.
- If an order appears incomplete or ambiguous to the physical therapist, clarify the order before beginning physical therapy.

Admission Note Format

The following outline summarizes the basic format of the initial admission note (often referred to as the "H&P," or History and Physical) written by a physician, physician's assistant, or nurse practitioner in the medical record.[17] The italicized items indicate the standard information the physical therapist should review before beginning an intervention.

I. History (subjective information)
   A. Data that identify the patient, including the source and degree of reliability of the information
   B. *History of present illness (HPI)*, including the chief complaint and a chronologic list of the problems associated with the chief complaint
   C. *Medical or surgical history*, *risk factors* for disease, and *allergies*
   D. Family health history, including age and health or age and cause of death for immediate family members as well as a relevant familial medical history

   E. Personal and social history, including *occupation, lifestyle, functional mobility status, the need for home or outpatient services*, and *architectural barriers at home*
   F. *Current medications*, including *level of compliance*
II. Physical examination (objective information). Negative (normal) or positive (abnormal) findings are described in detail according to the following:
   A. General information, including vital signs, laboratory findings, mental status, and appearance
   B. Skin
   C. Head, eyes, ears, nose, throat (HEENT), and neck
   D. Chest and back
   E. Heart (cor)
   F. Abdomen
   G. Genitalia/rectal exam
   H. Extremities
   I. Neurologic system
III. Assessment. The assessment is a statement of the condition and prognosis of the patient in regard to the chief complaint and medical-surgical status. If the etiology of the problem(s) is unclear, then differential diagnoses are listed.
IV. Plan. The plan of care includes further observation, tests, laboratory analysis, consultation with additional specialty services or providers, pharmacologic therapies, other interventions, and discharge planning.

Progress Notes

A progress note is a shortened version of the initial note with an emphasis on any new physical findings, an updated assessment, and plan. The progress note section in a written record is typically multidisciplinary, with documentation from all caregivers in chronologic order. The nursing staff documents its own admission assessment, problem list, and care plan(s). Medication reconciliation sheets, flow sheets, clinical pathways, consult service notes from other physicians and allied health professionals, and operative and procedural notes are also included in this section.

Reports

A variety of reports are filed chronologically in individual sections in the medical record (e.g., radiologic or laboratory reports). Each report includes an interpretation or normal reference ranges, or both, for various diagnostic or laboratory test results. Other types of reports include pulmonary function tests, electroencephalograms (EEGs), and stress testing.

References

1. Roach WH et al: Medical record entries. In Medical records and the law, ed 4, Boston, 2006, Jones and Bartlett, pp 51-61.
2. Monarch K: Documentation, part 1: principles for self-protection, AJN 107(7):58, 2007.
3. Centers for Medicare and Medicaid Services: CMS HER meaningful use overview (website): http://www.cms.gov/ EHRIncentivePrograms/30_Meaningful_ Use.asp#BOOKMARK1. Accessed March 20, 2012.
4. Blumenthal D, Tavenner M: The "meaningful use" regulation for electronic health records, N Engl J Med 363(6):501-504, 2010.

5. U.S. Department of Health and Human Services, The Office of the National Coordinator for Health Information Technology: Electronic health records and meaningful use (website): http://healthit.hhs.gov/portal/server.pt?open512&objID=2996&mode=2. Accessed March 20, 2012.

6. U.S. Department of Health and Human Services: Health information privacy (website): http://www.hhs.gov//ocr/privacy/hippa/understanding/coveredentities/index/html. Accessed March 20, 2012.

7. U.S. Department of Health and Human Services: Summary of the privacy rule (website): http//:www.hhs.gov/ocr/privacy/hippa/understanding/summary/privacysummary.pdf. Accessed March 20, 2012.

8. U.S. Department of Health and Human Services: Summary of the security rule (website): http:www.hhs.gov/ocr/privacy/hippa/understanding/srsummary.html. Accessed March 20, 2012.

9. Rutberg MP: Medical records confidentiality. In Weintraub MI, editor: Neurologic clinics: medical-legal issues facing neurologists, Neurol Clin 17:307-313, 1999.

10. Office for Civil Rights—HIPAA: Medical privacy—national standard to protect the privacy of personal health information (website): http//:www.hhs.gov/ocr/privacy/hipaa/administrative/privacyrule/index.html. Accessed March 20, 2012.

11. American Physical Therapy Association: Code of ethics for the physical therapist (website): http://www.apta.org. Accessed March 20, 2012.

11a. American Physical Therapy Association: Guide for professional conduct (website): http://www.apta.org. Accessed March 20, 2012.

12. American Physical Therapy Association. Guidelines: Physical therapy documentation of patient/client management BOD G03-05-16-41 (website): http://www.apta.org. Accessed March 20, 2012.

13. The Joint Commission: Official "do not use" list (website): http://www.jointcommission.org/topics/patient_safety.aspx. Accessed March 20, 2012.

14. American Physical Therapy Association:. Improving your clinical documentation: reflecting best practice (website): http://www.apta.org/Documentaion/DefensibleDocumentaion. Accessed March 20, 2012.

15. The Joint Commision: Comprehensive Accreditation Manual for Hospitals (CAMH), Update 2. September 2011.MM.04.01.01.

16. The Joint Commision: Comprehensive Accreditation Manual for Hospitals (CAMH), Update 2. September 2011. PC.02.01.03.10.

17. Surviving the wards: evaluating the patient (H&P). In Ferri FF, editor: Practical guide to the care of the medical patient, Philadelphia, 2010, Mosby, pp 1-3.

CHAPTER 3

Cardiac System

Sean M. Collins
Konrad J. Dias

CHAPTER OBJECTIVES

The objectives of this chapter are the following:

1. Provide a brief overview of the structure and function of the cardiovascular system
2. Give an overview of cardiac evaluation, including physical examination and diagnostic testing
3. Describe cardiac diseases and disorders, including clinical findings and medical and surgical management
4. Establish a framework on which to base physical therapy evaluation and intervention in patients with cardiovascular disease

PREFERRED PRACTICE PATTERNS

The most relevant practice patterns for the diagnoses discussed in this chapter, based on the American Physical Therapy Association's *Guide to Physical Therapist Practice*, second edition, are as follows:

- Primary Prevention/Risk Reduction for Cardiovascular/Pulmonary Disorders: 6A
- Impaired Aerobic Capacity/Endurance Associated with Deconditioning: 6B
- Impaired Aerobic Capacity/Endurance Associated with Cardiovascular Pump Dysfunction or Failure: 6D

Please refer to Appendix A for a complete list of the preferred practice patterns, as individual patient conditions are highly variable and other practice patterns may be applicable.

Physical therapists in acute care facilities commonly encounter patients with cardiac system dysfunction as either a primary morbidity or comorbidity. Recent estimates conclude that although the death rate associated with cardiovascular disease has declined in recent years, the overall burden of the disease remains high.[1] Based on current estimates, 82,500,000 (more than one in three) Americans have one or more types of cardiovascular disease (CVD).[1] In 2009 CVD ranked first among all disease categories and accounted for 6,165,000 hospital discharges.[1] In the acute care setting, the role of the physical therapist with this diverse group of patients remains founded in examination, evaluation, intervention, and discharge planning for the purpose of improving functional capacity and minimizing disability. The physical therapist must be prepared to safely accommodate for the effects of dynamic (pathologic, physiologic, medical, and surgical intervention) changes into his or her evaluation and plan of care.

The normal cardiovascular system provides the necessary pumping force to circulate blood through the coronary, pulmonary, cerebral, and systemic circulation. To perform work, such as during functional tasks, energy demands of the body increase, therefore increasing the oxygen demands of the heart. A variety of pathologic states can create impairments in the cardiac system's ability to meet these demands successfully, ultimately leading to functional limitations. To fully address these functional limitations, the physical therapist must understand normal and abnormal cardiac function, clinical tests, and medical and surgical management of the cardiovascular system.

Body Structure and Function

The heart and the roots of the great vessels (Figure 3-1) occupy the pericardium, which is located in the mediastinum. The sternum, the costal cartilages, and the medial ends of the third to fifth ribs on the left side of the thorax create the anterior border of the mediastinum. It is bordered inferiorly by the diaphragm, posteriorly by the vertebral column and ribs, and laterally by the pleural cavity (which contains the lungs). Specific cardiac structures and vessels and their respective functions are outlined in Tables 3-1 and 3-2.

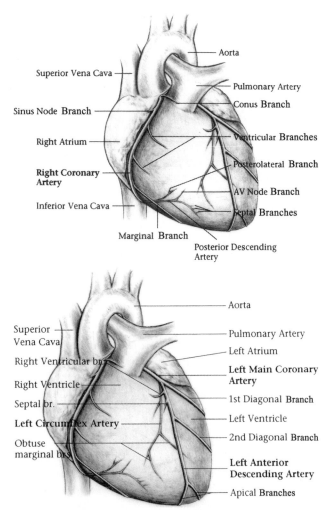

FIGURE 3-1

Anatomy of the right coronary artery and left coronary artery, including left main, left anterior descending, and left circumflex coronary arteries. (From Becker RC: Chest pain: the most common complaints series, Boston, 2000, Butterworth-Heinemann.)

Note: The mediastinum and the heart can be displaced from their normal positions with changes in the lungs secondary to various disorders. For example, a tension pneumothorax shifts the mediastinum away from the side of dysfunction (see Chapter 4 for a further description of pneumothorax).

The cardiovascular system must adjust the amount of nutrient- and oxygen-rich blood pumped out of the heart (cardiac output [CO]) to meet the spectrum of daily energy (metabolic) demands of the body.

The heart's ability to pump blood depends on the following characteristics[2]:

- Automaticity: The ability to initiate its own electrical impulse
- Excitability: The ability to respond to electrical stimulus
- Conductivity: The ability to transmit electrical impulse from cell to cell within the heart
- Contractility: The ability to stretch as a single unit and then passively recoil while actively contracting
- Rhythmicity: The ability to repeat the cycle in synchrony with regularity

Cardiac Cycle

Blood flow throughout the cardiac cycle depends on circulatory and cardiac pressure gradients. The right side of the heart is a low-pressure system with little vascular resistance in the pulmonary arteries, whereas the left side of the heart is a high-pressure system with high vascular resistance from the systemic circulation. The cardiac cycle is the period from the beginning of one contraction, starting with sinoatrial (SA) node depolarization, to the beginning of the next contraction. *Systole* is the period of contraction, whereas *diastole* is the period of relaxation. Systole and diastole can also be categorized into atrial and ventricular components:

- Atrial diastole is the period of atrial filling. The flow of blood is directed by the higher pressure in the venous circulatory system.
- Atrial systole is the period of atrial emptying and contraction. Initial emptying of approximately 70% of blood occurs as a result of the initial pressure gradient between the atria and the ventricles. Atrial contraction then follows, squeezing out the remaining 30%.[3] This is commonly referred to as the *atrial kick*.
- Ventricular diastole is the period of ventricular filling. It initially occurs with ease; then, as the ventricle is filled, atrial contraction is necessary to squeeze the remaining blood volume into the ventricle. The amount of stretch placed on the ventricular walls during diastole, referred to as left ventricular end diastolic pressure (LVEDP), influences the force of contraction during systole. (Refer to the Factors Affecting Cardiac Output section for a description of preload.)
- Ventricular systole is the period of ventricular contraction. The initial contraction is isovolumic (meaning it does not eject blood), which generates the pressure necessary to serve as the catalyst for rapid ejection of ventricular blood. The left ventricular ejection fraction (EF) represents the percent of end diastolic volume ejected during systole and is normally approximately 60%.[2]

TABLE 3-1 Primary Structures of the Heart

Structure	Description	Function
Pericardium	Double-walled sac of elastic connective tissue, a fibrous outer layer, and a serous inner layer	Protects against infection and trauma
Epicardium	Outermost layer of cardiac wall, covers surface of heart and great vessels	Protects against infection and trauma
Myocardium	Central layer of thick muscular tissue	Provides major pumping force of the ventricles
Endocardium	Thin layer of endothelium and connective tissue	Lines the inner surface of the heart, valves, chordae tendineae, and papillary muscles
Right atrium	Heart chamber	Receives blood from the venous system and is a primer pump for the right ventricle
Tricuspid valve	Atrioventricular valve between right atrium and ventricle	Prevents back flow of blood from the right ventricle to the atrium during ventricular systole
Right ventricle	Heart chamber	Pumps blood to the pulmonary circulation
Pulmonic valve	Semilunar valve between right ventricle and pulmonary artery	Prevents back flow of blood from the pulmonary artery to the right ventricle during diastole
Left atrium	Heart chamber	Acts as a reservoir for blood and a primer pump for the left ventricle
Mitral valve	Atrioventricular valve between left atrium and ventricle	Prevents back flow of blood from the left ventricle to the atrium during ventricular systole
Left ventricle	Heart chamber	Pumps blood to the systemic circulation
Aortic valve	Semilunar valve between left ventricle and aorta	Prevents back flow of blood from the aorta to the left ventricle during ventricular diastole
Chordae tendineae	Tendinous attachment of atrioventricular valve cusps to papillary muscles	Prevents valves from everting into the atria during ventricular systole
Papillary muscle	Muscle that connects chordae tendineae to floor of ventricle wall	Constricts and pulls on chordae tendineae to prevent eversion of valve cusps during ventricular systole

TABLE 3-2 Great Vessels of the Heart and Their Function

Structure	Description	Function
Aorta	Primary artery from the left ventricle that ascends and then descends after exiting the heart	Ascending aorta delivers blood to neck, head, and arms Descending aorta delivers blood to visceral and lower body tissues
Superior vena cava	Primary vein that drains into the right atrium	Drains venous blood from head, neck, and upper body
Inferior vena cava	Primary vein that drains into the right atrium	Drains venous blood from viscera and lower body
Pulmonary artery	Primary artery from the right ventricle	Carries blood to lungs

Cardiac Output

CO is the quantity of blood pumped by the heart in 1 minute. Regional demands for tissue perfusion (based on local metabolic needs) compete for systemic circulation, and total CO adjusts to meet these demands. Adjustment to CO occurs with changes in heart rate (HR—chronotropic) or stroke volume (SV—inotropic).[3] Normal resting CO is approximately 4 to 8 liters per minute (L/min), with a resting HR of 70 beats per minute (bpm); resting SV is approximately 71 ml/beat.[2] The maximum value of CO represents the functional capacity of the circulatory system to meet the demands of physical activity.

$$CO\ (L/min) = HR\ (bpm) \times SV\ (L)$$

CO also can be described relative to body mass as the cardiac index (CI), the amount of blood pumped per minute per square meter of body mass. Normal CI is between 2.5 and 4.2 L/min/m^2. This wide normal range makes it possible for cardiac output to decline by almost 40% and still remain within the normal limits. Although several factors interrupt a direct correlation between CI and functional aerobic capacity, a CI below 2.5 L/min/m^2 represents a marked disturbance in cardiovascular performance and is always clinically relevant.[4]

Factors Affecting Cardiac Output

Preload. Preload is the amount of tension on the ventricular wall before it contracts. It is related to venous return and affects SV by increasing left ventricular end diastolic volume in addition to pressure and therefore contraction.[2] This relationship is explained by the Frank-Starling mechanism and is demonstrated in Figure 3-2.

Frank-Starling Mechanism. The Frank-Starling mechanism defines the normal relationship between the length and tension of the myocardium.[5] The greater the stretch on the

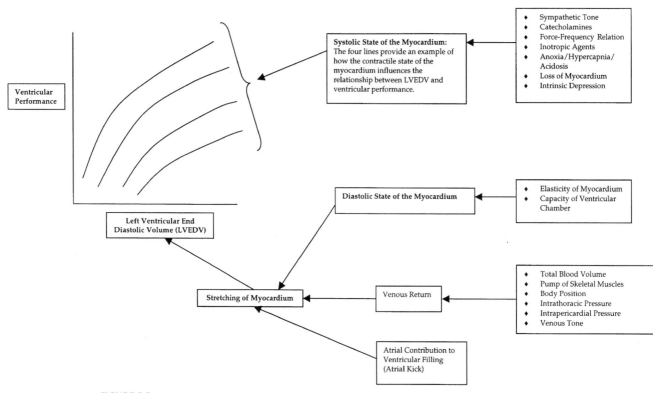

FIGURE 3-2

Factors affecting left ventricular function. (Modified from Braunwal E, Ross J, Sonnenblick E et al: Mechanisms of contraction of the normal and failing heart, ed 2, Boston, 1976, Little, Brown.)

myocardium before systole (preload), the stronger the ventricular contraction. The length-tension relationship in skeletal muscle is based on the response of individual muscle fibers; however, relationships between cardiac muscle length and tension consist of the whole heart. Therefore length is considered in terms of volume; tension is considered in terms of pressure. A greater volume of blood returning to the heart during diastole equates to greater pressures generated initially by the heart's contractile elements. Ultimately facilitated by elastic recoil, a greater volume of blood is ejected during systole. The effectiveness of this mechanism can be reduced in pathologic situations.[3]

Afterload. Afterload is the force against which a muscle must contract to initiate shortening.[5] Within the ventricular wall, this is equal to the tension developed across its wall during systole. The most prominent force contributing to afterload in the heart is blood pressure (BP), specifically vascular compliance and resistance. BP affects aortic valve opening and is the most obvious load encountered by the ejecting ventricle. An example of afterload is the amount of pressure in the aorta at the time of ventricular systole.[2]

Cardiac Conduction System

A schematic of the cardiac conduction system and a normal electrocardiogram (ECG) are presented in Figure 3-3. Normal conduction begins in the SA node and travels throughout the atrial myocardium (atrial depolarization) via intranodal pathways to the atrioventricular (AV) node, where it is delayed momentarily. It then travels to the bundle of His, to the bundle

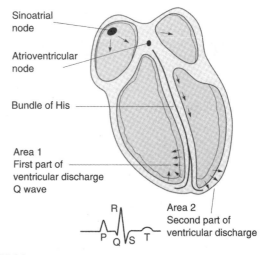

FIGURE 3-3

Schematic representation of the sequence of excitation in the heart. (From Walsh M, Crumbie A, Reveley S: Nurse practitioners: clinical skills and professional issues, Boston, 1999, Butterworth-Heinemann.)

branches, to the Purkinje fibers, and finally to the myocardium, resulting in ventricular contraction.[6] Disturbances in conduction can decrease CO (refer to the Health Conditions section for a discussion of rhythm and conduction disturbances).[7]

Neural Input. The SA node has its own inherent rate. However, neural input can influence HR, heart rate variability (HRV), and contractility through the autonomic nervous system.[2,8]

Parasympathetic system (vagal) neural input generally decelerates cardiac function, thus decreasing HR and contractility. Parasympathetic input travels through the vagus nerves. The right vagus nerve stimulates primarily the SA node and affects rate, whereas the left vagus nerve stimulates primarily the AV node and affects AV conduction.[2,8]

Sympathetic system neural input is through the thoracolumbar sympathetic system and increases HR and augment ventricular contractility, thus accelerating cardiac function.[2]

Endocrine Input. In response to physical activity or stress, a release in catecholamines increases HR, contractility, and peripheral vascular resistance for a net effect of increased cardiac function (Table 3-3).[2]

Local Input. Tissue pH, concentration of carbon dioxide (CO_2), concentration of oxygen (O_2), and metabolic products (e.g., lactic acid) can affect vascular tone.[2] During exercise, increased levels of CO_2, decreased levels of O_2, decreased pH, and increased levels of lactic acid at the tissue level dilate local blood vessels and therefore increase CO distribution to that area.

Cardiac Reflexes

Cardiac reflexes influence HR and contractility and can be divided into three general categories: baroreflex (pressure), Bainbridge reflex (stretch), and chemoreflex (chemical reflex).

Baroreflexes are activated through a group of mechanoreceptors located in the heart, great vessels, and intrathoracic and cervical blood vessels. These mechanoreceptors are most plentiful in the walls of the internal carotid arteries.[2] Mechanoreceptors are sensory receptors that are sensitive to mechanical changes such as pressure and stretch. Activation of the mechanoreceptors by high pressures results in an inhibition of the vasomotor center of the medulla that increases vagal stimulation. This chain of events is known as the *baroreflex* and results in vasodilation, decreased HR, and decreased contractility.

Mechanoreceptors located in the right atrial myocardium respond to stretch. An increased volume in the right atrium results in an increase in pressure on the atrial wall. This reflex, known as the *Bainbridge reflex*, stimulates the vasomotor center

of the medulla, which in turn increases sympathetic input and increases HR and contractility.[2] Respiratory sinus arrhythmia, an increased HR during inspiration and decreased HR during expiration, may be facilitated by changes in venous return and SV caused by changes in thoracic pressure induced by the respiratory cycle. At the beginning of inspiration when thoracic pressure is decreased, venous return is greater; therefore a greater stretch is exerted on the atrial wall.[9]

Chemoreceptors located on the carotid and aortic bodies have a primary effect on increasing rate and depth of ventilation in response to CO_2 levels, but they also have a cardiac effect. Changes in CO_2 during the respiratory cycle also may result in sinus arrhythmia.[2]

Coronary Perfusion

For a review of the major coronary arteries, refer to Figure 3-1. Blood is pumped to the large superficial coronary arteries during ventricular systole. At this time, myocardial contraction limits the flow of blood to the myocardium; therefore myocardial tissue is perfused during diastole.

Systemic Circulation

For a review of the distribution of systemic circulation, refer to Figure 3-4. Systemic circulation is affected by total peripheral resistance (TPR), which is the resistance to blood flow by the force created by the aorta and arterial system. Two factors that contribute to resistance are (1) vasomotor tone, in which vessels dilate and constrict, and (2) blood viscosity, in which greater pressure is required to propel thicker blood. TPR, also called *systemic vascular resistance*, and CO influence BP.[2] This relationship is illustrated in the following equation:

$$BP = CO \times TPR$$

Cardiac Evaluation

Cardiac evaluation consists of patient history, physical examination (which consists of observation, palpation, BP measurement,

TABLE 3-3 Cardiac Effects of Hormones

Hormone	Primary Site	Stimulus	Cardiac Effect
Norepinephrine	Adrenal medulla	Stress/exercise	Vasoconstriction
Epinephrine	Adrenal medulla	Stress/exercise	Coronary artery vasodilation
Angiotensin	Kidney	Decreased arterial pressure	Vasoconstriction, increased blood volume
Vasopressin	Posterior pituitary	Decreased arterial pressure	Potent vasoconstrictor
Bradykinin	Formed by polypeptides in blood when activated	Tissue damage/inflammation	Vasodilation, increased capillary permeability
Histamine	Throughout tissues of body	Tissue damage	Vasodilation, increased capillary permeability
Atrial natriuretic peptides	Atria of heart	Increased atrial stretch	Decreased blood volume
Aldosterone	Adrenal cortex	Angiotensin II (stimulated) by hypovolemia or decreased renal perfusion	Increased blood volume, kidneys excrete more potassium

Data from Guyton AC, Hall JE: Textbook of medical physiology, ed 12, Philadelphia, 2011, Saunders.

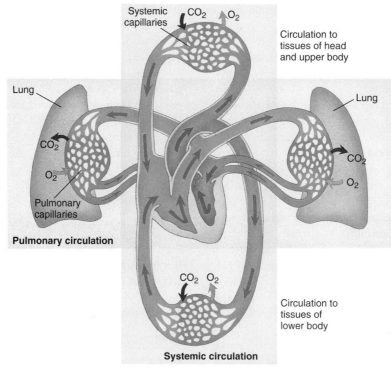

FIGURE 3-4

Schematic of systemic circulation. (From Thibodeau GA: Structure and function of the body, ed 13, St Louis, 2007, Mosby.)

BOX 3-1   Cardiac Risk Factors: Primary and Secondary Prevention

Major Independent Risk Factors	Predisposing Risk Factors	Conditional Risk Factors
Smoking	Physical inactivity	Elevated triglycerides
Hypertension	Obesity	Small LDL particles
Elevated serum cholesterol, total (and LDL)	Body mass index >30 kg/m^2	Elevated homocysteine
Decreased HDL cholesterol	Abdominal obesity (waist-hip ratio)	Elevated lipoprotein (a)
Diabetes mellitus	Men >40 in	Elevated inflammatory markers
Advancing age	Women >35 in	C-reactive protein
	Family history of premature heart disease	Fibrinogen
	Psychosocial factors	
	Job strain	
	Ethnic characteristics	

Data from Grundy SM, Pasternak R, Greenland P et al: Assessment of cardiovascular risk by use of multiple-risk-factor assessment equations: a statement for healthcare professionals from the American Heart Association and the American College of Cardiology, Circulation 100:1481-1492, 1999; Belkic KL, Landsbergis PA et al: Is job strain a major source of cardiovascular disease risk? Scand J Work Environ Health 30(2):85-128, 2004.

LDL, Low-density lipoprotein; *HDL,* high-density lipoprotein.

---

and heart sound auscultation), laboratory tests, and diagnostic procedures.

Patient History

In addition to the general chart review presented in Chapter 2 the following pertinent information about patients with cardiac dysfunction should be obtained before physical examination[3,10-12]:

- Presence of chest pain (see Chapter 17 for an expanded description of characteristics and etiology of chest pain)
  - Location and radiation
  - Character and quality (crushing, burning, numbing, hot)
  - Frequency

- Angina equivalents (what the patient feels as angina [e.g., jaw pain, shortness of breath, dizziness, lightheadedness, diaphoresis, burping, nausea, or any combination of these])
- Aggravating and alleviating factors
- Precipitating factors
- Medical treatment sought and its outcome
- Presence of palpitations
- Presence of cardiac risk factors (Box 3-1)
- Family history of cardiac disease
- History of dizziness or syncope
- Previous myocardial infarction (MI), cardiac studies, or procedures

Physical Examination

Observation

Key components of the observation portion of the physical examination include the following[3,7]:
- Facial color, skin color and tone, or the presence of diaphoresis
- Obvious signs of edema in the extremities
- Respiratory rate
- Signs of trauma (e.g., paddle burns or ecchymosis from cardiopulmonary resuscitation)
- Presence of jugular venous distention (JVD), which results from the backup of fluid into the venous system from right-sided congestive heart failure (CHF) (Figure 3-5)
  - Make sure the patient is in a semirecumbent position (45 degrees).
  - Have the patient turn his or her head away from the side being evaluated.
  - Observe pulsations in the internal jugular neck region. Pulsations are normally seen 3 to 5 cm above the sternum. Pulsations higher than this or absent pulsations indicate jugular venous distention.

Palpation

Palpation is the second component of the physical examination and is used to evaluate and identify the following:
- Pulses for circulation quality, HR, and rhythm (Table 3-4, Figure 3-6)
- Extremities for pitting edema bilaterally (Table 3-5)

When palpating HR, counting the pulse rate for 15 seconds and multiplying by 4 is sufficient with normal rates and rhythms. If rates are faster than 100 bpm or slower than 60 bpm, palpate the pulse for 60 seconds. If the rhythm is irregularly irregular (e.g., during atrial fibrillation) or regularly irregular (e.g., premature ventricular contractions [PVCs]), perform auscultation of heart sounds to identify the apical HR for a full minute. In these cases, palpation of pulse cannot substitute for ECG analysis to monitor the patient's rhythm, but it may alert the therapist to the onset of these abnormalities.

Blood Pressure

BP measurement with a sphygmomanometer (cuff) and auscultation is an indirect, noninvasive measurement of the force exerted against the arterial walls during ventricular systole (systolic blood pressure [SBP]) and during ventricular diastole (diastolic blood pressure). BP is affected by peripheral vascular resistance (blood volume and elasticity of arterial walls) and CO. Table 3-6 lists normal BP ranges. Occasionally, BP measurements can be performed only on certain limbs secondary to the presence of conditions such as a percutaneous inserted central catheter, arteriovenous fistula for hemodialysis, blood clots, scarring from brachial artery cutdowns, or lymphedema (e.g., status post mastectomy). BP of the upper extremity should be measured in the following manner:
1. Check for posted signs, if any, at the bedside that indicate which arm should be used in taking BP. BP variations of 5 to 10 mm Hg between the right and left upper extremity are considered normal. Patients with arterial compression or obstruction may have differences of more than 10 to 15 mm Hg.[12]
2. Use a properly fitting cuff. The inflatable bladder should have a width of approximately 40% and length of approximately 80% of the upper arm circumference.[13]

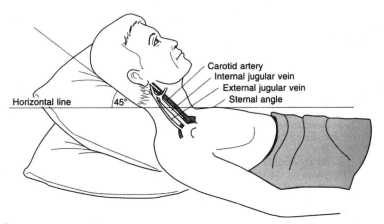

FIGURE 3-5
Measurement of jugular venous distention (JVD). The JVD reading is the maximum height, in centimeters, above the sternal angle at which venous pulsations are visible. (Modified from Thompson JM, McFarland GK, Hirsch JE et al: Mosby's clinical nursing, ed 5, St Louis, 2002, Mosby.)

TABLE 3-4 Pulse Amplitude Classification and Pulse Abnormalities

Pulse Amplitude Classification

Scale	Degree	Description
0	Absent pulse	No pulse—no circulation
1+	Diminished pulse	Reduced stroke volume and ejection fraction, increased vascular resistance
2+	Normal pulse	Normal resting conditions, no pathologies
3+	Moderately increased	Slightly increased stroke volume and ejection fraction
4+	Markedly increased (bounding)*	Increased stroke volume and ejection fraction, can be diminished with vasoconstriction

Pulse Abnormalities

Abnormality	Palpation	Description
Pulsus alternans	Regular rhythm with strong pulse waves alternating with weak pulse waves	Indicates left ventricular failure when present at normal heart rates
Bigeminal pulses	Every other pulse is weak and early	Result of premature ventricular contractions (bigeminy)
Pulsus paradoxus	Reduction in strength of the pulse with an abnormal decline in blood pressure during inspiration	May be caused by chronic obstructive lung disease, pericarditis, pulmonary emboli, restrictive cardiomyopathy, and cardiogenic shock

Data from Woods SL, Sivarajian-Froelicher ES, Underhill-Motzer S, editors: Cardiac nursing, ed 4, Philadelphia, 2000, Lippincott.
*Corrigan's pulse is a bounding pulse visible in the carotid artery that occurs with aortic regurgitation.

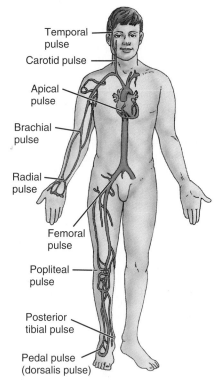

Temporal pulse
Carotid pulse
Apical pulse
Brachial pulse
Radial pulse
Femoral pulse
Popliteal pulse
Posterior tibial pulse
Pedal pulse (dorsalis pulse)

FIGURE 3-6
Arterial pulses. (From Pierson FM: Principles and techniques of patient care, ed 4, St Louis, 2008, Saunders.)

TABLE 3-5 Pitting Edema Scale

Scale	Degree	Description
1+ Trace	Slight	Barely perceptible depression
2+ Mild	0-0.6 cm	Easily identified depression (EID) (skin rebounds in <15 sec)
3+ Moderate	0.6-1.3 cm	EID (rebound 15-30 sec)
4+ Severe	1.3-2.5 cm	EID (rebound >30 sec)

Data from Woods SL, Sivarajian Froelicher ES, Underhill-Motzer S, editors: Cardiac nursing, ed 4, Philadelphia, 2000, Lippincott; Hillegass EA, Sadowsky HS, editors: Essentials of cardiopulmonary physical therapy, ed 2, Philadelphia, 2001, Saunders.

TABLE 3-6 Normal Blood Pressure Ranges

Age Ranges	Systolic	Diastolic
Age 8 years	85-114 mm Hg	52-85 mm Hg
Age 12 years	95-135 mm Hg	58-88 mm Hg
Adult	<120 mm Hg	<80 mm Hg
Prehypertension	120-139 mm Hg	80-89 mm Hg
Hypertension Stage 1	140-159 mm Hg	90-99 mm Hg
Stage 2	≥160 mm Hg	≥100 mm Hg
Normal exercise	Increases 5-12 mm Hg per MET increase in workload	±10 mm Hg

Data from Chobanian AV, Bakris GL et al: Seventh report of the Joint National Committee on prevention, detection, evaluation, and treatment of high blood pressure, Hypertension 42(6):1206-1252, 2003; American College of Sports Medicine, Armstrong LE, et al: ACSM's guidelines for exercise testing and prescription, Philadelphia, 2005, Lippincott Williams & Wilkins.
MET, Metabolic equivalent.

3. Position the cuff 2.5 cm above the antecubital crease.

4. Rest the arm at the level of the heart.

5. To determine how high to inflate the cuff, palpate the radial pulse, inflate until no longer palpable, and note the cuff inflation value. Deflate the cuff.

6. Place the bell of the stethoscope gently over the brachial artery.

7. Reinflate the cuff to 30 to 40 mm Hg greater than the value in step 5. Then slowly deflate the cuff. Cuff deflation should occur at approximately 2 to 3 mm Hg per second.[13]

8. Listen for the onset of tapping sounds, which represents blood flow returning to the brachial artery. This is the systolic pressure.

9. As the pressure approaches diastolic pressure, the sounds will become muffled and in 5 to 10 mm Hg will be completely absent. These sounds are referred to as *Korotkoff sounds* (Table 3-7).[12,13]

> ### ✎ CLINICAL TIP
>
> In situations when it is difficult to auscultate or discern a distinct diastolic pressure, the patient's blood pressure may be noted as systolic BP/P (i.e., "BP is 90 over palp") or systolic BP over 2 diastolic pressures (e.g., 140/85/62) denoting the onset of muffling sounds and the disappearance of sounds.[13]

Physical Therapy Considerations

- Recording preexertion, paraexertion, and postexertion BP is important for identification of BP responses to activity. During recovery from exercise, blood vessels dilate to allow for greater blood flow to muscles. In cardiac-compromised or very deconditioned individuals, total CO may be unable to support this increased flow to the muscles and may lead to decreased output to vital areas, such as the brain.

- If you are unable to obtain BP on the arm, the thigh is an appropriate alternative, with auscultation at the popliteal artery.

- Falsely high readings occur if the cuff is too small or applied loosely, or if the brachial artery is lower than the heart level.

- Evaluation of BP and HR in different postures can be used to monitor orthostatic hypotension with repeat measurements on the same arm 1 to 5 minutes after position changes. The symbols that represent patient position are shown in Figure 3-7.

- The same extremity should be used when serial BP recordings will be compared for an evaluation of hemodynamic response.

- A BP record is kept on the patient's vital sign flow sheet. This is a good place to check for BP trends throughout the day and, depending on your hospital's policy, to document BP changes during the therapy session.

- An auscultatory gap is the disappearance of sounds between phase 1 and phase 2 and is common in patients with high BP, venous distention, and severe aortic stenosis. Its presence can create falsely low systolic pressures if the cuff is not inflated enough (prevented by palpating for the disappearance of the pulse before measurement), or falsely high diastolic pressures if the therapist stops measurement during the gap (prevented by listening for the phase 3 to phase 5 transitions).[13]

Auscultation

Evaluation of heart sounds can yield information about the patient's condition and tolerance to medical treatment and physical therapy through the evaluation of valvular function, rate, rhythm, valvular compliance, and ventricular compliance.[3] To listen to heart sounds, a stethoscope with a bell and a

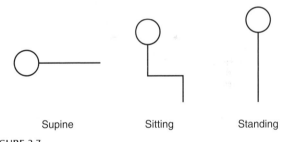

Supine   Sitting   Standing

FIGURE 3-7
Orthostatic blood pressure symbols.

TABLE 3-7 Korotkoff Sounds

Phase	Sound	Indicates
1	First sound heard, faint tapping sound with increasing intensity	Systolic pressure (blood starts to flow through compressed artery)
2	Start swishing sound	Blood flow continues to be heard; sounds are beginning to change because of the changing compression on the artery
3	Sounds increase in intensity with a distinct tapping	Blood flow is increasing as artery compression is decreasing
4	Sounds become muffled	Diastolic pressure in children <13 years of age and in adults who are exercising, pregnant, or hyperthyroid (see phase 5)
5	Disappearance	Diastolic pressure in adults—occurs 5-10 mm Hg below phase 4 in normal adults. In states of increased rate of blood flow, it may be >10 mm Hg below phase 4. In these cases, the phase 4 sound should be used as diastolic pressure in adults.

Data from Woods SL, Sivarajian-Froelicher ES, Underhill-Motzer S, editors: Cardiac nursing, ed 4, Philadelphia, 2000, Lippincott, 2000; Bickley LS, Szilagyi PG: Bates' guide to physical examination and history taking, Philadelphia, 2003, Lippincott Williams & Wilkins.

diaphragm is necessary. For a review of normal and abnormal heart sounds, refer to Table 3-8. The examination should follow a systematic pattern using the bell (for low-pitched sounds) and diaphragm (for high-pitched sounds) and should cover all auscultatory areas, as illustrated in Figure 3-8. Abnormal sounds should be noted with a description of the conditions in which they were heard (e.g., after exercise or during exercise).

Physical Therapy Considerations

- Always ensure proper function of a stethoscope by tapping the diaphragm before use with a patient.
- Avoid rubbing the stethoscope on extraneous objects because this can add noise and detract from the examination.
- Avoid auscultation of heart sounds over clothing, which can muffle the intensity of normal and abnormal sounds.
- If the patient has an irregular cardiac rhythm, determine HR through auscultation (apical HR). To save time, listen for the HR during a routine auscultatory examination with the stethoscope's bell or diaphragm in any of the auscultation locations (see Figure 3-8).
- Heart sounds can be heard online at the Auscultation Assistant, available at: http://www.med.ucla.edu/wilkes/intro.html.

Diagnostic and Laboratory Measures

The diagnostic and laboratory measures discussed in this section provide information used to determine medical diagnoses, guide interventions, and assist with determining prognoses. The clinical relevance of each test varies according to the pathology. This section is organized across a spectrum of least invasive to most invasive measures. When appropriate, the test results most pertinent to the physical therapist are detailed. For clinical decision making, physical therapists usually need information

TABLE 3-8 Normal and Abnormal Heart Sounds

Sound	Location	Description
S1 (normal)	All areas	First heart sound; signifies closure of atrioventricular valves and corresponds to onset of ventricular systole
S2 (normal)	All areas	Second heart sound; signifies closure of semilunar valves and corresponds with onset of ventricular diastole
S3 (abnormal)	Best appreciated at apex	Immediately following S2; occurs early in diastole and represents filling of the ventricle. In young, healthy individuals, it is considered normal and called a physiologic third sound. In the presence of heart disease, it results from decreased ventricular compliance (a classic sign of congestive heart failure)
S4 (abnormal)	Best appreciated at apex	Immediately preceding S1; occurs late in ventricular diastole; associated with increased resistance to ventricular filling; common in patients with hypertensive heart disease, coronary heart disease, pulmonary disease, or myocardial infarction, or following coronary artery bypass grafts
Murmur (abnormal)	Over respective valves	Indicates regurgitation of blood through valves; can also be classified as systolic or diastolic murmurs. Common pathologies resulting in murmurs include mitral regurgitation and aortic stenosis
Pericardial friction rub (abnormal)	Third or fourth intercostal space, anterior axillary line	Sign of pericardial inflammation (pericarditis), associated with each beat of the heart; sounds like a creak or leather being rubbed together

Data from Bickley LS, Szilagyi PG: Bates' guide to physical examination and history taking, Philadelphia, 2003, Lippincott Williams & Wilkins.

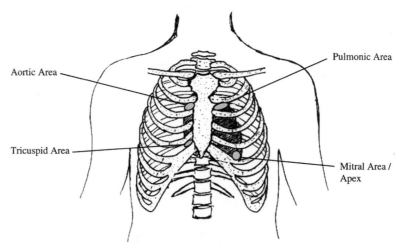

FIGURE 3-8
Areas for heart sound auscultation. (Courtesy Barbara Cocanour, PhD, University of Massachusetts, Lowell, Department of Physical Therapy.)

that helps identify indications for intervention, relative or absolute contraindications for intervention, possible complications during activity progression, and indicators of performance.

Oximetry

Oximetry (SaO_2) is used to evaluate indirectly the oxygenation of a patient and can be used to titrate supplemental oxygen. Refer to Chapter 4 for a further description of oximetry.

Electrocardiogram

An ECG provides a graphic analysis of the heart's electrical activity. The ECG commonly is used to detect arrhythmias, heart blocks, and myocardial perfusion. It also can detect atrial or ventricular enlargement. An ECG used for continuous monitoring of patients in the hospital typically involves a 3- to 5-lead system. A lead represents a particular portion, or "view," of the heart. The patient's rhythm usually is displayed in his or her room, in the hall, and at the nurses' station. Diagnostic ECG involves a 12-lead analysis, the description of which is beyond the scope of this book. For a review of basic ECG rate and rhythm analysis, refer to Table 3-9 and Figure 3-3.

Holter Monitoring. Holter monitoring is 24- or 48-hour ECG analysis conducted to detect cardiac arrhythmias and corresponding symptoms during a patient's daily activity.[12] Holter monitoring is different than telemetric monitoring because the ECG signal is recorded and later analyzed.

Indications for Holter monitoring include the evaluation of syncope, dizziness, shortness of breath with no other obvious cause, palpitations, antiarrhythmia therapy, pacemaker functioning, activity-induced silent ischemia, and risk of cardiac complications with the use of HRV.

Heart Rate Variability. HRV has been discussed in the literature to possibly reflect cardiac autonomic nervous system regulation. A common overall measure of HRV is the standard deviation of all RR intervals on an ECG during a 24-hour period (SDNN).[8] Evidence regarding the potential clinical utility of HRV for cardiology is growing; however, it continues to be used primarily in research.[14] In healthy populations, low HRV is a risk factor for all causes of cardiac mortality[15-17] and for new onset of hypertension.[18] Low HRV is also a risk for mortality in patients who have had an MI[19-21] or have coronary

artery disease[22] or CHF.[23] Evidence suggests that altered HRV during exercise may provide valuable information for risk assessment.[24] This is likely related to the increasingly accepted relationship between delayed heart rate recovery (HRR) after exercise and cardiac risk. Delayed HRR (<46 bpm) 3 minutes after an exercise test is a predictor of long-term (~15 years) mortality.[25] HRR is discussed further in the section on Physical Therapy Intervention.

Telemetric Electrocardiogram Monitoring. Telemetric ECG monitoring provides real-time ECG visualization via radiofrequency transmission of the ECG signal to a monitor. Benefits of telemetry include monitoring with no hardwire connection between the patient and the visual display unit and real-time graphic display of the ECG signal using the standard ECG monitor attachment.

> ✎ **CLINICAL TIP**
> Some hospitals use an activity log with Holter monitoring. If so, document physical therapy intervention on the log. If no log is available, record the time of day and physical therapy intervention in the medical record.

Complete Blood Cell Count

Relevant values from the complete blood cell count are hematocrit, hemoglobin, and white blood cell counts. Hematocrit refers to the number of red blood cells per 100 ml of blood and therefore fluctuates with changes in the total red blood cell count (hemoglobin) and with blood volume (i.e., reduced plasma volume results in relatively more red blood cells in 100 ml of blood). Elevated levels of hematocrit (which may be related to dehydration) indicate increased viscosity of blood that can potentially impede blood flow to tissues.[12] Hemoglobin is essential for the adequate oxygen-carrying capacity of the blood. A decrease in hemoglobin and hematocrit levels (10% below normal is called anemia) may decrease activity tolerance or make patients more susceptible to ischemia secondary to decreased oxygen-carrying capacity.[11,26] Slight decreases in hematocrit resulting from adaptations to exercise (with no change

TABLE 3-9 Electrocardiograph Interpretation

Wave/Segment	Duration (seconds)	Amplitude (mm)	Indicates
P wave	<0.10	1-3	Atrial depolarization
PR interval	0.12-0.20	Isoelectric line	Elapsed time between atrial depolarization and ventricular depolarization
QRS complex	0.06-0.10	25-30 (maximum)	Ventricular depolarization and atrial repolarization
ST segment	0.12	−½ to +1	Elapsed time between end of ventricular depolarization and beginning of repolarization
QT interval (QTc)	0.42-0.47	Varies	Elapsed time between beginning of ventricular repolarization and end of repolarization (QTc is corrected for heart rate)
T wave	0.16	5-10	Ventricular repolarization

Data from Meyers RS, editor: Saunders manual of physical therapy practice, Philadelphia, 1995, Saunders; Aehlert B, editor: ACLS quick review study guide, St Louis, 1994, Mosby; Davis D, editor: How to quickly and accurately master ECG interpretation, ed 2, Philadelphia, 1992, Lippincott Williams & Wilkins.

in hemoglobin) are related to increases in blood volume. The concomitant exercise-related decreases in blood viscosity may be beneficial to post-MI patients.[27]

Elevated white blood cell counts can indicate that the body is fighting infection, or they can occur with inflammation caused by cell death, such as in MI. Erythrocyte sedimentation rate (ESR), another hematologic test, is a nonspecific index of inflammation and commonly is elevated for 2 to 3 weeks after MI.[26] Refer to Chapter 7 for more information about these values.

Coagulation Profiles

Coagulation profiles provide information about the clotting time of blood. Patients who undergo treatment with thrombolytic therapy after the initial stages of MI or who are receiving anticoagulant therapy because of various cardiac arrhythmias require coagulation profiles to monitor anticoagulation in an attempt to prevent complications such as bleeding. The physician determines the patient's therapeutic range of anticoagulation using the prothrombin time (PT), partial thromboplastin time, and international normalized ratio.[26] Refer to Chapter 7 for details regarding these values and their significance to treatment.

Patients with low PT and partial thromboplastin time are at higher risk of thrombosis, especially if they have arrhythmias (e.g., atrial fibrillation) or valvular conditions (e.g., mitral regurgitation) that produce stasis of the blood. Patients with a PT greater than 2.5 times the reference range should not undergo physical therapy because of the potential for spontaneous bleeding. Likewise, an international normalized ratio of more than 3 warrants asking the physician if treatment should be withheld.[26]

Blood Lipids

Elevated total cholesterol levels in the blood are a significant risk factor for atherosclerosis and therefore ischemic heart disease.[28] Measuring blood cholesterol level is necessary to determine the risk for development of atherosclerosis and to assist in patient education, dietary modification, and medical management. Normal values can be adjusted for age; however, levels of total cholesterol more than 240 mg/dl are generally considered high, and levels of less than 200 mg/dl are considered normal.

A blood lipid analysis categorizes cholesterol into high-density lipoproteins (HDLs) and low-density lipoproteins (LDLs) and provides an analysis of triglycerides. HDLs are formed by the liver and are considered beneficial because they are readily transportable and do not adhere to the intimal walls of the vascular system. People with higher amounts of HDLs are at lower risk for coronary artery disease.[26,28] HDL levels of less than 33 mg/dl carry an elevated risk of heart disease. A more important risk for heart disease is an elevated ratio of total cholesterol to HDL. Normal ratios of total cholesterol to HDL range from 3 to 5.[12]

LDLs are formed by a diet excessive in fat and are related to a higher incidence of coronary artery disease. LDLs are not as readily transportable as HDLs because LDLs adhere to intimal

walls in the vascular system.[26] Normal LDL levels are below 100 mg/dl.[12]

Triglycerides are fat cells that are free floating in the blood. When not in use, they are stored in adipose tissue. A person's triglyceride levels increase after he or she eats foods high in fat and decrease with exercise. High levels of triglycerides are associated with a risk of coronary heart disease.[26]

> ### ✎ CLINICAL TIP
> Cholesterol levels may be elevated falsely after an acute MI; therefore preinfarction levels (if known) are used to guide risk factor modification. Values will not return to normal until at least 6 weeks post MI.

C-Reactive Protein

C-reactive protein (CRP) is a test that measures the amount of a protein in the blood that signals acute inflammation. To determine a person's risk for heart disease, a more sensitive CRP test called a *high-sensitivity C-reactive protein* (hs-CRP) assay is available. A growing number of studies have determined that high levels of hs-CRP consistently predict recurrent coronary events in patients with unstable angina (USA) and acute MI. In addition, elevated hs-CRP levels are associated with lower survival rates in these patients with cardiovascular disease.[29-31] Parameters for hs-CRP are as follows:

- hs-CRP lower than 1.0 mg/L indicates a low risk of developing cardiovascular disease
- hs-CRP between 1.0 and 3.0 mg/L indicates an average risk of developing cardiovascular disease
- hs-CRP higher than 3.0 mg/L indicates a high risk of developing cardiovascular disease

Biochemical Markers

After an initial myocardial insult, the presence of tissue necrosis can be determined by increased levels of biochemical markers. Levels of biochemical markers, such as serum enzymes (creatine kinase [CK]) and proteins (troponin I and T), also can be used to determine the extent of myocardial death and the effectiveness of reperfusion therapy. In patients presenting with specific anginal symptoms and diagnostic ECG, these biochemical markers assist with confirmation of the diagnosis of an MI (Table 3-10). Enzymes play a more essential role in medical assessment of many patients with nonspecific or vague symptoms and inconclusive ECG changes.[32] Such analysis also includes evaluation of isoenzyme levels.[33] Isoenzymes are different chemical forms of the same enzyme that are tissue specific and allow differentiation of damaged tissue (e.g., skeletal muscle vs. cardiac muscle).

CK (formally called *creatine phosphokinase*) is released after cell injury or cell death. CK has three isoenzymes. The CK-MB isoenzyme is related to cardiac muscle cell injury or death. The most widely used value is the CK-MB relative index calculated as 100% (CK-MB/Total CK).[32] Temporal measurements of the CK-MB relative index help physicians diagnose MI, estimate the size of infarction, and evaluate the occurrence of reperfusion

TABLE 3-10 Biochemical Markers

Enzyme or Marker	Isoenzyme	Normal Value	Onset of Rise (hours)	Time of Peak Rise	Return to Normal
Creatine kinase (CK)		55-71 IU	3-6	12-24 hours	24-48 hours
	CK-MB	0-3%	4-8	18-24 hours	72 hours
Troponin T (cTnT)		<0.2 pg/L	2-4	24-36 hours	10-14 days
Troponin I (cTnI)		<3.1 pg/L	2-4	24-36 hours	10-14 days

Data from Christenson RH, Azzazy HME: Biochemical markers of the acute coronary syndromes, Clin Chem 44:1855-1864, 1998; Kratz AK, Leqand-Rowski KB: Normal reference laboratory values, N Engl J Med 339:1063-1072, 1998.

  IU, International unit; *L,* liter; *pg,* picogram.

and possible infarct extension. An early CK-MB peak with rapid clearance is a good indication of reperfusion.[12] Values may increase from skeletal muscle trauma, cardiopulmonary resuscitation, defibrillation, and open-heart surgery. Postoperative coronary artery bypass surgery tends to elevate CK-MB levels secondary to the cross-clamp time in the procedure. Early postoperative peaks and rapid clearance seem to indicate reversible damage, whereas later peaks and longer clearance times with peak values exceeding 50 U/L may indicate an MI.[12] Treatment with thrombolytic therapy, such as streptokinase or a tissue plasminogen activator (tPa), has been shown to falsely elevate the values and may create a second peak of CK-MB, which strongly suggests successful reperfusion.[12,32]

Troponins are essential contractile proteins found in skeletal and cardiac muscle. Troponin I is an isotype found exclusively in the myocardium and is therefore 100% cardiac specific. Troponin T, another isotype, is sensitive to cardiac damage, but its levels also rise with muscle and renal failure.[32] These markers have emerged as sensitive and cardiac-specific clinical indicators for diagnosis of MI and for risk stratification.

✎ CLINICAL TIP

Wait for the final diagnosis of location, size, and type of MI before beginning active physical therapy treatment. This allows for rest and time for the control of possible post-MI complications. Withhold physical therapy geared toward testing functional capacity or increasing the patient's activity until cardiac enzyme levels have peaked and begin to fall.

Natriuretic Peptides

Three natriuretic peptides have been identified in humans. These include atrial natriuretic peptide (ANP), brain natriuretic peptide (BNP), and C-natriuretic peptide (CNP).[4] ANP is stored in the right atrium and released in response to increased atrial pressures. BNP is stored in the ventricles and released in response to increased ventricular distending pressures. ANP and BNP cause vasodilatation and natriuresis and counteract the water-retaining effects of the adrenergic and renin angiotensin system. CNP is located primarily in the vasculature. The physiologic role of CNP is not yet clarified.

Circulating levels of ANP and BNP are elevated in the plasma in patients with heart failure. In normal human hearts, ANP predominates in the atria, with a low-level expression of BNP and CNP. Patients with heart failure demonstrate an unchanged content of ANP in the atria with a marked increase in the concentrations of BNP. No level of BNP perfectly separates patients with and without heart failure. Normal levels include BNP less than 100 pg/ml . Values above 500 generally are considered to be positive. A diagnostic gray area exists between 100 and 500 pg/ml.[4,34]

Arterial Blood Gas Measurements

Arterial blood gas measurement may be used to evaluate the oxygenation (PaO_2), ventilation ($PaCO_2$), and pH in patients during acute MI and exacerbations of CHF in certain situations (i.e., obvious tachypnea, low SaO_2). These evaluations can help determine the need for supplemental oxygen therapy and mechanical ventilatory support in these patients. Oxygen is the first drug provided during a suspected MI. Refer to Chapters 4 and 18 for further description of arterial blood gas interpretation and supplemental oxygen, respectively.

Chest Radiography

Chest x-ray can be ordered for patients to assist in the diagnosis of CHF or cardiomegaly (enlarged heart). Patients in CHF have an increased density in pulmonary vasculature markings, giving the appearance of congestion in the vessels.[3,7] Refer to Chapter 4 for further description of chest x-rays.

Echocardiography

Transthoracic echocardiography, or "cardiac echo," is a noninvasive procedure that uses ultrasound to evaluate the function of the heart. Evaluation includes the size of the ventricular cavity, the thickness and integrity of the septum, valve integrity, and the motion of individual segments of the ventricular wall. Volumes of the ventricles are quantified, and EF can be estimated.[3]

Transesophageal echocardiography (TEE) is a newer technique that provides a better view of the mediastinum in cases of pulmonary disease, chest wall abnormality, and obesity, which make standard echocardiography difficult.[12,35] For this test, the oropharynx is anesthetized, and the patient is given enough sedation to be relaxed but still awake, because he or she needs to cooperate by swallowing the catheter. The catheter, a piezoelectric crystal mounted on an endoscope, is passed into the esophagus. Specific indications for TEE include bacterial endocarditis, aortic dissection, regurgitation through or around a prosthetic mitral or tricuspid valve, left atrial thrombus, intracardiac source of an embolus, and interarterial septal defect. Patients usually fast for at least 4 hours before the procedure.[35]

Principal indications for echocardiography are to assist in the diagnosis of pericardial effusion, cardiac tamponade, idiopathic or hypertrophic cardiomyopathy, a variety of valvular diseases, intracardiac masses, ischemic cardiac muscle, left ventricular aneurysm, ventricular thrombi, and a variety of congenital heart diseases.[12]

Transthoracic echocardiography (TTE) also can be performed during or immediately after bicycle or treadmill exercise to identify ischemia-induced wall motion abnormalities or during a pharmacologically induced exercise stress test (e.g., a dobutamine stress echocardiograph [DSE]). This stress echocardiograph adds to the information obtained from standard stress tests (ECGs) and may be used as an alternative to nuclear scanning procedures. Transient depression of wall motion during or after stress suggests ischemia.[36]

Contrast Echocardiograph. The ability of the echocardiograph to diagnose perfusion abnormalities and myocardial chambers is improved by using an intravenously injected contrast agent. The contrast allows greater visualization of wall motion and wall thickness and calculation of EF.[37]

Dobutamine Stress Echocardiograph. Dobutamine is a potent alpha-1 (α1) agonist and a beta-receptor agonist with prominent inotropic and less-prominent chronotropic effects on the myocardium. Dobutamine (which, unlike Persantine, increases contractility, HR, and BP in a manner similar to exercise) is injected in high doses into subjects as an alternative to exercise.[36] Dobutamine infusion is increased in a stepwise fashion similar to an exercise protocol. The initial infusion is 0.01 mg/kg and is increased 0.01 mg/kg every 3 minutes until a maximum infusion of 0.04 mg/kg is reached. Typically, the echocardiograph image of wall motion is obtained during the final minute(s) of infusion. This image can then be compared to baseline recordings.[36] If needed, atropine occasionally is added to facilitate a greater HR response for the test.[36] Low-dose DSE has the capacity to evaluate the contractile response of the impaired myocardium. Bellardinelli and colleagues[38] have demonstrated that improvements in functional capacity after exercise can be predicted by low-dose DSE. Patients with a positive contractile response to dobutamine were more likely to increase their $\dot{V}O_{2max}$ after a 10-week exercise program. Having a positive contractile response on the low-dose DSE had a positive predictive value of 84% and a negative predictive value of 59%.[38]

As this study indicates, research is beginning to demonstrate the prognostic value of certain medical tests for determining functional prognosis. Therefore physical therapists must be prepared to assess this area of literature critically to assist the medical team in determining the level of rehabilitative care for a patient during his or her recovery.

Exercise Testing

Exercise testing, or stress testing, is a noninvasive method of assessing cardiovascular responses to increased activity. The use of exercise testing in cardiac patients can serve multiple purposes, which are not mutually exclusive. The most widespread use of exercise testing is as a diagnostic tool for the presence of coronary artery disease. Other uses include determination of prognosis and severity of disease, evaluation of the effectiveness of treatment, early detection of labile hypertension, evaluation of CHF, evaluation of arrhythmias, and evaluation of functional capacity.[36] Exercise testing involves the systematic and progressive increase in intensity of activity (e.g., treadmill walking, bicycling, stair climbing, arm ergometry). These tests are accompanied by simultaneous ECG analysis, BP measurements, and subjective reports, commonly using Borg's Rating of Perceived Exertion (RPE).[39,40] Occasionally, the use of expired gas analysis can provide useful information about pulmonary function and maximal oxygen consumption.[36] Submaximal tests, such as the 12- and 6-minute walk tests, can be performed to assess a patient's function. For further discussion of the 6-minute walk test, refer to Chapter 23.

Submaximal tests differ from maximal tests in that the patient is not pushed to his or her maximum HR; instead the test is terminated at a predetermined end point, usually at 75% of the patient's predicted maximum HR.[41] For a comparison of two widely used exercise test protocols and functional activities, refer to Table 3-11. For a more thorough description of submaximal exercise testing, the reader is referred to Noonan and Dean.[41]

Contraindications to exercise testing include the following[42]:
- Recent MI (less than 48 hours earlier)
- Acute pericarditis
- Unstable angina (USA)
- Ventricular or rapid arrhythmias
- Untreated second- or third-degree heart block
- Decompensated CHF
- Acute illness

Exercise test results can be used for the design of an exercise prescription. Based on the results, the patient's actual or extrapolated maximum HR can be used to determine the patient's target HR range and safe activity intensity. RPE with symptoms during the exercise test also can be used to gauge exercise or activity intensity, especially in subjects on beta-blockers. (Refer to the Physical Therapy Intervention section for a discussion on the use of RPE.)

Any walk test that includes measurement of distance and time can be used to estimate metabolic equivalents (METs) and oxygen consumption with the following equations:

$$\dot{V}O_2 \, ml/kg/min = (mph)(26.83 \, m/min)(0.1 \, ml/kg/min) + 3.5 \, ml/kg/min$$
$$METs = \dot{V}O_2 \, ml/kg/min \div 3.5$$
$$MPH = (pace \, [feet/min] \times 60) \div 5280 \, (feet/mile)$$

A direct relationship exists between pace on a level surface and METs (oxygen consumption). A therapist can use walking pace to estimate oxygen consumption and endurance for other functional tasks that fall within a patient's oxygen consumption (aerobic functional capacity).

TABLE 3-11 Comparison of Exercise Test Protocols and Functional Tasks—Energy Demands

Oxygen Requirements (ml O_2/kg/min)	Metabolic Equivalents (METS)	Functional Tasks	Treadmill: Bruce Protocol 3-Minute Stages (mph/elevation)	Bike Ergometer: for 70 kg of Body Weight (kg/min)
52.5	15			
49.5	14			
45.5	13		4.2/16.0	1500
42.0	12			1350
38.5	11			1200
35.0	10	Jogging	3.4/14.0	1050
31.5	9			900
28.0	8			750
24.5	7		2.5/12.0	
21.0	6	Stair climbing		600
17.5	5		1.7/10.0	450
14.0	4	Walking (level surface)		300
10.5	3			150
7.0	2	Bed exercise (arm exercises in supine or sitting)		

Data from American Heart Association, Committee on Exercise: Exercise testing and training of apparently healthy individuals: a handbook for physicians, Dallas, 1972, The Association; Brooks GA, Fahey TD, White TP, editors: Exercise physiology: human bioenergetics and its applications, ed 2, Mountain View, Calif, 1996, Mayfield Publishing.

Figure 3-9 depicts the relationship between pace (feet/min) and METs for level surface ambulation. Bruce Protocol Stage 1 (because of its incline when at 1.7 mph) is similar to ambulation at 400 feet/min on a level surface. If a patient cannot sustain a particular pace for at least 10 minutes, it can be concluded that this pace exceeds the patient's anaerobic threshold. If the patient cannot sustain a pace for at least 1 minute, it can be concluded that the pace is close to the patient's maximal MET (oxygen consumption). Therefore continuous aerobic exercise programs should be at a walking pace below anaerobic threshold. For interval aerobic training, work periods at walking paces that can be sustained for 1 to 10 minutes would be appropriate with an equal period of rest. If a patient is required routinely to exceed maximal oxygen consumption during daily tasks, he or she is much more likely to experience signs of fatigue and exhaustion over time such as during repeated bouts of activity throughout the day.

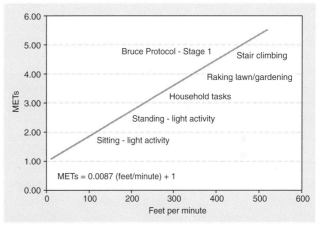

FIGURE 3-9

Relationship between walking pace, METs, and oxygen consumption on level surfaces. (Data from Fletcher GF, Balady GJ, Amsterdam EA et al: Exercise standards for testing and training: a statement for healthcare professionals from the American Heart Association, Circulation 104:1694-1740, 2001.)

> ✎ **CLINICAL TIP**
>
> Synonyms for exercise tests include exercise tolerance test (ETT) and graded exercise test (GXT).

Thallium Stress Testing. Thallium stress testing is a stress test that involves the injection of a radioactive nuclear marker for the detection of myocardial perfusion. The injection is given typically (via an intravenous line) during peak exercise or when symptoms are reported during the stress test. After the test, the subject is passed under a nuclear scanner to be evaluated for myocardial perfusion by assessment of the distribution of thallium uptake. The subject then returns 3 to 4 hours later to be reevaluated for myocardial reperfusion. This test appears to be more sensitive than stress tests without thallium for identifying patients with coronary artery disease.[12]

Persantine Thallium Stress Testing. Persantine thallium stress testing is the use of dipyridamole (Persantine) to dilate coronary arteries. Coronary arteries with atherosclerosis do not dilate; therefore dipyridamole shunts blood away from these areas. It is used typically in patients who are very unstable, deconditioned, or unable to ambulate or cycle for exercise-based stress testing.[36] Patients are asked to avoid all food and drugs containing methylxanthines (e.g., coffee, tea, chocolate, cola drinks) for at least 6 hours before the test in addition to phos-phodiesterase drugs, such as aminophylline, for 24 hours. While the patient is supine, an infusion of dipyridamole (0.56 ml/kg diluted in saline) is given intravenously over 4 minutes (using a large-vein intracatheter). Four minutes after the infusion is completed, the perfusion marker (thallium) is injected, and the patient is passed under a nuclear scanner to be evaluated for myocardial perfusion by assessment of the distribution of thallium uptake.[36]

Cardiac Catheterization

Cardiac catheterization, classified as either right or left, is an invasive procedure that involves passing a flexible, radiopaque catheter into the heart to visualize chambers, valves, coronary arteries, great vessels, cardiac pressures, and volumes to evaluate cardiac function (estimate EF, CO).

The procedure also is used in the following diagnostic and therapeutic techniques[12]:

- Angiography
- Percutaneous transluminal coronary angioplasty (PTCA)
- Electrophysiologic studies (EPSs)
- Cardiac muscle biopsy

Right-sided catheterization involves entry through a sheath that is inserted into a vein (commonly subclavian) for evaluation of right heart pressures; calculation of CO; and angiography of the right atrium, right ventricle, tricuspid valve, pulmonic valve, and pulmonary artery.[12] It also is used for continuous hemodynamic monitoring in patients with present or very recent heart failure to monitor cardiac pressures (see Chapter 18). Indications for right heart catheterization include an intra-cardiac shunt (blood flow between right and left atria or right and left ventricles), myocardial dysfunction, pericardial con-striction, pulmonary vascular disease, valvular heart disease, and status post heart transplant.

Left-sided catheterization involves entry through a sheath inserted into an artery (commonly femoral) to evaluate the aorta, left atrium, and left ventricle; left ventricular function; mitral and aortic valve function; and angiography of coronary arteries. Indications for left heart catheterization include aortic dissec-tion, atypical angina, cardiomyopathy, congenital heart disease, coronary artery disease, status post MI, valvular heart disease, and status post heart transplant.

Physical Therapy Considerations

- After catheterization, the patient is on bed rest for approxi-mately 4 to 6 hours when venous access is performed, or for 6 to 8 hours when arterial access is performed.[12]
- The sheaths typically are removed from the vessel 4 to 6 hours after the procedure, and pressure is applied constantly for 20 minutes after sheath removal.[12]
- The extremity should remain immobile with a sandbag over the access site to provide constant pressure to reduce the risk of vascular complications.[12]
- Some hospitals may use a knee immobilizer to assist with immobilizing the lower extremity.
- Physical therapy intervention should be deferred or limited to bedside treatment within the parameters of these precautions.

- During the precautionary period, physical therapy interven-tion such as bronchopulmonary hygiene or education may be necessary. Bronchopulmonary hygiene is indicated if pulmo-nary complications or risk of these complications exists. Edu-cation is warranted when the patient is anxious and needs to have questions answered regarding his or her functional mobility.
- After the precautionary period, normal mobility can progress to the limit of the patient's cardiopulmonary impairments; however, the catheterization results should be incorporated into the physical therapy treatment plan.

Angiography

Angiography involves the injection of radiopaque contrast material through a catheter to visualize vessels or chambers. Different techniques are used for different assessments (Table 3-12).

Electrophysiologic Studies

EPSs are performed to evaluate the electrical conduction system of the heart.[12] An electrode catheter is inserted through the femoral vein into the right ventricle apex. Continuous ECG monitoring is performed internally and externally. The elec-trode can deliver programmed electrical stimulation to evaluate conduction pathways, formation of arrhythmias, and the auto-maticity and refractoriness of cardiac muscle cells. EPSs evaluate the effectiveness of antiarrhythmic medication and can provide specific information about each segment of the conduction system.[12] In many hospitals, these studies may be combined with a therapeutic procedure, such as an ablation procedure (discussed in the Management section). Indications for EPSs include the following[12]:

- Sinus node disorders
- AV or intraventricular block
- Previous cardiac arrest
- Tachycardia at greater than 200 bpm
- Unexplained syncope

> ✎ **CLINICAL TIP**
> Patients undergoing EPSs should remain on bed rest for 4 to 6 hours after the test.

TABLE 3-12 Assessment Methods

Method	Region Examined
Aortography	Aorta and aortic valve
Coronary arteriography	Coronary arteries
Pulmonary angiography	Pulmonary circulation
Ventriculography	Right or left ventricle and AV valves

Data from Woods SL, Sivarajian Froelicher ES, Underhill-Motzer S, editors: Cardiac nursing, ed 6, Philadelphia, 2009, Lippincott Williams & Wilkins, Philadelphia.

AV, Atrioventricular.

Health Conditions

When disease and degenerative changes impair the heart's capacity to perform work, a reduction in CO occurs. If cardiac, renal, or central nervous system perfusion is reduced, a vicious cycle resulting in heart failure can ensue. A variety of pathologic processes can impair the heart's capacity to perform work. These pathologic processes can be divided into four major categories: (1) acute coronary syndrome, (2) rhythm and conduction disturbance, (3) valvular heart disease, and (4) myocardial and pericardial heart disease. CHF occurs when this failure to pump blood results in an increase in the fluid in the lungs, liver, subcutaneous tissues, and serous cavities.[5]

Acute Coronary Syndrome

When myocardial oxygen demand is higher than supply, the myocardium must use anaerobic metabolism to meet energy demands. This system can be maintained for only a short period of time before tissue ischemia will occur, which typically results in angina (chest pain). If the supply and demand are not balanced by rest, medical management, surgical intervention, or any combination of these, injury of the myocardial tissue will ensue, followed by infarction (cell death). This balance of supply and demand is achieved in individuals with normal coronary circulation; however, it is compromised in individuals with impaired coronary blood flow. The following pathologies can result in myocardial ischemia:

• Coronary arterial spasm is a disorder of transient spasm of coronary vessels that impairs blood flow to the myocardium. It can occur with or without the presence of atherosclerotic coronary disease. It results in variant angina (Prinzmetal angina).[12]

• Coronary atherosclerotic disease (CAD) is a multistep process of the deposition of fatty streaks, or plaques, on artery walls (atherosis). The presence of these deposits eventually leads to arterial wall damage and platelet and macrophage aggregation that then leads to thrombus formation and hardening of the arterial walls (sclerosis). The net effect is a narrowing of coronary walls. It can result in stable angina, unstable angina (USA), or MI.[3,5,12]

Clinical syndromes caused by these pathologies are as follows[7,12]:

• Stable (exertional) angina occurs with increased myocardial demand, such as during exercise; is relieved by reducing exercise intensity or terminating exercise; and responds well to nitroglycerin.

• Variant angina (Prinzmetal angina) is a less-common form of angina caused by coronary artery spasm. This form of angina tends to be prolonged, severe, and not readily relieved by nitroglycerin.

• USA is considered intermediate in severity between stable angina and MI. It usually has a sudden onset, occurs at rest or with activity below the patient's usual ischemic baseline, and may be different from the patient's usual anginal pattern. USA is not induced by activity or increased myocardial demand that cannot be met. It can be induced at rest, when supply is cut down with no change in demand. A common cause of USA is believed to be a rupture of an atherosclerotic plaque.

• MI occurs with prolonged or unmanaged ischemia (Table 3-13). It is important to realize that an evolution occurs from ischemia to infarction. Ischemia is the first phase of tissue response when the myocardium is deprived of oxygen. It is reversible if sufficient oxygen is provided in time. However, if oxygen deprivation continues, myocardial cells will become

TABLE 3-13   Myocardial Infarctions

Myocardial Infarction (MI)/Wall Affected	Possible Occluded Coronary Artery	Possible Complications
Anterior MI/anterior left ventricle	LCA	Left-sided CHF, pulmonary edema, bundle branch block, AV block, and ventricular aneurysm (which can lead to CHF, dysrhythmias, and embolism)
Inferior MI/inferior left ventricle	RCA	AV blocks (which can result in bradycardia) and papillary muscle dysfunction (which can result in valvular insufficiency and eventually CHF)
Anterolateral MI/anterolateral left ventricle	LAD, circumflex	Brady or tachyarrhythmias, acute ventricular septal defect
Anteroseptal MI/septal region—between left and right ventricles	LAD	Brady or tachyarrhythmias, ventricular aneurysm
Posterior MI/posterior heart	RCA, circumflex	Bradycardia, heart blocks
Right ventricular MI	RCA	Right ventricular failure (can lead to left ventricular failure and therefore cardiogenic shock), heart blocks, hepatomegaly, peripheral edema
Transmural MI (Q-wave MI)	Any artery	Full wall thickness MI, as above
Subendocardial MI (non–Q-wave MI)	Any artery	Partial wall thickness MI, as above, potential to extend to transmural MI

Data from Woods SL, Sivarajian-Froelicher ES, Underhill-Motzer S, editors: Cardiac nursing, ed 4, Philadelphia, 2000, Lippincott, 2000.
AV, Atrioventricular; *CHF,* congestive heart failure; *LAD,* left anterior descending; *LCA,* left coronary artery; *RCA,* right coronary artery.

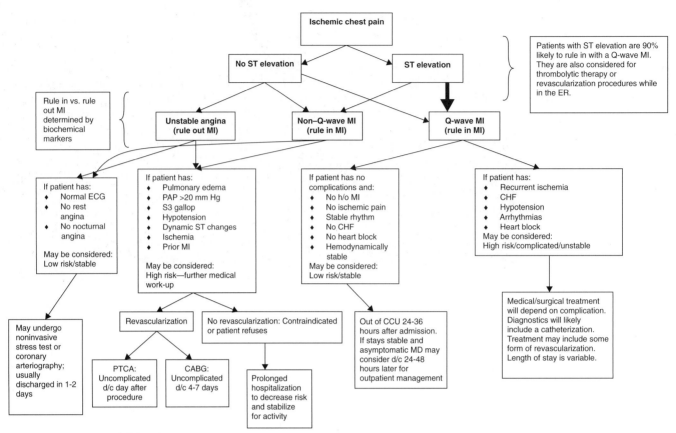

FIGURE 3-10

Possible clinical course of patients admitted with chest pain. *CABG*, Coronary artery bypass graft; *CHF*, congestive heart failure; *CC*, coronary care unit; *d/c*, discharge; *ECG*, electrocardiogram; *h/o*, history of; *MI*, myocardial infarction; *PAP*, pulmonary arterial pressure; *PTCA*, percutaneous transluminal coronary angioplasty; *ST elevation*, electrocardiogram that shows elevation of the ST segment. (Data from American College of Cardiology/American Heart Association: 1999 Update: ACC/AHA guidelines for the management of patients with acute myocardial infarction: executive summary and recommendations, Circulation 100:1016-1030, 1999; American College of Cardiology/American Heart Association: ACC/AHA guidelines for the management of patients with acute myocardial infarction, J Am Coll Cardiol 28:1328-1428, 1996; American College of Cardiology/American Heart Association: ACC/AHA guidelines for the management of patients with unstable angina [USA] and non-ST segment elevation myocardial infarction, J Am Coll Cardiol 36:971-1048, 2000.)

injured and eventually will die (infarct). The location and extent of cell death are determined by the coronary artery that is compromised and the amount of time that the cells are deprived. A clinical overview is provided in Figure 3-10.

✎ CLINICAL TIP

ST depression on a patient's ECG of approximately 1 to 2 mm generally is indicative of ischemia; ST elevation generally is indicative of myocardial injury or infarction.

Rhythm and Conduction Disturbance

Rhythm and conduction disturbances can range from minor alterations with no hemodynamic effects to life-threatening episodes with rapid hemodynamic compromise.[3,5,7] Refer to the tables in Chapter Appendix 3A for a description of atrial, ventricular, and junctional rhythms and AV blocks. Refer to

Chapter Appendix 3B for examples of common rhythm disturbances. Physical therapists must be able to identify abnormalities in the ECG to determine patient tolerance to activity. In particular, physical therapists should understand progressions of common ECG abnormalities so that they can identify, early on, when the patient is not tolerating an intervention. (Refer to the Physical Therapy Intervention section for a discussion on ECG.)

A common form of rhythm disturbance is a PVC, which also can be referred to as a ventricular premature beat. These abnormalities originate from depolarization of a cluster of cells in the ventricle (an ectopic foci), which results in ventricular depolarization. From the term *ectopic foci*, PVCs may be referred to as *ventricular ectopy*.

Valvular Heart Disease

Valvular heart disease encompasses valvular disorders of one or more of the four valves of the heart (Table 3-14). The following three disorders can occur[3,5]:

TABLE 3-14 Signs and Symptoms of Valvular Heart Disease

Disease	Symptoms	Signs
Aortic stenosis	Angina, syncope or near syncope, signs of left ventricle failure (dyspnea, orthopnea, cough)	Elevated left ventricular wall pressure, decreased subendocardial blood flow, systolic murmur, ventricular hypertrophy
Chronic aortic regurgitation	Angina, symptoms of left ventricular failure	Dilated aortic root, dilated left ventricle, diastolic murmur, left ventricular hypertrophy
Acute aortic regurgitation	Rapid progression of symptoms of left ventricular failure, pulmonary edema, angina	Sinus tachycardia to compensate for decreased stroke volume, loud S3, diastolic murmur, signs of ventricular failure
Mitral stenosis	Symptoms of pulmonary vascular congestion (dyspnea, orthopnea). If patient develops pulmonary hypertension (which can cause hypoxia, hypotension), he or she may have angina, syncope	Left atrial hypertrophy, pulmonary hypertension, atrial fibrillation, can have embolus formation (especially if in atrial fibrillation), long diastolic murmur
Chronic mitral regurgitation	Symptoms of pulmonary vascular congestion, angina, syncope, fatigue	Left atrial enlargement, atrial fibrillation, elevated left atrial pressure
Acute mitral regurgitation	Rapid progression of symptoms of pulmonary vascular congestion	Sinus tachycardia, presence of S3 or S4, pulmonary edema
Mitral valve prolapse	Most commonly asymptomatic, fatigue, palpitation	Systolic click, may have tachyarrhythmia syncope

Data from Woods SL, Sivarajian-Froelicher ES, Underhill-Motzer S, editors: Cardiac nursing, ed 4, Philadelphia, 2000, Lippincott; Cheitlin MD, Sokolow M, McIlroy MB: Clinical cardiology, ed 6, Norwalk, Conn, 1993, Appleton & Lange.

1. Stenosis involves narrowing of the valve.
2. Regurgitation, the back flow of blood through the valve, occurs with incomplete valve closure.
3. Prolapse involves enlarged valve cusps. The cusps can become floppy and bulge backward. This condition may progress to regurgitation.

Over time, these disorders can lead to pumping dysfunction and, ultimately, heart failure.

Myocardial and Pericardial Heart Disease

Myocardial heart disease affects the myocardial muscle tissue and also can be referred to as cardiomyopathy (Table 3-15); pericardial heart diseases affect the pericardium (Table 3-16).

Heart Failure

Heart failure, a decrease of CO, can be caused by a variety of cardiac pathologies. Because CO is not maintained, life cannot be sustained if heart failure continues without treatment. Heart failure results in the congestion of the pulmonary circulation and, in certain cases, even the systemic circulation. Therefore it is referred to commonly as congestive heart failure, or CHF. The most common pathologic etiology of CHF is some type of cardiomyopathy (see Table 3-15).

The following terms are used to classify the types of cardiac impairment in CHF[43]:

- Left-sided heart failure refers to failure of the left ventricle, resulting in back flow into the lungs.
- Right-sided failure refers to failure of the right side of the heart, resulting in back flow into the systemic venous system.
- High-output failure refers to heart failure that is secondary to renal system failure to filter off excess fluid. The renal system failure places a higher load on the heart, which cannot be maintained.

BOX 3-2 Signs and Symptoms of Congestive Heart Failure

Signs	Symptoms
Cold, pale, possibly cyanotic extremities	Dyspnea
Weight gain	Tachypnea
Peripheral edema	Paroxysmal nocturnal dyspnea
Hepatomegaly	Orthopnea
Jugular venous distention	Cough
Crackles (rales)	Fatigue
Tubular breath sounds and consolidation S3 heart sound	
Sinus tachycardia	
Decreased exercise tolerance and physical work capacity	

Adapted from Cahalin L: Cardiac muscle dysfunction. In Hillegass EA, Sadowsky HS: Essentials of cardiopulmonary physical therapy, ed 2, Philadelphia, 2001, Saunders.

- Low-output failure refers to the condition in which the heart is not able to pump the minimal amount of blood to support circulation.
- Systolic dysfunction refers to a problem with systole or the actual strength of myocardial contraction.
- Diastolic dysfunction refers to a problem during diastole or the ability of the ventricle to allow the filling of blood.

Possible signs and symptoms of CHF are described in Box 3-2. The American Heart Association revised the New York Heart Association (NYHA) Functional Classification of Heart Disease; this new classification is described in Table 3-17. Although the NYHA classification provides a good description of the patient's condition, it does not include management

TABLE 3-15 Myocardial Diseases—Cardiomyopathies

Functional Classification		
Cardiomyopathy	**Dysfunction**	**Description**
Dilated	Systolic	Ventricle is dilated, with marked contractile dysfunction of myocardium
Hypertrophic	Diastolic	Thickened ventricular myocardium, less compliant to filling, and therefore decreased filling during diastole
Restrictive	Systolic and diastolic	Endocardial scarring of ventricles, decreased compliance during diastole, and decreased contractile force during systole

Etiologic Classification	
Etiology	**Examples**
Inflammatory	Viral infarction, bacterial infarction
Metabolic	Selenium deficiency, diabetes mellitus
Fibroplastic	Carcinoid fibrosis, endomyocardial fibrosis
Hypersensitivity	Cardiac transplant rejection, methyldopa
Genetic	Hypertrophic cardiomyopathy, Duchenne's muscular dystrophy
Idiopathic	Idiopathic hypertrophic cardiomyopathy
Infiltrative	Sarcoidosis, neoplastic
Hematologic	Sickle cell anemia
Toxic	Alcohol, bleomycin
Physical agents	Heat stroke, hypothermia, radiation
Miscellaneous acquired	Postpartum cardiomyopathy, obesity

Data from Cahalin L: Cardiac muscle dysfunction. In Hillegass EA, Sadowsky HS, editors: Essentials of cardiopulmonary physical therapy, ed 2, Philadelphia, 2001, Saunders; Hare JM: The dilated, restrictive, and infiltrative cardiomyopathies. In Libby P, Bonow RO, Mann DL et al: Braunwald's heart disease: a textbook of cardiovascular medicine, ed 8, Philadelphia, 2008, Saunders.

TABLE 3-16 Signs and Symptoms of Pericardial Heart Diseases

Disease	Symptoms	Signs
Acute pericarditis	Retrosternal chest pain (worsened by supine and/or deep inspiration), dyspnea, cough, hoarseness, dysphagia, fever, chills, and weakness possible	Pericardial friction rub; diffuse ST segment elevation; decreased QRS voltage in all ECG leads if pericardial effusion also present
Constrictive pericarditis	Abdominal swelling, peripheral edema, fatigue, dyspnea, dizziness and/or syncope, signs of pulmonary venous congestion, vague nonspecific retrosternal chest pain	Jugular venous distention; QRS voltage diminished on ECG; occasionally atrial fibrillation
Chronic pericardial effusion (without tamponade)	May have vague fullness in anterior chest, cough, hoarseness, dysphagia	Muffled heart sounds; may have pericardial friction rub; QRS voltage diminished on ECG; chest x-ray with cardiomegaly without pulmonary congestion
Pericardial tamponade	Symptoms of low cardiac output (dyspnea, fatigue, dizziness, syncope); may have retrosternal chest pain; may have cough, hiccoughs, hoarseness	Jugular venous distention, cardiomegaly, diminished QRS voltage on ECG; becomes tamponade from effusion when right heart catheterization shows equal pressures in right atrium, ventricle, and capillary wedge (signifies left atria pressure), and left heart catheterization shows equal pressure on left side of heart to right side

Data from Woods SL, Sivarajian-Froelicher ES, Underhill-Motzer S, editors: Cardiac nursing, ed 4, Philadelphia, 2000, Lippincott; Cheitlin MD, Sokolow M, McIlroy MB: Clinical cardiology, ed 6, Norwalk, Conn, 1993, Appleton & Lange.

ECG, Electrocardiogram.

strategies based on patient severity. Therefore another classification system has been devised based on four stages (A to D)[44]:

- Stage A: Patients who are at high risk for developing left ventricular dysfunction. Treatment intervention is focused on risk factor modification.

- Stage B: Patients who have left ventricular dysfunction but are asymptomatic. Treatment intervention is focused on prevention of symptoms with risk factor modification.
- Stage C: Patients who have left ventricular dysfunction are symptomatic. Treatment intervention is centered around

TABLE 3-17   American Heart Association's Functional Capacity and Objective Assessment of Patients with Diseases of the Heart

	Class and Functional Capacity*	Objective Assessment†
Class I	Patients with cardiac disease but without resulting limitations of physical activity. Ordinary physical activity does not cause undue fatigue, palpitation, dyspnea, or anginal pain.	No objective evidence of cardiovascular disease
Class II	Patients with cardiac disease that results in a slight limitation of physical activity. Patients are comfortable at rest, but ordinary physical activity results in fatigue, palpitations, dyspnea, or anginal pain.	Objective evidence of minimal cardiovascular disease
Class III	Patients with cardiac disease that results in a marked limitation of physical activity. Patients are comfortable at rest, but less-than-ordinary activity causes fatigue, palpitations, dyspnea, or anginal pain.	Objective evidence of moderately severe cardiovascular disease
Class IV	Patients with cardiac disease that results in an inability to carry on any physical activity without discomfort. Fatigue, palpitations, dyspnea, or anginal pain may be present even at rest. If any physical activity is undertaken, symptoms increase.	Objective evidence of severe cardiovascular disease

From The Criteria Committee of the New York Heart Association: Nomenclature and criteria for diagnosis of diseases of the heart and great vessels, ed 9, Boston, 1994, Little, Brown & Co, pp 253-256.

*Functional capacity refers to subjective symptoms of the patient. This aspect of the classification is identical to the New York Heart Association's Classification.

†Objective assessment was added to the classification system by the American Heart Association in 1994. It refers to measurements such as electrocardiograms, stress tests, echocardiograms, and radiologic images.[42]

alleviating symptoms and slowing the progression of the disease.

- Stage D: Patients who have advanced-stage refractory heart failure. Treatment is based on specialized pharmacologic and surgical interventions such as ventricular assist devices (see Chapter 18, Appendix B) and possible transplantation (see Chapter 14).

Activity progression for patients hospitalized with CHF is based on the ability of medical treatments (e.g., diuresis, inotropes) to keep the patient out of heart failure. When a patient with CHF is medically stabilized, the heart is thought to be "compensated." Conversely, when the patient is unable to maintain adequate circulation, the heart would be "decompensated." Clinical examination findings allow the therapist to evaluate continuously the patient's tolerance to the activity progression. Although MET tables are not commonly used clinically, they do provide a method of progressively increasing a patient's activity level. As greater MET levels are achieved with an appropriate hemodynamic response, the next level of activity can be attempted. See Table 3-11 for MET levels for common activities that can be performed with patients.

Management

This section discusses surgical and nonsurgical procedures, pharmacologic interventions, and physical therapy interventions for patients with cardiac dysfunction.

Revascularization and Reperfusion of the Myocardium

Thrombolytic Therapy

Thrombolytic therapy has been established as an acute management strategy for patients experiencing an MI because of the high prevalence of coronary artery thrombosis during acute MI.

Thrombolytic agents, characterized as fibrin-selective and non-selective agents, are administered to appropriate candidates via intravenous access. The most common agents include streptokinase (nonselective), anisoylated plasminogen streptokinase activator complex (nonselective), and tissue plasminogen activator (t-PA) (fibrin-selective).[12] Fibrin-selective agents have a high velocity of clot lysis, whereas the nonselective agents have a slower clot lysis and more prolonged systemic lytic state.

The indication for thrombolytic therapy includes chest pain suggestive of myocardial ischemia and associated with acute ST segment elevation on a 12-lead ECG or a presumed new left ventricular bundle branch block. Hospital protocol regarding the time period to perform thrombolytic therapy usually varies because clinical trials have led to some controversy.[12] Some studies show benefits only if treatment is conducted within 6 hours of symptoms, whereas others have demonstrated improvement with treatment up to 24 hours after onset of symptoms.[12]

The contraindications to thrombolytic therapy generally include patients who are at risk for excessive bleeding. Because of the variability that can occur among patients, many contraindications are considered relative cautions, and the potential benefits of therapy are weighed against the potential risks. Thrombolytic therapy is used in conjunction with other medical treatments such as aspirin, intravenous heparin, intravenous nitroglycerin, lidocaine, atropine, and a beta-blocker. As previously discussed, early peaking of CK-MB is associated with reperfusion.[12]

Percutaneous Revascularization Procedures

Percutaneous revascularization procedures are used to return blood flow through coronary arteries that have become occlusive secondary to atherosclerotic plaques. The following list briefly describes three percutaneous revascularization procedures[12]:

1. Percutaneous transluminal coronary angioplasty (PTCA) is performed on atherosclerotic lesions that do not completely

occlude the vessel. PTCA can be performed at the time of an initial diagnostic catheterization, electively at some time after a catheterization, or urgently in the setting of an acute MI. Refer to the Diagnostic and Laboratory Measures section for a discussion on precautions after a catheterization procedure.

A sheath is inserted into the femoral, radial, or brachial artery, and a catheter is guided through the sheath into the coronary artery. A balloon system is then passed through the catheter to the lesion site. Inflations of variable pressure and duration may be attempted to reduce the lesion by at least 20% diameter with a residual narrowing of less than 50% in the vessel lumen.[12] Owing to some mild ischemia that can occur during the procedure, patients occasionally require temporary transvenous pacing, intraaortic balloon counterpulsation, or femorofemoral cardiopulmonary bypass circulatory support during PTCA.

The use of endoluminal stents prevents the major limitations of PTCA, which include abrupt closure (in up to 7.3% of patients), restenosis, anatomically unsuitable lesions, chronic total occlusions, and unsatisfactory results in patients with prior coronary artery bypass graft (CABG) surgery.[45] Endoluminal stents are tiny springlike tubes that can be placed permanently into the coronary artery to increase the intraluminal diameter. Stents are occasionally necessary when initial attempts at revascularization (e.g., angioplasty) have failed.[12]

2. Coronary laser angioplasty uses laser energy to create precise ablation of plaques without thermal injury to the vessel. The laser treatment results in a more pliable lesion that responds better to balloon expansion. The use of laser angioplasty is limited, owing to the expense of the equipment and a high restenosis rate (greater than 40%).[46]

3. Directional coronary atherectomy can be performed by inserting a catheter with a cutter housed at the distal end on one side of the catheter and a balloon on the other side.[12] The balloon inflates and presses the cutter against the atheroma (plaque). The cutter then can cut the atheroma and remove it from the arterial wall. This also can be performed with a laser on the tip of the catheter. Rotational ablation uses a high-speed rotating bur coated with diamond chips, creating an abrasive surface. This selectively removes atheroma because of its inelastic properties as opposed to the normal elastic tissue.[12] The debris emitted from this procedure is passed into the coronary circulation and is small enough to pass through the capillary beds. Commonly, PTCA is used as an adjunct to this procedure to increase final coronary diameter or to allow for stent placement.

Transmyocardial Revascularization

In transmyocardial revascularization, a catheter with a laser tip creates transmural channels from patent coronary arteries into an area of the myocardium thought to be ischemic. It is intended for patients with chronic angina who, because of medical reasons, cannot have angioplasty or CABG. Theoretically, ischemia is reduced by increasing the amount of oxygenated blood in ischemic tissue. Angiogenesis (the growth of new blood

vessels) also has been proposed as a mechanism of improvement after this procedure. Although therapists should expect improvements in functional capacity with decreased angina, the patient's risk status related to CAD or left ventricular dysfunction does not change.[47] Post-catheterization procedure precautions, as previously described, apply after this procedure.

Coronary Artery Bypass Graft

A CABG is performed when the coronary artery has become completely occluded or when it cannot be corrected by PTCA, coronary arthrectomy, or stenting. In this procedure a vascular graft is used to revascularize the myocardium. The saphenous vein, radial artery, left internal mammary artery (LIMA), or right internal mammary artery (RIMA) commonly is used as a vascular graft. CABG most commonly is performed through a median sternotomy, which extends caudally from just inferior to the suprasternal notch to below the xiphoid process and splits the sternum longitudinally.[12]

> ✎ **CLINICAL TIP**
>
> Because of the altered chest wall mechanics and the pain associated with a sternotomy, patients are at risk of developing pulmonary complications after a CABG. The physical therapist should be aware of postoperative complication risk factors and postoperative indicators of poor pulmonary function. Refer to Chapters 4 and 20 for further description of postoperative pulmonary complications.

Minimally Invasive Coronary Artery Bypass Graft Surgery. Advances in medicine have led to a set of minimally invasive cardiac surgical techniques using laparoscopic procedures and robotics to enter the thoracic cavity through small incisions in the chest in an effort to avoid a median sternotomy. These procedures aim to reduce complications associated with large surgical incisions and extensive periods on the cardiopulmonary bypass pump. Endoscopic robotic surgery involves the use of a computer-enhanced telemanipulation system to perform the grafting procedure.[48] The harvesting of the saphenous vein also can be achieved through minimal incision using video-based surgical techniques.[49] This minimally invasive procedure decreases morbidity associated with large leg incisions (pain and infection) in an effort to permit quicker recovery.[49]

Minimally invasive CABG techniques use a small thoracotomy incision as an alternate to median sternotomy.[50] Through the incision, the mammary arteries can be harvested and anastomosed thorascopically or with robotic assistance. These minimally invasive procedures performed through a small anterior thoracotomy are found to be best suited for occlusions within the anterior coronary vessels.[50] For multiple blocks located in multiple coronary arteries, surgeons may opt to perform a hybrid procedure involving the use of the minimally invasive CABG procedure coupled with a percutaneous transluminal coronary intervention procedure. The CABG procedure is used for restoring perfusion to the anterior vessel, specifically the left anterior descending artery, while the percutaneous procedure employs drug-eluting stents to the right coronary artery and circumflex artery.[51]

Off-Pump Coronary Artery Bypass Graft Procedure. The off-pump CABG procedure uses a standard median sternotomy and grafting of the coronary arteries under conditions of a beating, normothermic heart.[50] Regional ischemia is induced for 5- to 15-minute periods, during which each anastomosis must be constructed. The major advantage of the off-pump procedures is to reduce the complications associated with artificial perfusion induced by the cardiopulmonary bypass pump. Off-pump procedures reduce markers of inflammatory response and intraoperative troponin T release, thereby suggesting less myocyte injury.[52]

Median Sternotomy and Sternal Precautions. The primary premise for the use of sternal precautions is to reduce the possibility of sternal dehiscence. Interestingly, no direct evidence links the use of arm movements or activity to an increased risk of sternal complications after cardiothoracic surgery.[53] El-Ansary and colleagues found that patients with chronic sternal instability demonstrated the greatest sternal separation when pushing up from a chair with sit-to-stand transfers and least sternal separation when elevating both arms overhead.[54] In normal healthy individuals, the greatest amount of sternal skin movement was seen with sit-to-stand and supine-to-long-sitting transfers, and the least movement was noted when raising a unilateral weighted upper extremity (<8 lb) above shoulder height.[3,55] Patients with chronic sternal instability tend to experience greater pain when raising a unilateral loaded upper extremity as compared to raising bilateral loaded upper extremities.[54]

When prescribing sternal precautions for individuals after median sternotomy, consider the many risk factors that increase the potential for sternal dehiscence. Some of these risks include obesity, COPD, diabetes, repeat thoracotomy, smoking, peripheral vascular disease, and female gender with pendulous breasts. As the number of risk factors increase, the therapist must be more vigilant regarding sternal precautions. Sternal precautions usually are prescribed for at least 8 weeks to prevent wound dehiscence and preserve the integrity of sternal wiring. In managing the bariatric patient, physical therapists should evaluate the operative report as often the sternum is doubled wired during the surgical procedure to prevent dehiscence. In general, sternal precautions include restrictions for upper extremity lifting greater than 10 lb, pushing or pulling, scapular adduction, resistive exercises or loading of the upper extremity past 90 degrees of flexion and abduction, and minimal use of the arms for supine-to-sit and sit-to-stand transfers.[56]

> ✎ **CLINICAL TIP**
> To help patients understand the concept of lifting less than 10 lb, inform them that a gallon of milk weighs approximately 8½ lb.

Secondary Prevention After Revascularization

Improved medical and surgical interventions have reduced mortality resulting from cardiovascular disease; however, incidence and prevalence are still high.[1] After revascularization procedures, patients need education regarding cardiovascular disease risk factors. This ensures continued success of the procedures via secondary prevention of primary disease processes (refer to Box 3-1).

Ablation Procedure

Catheter ablation procedures are indicated for supraventricular tachycardia, AV nodal reentrant pathways, atrial fibrillation, atrial flutter, and certain types of ventricular tachycardia.[12] The procedure attempts to remove or isolate ectopic foci in an attempt to reduce the resultant rhythm disturbance. Radiofrequency ablation uses low-power, high-frequency AC current to destroy cardiac tissue and is the most effective technique for ablation.[12] After the ectopic foci are located under fluoroscopic guidance, the ablating catheter is positioned at the site to deliver a current for 10 to 60 seconds.

> ✎ **CLINICAL TIP**
> After an ablation procedure, the leg used for access (venous puncture site) must remain straight and immobile for 3 to 4 hours. If an artery was used, this time generally increases to 4 to 6 hours. (The exact time will depend on hospital policy.) Patients are sedated during the procedure and may require time after the procedure to recover. Most of the postintervention care is geared toward monitoring for complications. Possible complications include bleeding from the access site, cardiac tamponade from perforation, and arrhythmias. After a successful procedure (and the initial immobility to prevent vascular complications at the access site), usually activity is not restricted.

Maze Procedure

Surgical ablation of atrial fibrillation is accomplished by the maze procedure. This procedure was developed in 1990 and aims to surgically create a "maze" along the atria to best direct the electrical conduction appropriately to the AV node and the ventricles.[57] The procedure was named for the result of the surgical incisions, which often resembles a children's maze. The maze procedure is performed typically in conjunction with a CABG or valve replacement surgery.

The maze procedure has evolved over the last 20 years. It is currently the standard for nonpharmacologic treatment of atrial fibrillation.[58,59] The initial surgery (maze I or Cox maze) involved several small incisions around the SA node, the atrial-superior vena cava junction, and the sinus tachycardia region of the SA node.[60] The major complication after this procedure was chronotropic incompetence.[61] The procedure continues to be refined with the creation of the maze II and, most recently, the maze III procedure. Maze III reduces the frequency of chronotropic incompetence, improves atrial transport function, and involves a shorter procedure time.[62] It is important to note that atrial fibrillation may not reverse immediately after the procedure; it may take months for the arrhythmia to reverse.

Cardiac Pacemaker Implantation and Automatic Implantable Cardiac Defibrillator

Cardiac pacemaker implantation involves the placement of a unipolar or bipolar electrode on the myocardium. This electrode is used to create an action potential in the management of certain arrhythmias. Indications for cardiac pacemaker implantation include the following[12,63,64]:

- Sinus node disorders (bradyarrhythmias [HR lower than 60 bpm])
- Atrioventricular disorders (complete heart block, Mobitz type II block)
- Tachyarrhythmias (supraventricular tachycardia, frequent ectopy)
- Improving atrioventricular and/or biventricular synchrony

Temporary pacing may be performed after an acute MI to help control transient arrhythmias and after a CABG. Table 3-18 classifies various pacemakers.

One of the most critical aspects of pacer function for a physical therapist to understand is rate modulation. Rate modulation refers to the pacer's ability to modulate HR based on activity or physiologic demands. Not all pacers are equipped with rate modulation; therefore some patients have HRs that may not change with activity. In pacers with rate modulation, a variety of sensors are available to allow adjustment of HR. The type of sensor used may affect the ability of the pacer to respond to various exercise modalities. For more detail, refer to the review by Collins and Cahalin.[64]

An automatic implantable cardiac defibrillator (AICD) is used to manage uncontrollable, life-threatening ventricular arrhythmias by sensing the heart rhythm and defibrillating the myocardium as necessary to return the heart to a normal rhythm. Indications for AICD include ventricular tachycardia and ventricular fibrillation.[64]

Physical Therapy Considerations

- If the pacemaker does not have rate modulation, low-level activity with small increases in metabolic demand is preferred. An assessment of RPE, BP, and symptoms should be used to monitor tolerance.
- If the pacemaker does have rate modulation, then consider the type of rate modulation used.
  - With activity sensors, HR may respond sluggishly to activities that are smooth—such as on the bicycle ergometer.
  - For motion sensors, treadmill protocols should include increases in speed and grade because changes in only grade may not trigger an increase in HR.
  - QT sensors and ventilatory-driven sensors may require longer warm-up periods because of delayed responses to activity.
- Medication changes and electrolyte imbalance may affect responsiveness of HR with QT interval sensors.
- Know the upper limit of the rate modulation. When HR is at the upper limit of rate, monitor BP to maintain safe activity levels.
- In individuals who do not have rate-modulated pacers, BP response can be used to gauge intensity, as shown in the following equation:

$$\text{Training SBP} = (\text{SBP max} - \text{SBP rest})(\text{Intensity usually } 60\%\text{-}80\%) + \text{SBP rest}$$

- For example:

$$\text{Training SBP} = (180 - 120)(0.6 \text{ for lower limit to } 0.8 \text{ for upper limit}) + 120$$

  - Training SBP = 156-168 mm Hg

Life Vest

Recent developments in technology have resulted in the creation of a personal external defibrillator worn by patients at risk for sudden cardiac arrest. Life Vest is an external device that continuously monitors the patient's heart rhythm and delivers a shock in the event of a life-threatening arrhythmia. The two major components of the life vest include the garment and the monitor. The garment is worn under clothing and contains

TABLE 3-18 Pacemaker Classification

Position One Chamber(s) Paced	Position Two Chamber(s) Sensed	Position Three Response to a Sensed Event	Position Four Rate Modulation	Position Five Multisite Pacing
O = None	O = None	O = None	O = None	O = None
A = Atrium	A = Atrium	T = Triggered	R = Rate modulation in response to sensor technology	A = Atrium
V = Ventricle	V = Ventricle	I = Inhibited		V = Ventricle
D = Dual	D = Dual (atria and ventricles)	D = Dual (inhibited and triggered)		D = Dual (atrium and ventricle)
S = Manufacturer's designation for single (atrium or ventricle)	S = Manufacturer's designation for single (atrium or ventricle)			

Adapted from Bernstein A et al: The Revised NASPE/BPG (North American Society of Pacing and Electrophysiology/British Pacing and Electrophysiology Group) Generic Code for antibradycardic, adaptive-rate, and multisite pacing, Pacing Clin Electrophysiol 25(2):260-264.

Inhibited, Pending stimulus is inhibited when a spontaneous stimulation is detected. *Triggered,* Detection of stimulus produces an immediate stimulus in the same chamber. *Rate modulation,* Can adjust rate automatically based on one or more physiologic variables.

electrodes to pick up electrocardiographic readings. The monitor can be worn around the waist like a fanny pack or around the shoulder.

One advantage of this device is that it has the ability to sound an alarm to notify the patient of a dangerous arrhythmia before delivering the shock. If the patient is conscious, the patient has time to respond to the alarms by pressing two buttons to stop the treatment sequence in the event of a false alarm. If the patient is unconscious and does not respond, the device warns bystanders that a shock is to be delivered and then continues with the appropriate treatment sequence. Both the implantable defibrillator (ICD) and the Life Vest provide continuous protection to the patient. However, the Life Vest can be sought as a device to provide protection as a bridge to ICD implantation or cardiac transplantation. It also can be useful in higher-risk patients who are considered for ICD implantation but do not meet criteria for implantation.

Valve Replacement

Valve replacement is the most common surgical treatment for valvular disease. Patients with mitral and aortic stenosis, regurgitation, or both are the primary candidates for this surgery. Like the CABG, a median sternotomy is the route of access to the heart. Common valve replacements include mitral valve replacements (MVR) and aortic valve replacements (AVR). Prosthetic valves can be classified as mechanical (e.g., bi-leaflet and tilting disc valves) or biologic valves (i.e., derived from cadavers or porcine or bovine tissue).

Mechanical valves are preferred if the patient is younger than 65 years of age and is already on anticoagulation therapy (commonly because of history of atrial fibrillation or embolic cerebral vascular accident). The benefit of mechanical valves is their durability and long life.[12] Mechanical valves also tend to be thrombogenic and therefore require lifelong adherence to anticoagulation. For this reason, they may be contraindicated in patients who have a history of previous bleeding-related problems, wish to become pregnant, or have a history of poor medication compliance. These patients may benefit from biologic valves because anticoagulation therapy is not necessary. Biologic valves also may be preferred in patients older than 65 years of age.[12] Postoperative procedures and recovery from MVR and AVR surgeries are very similar to CABG.[12]

Percutaneous Aortic Valvotomy and Transcatheter Aortic Valve Implantation

For patients with aortic stenosis, the mainstay treatment involves an AVR executed through a median sternotomy. At times, this procedure entails substantial risks, especially if the patient has multiple comorbidities. Recent advances in medical technology have led to the development of catheter-based techniques for aortic valve implantation for the management of patients with symptomatic aortic stenosis.

Percutaneous aortic balloon valvotomy is a procedure in which a balloon is placed across the stenosed valve and inflated to relieve the stenosis.[65] Stenosis is ameliorated by stretching the annulus and fracturing calcific deposits within the leaflets of the valve. Despite reduction in transvalvular pressure and

overall reduction in symptoms after this procedure, patients continue to present with varying degrees of persistent aortic stenosis.[65] The 2006 American College of Cardiology/American Heart Association (ACC/AHA) guidelines state that this procedure is not a substitute for valve replacement but may be used as a bridge to surgery in hemodynamically unstable patients at high risk for an AVR.[66] In addition, the document demarcates the frequent use of this procedure in children with valvular aortic stenosis.

Another alternate to invasive open heart surgery involves a minimally invasive transcatheter aortic valve implantation procedure.[67] This procedure involves a replacement valve being fed through a small incision in the vascular system and progressed into the heart or through direct aortic access either via a mini-sternotomy or right anterior thoracotomy.[67] Two stent valve devices, including a balloon expandable valve (Edwards SAPIEN, Edwards Lifesciences LLC, Irvine, CA) and a self-expanding valve (Medtronic CoreValve, Minneapolis, MN), usually are implanted retrograde through an incision in the femoral artery.[68] The Medtronic CoreValve also can be inserted retrograde via the subclavian/axillary artery or through direct access to the heart by means of a mini-sternotomy or thoracotomy.[67]

Cardiac Transplantation

Cardiac transplantation is an acceptable intervention for the treatment of end-stage heart disease. A growing number of facilities are performing heart transplantation, and a greater number of physical therapists are involved in the rehabilitation of pretransplant and posttransplant recipients. Physical therapy intervention is vital for the success of heart transplantation; recipients have often survived a long period of convalescence before and after surgery, rendering them deconditioned. In general, heart transplant patients are immunosuppressed and are without neurologic input to their heart. These patients rely first on the Frank-Starling mechanism to augment SV and then on the catecholamine response to augment both HR and SV. Refer to Chapter 14 for information on heart and heart-lung transplantation.

Cardiac Medications

Cardiac medications are classified according to functional indications, drug classes, and mechanism of action. Cardiac drug classes occasionally are indicated for more than one clinical diagnosis. Chapter 19 lists the functional indications, mechanisms of action, side effects, and the generic (trade names) of these cardiac medications:
- Table 19-1: Antiarrhythmic agents
- Table 19-2: Anticoagulants
- Table 19-3: Antihypertensives
- Table 19-3a: Combination drugs for hypertension
- Table 19-4: Antiplatelet agents
- Table 19-5: Lipid-lowering agents
- Table 19-6: Positive inotropes (pressors)
- Table 19-7: Thrombolytics (also known as fibrinolytics)

Table 3-19 summarizes the presentation of digitalis toxicity.

TABLE 3-19 Signs and Symptoms of Digitalis Toxicity

System Affected	Effects
Central nervous system	Drowsiness, fatigue, confusion, visual disturbances
Cardiac system	Premature atrial and/or ventricular contractions, paroxysmal supraventricular tachycardia, ventricular tachycardia, high degrees of atrioventricular block, ventricular fibrillation
Gastrointestinal system	Nausea, vomiting, diarrhea

Data from Woods SL, Sivarajian-Froelicher ES, Underhill-Motzer S, editors: Cardiac nursing, ed 4, Philadelphia, 2000, Lippincott.

Physical Therapy Intervention

In the acute care setting, physical therapy intervention is indicated for patients with cardiac impairments that result from ACS, CHF, or status post invasive procedures such as CABG. However, a great majority of patients who receive physical therapy present with one or many other cardiac impairments or diagnoses. Given the prevalence of cardiac disease in the older adult population and number of hospital admissions for older adults, there is a high likelihood that physical therapists will manage patients who have cardiac impairment. This section discusses basic treatment guidelines for physical therapists working with patients who have present or past cardiac impairments.

Goals

The primary goals in treating patients with primary or secondary cardiac pathology are the following[69]:
- Assess hemodynamic response in conjunction with medical or surgical management during self-care activities and functional mobility.
- Maximize activity tolerance.
- Provide patient and family education regarding behavior modification and risk factor reduction (especially in patients with CAD, status post MI, PTCA, CABG, or cardiac transplant).

Concepts for the Management of Patients with Cardiac Dysfunction

The patient's medical or surgical status must be considered in intervention planning because it is inappropriate to treat a hemodynamically unstable patient. A hemodynamically unstable patient is a patient who clearly requires medical intervention to stabilize a life-threatening condition. A patient's status may fluctuate on a daily or hourly basis. Box 3-3 provides general guidelines of when to withhold physical therapy (i.e., instances in which further medical care should precede physical therapy).[70] These are provided as absolute and relative indications of instability. Relative indications of instability should be considered on a case-by-case basis.

Once it is determined that a patient is stable at rest, the physical therapist is able to proceed with activity or an exercise program, or both. Figure 3-11 provides a general guide to

BOX 3-3 Indications of Patient Instability

Absolute Indications That Patient Is Unstable and Treatment Should Be Withheld	Relative Indications That Patient Is Unstable and Treatment Should Be Modified or Withheld
Decompensated congestive heart failure	Resting heart rate >100 bpm
Second-degree heart block coupled with premature ventricular contractions (PVCs) of ventricular tachycardia at rest	Hypertensive resting BP (systolic >160 mm Hg, diastolic >90 mm Hg)
Third-degree heart block	Hypotensive resting BP (systolic <80 mm Hg)
More than 10 PVCs per minute at rest	Myocardial infarction or extension of infarction within the previous 2 days
Multifocal PVCs, unstable angina pectoris with recent changes in symptoms (less than 24 hr), and electrocardiographic changes associated with ischemia/injury	Ventricular ectopy at rest
Dissecting aortic aneurysm	Atrial fibrillation with rapid ventricular response at rest (HR >100 bpm)
New onset (less than 24 hours) of atrial fibrillation with rapid ventricular response at rest (HR >100 bpm)	Uncontrolled metabolic diseases
Chest pain with new ST segment changes on ECG	Psychosis or other unstable psychologic condition

Data from Cahalin LP: Heart failure, Phys Ther 76:520, 1996; Ellestad MH: Stress testing: principles and practice, ed 4, Philadelphia, 1996, FA Davis; Wegener NK: Rehabilitation of the patient with coronary heart disease. In Schlant RC, Alexander RW, editors: Hurst's the heart, ed 8, New York, 1994, McGraw-Hill p 1227.

BP, Blood pressure; *bpm,* beats per minute; *ECG,* electrocardiogram; *HR,* heart rate.

determining whether a patient's response to activity is stable or unstable.

Everything the physical therapist asks a patient to do is an activity that requires energy and therefore must be supported by the cardiac system. Although an activity can be thought of in terms of absolute energy requirements (i.e., metabolic equivalents [see Table 3-11]), an individual's response to that activity is relative to that individual's capacity. Therefore, although MET levels can be used to help guide the progression of activity, the physical therapist must be aware that even the lowest MET levels may represent near-maximal exertion for a patient or may result in an unstable physiologic response.

Unstable responses indicate that the patient is not able to meet physiologic demands because of the pathologic process for the level of work that the patient is performing. In this situation, the physical therapist needs to consider the patient's response to other activities and determine whether these activities create a stable response. If it is stable, can the patient function independently doing that level of work? For example, some patients may be stable walking 10 feet to the bathroom without stopping; however, this activity may require maximal exertion for the patient and therefore should be considered too much for the patient to continue to do independently throughout the day.

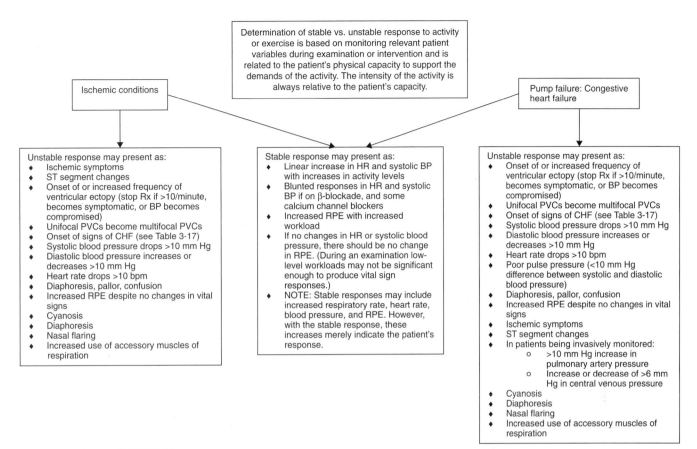

Determination of stable vs. unstable response to activity or exercise is based on monitoring relevant patient variables during examination or intervention and is related to the patient's physical capacity to support the demands of the activity. The intensity of the activity is always relative to the patient's capacity.

Ischemic conditions

Pump failure: Congestive heart failure

Unstable response may present as:
- Ischemic symptoms
- ST segment changes
- Onset of or increased frequency of ventricular ectopy (stop Rx if >10/minute, becomes symptomatic, or BP becomes compromised)
- Unifocal PVCs become multifocal PVCs
- Onset of signs of CHF (see Table 3-17)
- Systolic blood pressure drops >10 mm Hg
- Diastolic blood pressure increases or decreases >10 mm Hg
- Heart rate drops >10 bpm
- Diaphoresis, pallor, confusion
- Increased RPE despite no changes in vital signs
- Cyanosis
- Diaphoresis
- Nasal flaring
- Increased use of accessory muscles of respiration

Stable response may present as:
- Linear increase in HR and systolic BP with increases in activity levels
- Blunted responses in HR and systolic BP if on β-blockade, and some calcium channel blockers
- Increased RPE with increased workload
- If no changes in HR or systolic blood pressure, there should be no change in RPE. (During an examination low-level workloads may not be significant enough to produce vital sign responses.)
- NOTE: Stable responses may include increased respiratory rate, heart rate, blood pressure, and RPE. However, with the stable response, these increases merely indicate the patient's response.

Unstable response may present as:
- Onset of or increased frequency of ventricular ectopy (stop Rx if >10/minute, becomes symptomatic, or BP becomes compromised)
- Unifocal PVCs become multifocal PVCs
- Onset of signs of CHF (see Table 3-17)
- Systolic blood pressure drops >10 mm Hg
- Diastolic blood pressure increases or decreases >10 mm Hg
- Heart rate drops >10 bpm
- Poor pulse pressure (<10 mm Hg difference between systolic and diastolic blood pressure)
- Diaphoresis, pallor, confusion
- Increased RPE despite no changes in vital signs
- Ischemic symptoms
- ST segment changes
- In patients being invasively monitored:
    o >10 mm Hg increase in pulmonary artery pressure
    o Increase or decrease of >6 mm Hg in central venous pressure
- Cyanosis
- Diaphoresis
- Nasal flaring
- Increased use of accessory muscles of respiration

FIGURE 3-11
Determination of stable vs. unstable responses to activity/exercise. *BP,* Blood pressure; *CHF,* congestive heart failure; *HR,* heart rate; *PVC,* premature ventricular contraction; *RPE,* rating of perceived exertion; *Rx,* treatment.

If the patient's response is not stable, then the therapist should try to discern why and find out if anything can be done to make the patient stable (i.e., medical treatment may stabilize this response). In addition, the therapist should find the level of function that a patient could perform with a stable response. However, at times, patients will not be able to be stabilized to perform activity. In these cases, physical therapists must determine whether a conditioning program would allow the patient to meet the necessary energy demands without becoming unstable. Proceeding with therapy at a lower level of activity is based on the premise that conditioning will improve the patient's response. The cardiac system supports the body in its attempt to provide enough energy to perform work. Often becoming stronger—increased peripheral muscle strength and endurance—will reduce the demands on the heart at a certain absolute activity (work) level. Figure 3-12 provides a general guide to advancing a patient's activity while considering his or her response to activity.

Physical therapy intervention should include a warm-up phase to prepare the patient for activity. This usually is performed at a level of activity lower than the expected exercise program. For example, it may consist of supine, seated, or standing exercises. A conditioning phase follows the warm-up period. Very often in the acute care hospital, this conditioning phase is part of the patient's functional mobility training. With patients who are independent with functional mobility, an aerobic-based conditioning program of walking or stationary cycling may be used for conditioning. Finally, a cool-down, or relaxation, phase of deep breathing and stretching ends the physical therapy session.

> ✎ **CLINICAL TIP**
> Patients should be encouraged to report any symptom(s), even those they consider trivial.

Listed below are various ways to monitor the patient's activity tolerance.
1. HR: HR is the primary means of determining the exercise intensity level for patients who are not taking beta-blockers or who have rate-responsive pacemakers.
   - A linear relationship exists between HR and work.
   - In general, a 20- to 30-beat increase from the resting value during activity is a safe intensity level in which a patient can exercise.
   - If a patient has undergone an exercise stress test during the hospital stay, a percentage (e.g., 60% to 80%) of the maximum HR achieved during the test can be calculated to determine the exercise intensity.[71]

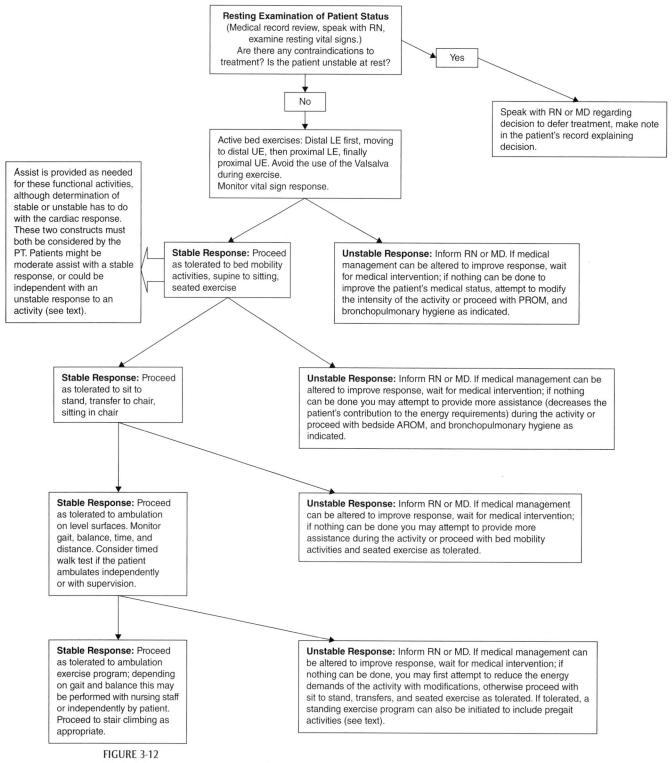

FIGURE 3-12

Physical therapy activity examination algorithm. *AROM,* Active range of motion; *LE,* lower extremity; *PROM,* passive range of motion; *UE,* upper extremity.

- An example of a disproportionate HR response to low-level activity (bed or seated exercises or ambulation in room) is an HR of more than 120 bpm or less than 50 bpm.[71]
- HR recovery (HRR), which provides an indication of reduced parasympathetic activity and an indicator of

all-cause mortality, can be used to document improvement of tolerance to functional demands.[72] HRR is the absolute difference between peak HR achieved with exercise minus the HR at 60 seconds after the completion of exercise (HRR60sec).[73] An abnormal HRR at 1 minute, after a treadmill test, is reported to be a decrease of

12 bpm or less with a cool-down period and less than 18 bpm without a cool-down period.[74]

- When prescribing activity intensity for a patient taking beta-blockers, consider that the HR should not exceed 20 beats above resting HR.
- If prescribing activity intensity using HR for patients with an AICD, remember that the exercise target HR should be 20 to 30 beats below the threshold rate on the defibrillator.[71]
- HR cannot be used to prescribe exercise status post heart transplant secondary to denervation of the heart during transplantation.
- Baseline HR and recent changes in medications always should be considered before beginning an exercise session.

2. BP: Refer to the Cardiac Evaluation section regarding BP measurements and Table 3-6 for BP ranges. A clearly disproportionate response to exercise includes a systolic pressure decrease of 10 mm Hg below the resting value, a hypertensive systolic response of more than 180 mm Hg, or a hypertensive diastolic response of more than 110 mm Hg.[71] A normotensive systolic blood response should increase 5 to 12 mm Hg per increase in METs.[75]

- If the patient is on a pacemaker that does not have rate modulation, BP response can be used to gauge intensity. Refer to the Cardiac Pacemaker Implantation and Automatic Implantable Cardiac Defibrillator section for a discussion on pacemakers.

3. The "Borg RPE Scale" (6-20), the "Borg CR10 Scale", and the Borg CR100 (centiMax) Scale:

- The "Borg RPE Scale" (6-20) is used mainly for "overall ratings (R) of perceived (P) exertion (E)"[76] during physical training and rehabilitation and has evolved to be the classic means of objectively documenting subjective feelings of exercise intensity. This scale also can be used for breathlessness and muscle fatigue.[76,77]
- The Borg CR10 Scale and the Borg CR100 (centiMax) Scale are general scales for measuring intensities of most kinds of perceptions, experiences, and feelings.[76,77]
- The Borg CR10 Scale also is used to measure ratings of perceived exertion (RPE).
- The Borg CR100 (centiMax) Scale was developed because a more finely graded scale became necessary in certain situations.[77]
- These scales easily can be used to monitor exercise intensity for the purpose of exercise prescription in a variety of patient populations. They are the preferred method of prescribing exercise intensity for a patient taking beta-blockers.
- A general guideline for everyone is to exercise to a point no greater than 5 on the 10-point scale and no greater than 13 on the 6-20 scale.[71]
- For the scales to be used in the most safe, reliable, and valid manner, complete instructions regarding the scale and its use must be provided to the patient before its implementation. These instructions are included with the scales and should be followed exactly as designed and not be modified.[76,77]

4. Rate pressure product (RPP) is HR × SBP and is an indication of myocardial oxygen demand.

- If a patient undergoes maximal exercise testing and has myocardial ischemia, RPP can be calculated at the point when ischemia is occurring to establish the patient's ischemic threshold.
- This RPP value can then be used during exercise to provide a safe guideline of exercise intensity.

5. Heart sounds: Refer to the section on Auscultation and Table 3-8 for normal and abnormal heart sounds.

- The onset of murmurs, S3 heart sounds, or S4 heart sounds during treatment may be detected and could indicate a decline in cardiac function during activity. This finding should be brought to the attention of the nurse and physician.

6. Breath sounds: Refer to Chapter 4 for a discussion of lung auscultation and the interpretation of breath sounds.

- The presence of or increase in bibasilar crackles during activity may be indicative of acute CHF. Activity should be terminated and the nurse and physician notified.

7. ECG rhythm: Refer to the Electrocardiogram and the Rhythm and Conduction Disturbance sections.

- When treating patients who are being continuously monitored by an ECG, know their baseline rhythm, the most recently observed rhythm, what lead is being monitored, and the reason for monitoring.
- Recognizing their normal rhythm and any deviations from this norm in addition to changes that could indicate a decline in cardiac status is important. Examples of declining cardiac status include the following:
  - Onset of ST changes (elevation or depression of more than 1 mm), which could indicate ischemia
  - Increased frequency of PVCs (trigeminy to bigeminy or couplets)
  - Unifocal PVCs to multifocal PVCs
  - Premature atrial contractions to atrial flutter or atrial fibrillation
  - Atrial flutter to atrial fibrillation
  - Any progression in heart blocks (first degree to Mobitz I)
  - Loss of pacer spike capturing (pacer spike without resultant QRS complex on ECG)
- Be able to recognize signs and symptoms of cardiac decompensation and immediately notify the physician if any develop (see Figure 3-11). Record any signs noted during activity and other objective data at that time. Other signs and symptoms include weakness, fatigue, dizziness, lightheadedness, angina, palpitations, and dyspnea. Record any symptoms reported by the patient and any objective information at that time (e.g., ECG readings; BP, HR, and RPP measurements; breath sounds).

References

1. Roger V, Go AG et al: Heart disease and stroke statistics—2012 update: a report from the American Heart Association, Circulation 125:e2-e220, 2012.
2. Guyton AC, Hall JE: In Textbook of medical physiology, ed 12, Philadelphia, 2011, Saunders.
3. Cheitlin MD, Sokolow M, McIlroy MB, editors: Clinical cardiology, ed 6, Norwalk, Conn, 1993, Appleton & Lange.
4. Braunwald E, Zipes DP, Libby P, editors: Heart disease: a textbook of cardiovascular medicine, ed 6, St Louis, 2001, Saunders.
5. Braunwald E, editor: Heart disease: a textbook of cardiovascular medicine, ed 4, Philadelphia, 1992, Saunders.
6. Davis D, editor: Quick and accurate 12 lead ECG interpretation, ed 4, Philadelphia, 2004, Lippincott Williams & Wilkins.
7. Hillis LD, Firth BG, Willerson JT, editors: Manual of clinical problems in cardiology, Boston, 1984, Little, Brown.
8. Task Force of the European Society of Cardiology and the North American Society of Pacing and Electrophysiology: Heart rate variability: standards of measurement, physiological interpretation, and clinical use, Circulation 93:1043-1065, 1996.
9. Bernston G, Cacioppo JT, Quigley KS: Autonomic determinism: the modes of autonomic control, the doctrine of autonomic space, and the laws of autonomic constraint, Psychol Rev 98: 459-487, 1991.
10. Urden LD, Davie JK, Thelan LA, editors: Essentials of critical care nursing, St Louis, 1992, Mosby.
11. Cohen M, Michel TH, editors: Cardiopulmonary symptoms in physical therapy practice, New York, 1988, Churchill Livingstone.
12. Woods SL, Sivarajian Froelicher ES, Underhill-Motzer S, editors: Cardiac nursing, ed 6, Philadelphia, 2009, Lippincott Williams & Wilkins.
13. Bickley LS: In Bates' guide to physical examination and history taking, ed 10, Philadelphia, 2010, Lippincott Williams & Wilkins.
14. Kleiger RE, Stein PK et al: Heart rate variability: measurement and clinical utility, Ann Noninvasive Electrocardiol 10(1):88-101, 2005.
15. Algra A: Heart rate variability from 24-hour Holter ECG and the 2 year risk for sudden death, Circulation 88:180-185, 1993.
16. Dekker JM: Heart rate variability from short electrocardiographic recordings predicts mortality from all causes in middle aged and elderly men, Am J Epidemiol 145:899-908, 1997.
17. Tusji H, Larson MG: Impact of reduced HRV on risk for cardiac events: the Framingham Heart Study, Circulation 94:2850-2855, 1996.
18. Singh JP, Larson MG, Tsuji H et al: Reduced heart rate variability and new onset hypertension, Hypertension 32:293-297, 1998.
19. Bigger JT, La Rovere RT, Marcus FI et al: Baroreflex sensitivity and heart rate variability in prediction of total cardiac mortality after MI, Lancet 351:478-484, 1998.
20. Bigger JT: Frequency domain measures of heart period variability and mortality after myocardial infarction, Circulation 85:164-171, 1992.
21. Doulalas A, Flather MD, Pipilis A et al: Evolutionary pattern and prognostic importance of heart rate variability during the early phase of acute myocardial infarction, Int J Cardiol 77:169-179, 2001.
22. Van Boven AJ, Crijns H, Haaksma J et al: Depressed heart rate variability is associated with events in patients with stable coronary artery disease and preserved left ventricular dysfunction, Am Heart J 135:571-576, 1998.
23. Galinier M, Pathak A, Fourcade J et al: Depressed low frequency power of heart rate variability as an independent predictor of sudden cardiac death in chronic heart failure, Eur Heart J 21:475-482, 2000.
24. Dewey FE, Freeman JV, Engel G et al: Novel predictor of prognosis from exercise stress testing: heart rate variability response to the exercise treadmill test, Am Heart J 153(2):281-288, 2007.
25. Gayda M, Bourassa MG, Tardiff JC et al: Heart rate recovery after exercise and long term prognosis in patients with coronary artery disease, Can J Cardiol 28:201-207, 2012.
26. Polich S, Faynor SM: Interpreting lab test values, PT Magazine 3:110, 1996.
27. Suzuki T, Yamauchi K, Yamada Y: Blood coaguability and fibrinolytic activity before and after physical training during the recovery phase of acute myocardial infarction, Clin Cardiol 15:358-364, 1992.
28. Grundy SM, Pasternak R, Greenland P et al: Assessment of cardiovascular risk by use of multiple-risk-factor assessment equations: a statement for healthcare professionals from the American Heart Association and the American College of Cardiology, Circulation 100:1481-1492, 1999.
29. Danesh MB, Phil D, Wheeler JG et al: C reactive protein and other circulating markers of inflammation in the prediction of coronary heart disease, N Engl J Med 350(14):1387-1397, 2004.
30. Ridker PAM, Charles HH, Bering JE: C reactive protein and other markers of inflammation in the prediction of cardiovascular disease in women, N Engl J Med 342(12):836-843, 2000.
31. Liuzzo G, Biasucci LM, Gallimore JR et al: The prognostic value of C reactive protein in severe unstable angina, N Engl J Med 331(7):417-424, 1994.
32. Christenson RH, Azzazy HME: Biochemical markers of the acute coronary syndromes, Clin Chem 44:1855-1864, 1998.
33. Kratz AK, Leqand-Rowski KB: Normal reference laboratory values, N Engl J Med 339:1063-1072, 1998.
34. Januzzi JL Jr: Natriuretic peptide testing: a window into the diagnosis and prognosis of heart failure, Cleve Clin J Med 73(2):149-152, 155-157, 2006.
35. Fisher EA, Stahl JA, Budd JH et al: Transesophageal echocardiography: procedures and clinical application, J Am Coll Cardiol 18:1333-1348, 1991.
36. Ellestad MH, editor: Stress testing: principles and practice, ed 5, New York, 2003, Oxford University Press.
37. Perez JE: Current role of contrast echocardiography in the diagnosis of cardiovascular disease, Clin Cardiol 20:31-38, 1997.
38. Bellardinelli R, Geordiou D, Prucaro A: Low dose dobutamine echocardiography predicts improvement in functional capacity after exercise training in patients with ischemic cardiomyopathy: prognostic implications, J Am Coll Cardiol 31(5):1027-1034, 1998.
39. American Heart Association, Committee on Exercise: In Exercise testing and training of apparently healthy individuals: a handbook for physicians, Dallas, 1972, The Association.
40. Brooks GA, Fahey TD, White TP, editors: Exercise physiology: human bioenergetics and its applications, ed 4, New York, 2004, McGraw Hill.
41. Noonan V, Dean E: Submaximal exercise testing: clinical applications and interpretation, Phys Ther 80:782-807, 2000.
42. American College of Cardiology/American Heart Association: 1999 update: ACC/AHA guidelines for the management of patients with acute myocardial infarction: executive summary and recommendations, Circulation 100:1016-1030, 1999.
43. Cahalin LP: Heart failure, Phys Ther 76:520, 1996.

44. Dekerlegand J: Congestive heart failure. In Cameron MH, Monroe LG, editors: Physical rehabilitation: evidence-based examination, evaluation, and intervention, St Louis, 2007, Saunders, pp 677-678.

45. Detre KM, Holmes DR, Holudrov R et al: Incidence and consequences of periprocedural occlusion, Circulation 82:739, 1990.

46. Litzak F, Margilis J, Cumins R: Excimer Laser Coronary (ECLA) Registry: report of the first 2080 patients, J Am Coll Cardiol 19:276A, 1992.

47. Humphrey R, Arena R: Surgical innovations for chronic heart failure in the context of cardiopulmonary rehabilitation, Phys Ther 80:61-69, 2000.

48. Dogan S, Aybek T, Andressen E et al: Totally endoscopic coronary artery bypass grafting on cardiopulmonary bypass with robotically enhanced telemanipulation: report of forty-five cases, J Thorac Cardiovasc Surg 123:1125, 2002.

49. Black EA, Guzik TJ, West NE et al: Minimally invasive saphenous vein harvesting: effects on endothelial and smooth muscle function, Ann Thorac Surg 71:1503, 2001.

50. Isomura T, Suma H, Horii T et al: Minimally invasive coronary artery revascularization: off-pump bypass grafting and they hybrid procedure, Ann Thorac Surg 70:2017, 2000.

51. DeRose JJ: Current state of integrated "hybrid" coronary revascularization, Semin Thorac Cardiovasc Surg 21:229, 2009.

52. Struber M, Cremer JT, Gohrbandt B et al: Human cytokine responses to coronary artery bypass grafting with and without cardiopulmonary bypass, Ann Thorac Surg 68:1330, 1999.

53. Cahalin LP, LaPier TK, Shaw DK: Sternal precautions: Is it time for change? Precautions versus restrictions—a review of the literature and recommendations for revision, Cardiopulm Phys Ther J 22(1):5-15, 2011.

54. El-Ansary D, Waddington G, Adams R: Measurement of non-physiological movement in sternal instability by ultrasound, Ann Thorac Surg 83:1513-1517, 2007.

55. Irion G: Effect of upper extremity movement on sternal skin stress, Acute Care Perspect 15:3-6, 2006.

56. Irion GL, Boyte B, Ingram J et al: Sternal skin stress produced by functional upper extremity movements, Acute Care Perspect 16(3):1-5, 2007.

57. Gillinov AM, Bhavani S, Blackstone EH et al: Surgery for permanent atrial fibrillation: impact of patient factors and lesion set, Ann Thorac Surg 82:502, 2006.

58. Sundt T: The maze procedure. The Society of Thoracic Surgeons patient information, 2000 (website): http://www.sts.org/doc/4511. Accessed March 13, 2008.

59. Schuessler RB: Do we need a map to get through the maze? (editorial), Thorac Cardiovasc Surg 127:627-628, 2004.

60. Cox JL: The surgical treatment of atrial fibrillation. IV. Surgical technique, J Thorac Cardiovasc Surg 101:584, 1991.

61. Lonnerholm S, Blomstrom P, Nilsson L et al: Effects of the maze operation on health-related quality of life in patients with atrial fibrillation, Circulation 101:2607, 2000.

62. Doty JR, Doty DB, Jones KW et al: Comparison of standard Maze III and radiofrequency Maze operations for treatment of atrial fibrillation, J Thorac Cardiovasc Surg 133:1037, 2007.

63. Bernstein AD, Camm AJ, Fletcher RD et al: The NASPE/BPEG generic pacemaker code for antibradyarrhythmia and adaptive pacing and anti-tachyarrhythmia devices, PACE 10:795, 1987.

64. Collins SM, Cahalin LP: Acute care physical therapy in patients with pacemakers, Acute Care Perspect 14(5):9-14, 2005.

65. Nietlispach F, Wijesinghe N, Wood D et al: Current balloon-expandable transcatheter heart valve and delivery systems, Catheter Cardiovasc Inter 75:295, 2010.

66. Bonow RO, Carabello BA, Chatterjee K et al: 2008 Focused update incorporated into the ACC/AHA 2006 guidelines for the management of patients with valvular heart disease: a report of the American College of Cardiology/American Heart Association Task Force on Practice Guidelines (Writing Committee to Revise the 1998 Guidelines for the Management of Patients with Valvular Heart Disease): endorsed by the Society of Cardiovascular Anesthesiologists, Society for Cardiovascular Angiography and Interventions, and Society of Thoracic Surgeons, Circulation 118:e523, 2008.

67. Petronio AS, De Carlo M, Bedongni F et al: Safety and efficacy of the subclavian approach for transcatheter aortic valve implantation with the CoreValve revalving system, Circ Cardiovasc Interv 3:359, 2010.

68. Thomas M, Schymik G, Walther T et al: Thirty-day results of the SAPIEN aortic bioprosthesis european outcome (SOURCE) registry: a European registry of transcatheter aortic valve implantation using the Edwards SAPIEN valve, Circulation 122:62, 2010.

69. Cahalin LP, Ice RG, Irwin S: Program planning and implementation. In Irwin S, Tecklin JS, editors: Cardiopulmonary physical therapy, ed 4, St Louis, 2004, Mosby, p 144.

70. Grimes K, Cohen M: Cardiac medications. In Hillegass EA, Sadowsky HS, editors: Essentials of cardiopulmonary physical therapy, ed 3, Philadelphia, 2010, Saunders, pp 537-585.

71. Wegener NK: Rehabilitation of the patient with coronary heart disease. In Fuster V, Walsh RA, Harrington RA, editors: Hurst's the heart, ed 13, New York, 2010, McGraw-Hill.

72. Huang PH, Leu HB et al: Heart rate recovery after exercise and endothelial function—two important factors to predict cardiovascular events, Prevent Cardiol 8(3):167, 2005.

73. Buchheit M, Papelier Y et al: Noninvasive assessment of cardiac parasympathetic function: postexercise heart rate recovery or heart rate variability? Am J Physiol Heart Circ Physiol 293(1):H8-H10, 2007.

74. MacMillan JS, Davis LL, Durham CF et al: Exercise and heart rate recovery, Heart Lung 35(6):383-390, 2006.

75. ACSM's guidelines for exercise testing and prescription, ed 8, Philadelphia, 2009, Lippincott Williams & Wilkins.

76. Borg G: The usage of "Borg Scales." http://fysio.dk/upload/graphics/PDF-filer/Maaleredskaber/The_usage_of_%27Borg_scale_16.pdf, Accessed March 7, 2013.

77. The Borg CR Scales Folder: Methods for measuring intensity of experience, Hasselby, Sweden, 2004, 2007, Borg Perception.

APPENDIX 3A DESCRIPTION OF ECG CHARACTERISTICS AND ASSOCIATED CAUSES

TABLE 3A-1 Electrocardiographic (ECG) Characteristics and Causes of Atrial Rhythms

Name	ECG Characteristics	Common Causes	PT Consideration
Supraventricular tachycardia	Regular rhythm; rate of 160-250 bpm; may originate from any location above atrioventricular node; can be paroxysmal (comes and goes without reason)	Rheumatoid heart disease (RHD), mitral valve prolapse, cor pulmonale, digitalis toxicity	May produce palpitations, chest tightness, dizziness, anxiety, apprehension, weakness; PT would not treat if in supraventricular tachycardia until controlled
Atrial flutter	Regular or irregular rhythm; atrial rate of 250-350; ventricular rate is variable and depends on the conduction ratio (atrial : ventricular, e.g., atrial rate = 250, ventricular rate = 125; 2 : 1 classic saw tooth P waves)	Mitral stenosis, CAD, hypertension	Signs and symptoms depend on presence or absence of heart disease but can lead to CHF, palpitations, angina, and syncope if cardiac output decreases far enough to reduce myocardial and cerebral blood flow; PT treatment would depend on tolerance to the rhythm
Atrial fibrillation (AF)	Irregular rhythm; atrial has no rate (just quivers); ventricular rate varies	One of most commonly encountered rhythms, CHF, CAD, RHD, hypertension, cor pulmonale	Can produce CHF, syncope secondary to no "atrial kick"; if new diagnosis, hold PT until medical treatment; if chronic and not in CHF, would treat with caution
Premature atrial contractions	Irregular rhythm (can be regularly irregular, i.e., skip every third beat); rate normal 60-100	Normal people with caffeine, smoking, emotional disturbances; abnormal with CAD, CHF, electrolyte disturbances	Usually asymptomatic but needs to be considered with other cardiac issues at time of treatment; can proceed with treatment with close monitoring; if they are consistent and increasing, can progress to AF

Data from Aehlert B: ACLS quick review study guide, St Louis, 1993, Mosby; Chung EK: Manual of cardiac arrhythmias, Boston, 1986, Butterworth-Heinemann.
AF, Atrial fibrillation; *CAD,* coronary artery disease; *CHF,* congestive heart failure; *RHD,* rheumatoid heart disease.

TABLE 3A-2 Electrocardiographic Characteristics and Causes of Ventricular Rhythms

Name	ECG Characteristics	Common Causes	PT Considerations
Agonal rhythm	Irregular rhythm, rate <20, no P wave	Near death	Do not treat.
Ventricular tachycardia (VT)	Usually regular rhythm, rate >100, no P wave or with retrograde conduction and appears after the QRS complex	CAD most common after acute MI; may occur in rheumatoid heart disease, cardiomyopathy, hypertension	Do not treat; patient needs immediate medical assistance; patient may be stable (maintain CO) for a short while but can progress quickly to unstable (no CO)—called pulseless VT.
Multifocal VT (torsades de pointes)	Irregular rhythm, rate >150, no P waves	Drug induced with antiarrhythmic medicines (quinidine, procainamide); hypokalemia; hypomagnesemia; MI; hypothermia	Do not treat; patient needs immediate medical assistance.
Premature ventricular contractions (PVCs) (focal = one ectopic foci and all look the same; multifocal = more than one ectopic foci and will have different waveforms)	Irregular rhythm, (can be regularly irregular, i.e., skipped beat every fourth beat); rate varies but is usually normal 60-100; couplet is 2 in a row; bigeminy is every other beat; trigeminy is every third beat	In normal individuals, secondary to caffeine, smoking, emotional disturbances, CAD, MI, cardiomyopathy, MVP, digitalis toxicity	Frequency will dictate effect on CO; monitor electrocardiograph with treatment; can progress to VT; more likely if multifocal in nature or if >6 per minute; stop treatment or rest if change in frequency or quality.
Ventricular fibrillation	Chaotic	Severe heart disease most common after acute MI, hyperkalemia or hypokalemia, hypercalcemia, electrocution	Do not treat; patient needs immediate medical assistance.
Idioventricular rhythm	Essentially regular rhythm, rate 20-40	Advanced heart disease; high degree of atrioventricular block; usually a terminal arrhythmia	CHF is common secondary to slow rates; do not treat unless rhythm well tolerated.

Data from Aehlert B: ACLS quick review study guide, St Louis, 1994, Mosby; Chung EK: Manual of cardiac arrhythmias, Boston, 1986, Butterworth-Heinemann.
CAD, Coronary artery disease; *CHF*, congestive heart failure; *CO*, cardiac output; *ECG*, echocardiographic; *MI*, myocardial infarction; *MVP*, mitral valve prolapse; *VT*, ventricular tachycardia.

TABLE 3A-3 Electrocardiographic (ECG) Characteristics and Causes of Junctional Rhythms

Name	ECG Characteristics	Common Causes	PT Considerations
Junctional escape rhythm	Regular rhythm, rate 20-40; inverted P wave before or after QRS complex; starts with ectopic foci in AV junction tissue	Usual cause is physiologic to control the ventricles in AV block, sinus bradycardia, AF, sinoatrial block, drug intoxication	If occasional and intermittent during bradycardia or chronic AF, usually insignificant and can treat (with close watch of possible worsening condition via symptoms and vital signs); if consistent and present secondary to AV block, acute myocardial infarction, or drug intoxication, can be symptomatic with CHF (see Box 3-2).
Junctional tachycardia	Regular rhythm; rate 100-180; P wave as above	Most common with chronic AF; also with coronary artery disease, rheumatoid heart disease, and cardiomyopathy	May produce or exacerbate symptoms of CHF or angina secondary to decreased cardiac output; PT treatment depends on patient tolerance—if new onset, should wait for medical treatment.

Data from Aehlert B: ACLS quick review study guide, St Louis, 1994, Mosby; Chung EK: Manual of cardiac arrhythmias, Boston, 1986, Butterworth-Heinemann.
AF, Atrial fibrillation; *AV*, atrioventricular; *CHF*, congestive heart failure.

TABLE 3A-4 Electrocardiographic Characteristics and Causes of Atrioventricular Blocks

Name	ECG Characteristics	Common Causes	PT Considerations
First-degree AV block	Regular rhythm, rate normal 60-100, prolonged PR interval >0.2 (constant).	Elderly with heart disease, acute myocarditis, acute MI	If chronic, need to be more cautious of underlying heart disease; if new onset, monitor closely for progression to higher level block.
Second-degree AV block type I (Wenckebach, Mobitz I)	Irregular rhythm, atrial rate > ventricular rate, usually both 60-100; PR interval lengthens until P wave appears without a QRS complex.	Acute infection, acute MI	Symptoms are uncommon, as above.
Second-degree AV block type II (Mobitz II)	Irregular rhythm, atrial rate > ventricular rate, PR interval may be normal or prolonged but is constant for each conducted QRS.	Anteroseptal MI	CHF is common; can have dizziness, fainting, complete unconsciousness; may need pacing and PT treatment; should be held for medical management.
Third-degree AV block (complete heart block)	Regular rhythm, atrial rate > ventricular rate	Anteroseptal MI, drug intoxication, infections, electrolyte imbalances, coronary artery disease, degenerative sclerotic process of AV conduction system	Severe CHF; patient will need medical management; a pacer (temporary or permanent, depending on reversibility of etiology) is almost always necessary.

Data from Aehlert B: ACLS quick review study guide, St Louis, 1994, Mosby; Chung EK: Manual of cardiac arrhythmias, Boston, 1986, Butterworth-Heinemann. *AV,* Atrioventricular; *CHF,* congestive heart failure; *MI,* myocardial infarction.

APPENDIX 3B COMMON RHYTHM DISTURBANCES

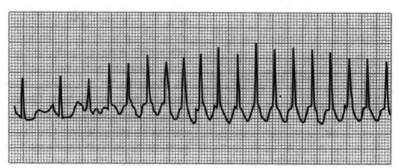

FIGURE 3B-1
Paroxysmal supraventricular tachycardia. Note development from normal sinus rhythm. (From Walsh M, Crumbie A, Reveley S: Nurse practitioners: clinical skills and professional issues, Boston, 1993, Butterworth-Heinemann.)

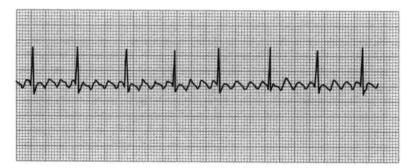

FIGURE 3B-2
Atrial flutter. Note regular rhythm (P waves), but ventricular rhythm depends on conduction pattern. (From Walsh M, Crumbie A, Reveley S: Nurse practitioners: clinical skills and professional issues, Boston, 1993, Butterworth-Heinemann.)

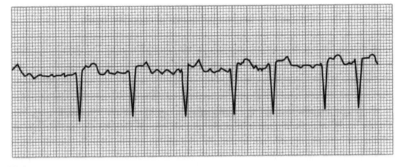

FIGURE 3B-3
Atrial fibrillation. Note the irregular rhythm and absence of normal P waves. (From Walsh M, Crumbie A, Reveley S: Nurse practitioners: clinical skills and professional issues, Boston, 1993, Butterworth-Heinemann.)

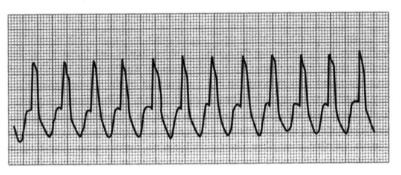

FIGURE 3B-4
Ventricular tachycardia. Rate 100-170 beats per minute. No P waves, broad electrocardiographic wave complexes. (From Walsh M, Crumbie A, Reveley S: Nurse practitioners: clinical skills and professional issues, Boston, 1993, Butterworth-Heinemann.)

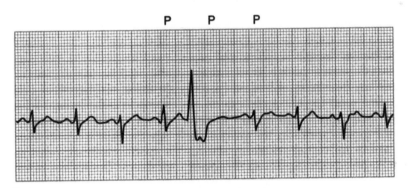

FIGURE 3B-5
Ventricular ectopy with refractory period afterward. (From Walsh M, Crumbie A, Reveley S: Nurse practitioners: clinical skills and professional issues, Boston, 1993, Butterworth-Heinemann.)

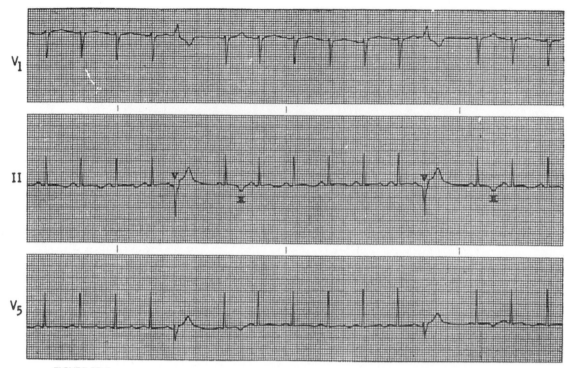

FIGURE 3B-6
Sinus rhythm with premature ventricular contractions. (From Chung EK: Manual of cardiac arrhythmias, Boston, 1986, Butterworth-Heinemann.)

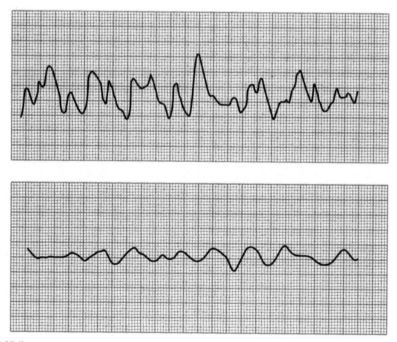

FIGURE 3B-7
Ventricular fibrillation. (From Walsh M, Crumbie A, Reveley S: Nurse practitioners: clinical skills and professional issues, Boston, 1993, Butterworth-Heinemann.)

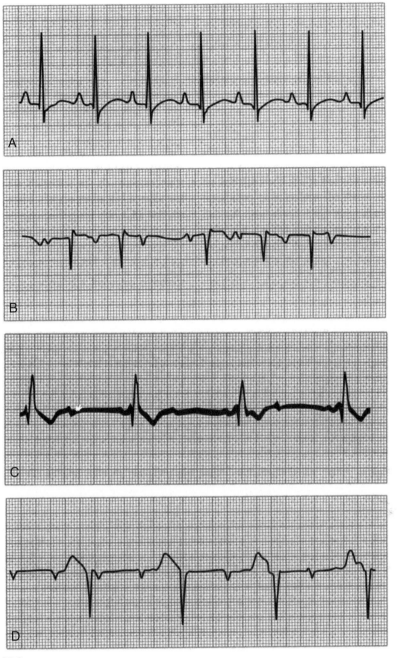

FIGURE 3B-8
Degrees of heart block. (From Walsh M, Crumbie A, Reveley S: Nurse practitioners: clinical skills and professional issues, Boston, 1993, Butterworth-Heinemann.)

Pulmonary System

Paul E.H. Ricard

CHAPTER OBJECTIVES

The objectives of this chapter are the following:

1. Provide a brief review of the structure and function of the pulmonary system
2. Give an overview of pulmonary evaluation, including physical examination and diagnostic testing
3. Describe pulmonary diseases and disorders, including clinical findings, medical-surgical management, and physical therapy intervention

PREFERRED PRACTICE PATTERNS

The most relevant practice patterns for the diagnoses discussed in this chapter, based on the American Physical Therapy Association's *Guide to Physical Therapist Practice*, second edition, are as follows:

- Impaired Aerobic Capacity/Endurance Associated with Deconditioning: 6B
- Impaired Ventilation, Respiration/Gas Exchange, and Aerobic Capacity/Endurance Associated with Airway Clearance Dysfunction: 6C
- Impaired Ventilation and Respiration/Gas Exchange Associated with Ventilatory Pump Dysfunction or Failure: 6E
- Impaired Ventilation and Respiration/Gas Exchange Associated with Respiratory Failure: 6F
- Impaired Ventilation, Respiration/Gas Exchange, and Aerobic Capacity/Endurance Associated with Respiratory Failure in the Neonate: 6G

Please refer to Appendix A for a complete list of the preferred practice patterns, as individual patient conditions are highly variable and other practice patterns may be applicable.

To safely and effectively provide exercise, bronchopulmonary hygiene program(s), or both to patients with pulmonary system dysfunction, physical therapists require an understanding of the pulmonary system and of the principles of ventilation and gas exchange. *Ventilation* is defined as gas (oxygen [O_2] and carbon dioxide [CO_2]) transport into and out of lungs, and *respiration* is defined as gas exchange across the alveolar-capillary and capillary-tissue interfaces. The term *pulmonary* primarily refers to the lungs, their airways, and their vascular system.[1]

Body Structure and Function

Structure

The primary organs and muscles of the pulmonary system are outlined in Tables 4-1 and 4-2, respectively. A schematic of the pulmonary system within the thorax is presented in Figure 4-1.

Function

To accomplish ventilation and respiration, the pulmonary system is regulated by many neural, chemical, and nonchemical mechanisms, which are discussed in the sections that follow.

Neural Control

Ventilation is regulated by two separate neural mechanisms: one controls automatic ventilation, and the other controls voluntary ventilation. The medullary respiratory center in the

TABLE 4-1 Structure and Function of Primary Organs of the Pulmonary System

Structure	Description	Function
Nose	Paired mucosal-lined nasal cavities supported by bone and cartilage	Conduit that filters, warms, and humidifies air entering lungs
Pharynx	Passageway that connects nasal and oral cavities to larynx, and oral cavity to esophagus Subdivisions naso-, oro-, and laryngopharynx	Conduit for air and food Facilitates exposure of immune system to inhaled antigens
Larynx	Passageway that connects pharynx to trachea Opening (glottis) covered by vocal folds or by the epiglottis during swallowing	Prevents food from entering the lower pulmonary tract Voice production
Trachea	Flexible tube composed of C-shaped cartilaginous rings connected posteriorly to the trachealis muscle Divides into the left and right main stem bronchi at the carina	Cleans, warms, and moistens incoming air
Bronchial tree	Right and left main stem bronchi subdivide within each lung into secondary bronchi, tertiary bronchi, and bronchioles, which contain smooth muscle	Warms and moistens incoming air from trachea to alveoli Smooth muscle constriction alters airflow
Lungs	Paired organs located within pleural cavities of the thorax The right lung has three lobes, and the left lung has two lobes	Contains air passageways distal to main stem bronchi, alveoli, and respiratory membranes
Alveoli	Microscopic sacs at end of bronchial tree immediately adjacent to pulmonary capillaries Functional unit of the lung	Primary gas exchange site Surfactant lines the alveoli to decrease surface tension and prevent complete closure during exhalation
Pleurae	Double-layered, continuous serous membrane lining the inside of the thoracic cavity Divided into parietal (outer) pleura and visceral (inner) pleura	Produces lubricating fluid that allows smooth gliding of lungs within the thorax Potential space between parietal and visceral pleura

Data from Marieb E: Human anatomy and physiology, ed 3, Redwood City, Calif, 1995, Benjamin-Cummings; Moldover JR, Stein J, Krug PG: Cardiopulmonary physiology. In Gonzalez EG, Myers SJ, Edelstein JE et al: Downey & Darling's physiological basis of rehabilitation medicine, ed 3, Philadelphia, 2001, Butterworth-Heinemann.

TABLE 4-2 Primary and Accessory Ventilatory Muscles with Associated Innervation

	Pulmonary Muscles	Innervation
Primary inspiratory muscles	Diaphragm External intercostals	Phrenic nerve (C3-C5) Spinal segments T1-T9
Accessory inspiratory muscles	Trapezius Sternocleidomastoid Scalenes Pectorals Serratus anterior Latissimus dorsi	Cervical nerve (C1-C4), spinal part of cranial nerve XI Spinal part of cranial nerve XI Cervical/brachial plexus branches (C3-C8, T1) Medial/lateral pectoral nerve (C5-C8, T1) Long thoracic nerve (C5-C7) Thoracodorsal nerve (C5-C8)
Primary expiratory muscles	Rectus abdominis External obliques Internal obliques Internal intercostals	Spinal segments T5-T12 Spinal segments T7-T12 Spinal segments T8-T12 Spinal segments T1-T9
Accessory expiratory muscles	Latissimus dorsi	Thoracodorsal nerve (C5-C8)

Data from Kendall FP, McCreary EK, editors: Muscles: testing and function, ed 3, Baltimore, 1983, Lippincott, Williams, and Wilkins; Rothstein JM, Roy SH, Wolf SL: The rehabilitation specialist's handbook, ed 2, Philadelphia, 1998, FA Davis; DeTurk WE, Cahalin LP: Cardiovascular and pulmonary physical therapy: an evidence-based approach, New York, 2004, McGraw-Hill Medical Publishing Division.

brain stem, which is responsible for the rhythmicity of breathing, controls automatic ventilation. The pneumotaxic center, located in the pons, controls ventilation rate and depth. The cerebral cortex, which sends impulses directly to the motor neurons of ventilatory muscles, mediates voluntary ventilation.[3]

Chemical Control

Arterial levels of CO_2 (P_{CO_2}), hydrogen ions (H^+), and O_2 (P_{O_2}) can modify the rate and depth of respiration. To maintain homeostasis in the body, specialized chemoreceptors on the carotid arteries and aortic arch (carotid and aortic bodies, respectively) respond to either a rise in P_{CO_2} and H^+ or a fall in P_{O_2}.

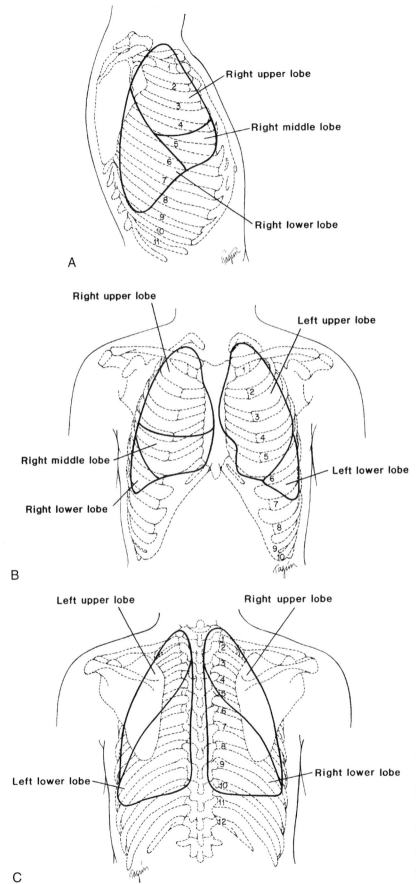

FIGURE 4-1

A, Right lung positioned in the thorax. Bony landmarks assist in identifying normal right lung configuration. B, Anterior view of the lungs in the thorax in conjunction with bony landmarks. Left upper lobe is divided into apical and left lingula, which match the general position of the right upper and middle lobes. C, Posterior view of the lungs in conjunction with bony landmarks. (From Ellis E, Alison J, editors: Key issues in cardiorespiratory physiotherapy, Oxford, 1992, Butterworth-Heinemann, p 12.)

Stimulation of these chemoreceptors results in transmission of impulses to the respiratory centers to increase or decrease the rate or depth, or both, of respiration. For example, an increase in P_{CO_2} would increase the ventilation rate to help increase the amount of CO_2 exhaled and ultimately lower the P_{CO_2} levels in arterial blood. The respiratory center found in the medulla primarily responds to a rise in P_{CO_2} and H^+.[4,5]

Nonchemical Influences

Coughing, bronchoconstriction, and mucus secretion occur in the lungs as protective reflexes to irritants such as smoke or dust. Emotions, stressors, pain, and visceral reflexes from lung tissue and other organ systems also can influence ventilation rate and depth.

Mechanics of Ventilation

Ventilation occurs as a result of changes in the potential space (volume) and subsequent pressures within the thoracic cavity created by the muscles of ventilation. The largest primary muscle of inhalation, the diaphragm, compresses the contents of the abdominal cavity as it contracts and descends, increasing the volume of the thoracic cavity.

> ✎ **CLINICAL TIP**
>
> The compression of the abdominal contents can be observed with the protrusion of the abdomen. Clinicians use the term "belly breathing" to facilitate diaphragmatic breathing.

The contraction of the intercostal muscles results in two motions simultaneously: bucket and pump handle. The combined motions further increase the volume of the thorax. The overall increase in the volume of the thoracic cavity creates a negative intrathoracic pressure compared with outside the body. As a result, air is pulled into the body and lungs via the pulmonary tree, stretching the lung parenchyma, to equalize the pressures within the thorax with those outside the body.

Accessory muscles of inspiration, noted in Table 4-2, are generally not active during quiet breathing. Although not the primary actions of the individual muscles, their contractions can increase the depth and rate of ventilation during progressive activity by increasing the expansion of the thorax. Increased expansion results in greater negative pressures being generated and subsequent larger volumes of air entering the lungs.

> ✎ **CLINICAL TIP**
>
> In healthy lungs, depth of ventilation generally occurs before increases in rate.

Although inhalation is an active process, exhalation is a generally passive process. The muscles relax, causing a decrease in the thoracic volume while the lungs deflate to their natural resting state. The combined effects of these actions result in an increase of intrathoracic pressure and flow of air out of the lungs. Contraction of the primary and accessory muscles of exhalation, found in Table 4-2, results in an increase in intrathoracic pressure and a faster rate of decrease in thoracic size, which forces air out of the lungs. These motions are outlined schematically in Figure 4-2.[6,7]

In persons with primary or secondary chronic pulmonary health conditions, changes in tissue and mechanical properties in the pulmonary system can result in accessory muscle use being observed earlier in activity or may even be present at rest. Determination of the impairment(s) resulting in the observed activity limitation can help a clinician focus a plan of care. In addition, clinicians should consider the reversibility, or the degree to which the impairment can be improved, when determining a patient's prognosis for improvement with physical therapy. If reversing a patient's ventilatory impairments is unlikely, facilitation of accessory muscle use can be promoted during functional activities and strengthening of these accessory muscles (e.g., use of a four-wheeled rolling walker with a seat and accompanying arm exercises).

> ✎ **CLINICAL TIP**
>
> Patients with advanced pulmonary conditions may automatically assume positions to optimize accessory muscle use, such as forward leaning on their forearms (i.e., tripod posturing).

Gas Exchange. Once air has reached the alveolar spaces, respiration or gas exchange can occur at the alveolar-capillary membrane. Diffusion of gases through the membrane is affected by the following:

- A concentration gradient in which gases will diffuse from areas of high concentration to areas of low concentration:

$$\text{Alveolar } O_2 = 100 \text{ mm Hg} \rightarrow \text{Capillary } O_2 = 40 \text{ mm Hg}$$

- Surface area, or the total amount of alveolar-capillary interface available for gas exchange (e.g., the breakdown of alveolar membranes that occurs in emphysema will reduce the amount of surface area available for gas exchange)
- The thickness of the barrier (membrane) between the two areas involved (e.g., retained secretions in the alveolar spaces will impede gas exchange through the membrane)

Ventilation and Perfusion Ratio. Gas exchange is optimized when the ratio of air flow (ventilation $\dot{V}$) to blood flow (perfusion $\dot{Q}$) approaches a $1:1$ relationship. However, the actual $\dot{V}/\dot{Q}$ ratio is 0.8 because alveolar ventilation is approximately equal to 4 L per minute and pulmonary blood flow is approximately equal to 5 L per minute.[2,8,9]

Gravity, body position, and cardiopulmonary dysfunction can influence this ratio. Ventilation is optimized in areas of least resistance. For example, when a person is in a sitting position, the upper lobes initially receive more ventilation than the lower lobes; however, the lower lobes have the largest net change in ventilation.

Perfusion is greatest in gravity-dependent areas. For example, when a person is in a sitting position, perfusion is the greatest at the base of the lungs; when a person is in a left side-lying position, the left lung receives the most blood.

A $\dot{V}/\dot{Q}$ mismatch (inequality in the relationship between ventilation and perfusion) can occur in certain situations. Two

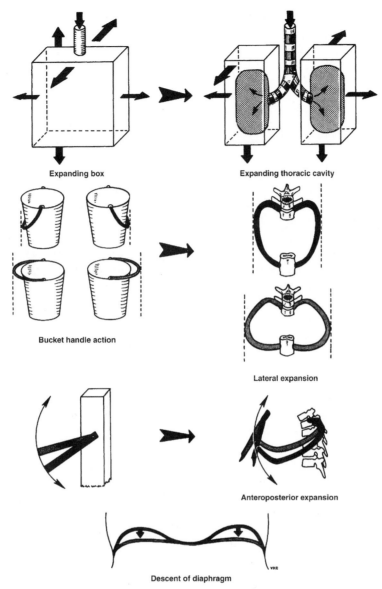

FIGURE 4-2
Respiratory mechanics (bucket and pump handle motions). (From Snell RS, editor: Clinical anatomy by regions, ed 9, Baltimore, 2012, Lippincott, Williams & Wilkins.)

terms associated with $\dot{V}/\dot{Q}$ mismatch are *dead space* and *shunt*. Dead space occurs when ventilation is in excess of perfusion, as with a pulmonary embolus. A shunt occurs when perfusion is in excess of ventilation, as in alveolar collapse from secretion retention. These conditions are shown in Figure 4-3.

Gas Transport. O_2 is transported away from the lungs to the tissues in two forms: dissolved in plasma (PO_2) or chemically bound to hemoglobin on a red blood cell (oxyhemoglobin). As a by-product of cellular metabolism, CO_2 is transported away from the tissues to the lungs in three forms: dissolved in plasma (PCO_2), chemically bound to hemoglobin (carboxyhemoglobin), and as bicarbonate.

Approximately 97% of O_2 transported from the lungs is carried in chemical combination with hemoglobin. The majority of CO_2 transport, 93%, occurs in the combined forms of carbaminohemoglobin and bicarbonate. A smaller percentage, 3% of O_2 and 7% of CO_2, is transported in dissolved forms.[10]

Dissolved O_2 and CO_2 exert a partial pressure within the plasma and can be measured by sampling arterial, venous, or mixed venous blood.[11] See the Arterial Blood Gas section for further description of this process.

Evaluation

Pulmonary evaluation is composed of patient history, physical examination, and interpretation of diagnostic test results.

Patient History

In addition to the general chart review presented in Chapter 2, other relevant information regarding pulmonary dysfunction that should be ascertained from the chart review or patient interview is listed as follows[11-13]:

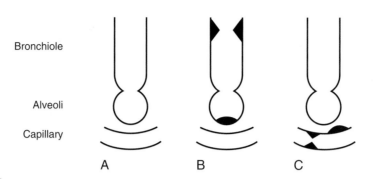

FIGURE 4-3
Ventilation and perfusion mismatch. **A,** Normal alveolar ventilation. **B,** Capillary shunt. **C,** Alveolar dead space.

- History of smoking, including packs per day or pack years (packs per day × number of years smoked) and the amount of time that smoking has been discontinued (if applicable)
- Presence, history, and amount of O_2 therapy at rest, with activity and at night
- Exposure to environmental or occupational toxins (e.g., asbestos)
- History of pneumonia, thoracic procedures, or surgery
- History of assisted ventilation or intubation with mechanical ventilation
- History or current reports of dyspnea either at rest or with exertion. Dyspnea is the subjective complaint of difficulty with respiration, also known as shortness of breath. A visual analog scale or ratio scale (Modified Borg scale) can be used to obtain a measurement of dyspnea. The American Thoracic Society Dyspnea Scale can be found in Table 4-3. Note: The abbreviation *DOE* represents "dyspnea on exertion"
- Level of activity before admittance
- History of baseline sputum production, including color (e.g., yellow, green), consistency (e.g., thick, thin), and amount. Familiar or broad terms can be applied as units of measure for sputum (e.g., quarter-sized, tablespoon, or copious)
- Sleeping position and number of pillows used

> ✎ **CLINICAL TIP**
>
> Dyspnea also may be measured by counting the number of words a person can speak per breath. For example, a patient with one- to two-word dyspnea is noticeably more dyspneic than a person who can speak a full sentence per breath. Measurement of dyspnea can be used in goal writing (e.g., "Patient will ascend/descend 10 stairs with one rail with reported dyspnea < 2/10.").

Physical Examination

The physical examination of the pulmonary system consists of inspection, auscultation, palpation, mediate percussion, and cough examination. Suggested guidelines for physical therapy intervention(s) that are based on examination findings and diagnostic test results are found at the end of this chapter.

TABLE 4-3 American Thoracic Society Dyspnea Scale

Grade	Degree	
0	None	Not troubled with breathlessness except with strenuous exercise
1	Slight	Troubled by shortness of breath when hurrying on the level or walking up a slight hill
2	Moderate	Walks slower than people of the same age on the level because of breathlessness, or has to stop for breath when walking at own pace on the level
3	Severe	Stops for breath after walking about 100 yards or after a few minutes on the level
4	Very severe	Too breathless to leave the house or breathless when dressing or undressing

From Brooks SM: Surveillance for respiratory hazards, ATS News 8:12-16, 1982.

Inspection

A wealth of information can be gathered by simple observation of the patient at rest and with activity. Physical observation should proceed in a systematic fashion and include the following:

- General appearance and level of alertness
- Ease of phonation
- Skin color
- Posture and chest shape
- Ventilatory or breathing pattern
- Presence of digital clubbing
- Presence of supplemental O_2 and other medical equipment (refer to Chapter 18)
- Presence and location of surgical incisions

Observation of Breathing Patterns

Breathing patterns vary among individuals and may be influenced by pain, emotion, body temperature, sleep, body position, activity level, and the presence of pulmonary, cardiac, metabolic, or nervous system disease (Table 4-4). The optimal time, clinically, to examine a patient's breathing pattern is when he

TABLE 4-4 Description of Breathing Patterns and Their Associated Conditions

Breathing Pattern	Description	Associated Conditions
Apnea	Lack of airflow to the lungs for >15 seconds	Airway obstruction, cardiopulmonary arrest, alterations of the respiratory center, narcotic overdose
Biot's respirations	Constant increased rate and depth of respiration followed by periods of apnea of varying lengths	Elevated intracranial pressure, meningitis
Bradypnea	Ventilation rate <12 breaths per minute	Use of sedatives, narcotics, or alcohol; neurologic or metabolic disorders; excessive fatigue
Cheyne-Stokes respirations	Increasing depth of ventilation followed by a period of apnea	Elevated intracranial pressure, CHF, narcotic overdose
Hyperpnea	Increased depth of ventilation	Activity, pulmonary infections, CHF
Hyperventilation	Increased rate and depth of ventilation resulting in decreased P_{CO_2}	Anxiety, nervousness, metabolic acidosis
Hypoventilation	Decreased rate and depth of ventilation resulting in increased P_{CO_2}	Sedation or somnolence, neurologic depression of respiratory centers, overmedication, metabolic alkalosis
Kussmaul respirations	Increased regular rate and depth of ventilation	Diabetic ketoacidosis, renal failure
Orthopnea	Dyspnea that occurs in a flat supine position. Relief occurs with more upright sitting or standing	Chronic lung disease, CHF
Paradoxic ventilation	Inward abdominal or chest wall movement with inspiration and outward movement with expiration	Diaphragm paralysis, ventilation muscle fatigue, chest wall trauma
Sighing respirations	The presence of a sigh >2-3 times per minute	Angina, anxiety, dyspnea
Tachypnea	Ventilation rate >20 breaths per minute	Acute respiratory distress, fever, pain, emotions, anemia
Hoover's sign*	The inward motion of the lower rib cage during inhalation	Flattened diaphragm often related to decompensated or irreversible hyperinflation of the lungs

Data from Kersten LD: Comprehensive respiratory nursing: a decision-making approach, Philadelphia, 1989, Saunders; DesJardins T, Burton GG: Clinical manifestations and assessment of respiratory disease, ed 3, St Louis, 1995, Mosby;

  *Hoover's sign has been reported to have a sensitivity of 58% and specificity of 86% for detection of airway obstruction. Hoover's sign is associated with a patient's body mass index, severity of dyspnea, and frequency of exacerbations and is seen in up to 70% of patients with severe obstruction.†

  †Data from Johnson CR, Krishnaswamy N, Krishnaswamy G: The Hoover's sign of pulmonary disease: molecular basis and clinical relevance, Clin Mol Allergy 6:8, 2008.

  CHF, Congestive heart failure; *P_{CO_2}*, partial pressure of carbon dioxide.

or she is unaware of the inspection because knowledge of the physical examination can influence the patient's respiratory pattern.

Observation of breathing pattern should include an assessment of rate (12 to 20 breaths per minute is normal), depth, ratio of inspiration to expiration (one to two is normal), sequence of chest wall movement during inspiration and expiration, comfort, presence accessory muscle use, and symmetry.

> ✎ **CLINICAL TIP**
>
> If possible, examine a patient's breathing pattern when he or she is unaware of the inspection because knowledge of the physical examination can influence the patient's respiratory pattern. Objective observations of ventilation rate may not always be consistent with a patient's subjective complaints of dyspnea. For example, a patient may complain of shortness of breath but have a ventilation rate within normal limits. Therefore the patient's subjective complaints, rather than the objective observations, may be a more accurate measure of treatment intensity.

Auscultation

Auscultation is the process of listening to the sounds of air passing through the tracheobronchial tree and alveolar spaces. The sounds of airflow normally dissipate from proximal to distal airways, making the sounds less audible in the periphery than the central airways. Alterations in airflow and ventilation effort result in distinctive sounds within the thoracic cavity that may indicate pulmonary disease or dysfunction.

Auscultation proceeds in a systematic, side-to-side, and cephalocaudal fashion. Breath sounds on the left and right sides are compared in the anterior, lateral, and posterior segments of the chest wall, as shown in Figure 4-4. The diaphragm (flat side) of the stethoscope should be used for auscultation. The patient should be seated or lying comfortably in a position that allows access to all lung fields. Full inspirations and expirations are performed by the patient through the mouth, as the clinician listens to the entire cycle of respiration before moving the stethoscope to another lung segment.

All of the following ensure accurate auscultation:
* Make sure stethoscope earpieces are pointing up and inward (toward your patient) before placing in the ears.

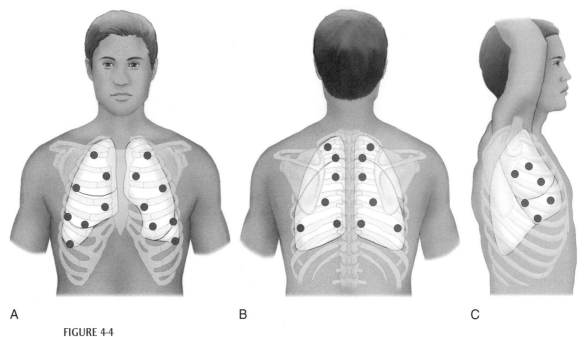

A   B   C

FIGURE 4-4
Landmarks for lung auscultation on (**A**) anterior, (**B**) posterior, and (**C**) lateral aspects of the chest wall. (Courtesy Peter P. Wu.)

- Long stethoscope tubing may dampen sound transmission. Length of tubing should be approximately 30 cm (12 in) to 55 cm (21 to 22 in).[12]
- Always check proper function of the stethoscope before auscultating by listening to finger tapping on the diaphragm while the earpieces are in place.
- Apply the stethoscope diaphragm firmly against the skin so that it lays flat.
- Observe chest wall expansion and breathing pattern while auscultating to help confirm palpatory findings of breathing pattern (e.g., sequence and symmetry). For example, decreased chest wall motion palpated earlier in the left lower lung field may present with decreased breath sounds in that same area.

Breath sounds may be normal or abnormal (adventitious or added) breath sounds; all breath sounds should be documented according to the location and the phase of respiration (i.e., inspiration, expiration, or both) and in comparison with the opposite lung. Several strategies can be used to reduce the chance of false-positive adventitious breath sound findings, including the following:

- Ensure full, deep inspirations (decreased effort can be misinterpreted as decreased breath sounds).
- Be aware of the stethoscope tubing's touching other objects (especially ventilator tubing) or chest hair.
- Periodically lift the stethoscope off the chest wall to help differentiate extraneous sounds (e.g., chest or nasogastric tubes, patient snoring) that may appear to originate from the thorax.

To maximize patient comfort, allow periodic rest periods between deep breaths to prevent hyperventilation and dizziness.

Normal Breath Sounds. Clinically, tracheal or bronchial and vesicular breath sounds generally are documented as "normal" or "clear" breath sounds; however, the use of tracheal or vesicular breath sounds is more accurate.

Tracheal, Bronchial, or Bronchovesicular Sounds. Normal tracheal or bronchial breath sounds are loud tubular sounds heard over the proximal airways, such as the trachea and main stem bronchi. A pause is heard between inspiration and expiration; the expiratory phase is longer than the inspiratory phase. Normal bronchovesicular sounds are similar to bronchial breath sounds; however, no pause occurs between inspiration and expiration.[11,12]

Vesicular Sounds. Vesicular sounds are soft rustling sounds heard over the more distal airways and lung parenchyma. Inspiration is longer and more pronounced than expiration because a decrease in airway lumen during expiration limits transmission of airflow sounds.[11,12]

Note: In most reference books, a distinction between normal bronchial and bronchovesicular sounds is made to help with standardization of terminology. Often, however, this distinction is not used in the clinical setting.

> ✎ **CLINICAL TIP**
> The abbreviation CTA stands for "clear to auscultation."

Abnormal Breath Sounds. Breath sounds are abnormal if they are heard outside their usual location in the chest or if they are qualitatively different from normal breath sounds.[14] Despite efforts to make the terminology of breath sounds more

TABLE 4-5 Possible Sources of Abnormal Breath Sounds

Sound	Possible Etiology
Bronchial (abnormal if heard in areas where vesicular sounds should be present)	Fluid or secretion consolidation (airlessness) that could occur with pneumonia
Decreased or diminished (less audible)	Hypoventilation, severe congestion, or emphysema
Absent	Pneumothorax or lung collapse

consistent, terminology may still vary from clinician to clinician and facility to facility. Always clarify the intended meaning of the breath sound description if your findings differ significantly from what has been documented or reported. Abnormal breath sounds with possible sources are outlined in Table 4-5.

Adventitious Breath Sounds. Adventitious breath sounds occur from alterations or turbulence in airflow through the tracheobronchial tree and lung parenchyma. These sounds can be divided into continuous (wheezes and rhonchi) or discontinuous (crackles) sounds.[12,14]

The American Thoracic Society and American College of Chest Physicians have discouraged use of the term *rhonchi*, recommending instead that the term *wheezes* be used for all continuous adventitious breath sounds.[15] Many academic institutions and hospitals continue to teach and practice use of the term *rhonchi*; therefore it is mentioned in this section.

Continuous Sounds

Wheeze. Wheezes occur most commonly with airway obstruction from bronchoconstriction or retained secretions and commonly are heard on expiration. Wheezes also may be present during inspiration if the obstruction is significant enough. Wheezes can be high pitched (usually from bronchospasm or constriction, as in asthma) or low pitched (usually from secretions, as in pneumonia).

STRIDOR. Stridor is an extremely high-pitched wheeze that occurs with significant upper airway obstruction and is present during inspiration and expiration. The presence of stridor indicates a medical emergency. Stridor is also audible without a stethoscope.

> ✎ **CLINICAL TIP**
> Acute onset of stridor during an intervention session warrants immediate notification of the nursing and medical staff.

Rhonchi. Low-pitched or "snoring" sounds that are continuous characterize rhonchi. These sounds generally are associated with large airway obstruction, typically from secretions lining the airways.

Discontinuous Sounds

Crackles. Crackles are bubbling or popping sounds that represent the presence of fluid or secretions, or the sudden opening of closed airways. Crackles that result from fluid (pulmonary edema) or secretions (pneumonia) are described as "wet" or

"coarse," whereas crackles that occur from the sudden opening of closed airways (atelectasis) are referred to as "dry" or "fine."

> ✎ **CLINICAL TIP**
> Wet crackles also can be referred to as *rales,* but the American Thoracic Society–American College of Chest Physicians has moved to eliminate this terminology for purposes of standardization.[15]

Extrapulmonary Sounds. These sounds are generated from dysfunction outside of the lung tissue. The most common sound is the pleural friction rub. This sound is heard as a loud grating sound, generally throughout both phases of respiration, and almost always is associated with pleuritis (inflamed pleurae rubbing on one another).[12,14] The presence of a chest tube inserted into the pleural space also may cause a sound similar to a pleural rub.

> ✎ **CLINICAL TIP**
> Asking the patient to hold his or her breath can help differentiate a true pleural friction rub from a sound artifact or a pericardial friction rub.

Voice Sounds. Normal phonation is audible during auscultation, with the intensity and clarity of speech also dissipating from proximal to distal airways. Voice sounds that are more or less pronounced in distal lung regions, where vesicular breath sounds should occur, may indicate areas of consolidation or hyperinflation, respectively. The same areas of auscultation should be used when assessing voice sounds. The following three types of voice sound tests can be used to help confirm breath sound findings:

1. Whispered pectoriloquy. The patient whispers "one, two, three." The test is positive for consolidation if phrases are clearly audible in distal lung fields. This test is positive for hyperinflation if the phrases are less audible in distal lung fields.
2. Bronchophony. The patient repeats the phrase "ninety-nine." The results are similar to whispered pectoriloquy.
3. Egophony. The patient repeats the letter *e*. If the auscultation in the distal lung fields sound like *a*, then fluid in the air spaces or lung parenchyma is suspected.

Palpation

The third component of the physical examination is palpation of the chest wall, which is performed in a cephalocaudal direction. Figure 4-5 demonstrates hand placement for chest wall palpation of the upper, middle, and lower lung fields. Palpation is performed to examine the following:

- Presence of fremitus (a vibration caused by the presence of secretions or voice production, which is felt through the chest wall) during respirations[11]

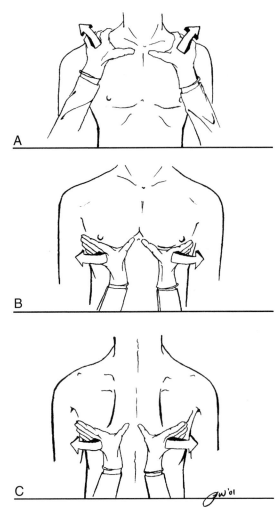

FIGURE 4-5
Palpation of (A) upper, (B) middle, and (C) lower chest wall motion. (Courtesy Peter P. Wu.)

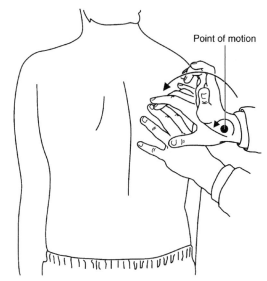

FIGURE 4-6
Demonstration of mediate percussion technique. (From Hillegass EA, Sadowsky HS: Essentials of cardiopulmonary physical therapy, ed 2, Philadelphia, 2001, Saunders.)

- Presence, location, and reproducibility of pain, tenderness, or both
- Skin temperature
- Presence of bony abnormalities, rib fractures, or both
- Chest expansion and symmetry
- Presence of subcutaneous emphysema (palpated as bubbles popping under the skin from the presence of air in the subcutaneous tissue). This finding is abnormal and represents air that has escaped or is escaping from the lungs. Subcutaneous emphysema can occur from a pneumothorax (PTX), a complication from central line placement, or after thoracic surgery[1]

> ✎ **CLINICAL TIP**
> To decrease patient fatigue while palpating each of the chest wall segments for motion, all of the items listed above can be examined simultaneously.

Chest Wall and Abdominal Excursion. Direct measurement of chest wall expansion can be used for objective data collection, intervention, or goal setting. Begin by placing a tape measure snugly around the circumference of the patient's chest wall at three levels:

1. Angle of Louis
2. Xyphoid process
3. Umbilicus

Measure the change in circumference in each of these areas with normal breathing and then deep breathing. The resulting values can be used to describe breathing patterns or identify ventilation impairments. Changes in these values after an intervention may indicate improvements in breathing patterns and can be used to evaluate treatment efficacy. Normal changes in breathing patterns exist in supine, sitting, and standing.

> ✎ **CLINICAL TIP**
> By placing your thumb tips together on the spinous processes or xyphoid process, you can estimate the distance of separation between your thumb tips to qualitatively measure chest wall motion.

Mediate Percussion. Mediate percussion can evaluate tissue densities within the thoracic cage and indirectly measure diaphragmatic excursion during respirations. Mediate percussion also can be used to confirm other findings in the physical examination. The procedure is shown in Figure 4-6 and is performed by placing the palmar surface of the index finger, middle finger, or both from one hand flatly against the surface of the chest wall within the intercostal spaces. The tip(s) of the other index finger, middle finger, or both then strike(s) the distal third of the fingers resting against the chest wall. The clinician proceeds from side to side in a cephalocaudal fashion, within the intercostal spaces, for anterior and posterior aspects of the chest wall. Mediate percussion is a difficult skill and is performed most proficiently by experienced clinicians; mediate percussion also can be performed over the abdominal cavity to assess tissue densities, which is described further in Chapter 8.

Sounds produced from mediate percussion can be characterized as one of the following:

- Resonant (over normal lung tissue)
- Hyperresonant (over emphysematous lungs or PTX)
- Tympanic (over gas bubbles in abdomen)
- Dull (from increased tissue density or lungs with decreased air)
- Flat (extreme dullness over very dense tissues, such as the thigh muscles)[12]

To evaluate diaphragmatic excursion with mediate percussion, the clinician first delineates the resting position of the diaphragm by percussing down the posterior aspect of one side of the chest wall until a change from resonant to dull (flat) sounds occurs. The clinician then asks the patient to inspire deeply and repeats the process, noting the difference in landmarks when sound changes occur. The difference is the amount of diaphragmatic excursion. The other also is examined, and a comparison then can be made of the hemidiaphragms.

> ✎ **CLINICAL TIP**
>
> Do not confuse this examination technique with the intervention technique of percussion, which is used to help mobilize bronchopulmonary secretions in patients.

Cough Examination. An essential component of bronchopulmonary hygiene is cough effectiveness. The cough mechanism can be divided into four phases: (1) full inspiration, (2) closure of the glottis with an increase of intrathoracic pressure, (3) abdominal contraction, and (4) rapid expulsion of air. The inability to perform one or more portions of the cough mechanism can lead to pulmonary secretion clearance. Cough examination includes the following components[11,12]:

- Effectiveness (ability to clear secretions)
- Control (ability to start and stop coughs)
- Quality (wet, dry, bronchospastic)
- Frequency (how often during the day and night cough occurs)
- Sputum production (color, quantity, odor, and consistency)

The effectiveness of a patient's cough can be examined directly by simply asking the patient to cough or indirectly by observing the above components when the patient coughs spontaneously.

Hemoptysis. Hemoptysis, the expectoration of blood during coughing, may occur for many reasons. Hemoptysis is usually benign postoperatively if it is not sustained with successive coughs. The therapist should note whether the blood is dark red or brownish in color (old blood) or bright red (new or frank blood). The presence of new blood in sputum should be documented and the nurse or physician notified.

Patients with cystic fibrosis may have periodic episodes of hemoptysis with streaking or larger quantities of new blood.

During these episodes airway clearance techniques (ACT) may need to be modified. Current recommendations for patients who have scant hemoptysis (<5 ml) are to continue with all ACT, and those with massive hemoptysis should discontinue all ACT. For persons with mild to moderate hemoptysis (≥5 ml), no clear recommendations exist for continuing or discontinuing ACT. However, expert consensus is that autogenic drainage or active cycle of breathing techniques are least likely to exacerbate hemoptysis while maintaining the needs of assisted sputum clearance.[16]

Diagnostic Testing

Oximetry

Pulse oximetry is a noninvasive method of determining arterial oxyhemoglobin saturation (SaO_2) through the measurement of the saturation of peripheral oxygen (SpO_2). It also indirectly examines the partial pressure of O_2. Finger or ear sensors generally are applied to a patient on a continuous or intermittent basis. O_2 saturation readings can be affected by poor circulation (cool digits), movement of sensor cord, cleanliness of the sensors, nail polish, intense light, increased levels of carboxyhemoglobin ($HbCO_2$), jaundice, skin pigmentation, shock states, cardiac dysrhythmias (e.g., atrial fibrillation), and severe hypoxia.[17,18]

> ✎ **CLINICAL TIP**
>
> To ensure accurate O_2 saturation readings, (1) check for proper waveform or pulsations, which indicate proper signal reception, and (2) compare pulse readings on an O_2 saturation monitor with the patient's peripheral pulses or electrocardiograph readings (if available).

Oxyhemoglobin saturation is an indication of pulmonary reserve and is dependent on the PO_2 level in the blood. Figure 4-7 demonstrates the direct relationship of oxyhemoglobin saturation and partial pressures of O_2. As shown on the steep portion of the curve, small changes in PO_2 levels below

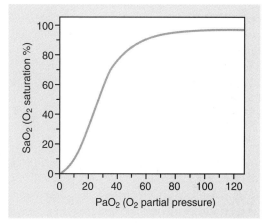

FIGURE 4-7

The oxyhemoglobin dissociation curve. (Courtesy Marybeth Cuaycong.)

TABLE 4-6 Relationship Between Oxygen Saturation, the Partial Pressure of Oxygen, and the Signs and Symptoms of Hypoxemia

Oxyhemoglobin Saturation (SaO_2) (%)	Oxygen Partial Pressure (PaO_2) (mm Hg)	Signs and Symptoms of Hypoxemia
97-99	90-100	None
95	80	Tachypnea Tachycardia
90	60	As above Restlessness Malaise Impaired judgment Incoordination Vertigo Nausea
85	50	As above Labored respiration Cardiac dysrhythmia Confusion
80	45	As above
75	40	As above

From Frownfelter DL, Dean E: Principles and practice of cardiopulmonary physical therapy, ed 4, St Louis, 2006, Mosby.

TABLE 4-7 Causes of Acid-Base Imbalances

	Respiratory	Metabolic

Acidosis	Chronic obstructive pulmonary disease
	Sedation
	Head trauma
	Drug overdose
	Pneumothorax
	Central nervous system disorders
	Pulmonary edema
	Sleep apnea
	Chest wall trauma
		Lactic acidosis
		Ketoacidosis:
		  Diabetes
		  Starvation
		  Alcoholism
		  Diarrhea
		  Parenteral nutrition

Alkalosis	Pulmonary embolism Pregnancy Anxiety/fear Hypoxia Pain Fever Sepsis Congestive heart failure Pulmonary edema Asthma Acute respiratory distress syndrome	Vomiting Nasogastric suction Diuretics Steroids Hypokalemia Excessive ingestion of antacids Administration of HCO_3 Banked blood transfusions Cushing's syndrome

From George-Gay B, Chernecky CC, editors: Clinical medical-surgical nursing: a decision-making reference, Philadelphia, 2002, WB Saunders.

60 mm Hg result in large changes in oxygen saturation, which is considered moderately hypoxic.[11] The relationship between oxygen saturation and PO_2 levels is further summarized in Table 4-6. The affinity or binding of O_2 to hemoglobin is affected by changes in pH, PCO_2, temperature, and 2,3-diphosphoglycerate (a by-product of red blood cell metabolism) levels. Note that pulse oximetry can measure only changes in oxygenation (PO_2) indirectly and cannot measure changes in ventilation (PCO_2). Changes in ventilation must be measured by arterial blood gas (ABG) analysis.[19]

Blood Gas Analysis

Arterial Blood Gases. ABG analysis examines acid-base balance (pH), ventilation (CO_2 levels), and oxygenation (O_2 levels) and guides medical or therapy interventions, such as mechanical ventilation settings or breathing assist techniques.[11] For proper cellular metabolism to occur, acid-base balance must be maintained. Disturbances in acid-base balance can be caused by pulmonary or metabolic dysfunction (Table 4-7). Normally, the pulmonary and metabolic systems work in synergy to help maintain acid-base balance. Clinical presentation of carbon dioxide retention, which can occur in patients with lung disease, is outlined in Box 4-1.

The ability to interpret ABGs provides the physical therapist with valuable information regarding the current medical status of the patient, the appropriateness for bronchopulmonary hygiene or exercise treatments, and the outcomes of medical and physical therapy intervention.

ABG measurements usually are performed on a routine basis, which is specified according to need in the critical care setting. For the critically ill patient, ABG sampling may occur every 1 to 3 hours. In contrast, ABGs may be sampled one or two times

BOX 4-1 Clinical Presentation of Carbon Dioxide Retention and Narcosis

- Altered mental status
- Lethargy
- Drowsiness
- Coma
- Headache
- Tachycardia
- Hypertension
- Diaphoresis
- Tremor
- Redness of skin, sclera, or conjunctiva

From Kersten LD: Comprehensive respiratory nursing: a decision-making approach, Philadelphia, 1989, Saunders, p 351.

a day in a patient whose pulmonary or metabolic status has stabilized. Unless specified, arterial blood is sampled from an indwelling arterial line. Other sites of sampling include arterial puncture, venous blood from a peripheral venous puncture or catheter, and mixed venous blood from a pulmonary artery catheter. Chapter 18 describes vascular monitoring lines in more detail.

Terminology. The following terms are frequently used in ABG analysis:
- PaO_2 (PO_2): Partial pressure of dissolved O_2 in plasma
- $PaCO_2$ (PCO_2): Partial pressure of dissolved CO_2 in plasma
- pH: Degree of acidity or alkalinity in blood
- HCO_3: Level of bicarbonate in the blood

- Percentage of SaO_2 (O_2 saturation): A percentage of the amount of hemoglobin sites filled (saturated) with O_2 molecules (PaO_2 and SaO_2 are intimately related but are not synonymous)

Normal Values. The normal ranges for ABGs are as follows[20]:

PaO_2	Greater than 80 mm Hg
$PaCO_2$	35 to 45 mm Hg
pH	7.35 to 7.45
HCO_3	22 to 26 mEq/liter

ABGs generally are reported in the following format: pH/$Paco_2$/Pao_2/HCO_3 (e.g., 7.38/42/90/26).

Interpretation. Interpretation of ABGs includes the ability to determine any deviation from normal values and hypothesize a cause (or causes) for the acid-base disturbance in relation to the patient's clinical history. Acid-base balance—or pH—is the most important ABG value for the patient to have within normal limits (Figure 4-8). It is important to relate ABG values with medical history and clinical course. ABG values and vital signs generally are documented on a daily flow sheet, an invaluable source of information. Because changes in ABG are not immediately available in most circumstances, the value of this test is to observe changes over time. Single ABG readings should be correlated with previous ABG readings, medical status, supplemental O_2 or ventilator changes, and medical procedures. Be sure to note if an ABG sample is drawn from mixed venous blood, as the normal O_2 value is lower. Po_2 of mixed venous blood is 35 to 40 mm Hg.

Acid-base disturbances that occur clinically can arise from pulmonary and metabolic disorders; therefore interpretation of the ABG results may not prove to be as straightforward as shown in Figure 4-8. Therefore the clinician must use this information as part of a complete examination process to gain full understanding of the patient's current medical status.

Venous Blood Gas Analysis. Although not as common as ABGs, venous or mixed venous blood gases (VBGs) also can provide important information to the clinician. VBGs CO_2 (S_vCO_2) and O_2 (S_vO_2) values represent the body's metabolic workload and efficiency for any given state. Large increases in S_vCO_2 values can represent inefficient/deconditioned peripheral muscles or overall deconditioning associated with acute/chronic illness.

S_vCO_2 and cardiac output (estimated) values can be observed in patients with central catheters and may be continuously monitored in those receiving tailored therapy for advanced heart failure. Direct monitoring of S_vCO_2 values and cardiac output during an exercise session can drive your treatment and recommendations.

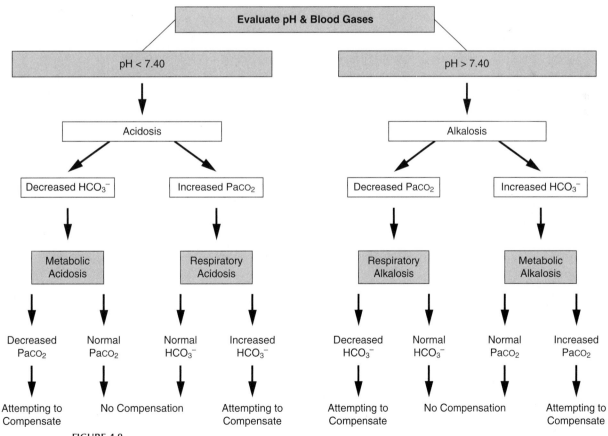

FIGURE 4-8
Methods to analyze arterial blood gases. (From Cahalin LP: Pulmonary evaluation. In DeTurk WE, Cahalin LP, editors: Cardiovascular and pulmonary physical therapy, ed 2, New York, 2011, McGraw Hill, p 265.)

Chest X-Rays

Radiographic information of the thoracic cavity in combination with a clinical history provides critical assistance in the differential diagnosis of pulmonary conditions. Diagnosis cannot be made by CXR alone; the therapist should use CXR reports as a guide for decision making and not as an absolute parameter for bronchopulmonary hygiene evaluation and treatment.

✎ CLINICAL TIP

CXRs sometimes lag behind significant clinical presentation (e.g., symptoms of pulmonary infection may resolve clinically, whereas CXR findings remain positive for infection). CXR also can be a helpful tool pre-and post-physical therapy sessions for bronchopulmonary hygiene to determine the effectiveness of the treatment. This is more common in the ICU setting or in hospital units where patients receive daily CXR.

Indications for CXRs are as follows[21,22]:

- Assist in the clinical diagnosis and monitor the progression or regression of the following:
  - Airspace consolidation (pulmonary edema, pneumonia, adult respiratory distress syndrome [ARDS], pulmonary hemorrhage, and infarctions)
  - Large intrapulmonary air spaces and presence of mediastinal or subcutaneous air, as well as PTX
  - Lobar atelectasis
  - Other pulmonary lesions, such as lung nodules and abscesses
  - Rib fractures
- Determine proper placement of endotracheal tubes, central lines, chest tubes, or nasogastric tubes
- Evaluate structural features, such as cardiac or mediastinal size and diaphragmatic shape and position

CXRs are classified according to the direction of radiographic beam projection. The first word describes where the beam enters the body, and the second word describes the exit. Common types of CXRs include the following:

- Posterior-anterior (P-A): Taken while the patient is upright sitting or standing
- Anterior-posterior (A-P): Taken while the patient is upright sitting or standing, semireclined, or supine
- Lateral: Taken while the patient is upright sitting or standing, or decubitus (lying on the side)

Upright positions are preferred to allow full expansion of lungs without hindrance of the abdominal viscera and to visualize gravity-dependent fluid collections. Lateral films aid in three-dimensional, segmental localization of lesions and fluid collections not visible in P-A or A-P views.

The appearance of various chest structures on CXR depends on the density of the structure. For example, bone appears white on CXR because of absorption of the x-ray beams, whereas air appears black. Moderately dense structures such as the heart, aorta, and pulmonary vessels appear gray, as do fluids such as pulmonary edema and blood.[2] Figure 4-9 outlines the anatomic structures used for chest x-ray (CXR) interpretation.

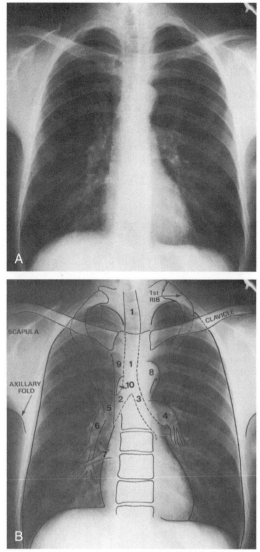

FIGURE 4-9
A, Normal chest radiograph (posteroanterior view). **B,** Same radiograph as in **A** with normal anatomic structures labeled or numbered. (*1,* Trachea; *2,* right main stem bronchus; *3,* left main stem bronchus; *4,* left pulmonary artery; *5,* pulmonary vein to the right upper lobe; *6,* right interlobar artery; *7,* vein to right middle and lower lobes; *8,* aortic knob; *9,* superior vena cava; *10,* ascending aorta.) (From Fraser RS, Müller NL, Colman N, Paré MD: Diagnosis of diseases of the chest, ed 4, Philadelphia, 1999, Saunders.)

A systematic approach to a basic CXR interpretation is important. First, assess the densities of the various structures to identify air, bone, tissue, and fluid. Next, determine if the findings are normal or abnormal and if they are consistent on both sides of the lungs. Common CXR findings with various pulmonary diagnoses are discussed in the Health Conditions section of this chapter.

Sputum Analysis

Analysis of sputum includes culture and Gram stain to isolate and identify organisms that may be present in the lower respiratory tract. Refer to Chapter 13 for more details on culture and Gram stain. After the organisms are identified, appropriate antibiotic therapy can be instituted. Sputum specimens are collected when the patient's temperature rises or the color or consistency of sputum changes. They also can be used to evaluate the efficacy of antibiotic therapy. Sputum analysis can be inaccurate if a sterile technique is not maintained during sputum collection or if the specimen is contaminated with too much saliva, as noted microscopically by the presence of many squamous epithelial cells. Therapists involved in bronchopulmonary hygiene and collecting sputum samples should have sterile sputum collection containers and equipment on hand before beginning the treatment session to ensure successful sputum collection.

> ### ✎ CLINICAL TIP
> Patients who present with a sputum analysis negative for active infection may still have retained secretions that could hinder gas exchange and tolerance to activity. Therefore therapists must evaluate clinically the need for secretion clearance techniques.

Flexible Bronchoscopy

A flexible, fiberoptic tube is used as a diagnostic and interventional tool to visualize directly and aspirate (suction) the bronchopulmonary tree. If a patient is mechanically ventilated, the bronchoscope is inserted through the endotracheal or tracheal tube. Refer to Chapter 18 for more information on mechanical ventilation and endotracheal and tracheal tubes. If the patient is spontaneously breathing, a local anesthetic is applied and light sedation via intravenous access is given before the bronchoscope is inserted through one of the patient's nares.

> ### ✎ CLINICAL TIP
> Bronchoscopy also can be performed with a rigid bronchoscope. This is primarily an operative procedure.[22-24]

Box 4-2 summarizes the diagnostic and therapeutic indications of bronchoscopy.

Ventilation-Perfusion Scan

The $\dot{V}/\dot{Q}$ scan is used to rule out the presence of pulmonary embolism (PE) and other acute abnormalities of oxygenation and gas exchange and as preoperative and postoperative evaluation of lung transplantation.

During a ventilation scan, inert radioactive gases or aerosols are inhaled, and three subsequent projections (i.e., after first breath, at equilibrium, and during washout) of airflow are recorded.

During a perfusion lung scan, a radioisotope is injected intravenously into a peripheral vessel, and six projections are taken (i.e., anterior, posterior, both laterals, and both posterior obliques). The scan is sensitive to diminished or absent blood flow, and lesions of 2 cm or greater are detected.

Perfusion defects can occur with pulmonary embolus, asthma, emphysema, and virtually all alveolar filling, destructive or space-occupying lesions in lung, and hypoventilation. A

> ### BOX 4-2   Diagnostic and Therapeutic Indications for Flexible Bronchoscopy
>
> | Diagnostic Indications | Therapeutic Indications |
> |---|---|
> | Evaluation of neoplasms (benign or malignant) in air spaces and mediastinum, tissue biopsy | Removal of retained secretions, foreign bodies, and/or obstructive endotracheal tissue |
> | Evaluation of the patient before and after lung transplantation | Intubation or stent placement |
> | Endotracheal intubation | Bronchoalveolar lavage |
> | Infection, unexplained chronic cough, or hemoptysis | Aspiration of cysts or drainage of abscesses |
> | Tracheobronchial stricture and stenosis | Pneumothorax or lobar collapse |
> | Hoarseness or vocal cord paralysis | Thoracic trauma |
> | Fistula or unexplained pleural effusion | Airway maintenance (tamponade for bleeding) |
> | Localized wheezing or stridor | |
> | Chest trauma or persistent pneumothorax | |
> | Postoperative assessment of tracheal, tracheobronchial, bronchial, or stump anastomosis | |

Data from Hetzed MR: Minimally invasive techniques in thoracic medicine and surgery, London, 1995, Chapman & Hall; Rippe JM, Irwin RS, Fink MP et al: Procedures and techniques in intensive care medicine, Boston, 1994, Little, Brown; Malarkey LM, McMorrow ME: Nurse's manual of laboratory tests and diagnostic procedures, ed 2, Philadelphia, 2000, Saunders.

CXR a few hours after the perfusion scan helps the differential diagnosis.

Ventilation scans are performed first, followed by perfusion scan. The two scans are then compared to determine extent of $\dot{V}/\dot{Q}$ matching. As described earlier, in the Ventilation and Perfusion Ratio section, average reference $\dot{V}/\dot{Q}$ ratio is approximately equal to 0.8.[23,25]

Computed Tomographic Pulmonary Angiography

Computed tomographic pulmonary angiography (CT-PA) is a minimally invasive test that allows direct visualization of the pulmonary artery and subsequently facilitates rapid detection of a thrombus. CT-PA is most useful for detecting a clot in the main or segmental vasculature. In recent years, CT-PA has become the preferred method to diagnose acute PE, rather than $\dot{V}/\dot{Q}$ scanning.[26,27] Benefits of CT-PA include its wide availability for testing, high sensitivity, and rapid reporting. The test is also useful in determining other pulmonary abnormalities that may be contributing to a patient's symptoms. The American and European Thoracic Societies have incorporated CT-PA into their algorithms for diagnosing PE.[28,29] Prospective Investigation of Pulmonary Embolism Diagnosis (PIOPED II) investigators also recommend CT-PA as a first-line imaging test to diagnose PE.[30]

Pulmonary Function Tests

Pulmonary function tests (PFTs) consist of measuring a patient's lung volumes and capacities, in addition to inspiratory and expiratory flow rates. Lung capacities are composed of two or more lung volumes. Quantification of these parameters helps to distinguish obstructive from restrictive respiratory patterns, in addition to determining how the respiratory system contributes to physical activity limitations. The respiratory system's volumes and capacities are shown in Figure 4-10. Alterations in volumes and capacities occur with obstructive and restrictive diseases; these changes are shown in Figure 4-11. Volume, flow, and gas dilution spirometers and body plethysmography are the measurement tools used for PFTs. A flow-volume loop also is included as part of the patient's PFTs and is shown in Figure 4-12. A comprehensive assessment of PFT results includes comparisons with normal values and prior test results. PFT results may be skewed according to a patient's effort. Table 4-8 outlines the measurements performed during PFTs. FEV_1, FVC, and the FEV_1/FVC ratio are the most commonly interpreted PFT values. These measures represent the degree of airway patency during expiration, which affects airflow in and out of the lung.

The normal range of values for PFTs is variable and is based on a person's age, gender, height, ethnic origin, and weight (body surface area). Normal predicted values can be extrapolated from a nomogram or calculated from regression (prediction) equations obtained from statistical analysis.

> ### ✎ CLINICAL TIP
> Predicted normal values for a person's given age, gender, and height are provided in the PFT report for reference to the person's actual PFT result.

For example, based on a nomogram, the following predicted values for forced vital capacity (FVC) and forced expiratory volume in 1 second (FEV_1) would be approximately the following[31]:

- FVC = 4.1 L, FEV_1 = 3 L for a man who is 55 years old and 66 inches tall
- FVC = 2.95 L, FEV_1 = 2.2 L for a woman who is 55 years old and 62 inches tall

Because results can vary from person to person, compare a person's PFT results from his or her previous tests. Indications for PFTs are as follows[31-33]:

- Detection and quantification of respiratory disease
- Evaluation of pulmonary involvement in systemic diseases
- Assessment of disease progression
- Evaluation of impairment, activity limitation, or disability
- Assessment for bronchodilator therapy or surgical intervention, or both, along with subsequent response to the respective intervention
- Preoperative evaluation (high-risk patient identification)

Health Conditions

Respiratory disorders can be classified as obstructive or restrictive. A patient may present with single or multiple obstructive and restrictive processes, or with a combination of both as a result of environmental, traumatic, orthopedic, neuromuscular, nutritional, or drug-induced factors. These disorders may be infectious, neoplastic, or vascular or involve the connective tissue of the thorax.[11]

Common terminology often used to describe respiratory dysfunction is listed below:

- *Air trapping:* Retention of gas in the lung as a result of partial or complete airway obstruction

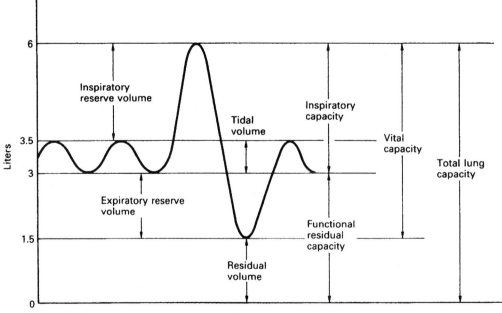

FIGURE 4-10
Lung volumes. (From Yentis SM, Hirsch NP, Smith GB, editors: Anaesthesia and intensive care a-z: an encyclopedia of principles and practice, ed 2, Oxford, 2000, Butterworth-Heinemann, p 340.)

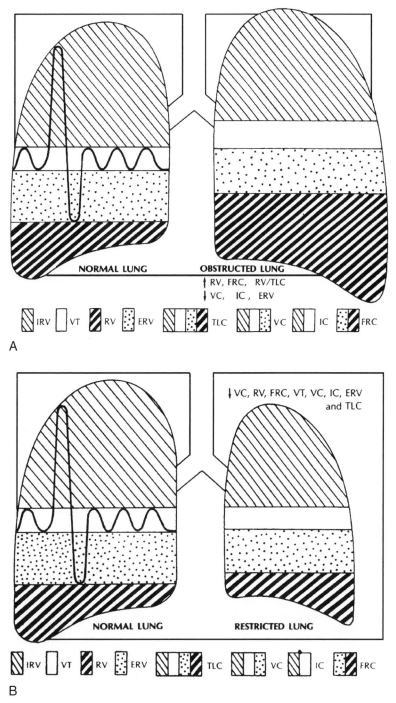

FIGURE 4-11

A, How obstructive lung disorders alter lung volumes and capacities. **B,** How restrictive lung disorders alter lung volumes and capacities. *ERV,* Expiratory reserve volume; *FRC,* functional residual capacity; *IC,* inspiratory capacity; *IRV,* inspiratory reserve volume; *RV,* residual volume; *TLC,* total lung capacity; *VC,* vital capacity; *VT,* tidal volume. (From Des Jardins T, Burton GC, editors: Clinical manifestations and assessment of respiratory disease, ed 3, St Louis, 1995, Mosby, pp 40, 49.)

- *Bronchospasm:* Smooth muscle contraction of the bronchi and bronchiole walls resulting in a narrowing of the airway lumen
- *Consolidation:* Transudate, exudate, or tissue replacing alveolar air
- *Hyperinflation:* Overinflation of the lungs at resting volume as a result of air trapping

- *Hypoxemia:* A low level of oxygen in the blood, usually a PaO_2 less than 60 to 80 mm Hg
- *Hypoxia:* A low level of oxygen in the tissues available for cell metabolism
- *Respiratory distress:* The acute or insidious onset of dyspnea, respiratory muscle fatigue, abnormal respiratory pattern and rate, anxiety, and cyanosis related to inadequate gas exchange;

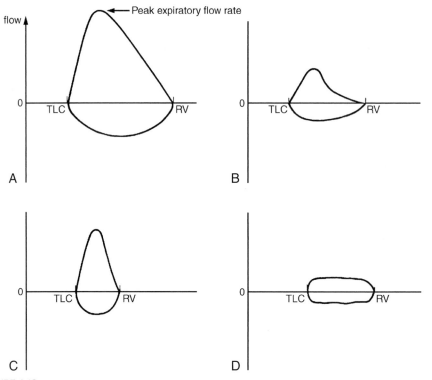

FIGURE 4-12
Characteristic flow-volume loops: **(A)** normal, **(B)** obstructive lung disease, **(C)** restrictive lung disease, **(D)** tracheal/laryngeal obstruction. *RV,* Residual volume; *TLC,* total lung capacity. (From Yentis SM, Hirsch NP, Smith GB, editors: Anaesthesia and intensive care a-z: an encyclopedia of principles and practice, ed 2, Oxford, 2000, Butterworth-Heinemann.)

TABLE 4-8 Description and Clinical Significance of Pulmonary Function Tests

Test	Description	Significance
Lung Volume Tests		
Tidal volume (VT)	The volume of air inhaled or exhaled during a single breath in a resting state	Decreased tidal volume could be indicative of atelectasis, fatigue, restrictive lung disorders, and tumors.
Inspiratory reserve volume (IRV)	The maximum amount of air that can be inspired following a normal inspiration	Decreased IRV could be indicative of obstructive pulmonary disease.
Expiratory reserve volume (ERV)	The maximum amount of air that can be exhaled after a normal exhalation	ERV is necessary to calculate residual volume and FRC. Decreased values could be indicative of ascites, pleural effusion, or pneumothorax.
Residual volume (RV)	The volume of air remaining in the lungs at the end of maximal expiration that cannot be forcibly expelled	RV helps to differentiate between obstructive and restrictive disorders. An increased RV indicates an obstructive disorder, and a decreased RV indicates a restrictive disorder.
Total lung capacity (TLC)	The volume of air contained in the lung at the end of maximal inspiration (TLC = VT + IRV + ERV + RV)	TLC helps to differentiate between obstructive and restrictive disorders. An increased TLC indicates an obstructive disorder; a decreased TLC indicates a restrictive disorder.
Vital capacity (VC)	The maximum amount of air that can be expired slowly and completely following a maximal inspiration (VC = VT + IRV + ERV)	A decreased VC can result from a decrease in lung tissue distensibility or depression of the respiratory centers in the brain.
Functional residual capacity (FRC)	The volume of air remaining in the lungs at the end of a normal expiration. Calculated from body plethysmography (FRC = ERV + RV)	FRC values help differentiate between obstructive and restrictive respiratory patterns. An increased FRC indicates an obstructive respiratory pattern, and a decreased FRC indicates a restrictive respiratory pattern.

TABLE 4-8 Description and Clinical Significance of Pulmonary Function Tests—cont'd

Test	Description	Significance
Inspiratory capacity (IC)	The largest volume of air that can be inspired in one breath from the resting expiratory level (IC = VT + IRV)	Changes in IC usually parallel changes in VC. Decreased values could be indicative of restrictive disorders.
Residual volume to total lung capacity ratio (RV : TLC × 100)	The percentage of air that cannot be expired in relation to the total amount of air that can be brought into the lungs	Values >35% are indicative of obstructive disorders.
Ventilation Tests		
Minute volume (VE) or minute ventilation	The total volume of air inspired or expired in 1 minute (VE = VT × respiratory rate)	VE is most commonly used in exercise or stress testing. VE can increase with hypoxia, hypercapnia, acidosis, and exercise.
Respiratory dead space (VD)	The volume of air in the lungs that is ventilated but not perfused in conducting airways and nonfunctioning alveoli	VD provides information about available surface area for gas exchange. Increased dead space = decreased gas exchange
Alveolar ventilation (VA)	The volume of air that participates in gas exchange Estimated by subtracting dead space from tidal volume (VA = VT − VD)	VA measures the amount of oxygen available to tissue, but it should be confirmed by arterial blood gas measurements.
Pulmonary Spirometry Tests		
Forced vital capacity (FVC)	The volume of air that can be expired forcefully and rapidly after a maximal inspiration	FVC is normally equal to VC, but FVC can be decreased in obstructive disorders.
Forced expiratory volume timed (FEVt)	The volume of air expired over a time interval during the performance of an FVC maneuver The interval is usually 1 second (FEV_1) After 3 seconds, FEV should equal FVC	A decrease in FEV_1 can indicate either obstructive or restrictive airway disease. With obstructive disease, a decreased FEV_1 results from increased resistance to exhalation. With restrictive disease, a subsequent decrease in FEV_1 results from a decreased ability to initially inhale an adequate volume of air.
FEV% (usually FEV_1/FVC × 100)	The percent of FVC that can be expired over a given time interval, usually 1 second	FEV% is a better discriminator of obstructive and restrictive disorders than FEVt. An increase in FEV_1/FVC indicates a restrictive disorder, and a decrease in FEV_1/FVC indicates an obstructive disorder.
Forced expiratory flow 25%-75% ($FEF_{25\%-75\%}$)	The average flow of air during the middle 50% of an FEV maneuver Used in comparison with VC Represents peripheral airway resistance	A decrease in ($FEF_{25\%-75\%}$) generally indicates obstruction in the medium-sized airways.
Peak expiratory flow rate (PEFR)	The maximum flow rate attainable at any time during an FEV	PEFR can assist with diagnosing obstructive disorders such as asthma.
Maximum voluntary ventilation (MVV)	The largest volume of air that can be breathed per minute by maximal voluntary effort Test lasts 10 or 15 seconds and is multiplied by 6 to 4, respectively, to determine the amount of air that can be breathed in a minute (liters/min)	MVV measures status of respiratory muscles, the resistance offered by airways and tissues, and the compliance of the lung and thorax.
Flow-volume loop (F-V loop)	A graphic analysis of the maximum forced expiratory flow volume followed by a maximum inspiratory flow volume	The distinctive curves of the F-V loop are created according to the presence or absence of disease. Restrictive disease demonstrates an equal reduction in flow and volume, resulting in a vertical oval loop. Obstructive disease demonstrates a greater reduction in flow compared with volume, resulting in a horizontal tear-shaped loop.
Gas Exchange		
Diffusing capacity of carbon monoxide (DLCO)	A known mixture of carbon monoxide and helium gas inhaled and then exhaled after 10 seconds, and the amount of gases are remeasured	DLCO assesses the amount of functioning pulmonary capillary bed in contact with functioning alveoli (gas exchange area).

Adapted from Thompson JM, McFarland GK, Hirsch JE, et al, editors: Clinical nursing practice, ed 5, St. Louis, 2002, Mosby; and data from Malarkey LM, Morrow ME, editors: Nurse's manual of laboratory tests and diagnostic procedures, ed 2, Philadelphia, 2000, Saunders, pp 293-297.

the clinical presentation that usually precedes respiratory failure

- *Respiratory failure:* The inability of the pulmonary system to maintain an adequate exchange of oxygen and carbon dioxide (see Chapter 18)

Obstructive Pulmonary Conditions

Obstructive lung diseases or conditions may be described by onset (acute or chronic), severity (mild, moderate, or severe), and location (upper or lower airway). Obstructive pulmonary patterns are characterized by decreased airflow out of the lungs as a result of narrowing of the airway lumen. This causes increased dead space and decreased surface area for gas exchange.

Chronic obstructive pulmonary disease (COPD) describes airflow limitation that is not fully reversible. The Global Initiative for Obstructive Lung Disease (GOLD) states that the airflow limitation in COPD is usually progressive and associated with an abnormal inflammatory response to noxious particles or gases.[34] The diagnosis of COPD is confirmed with spirometric testing. Patients with COPD typically have a combination of chronic bronchitis, emphysema, and small airway obstruction.[35] Table 4-9 outlines obstructive disorders, their general physical and diagnostic findings, and their general clinical management.

Asthma

Asthma is an immunologic response that can result from allergens (e.g., dust, pollen, smoke, pollutants), food additives, bacterial infection, gastroesophageal reflux, stress, cold air, and exercise.[8] The asthmatic exacerbation may be immediate or delayed, resulting in air entrapment and alveolar hyperinflation during the episode with symptoms disappearing between attacks. The primary characteristics of an asthma exacerbation are as follows:

- Bronchial smooth muscle constriction
- Mucus production (without infection) resulting from the increased presence of leukocytes, such as eosinophils
- Bronchial mucosa inflammation and thickening resulting from cellular and fluid infiltration[36]

Admission to a hospital occurs if signs and symptoms of an asthma exacerbation do not improve after several hours of medical therapy, especially if FEV_1 is less than 50% of normal.[37] Status asthmaticus is a severe, life-threatening airway obstruction with the potential for cardiopulmonary complications, such as arrhythmia, heart failure, and cardiac arrest. Status asthmaticus is not responsive to basic medical therapies and is characterized by severe hypoxemia and hypercarbia that require assisted or mechanical ventilation.[38]

Chronic Bronchitis

Chronic bronchitis is the presence of cough and pulmonary secretion expectoration for at least 3 months, 2 years in a row.[20,39] Chronic bronchitis usually is linked to cigarette smoking or, less likely, to air pollution or infection. It begins with the following[8]:

- Narrowing of large, then small, airways because of inflammation of bronchial mucosa

- Bronchial mucous gland hyperplasia and bronchial smooth muscle cell hypertrophy
- Decreased mucociliary function

These changes result in air trapping, hyperinflated alveoli, bronchospasm, and excess secretion retention.

The definition of an acute exacerbation of chronic bronchitis is vague.[40] The patient often describes (1) worsened dyspnea at rest or with activity, with a notable inability to ambulate, eat, or sleep; (2) fatigue; and (3) abnormal sputum production or inability to clear sputum. On clinical examination, the patient may have hypoxemia, hypercarbia, pneumonia, cor pulmonale, or worsening of comorbidities. Hospital admission is determined by the degree of respiratory failure, hemodynamic stability, the number of recent physician visits, home oxygen use, and doses of pulmonary medications.[40]

Emphysema

Emphysema may be genetic (α1-antitrypsin protein deficiency), in which the lack of proteolytic inhibitors allows the alveolar interstitium to be destroyed, or it may be caused by cigarette smoking, air pollutants, or infection. Three types of emphysema occur: centrilobular (centriacinar), panlobular (panacinar), and paraseptal. Centrilobular emphysema affects the respiratory bronchioles and the proximal acinus, mostly within the upper lobes. Panlobular emphysema affects the respiratory bronchioles, alveolar ducts and sacs, and alveoli. Paraseptal emphysema affects the distal acinus and can be associated with bullae formation and pneumothorax.[41]

Emphysema leads to progressive destruction of alveolar walls and adjacent capillaries secondary to the following[8]:

- Decreased pulmonary elasticity
- Premature airway collapse
- Bullae formation (a bulla is a pocket of air surrounded by walls of compressed lung parenchyma)

These changes result in decreased lung elasticity, air trapping, and hyperinflation.[42] Reasons for hospital admission are similar to those of a patient with chronic bronchitis, except cor pulmonale does not develop until the late stages of emphysema. A spontaneous PTX is a sequela of emphysema in which a bleb (a pocket of air between the two layers of visceral pleura) ruptures to connect with the pleural space.

Cystic Fibrosis

Cystic fibrosis (CF) is a lethal, autosomal-recessive trait (chromosome 7) that affects exocrine glands of the entire body, particularly of the respiratory, gastrointestinal, and reproductive systems. Soon after birth, an initial pulmonary infection occurs that leads to the following changes throughout life[8]:

- Bronchial and bronchiolar walls become inflamed.
- Bronchial gland and goblet cells hypertrophy to create tenacious pulmonary secretions.
- Mucociliary clearance is decreased.

These changes result in bronchospasm, atelectasis, $\dot{V}/\dot{Q}$ mismatch, increased airway resistance, hypoxemia, and recurrent pulmonary infections.[42] Hospitalization may be indicated if there is increased sputum production or cough for longer than

TABLE 4-9 Characteristics and General Management of Obstructive Disorders

Disorder	Observation	Palpation	Auscultation	Cough	Chest X-Ray	Management
Asthma (exacerbation)	Tachypnea Fatigue Anxiety Pursed lip breathing Active expiration Cyanosis, if severe Accessory muscle use	Tachycardia with weak pulse on inspiration Increased A-P chest diameter Decreased tactile and vocal fremitus Hyperresonant percussion Pulsus paradoxus (systolic blood pressure decreases on inspiration), if severe	Polyphonic wheezing on expiration >inspiration Diminished breath sounds	Tight, usually nonproductive, then slightly productive of benign sputum	During exacerbation: translucent lung fields, flattened diaphragms, increased A-P diameter of chest, more horizontal ribs Chest x-ray normal between asthma exacerbations	Removal of causative agent Bronchodilators Corticosteroids Supplemental O_2 IV fluid administration
Chronic bronchitis	"Blue bloater" with stocky build and dependent edema Tachypnea with prolonged expiratory phase Pursed lip breathing Accessory muscle use, often with fixed upper extremities Elevated shoulders Barrel chest Fatigue Anxiety	Tachycardia Hypertension Decreased tactile and vocal fremitus Hyperresonant percussion Increased A-P chest diameter	Rhonchi Diminished breath sounds Crackles	Spasmodic cough Sputum ranges from clear to purulent Often most productive in the morning	Translucent lung fields Flattened diaphragms ± Cardiomegaly with increased bronchovascular markings	Smoking cessation Bronchodilator Steroids Expectorants Antibiotics if infection exists Diuretics if cor pulmonale present Supplemental O_2 Bronchopulmonary hygiene Assisted or mechanical ventilation, if severe
Emphysema	"Pink puffer" with cachexia Otherwise, see Chronic bronchitis, above	See Chronic bronchitis, above	Very diminished breath sounds Wheeze Crackles	Usually absent and nonproductive	Translucent lung fields Flattened diaphragms Bullae. ± Small heart with decreased vascular markings	Bronchodilators Supplemental O_2 Nutritional support
Cystic fibrosis	Tachypnea Fatigue Accessory muscle use Barrel chest Cachexia Clubbing	See Chronic bronchitis, above	Crackles Diminished breath sounds Rhonchi	Cough likely tight, either controlled or spasmodic Usually very viscous, greenish sputum ± blood streaks	Translucent lung fields Flattened diaphragms Fibrosis Atelectasis Enlarged right ventricle Linear opacities	Antibiotics Bronchodilators Mucolytics Supplemental O_2 Bronchopulmonary hygiene Nutritional support Psychosocial support Lung transplantation
Bronchiectasis	See Cystic fibrosis, above	See Chronic bronchitis, above	See Cystic fibrosis, above	Purulent, odorous sputum ± Hemoptysis	Patchy infiltrates ± Atelectasis + Honeycombing, if advanced Increased vascular markings Crowded bronchial markings	Antibiotics Bronchodilators Corticosteroids Supplemental O_2 IV fluid administration Nutritional support Bronchopulmonary hygiene ± Pain control for pleuritic pain Lung transplantation

±, With or without; A-P, anterior-posterior.

2 weeks; worsened dyspnea or pulmonary function; weight loss; or the development of hemoptysis, PTX, or cor pulmonale.[43]

> ✎ **CLINICAL TIP**
>
> Periodic admissions for infections are referred to as "cleanouts." A progressive exercise program in conjunction with bronchopulmonary hygiene during a cleanout has been shown to significantly improve secretion expectoration and increase muscle strength and aerobic capacity, lasting up to 1 month after discharge.[44,45]

Bronchiectasis

Bronchiectasis is an obstructive, restrictive disorder characterized by the following[8]:

- Destruction of the elastic and muscular bronchiole walls
- Destruction of the mucociliary escalator (in which normal epithelium is replaced by nonciliated mucus-producing cells)
- Bronchial dilatation
- Bronchial artery enlargement

Bronchiectasis is defined as the permanent dilatation of airways that have a normal diameter of greater than 2 mm.[46] Bronchiectasis results in fibrosis and ulceration of bronchioles, chronically retained pulmonary secretions, atelectasis, and infection. The etiology of bronchiectasis includes previous bacterial respiratory infection, CF, tuberculosis, and immobile cilia syndromes.[46] In order of frequency, bronchiectatic changes occur in the left lower lobe, right middle lobe, lingula, entire left lung, right lower lobe, and entire right lung.[46] Hospitalization usually occurs when complications of bronchiectasis arise, including hemoptysis, pneumonia, PTX, empyema, or cor pulmonale.

Restrictive Pulmonary Conditions

Restrictive lung diseases or conditions may be described by onset (acute or chronic) or location (pulmonary or extrapulmonary). Restrictive patterns are characterized by low lung volumes that result from decreased lung compliance and distensibility and increased lung recoil. The result is increased work of breathing. Table 4-10 outlines restrictive disorders, their general physical and diagnostic findings, and their general clinical management.

Atelectasis

Atelectasis involves the partial or total collapse of alveoli, lung segment(s), or lobe(s). It most commonly results from hypoventilation or ineffective pulmonary secretion clearance. The following conditions also may contribute to atelectasis:

- Inactivity
- Upper abdominal or thoracic incisional pain
- Compression of lung parenchyma
- Diaphragmatic restriction from weakness or paralysis
- Postobstructive pneumonia
- Presence of a foreign body

The result is hypoxemia from $\dot{V}/\dot{Q}$ mismatch, transpulmonary shunting, and pulmonary vasoconstriction of variable severity depending on the amount of atelectasis.[8] General risks for the development of atelectasis include cigarette smoking or pulmonary disease, obesity, and increased age. Perioperative or postoperative risk factors include altered surfactant function from anesthesia, emergent or extended operative time, altered consciousness or prolonged narcotic use, hypotension, and sepsis.

Pneumonia

Pneumonia is the multistaged inflammatory reaction of the distal airways from the inhalation of bacteria, viruses, microorganisms, foreign substances, gastric contents, dusts, or chemicals, or as a complication of radiation therapy.[8] Pneumonia often is described as community or hospital (nosocomial) acquired. Hospital-acquired pneumonia is defined as pneumonia occurring after 48 hours within a hospital stay and is associated with ventilator use, contaminated equipment, or poor hand washing.[47,48] The consequences of pneumonia are $\dot{V}/\dot{Q}$ mismatch and hypoxemia. The phases of pneumonia are the following[46]:

1. Alveolar edema with exudate formation (0 to 3 days)
2. Alveolar infiltration with bacterial colonization, red and white blood cells, and macrophages (2 to 4 days)
3. Alveolar infiltration and consolidation with dead bacteria, white blood cells, and fibrin (4 to 8 days)
4. Resolution with expectoration or enzymatic digestion of infiltrative cells (after 8 days)
5. Pneumonia may be located in single or multiple lobes either unilaterally or bilaterally. The complete clearance of pneumonia can take up to 6 weeks.[47] Resolution of pneumonia is slower with increased age, previous pneumonia, positive smoking history, poor nutritional status, or coexisting illness.

> ✎ **CLINICAL TIP**
>
> Viral pneumonias may not produce the same quantity of secretions as bacterial pneumonias. Necessity and efficacy of bronchopulmonary clearance techniques should be considered before providing these interventions to patients with viral pneumonias.

Pulmonary Edema

The etiology of pulmonary edema can be categorized as either cardiogenic or noncardiogenic. Cardiogenic pulmonary edema is an imbalance of hydrostatic and oncotic pressures within the pulmonary vasculature that results from backflow of blood from the heart.[8] This backflow increases the movement of fluid from the pulmonary capillaries to the alveolar spaces. Initially, the fluid fills the interstitium and then progresses to the alveolar spaces, bronchioles, and, ultimately, the bronchi. A simultaneous decrease in the lymphatic drainage of the lung may occur, exacerbating the problem. Cardiogenic pulmonary edema can occur rapidly (flash pulmonary edema) or insidiously in association with left ventricular hypertrophy, mitral regurgitation, or aortic stenosis. Cardiogenic pulmonary edema results in atelectasis, $\dot{V}/\dot{Q}$ mismatch, and hypoxemia.[8]

TABLE 4-10 Characteristics and General Management of Restrictive Disorders

Disorder	Observation	Palpation	Auscultation	Cough	Chest X-Ray	Management
Atelectasis	± Tachypnea ± Fever ± Shallow respirations	± Tachycardia Decreased tactile fremitus and vocal resonance	Crackles at involved site Diminished breath sounds If lobar collapse exists, absent or bronchial breath sounds	Dry or wet Sputum ranges in color, depending on reason for atelectasis	Linear opacity of involved area If lobar collapse exists, white triangular density Fissure and diaphragmatic displacement	Incentive spirometry Supplemental O_2 Functional mobilization Bronchopulmonary hygiene
Pneumonia	See Atelectasis Fatigue ± Accessory muscle use	See Atelectasis Decreased chest wall expansion at involved site Dull percussion	Crackles Rhonchi Bronchial breath sounds over area of consolidation	Initially dry to more productive Sputum may be yellow, tan, green, or rusty	Well-defined density at the involved lobe(s) ± Air bronchogram ± Pleural effusion	Antibiotics Supplemental O_2 IV fluid administration Functional mobilization Bronchopulmonary hygiene
Pulmonary edema	Tachypnea Orthopnea Anxiety Accessory muscle use	Increased tactile and vocal fremitus	Symmetric wet crackles, especially at bases ± Wheeze	Sputum may be thin, frothy, clear, white, or pink	Increased hilar vascular markings Kerley's B lines (short, horizontal lines at lung field periphery) ± Pleural effusion Left ventricular hypertrophy Cardiac silhouette Fluffy opacities	Diuretics Other medications, dependent on etiology Supplemental O_2 Hemodynamic monitoring
Adult respiratory distress syndrome (ARDS)	Labored breathing and altered mental status at onset Tachypnea Increased PA pressure	Hypotension Tachycardia or bradycardia Decreased bilateral chest wall expansion Dull percussion	Diminished breath sounds Crackles Wheeze Rhonchi (rare)	Generally without sputum, although sputum may be present if infection exists or from the presence of an endotracheal tube	Pulmonary edema with diffuse bilateral patchy opacities "Ground glass" appearance	Mechanical ventilation Hemodynamic monitoring IV fluid administration Prone positioning Nitrous oxide therapy
Pulmonary embolism (PE)	Rapid onset of tachypnea ± Chest pain Anxiety Dysrhythmia Lightheadedness	Hypotension Tachycardia Decreased chest wall expansion at involved site	Diminished or absent breath sounds distal to PE Wheeze Crackles	Usually absent	Nondiagnostic for PE May show density at infarct site with lucency distal to the infarct Decreased lung volume Dilated PA with increased vascular markings ± Atelectasis	Anticoagulation Hemodynamic stabilization Supplemental O_2 or mechanical ventilation Inferior vena cava filter placement Thrombolysis Embolectomy
Lung contusion	Tachypnea Chest wall ecchymosis Cyanosis, if severe	Hypotension Tachycardia Crepitus resulting from rib fracture	Wet crackles Diminished or absent breath sounds at involved site	Weak cough if pain present, dry or wet Sputum may be clear, white, or blood-tinged	Patchy, irregular opacities localized to a segment or lobe ± Consolidation	Pain management Supplemental O_2 Mechanical ventilation IV fluid administration

Data from Thompson JM, McFarland GK, Hirsch JE et al, editors: Clinical nursing practice, St Louis, 1993, Mosby; Malarkey LM, McMorrow ME, editors: Nurse's manual of laboratory tests and diagnostic procedures, ed 2, Philadelphia, 2000, Saunders.
±, With or without; PA, pulmonary artery.

Noncardiogenic pulmonary edema can result from alterations in capillary permeability (as in adult respiratory distress syndrome [ARDS] or pneumonia), intrapleural pressure from airway obstruction(s), or lymph vessel obstruction. The results are similar to those of cardiogenic pulmonary edema.

> ✎ **CLINICAL TIP**
>
> Beware of a flat position in bed or other positions that worsen dyspnea during physical therapy intervention in patients with pulmonary edema.

Adult Respiratory Distress Syndrome

ARDS is an acute inflammation of the lung generally associated with aspiration, drug toxicity, inhalation injury, pulmonary trauma, shock, systemic infections, and multisystem organ failure.[49] It is considered a critical illness and has a lengthy recovery and a high mortality rate. Characteristics of ARDS include the following:

- An exudative phase (hours to days), characterized by increased capillary permeability, interstitial and alveolar edema, hemorrhage, and alveolar consolidation with leukocytes and macrophages
- A proliferative stage (days to weeks) characterized by hyaline formation on alveolar walls and intraalveolar fibrosis resulting in atelectasis, $\dot{V}/\dot{Q}$ mismatch, severe hypoxemia, and pulmonary hypertension

Latent pulmonary sequelae of ARDS are variable and range from no impairments to mild exertional dyspnea to mixed obstructive-restrictive abnormalities.[50]

> ✎ **CLINICAL TIP**
>
> Prone positioning can be used in the ICU setting as a treatment strategy in patients with ARDS. Prone positioning facilitates improved aeration to dorsal lung segments, improved $\dot{V}/\dot{Q}$ matching, and improved secretion drainage.[51,52] Prone positioning should be performed only by experienced clinicians and with proper equipment (specialty frames or beds).

Pulmonary Embolism

PE is the partial or full occlusion of the pulmonary vasculature by one large or multiple small emboli from one or more of the following possible sources: thromboembolism originating from the lower extremity (more than 90% of the time),[53] air entering the venous system through catheterization or needle placement, fat droplets from traumatic origin, or tumor fragments.

> ✎ **CLINICAL TIP**
>
> PT intervention should be discontinued if the signs and symptoms of PE arise during treatment (see Table 4-10). Seat or lay the patient down, and call for help immediately.

A PE results in the following[54]:
- Decreased blood flow to the lungs distal to the occlusion
- Atelectasis and focal edema
- Bronchospasm from the release of humeral agents
- Possible parenchymal infarction

Emboli size and location determine the extent of $\dot{V}/\dot{Q}$ mismatch, pulmonary shunt, and thus the degree of hypoxemia and hemodynamic instability.[53] The onset of a PE is usually acute and may be a life-threatening emergency, especially if a larger artery is obstructed.

> ✎ **CLINICAL TIP**
>
> If you are evaluating the patient for the first time since a PE, make sure the patient has received a therapeutic level of anticoagulation medicine or that other medical treatment has been completed. Refer to Chapter 7 for more information on anticoagulation.

Interstitial Lung Disease

Interstitial lung disease (ILD) is a general term for the destruction of the respiratory membranes in multiple lung regions. This destruction occurs after an inflammatory phase, in which the alveoli become infiltrated with macrophages and mononuclear cells, followed by a fibrosis phase, in which the alveoli become scarred with collagen.[46] Fibrotic changes may extend proximally toward the bronchioles. More than 100 suspected predisposing factors exist for ILD, such as infectious agents, environmental and occupational inhalants, and drugs; however, no definite etiology is known.[8,55] Clinically, the patient presents with exertional dyspnea and bilateral diffuse chest radiograph changes and without pulmonary infection or neoplasm.[56] ILD has a variety of clinical features and patterns beyond the scope of this text; however, the general sequela of ILD is a restrictive pattern with $\dot{V}/\dot{Q}$ mismatch.

Lung Contusion

Lung contusion is the result of a sudden compression and decompression of lung tissue against the chest wall from a direct blunt (e.g., fall) or blast (e.g., air explosion) trauma. The compressive force causes shearing of the alveolar-capillary membrane and results in microhemorrhage, whereas the decompressive force causes a rebound stretching of the parenchyma.[57] A diffuse accumulation of blood and fluid in the alveoli and interstitium causes alveolar shunting, decreased lung compliance, and increased pulmonary vascular resistance.[58] The resultant degree of hypoxemia is dependent on the size of contused tissue. Lung contusion usually is located below rib fracture(s) and is associated with PTX and flail chest.

Restrictive Extrapulmonary Conditions

Disorders or trauma occurring outside of the visceral pleura also may affect pulmonary function. Table 4-11 outlines restrictive extrapleural disorders, their general physical findings, and their general medical management.

TABLE 4-11 Characteristics and General Management of Extrapleural Disorders

Disorder	Observation	Palpation	Auscultation	Cough	Chest X-Ray	Management
Pleural effusion	Tachypnea ± Discomfort from pleuritis Decreased chest expansion on involved side	± Tachycardia Decreased tactile fremitus Dull percussion	Normal to decreased breath sounds or bronchial breath sounds at the level of the effusion	Usually absent	Homogenous density in dependent lung Fluid obscures diaphragm and fills costophrenic angle Fluid shifts with change in patient position Mediastinal shift to opposite side, if severe	If effusion is small and respiratory status is stable, monitor only Supplemental O$_2$ Chest tube placement for moderate or large effusion Thoracocentesis if persistent Pleurodesis Diuretics Workup to determine cause if unknown Pain management if pleuritic pain present
Pneumothorax (PTX)	See Pleural effusion, above	See Pleural effusion, above	Diminished breath sounds near involved site Absent if tension PTX	Usually absent	Translucent area usually at apex of lung ± Associated depressed diaphragm, atelectasis, lung collapse, mediastinal shift, if severe Visceral pleura can be seen as thin white line	If PTX is small and respiratory status is stable, monitor only If PTX is moderate-sized or large, chest tube placement Supplemental O$_2$ Pain management if pleuritic pain present
Hemothorax	See Pneumothorax, above	See Pleural effusion, above	See Pneumothorax, above	Usually absent, unless associated with significant lung contusion in which hemoptysis may occur	See Pleural effusion, above	Supplemental O$_2$ Chest tube placement Pain management if pleuritic pain present Monitor and treat for shock Blood transfusion, as needed

±, With or without.

Pleural Effusion

A pleural effusion is the presence of transudative or exudative fluid in the pleural space. Transudative fluid results from a change in the hydrostatic/oncotic pressure gradient of the pleural capillaries, which is associated with congestive heart failure, cirrhosis, PE, and pericardial disease.[59] Exudative fluid (containing cellular debris) occurs with pleural or parenchymal inflammation or altered lymphatic drainage, which is associated with neoplasm, tuberculosis (TB), pneumonia, pancreatitis, rheumatoid arthritis, and systemic lupus erythematosus.[59,60] Pleural effusions may be unilateral or bilateral, depending on the cause of the effusion, and may result in compressive atelectasis.

Pneumothorax

PTX is the presence of air in the pleural space that can occur from (1) visceral pleura perforation with movement of air from within the lung (spontaneous pneumothorax), (2) chest wall and parietal pleura perforation with movement of air from the atmosphere (traumatic or iatrogenic pneumothorax), or (3) formation of gas by microorganisms associated with empyema. Spontaneous PTX can be a complication of chronic obstructive pulmonary disease or TB, or it can occur idiopathically in tall persons secondary to elevated intrathoracic pressures in the upper lung zones.[8] Traumatic PTX results from rib fracture, chest wounds, or other penetrating chest trauma. Complications of mechanical ventilation and central line placement are two examples of iatrogenic PTX. Pneumothoraces also may be described as follows:

- Closed: Without air movement into the pleural space during inspiration and expiration (chest wall intact)
- Open: With air moving in and out of the pleural space during inspiration and expiration (pleural space in contact with the atmosphere)
- Tension: With air moving into the pleural space only during inspiration

PTX is usually unilateral. Complications of PTX include atelectasis and $\dot{V}/\dot{Q}$ mismatch. A large or tension PTX can result in lung collapse, mediastinal shift (displacement of the mediastinum) to the contralateral side, and cardiac tamponade (altered cardiac function secondary to decreased venous return to the heart from compression).[8]

Hemothorax

Hemothorax is characterized by the presence of blood in the pleural space from damage to the pleura and great or smaller vessels (e.g., interstitial arteries). Causes of hemothorax are penetrating or blunt chest wall injury, draining aortic aneurysms, pulmonary arteriovenous malformations, and extreme coagulation therapy. Blood and air together in the pleural space, common after trauma, is a hemopneumothorax.

Flail Chest

Flail chest is caused by the double fracture of three or more adjacent ribs, resulting from a crushing chest injury or vigorous cardiopulmonary resuscitation. The sequelae of this injury are as follows[8]:

- A paradoxic breathing pattern, with the discontinuous ribs moving inward on inspiration and outward on expiration as a result of alterations in atmospheric and intrapleural pressure gradients
- Contused lung parenchyma under the flail portion
- In severe cases, mediastinal shift to the contralateral side as air from the involved side is shifted and rebreathed (pendelluft)

Empyema

Empyema is the presence of anaerobic bacterial pus in the pleural space, resulting from underlying infection (e.g., pneumonia, lung abscess), which crosses the visceral pleura or chest wall and parietal pleura penetration from trauma, surgery, or chest tube placement. Empyema formation involves pleural swelling and exudate formation, continued bacterial accumulation, fibrin deposition on pleura, and chronic fibroblast formation.

Chest Wall Restrictions

A restrictive respiratory pattern may be caused by abnormal chest wall movement not directly related to pulmonary pathology. Musculoskeletal changes of the thoracic cage can occur with diseases such as ankylosing spondylitis, rheumatoid arthritis, and kyphoscoliosis, or with conditions such as pregnancy and obesity. Neurologic diagnoses, such as cervical/thoracic spinal cord injury or Guillain-Barré syndrome, also can create restrictive breathing patterns depending on the level of respiratory muscle weakness or paralysis. Refer to Chapter 6 for more information on neurologic disorders. Kyphoscoliosis and obesity are discussed in further detail because of their frequency in the clinical setting. Kyphoscoliosis can result in atelectasis from decreased thoracic cage mobility, respiratory muscle insufficiency, and parenchymal compression. Other consequences of kyphoscoliosis are progressive alveolar hypoventilation, increased dead space, hypoxemia with eventual pulmonary artery hypertension, cor pulmonale, or mediastinal shift (in very severe cases) toward the direction of the lateral curve of the spine.[8]

Obesity (defined as body weight 20% to 30% above age-predicted and gender-predicted weight) can cause an abnormally elevated diaphragm position secondary to the upward displacement of abdominal contents, inefficient respiratory muscle use, and a noncompliant chest wall. These factors result in early airway closure (especially in dependent lung areas), tachypnea, altered respiratory pattern, $\dot{V}/\dot{Q}$ mismatch, and secretion retention. Refer to Chapter 8 for more information on obesity management with bariatric procedures.

Management

Pharmacologic Agents

The pharmacologic agents commonly used for the management of respiratory dysfunction include adrenocortical steroids (glucocorticoids) (see Table 19-8), antihistamines (see Table 19-9), bronchodilators (see Table 19-10), leukotriene modifiers (see Table 19-11), and mast cell stabilizers (see Table 19-12).

Generally, nebulized medications are optimally active 15 to 20 minutes after administration, so therapy sessions should be timed to coincide with maximal medication benefit.

✎ CLINICAL TIP

Be aware of respiratory medication changes, especially the addition or removal of medications from the regimen. If a patient has an inhaler, it may be beneficial for the patient to bring it to physical therapy sessions in case of activity-induced bronchospasm.

Thoracic Procedures

The most common thoracic operative and nonoperative procedures for respiratory disorders are described below in alphabetic order.[2,61,62] Lung transplantation is described separately in Chapter 14 in addition to other transplant procedures. Illustrations of many of the procedures described below are shown in Figure 4-13.

- *Bronchoplasty:* Also called a *sleeve resection.* Resection and reanastomosis (reconnection) of a bronchus; most commonly performed for bronchial carcinoma (a concurrent pulmonary resection also may be performed)
- *Laryngectomy:* The partial or total removal of one or more vocal cords; most commonly performed for laryngeal cancer
- *Laryngoscopy:* Direct visual examination of the larynx with a fiberoptic scope; most commonly performed to assist with differential diagnosis of thoracic pathology or to assess the vocal cords
- *Lobectomy:* Resection of one or more lobes of the lung; most commonly performed for isolated lesions
- *Lung volume reduction:* The unilateral or bilateral removal of one or more portions of emphysematous lung parenchyma, resulting in increased alveolar surface area
- *Mediastinoscopy:* Endoscopic examination of the mediastinum; most commonly performed for precise localization and biopsy of a mediastinal mass or for the removal of lymph nodes
- *Pleurodesis:* The obliteration of the pleural space; most commonly performed for persistent pleural effusions or pneumothoraces. A chemical agent is introduced into the pleural space via thoracostomy (chest) tube or with a thoracoscope
- *Pneumonectomy:* Removal of an entire lung; most commonly performed as a result of bronchial carcinoma, emphysema, multiple lung abscesses, bronchiectasis, or TB
- *Rib resection:* Removal of a portion of one or more ribs for accessing underlying pulmonary structures as a treatment for thoracic outlet syndrome or for bone grafting
- *Segmentectomy:* Removal of a segment of a lung; most commonly performed for a peripheral bronchial or parenchymal lesion
- *Thoracentesis:* Therapeutic or diagnostic removal of pleural fluid via percutaneous needle aspiration

Procedure	Definition	Indications
Pneumonectomy	Removal of entire lung with or without resection of the mediastinal lymph nodes	Malignant lesions
		Unilateral tuberculosis
		Extensive unilateral bronchiectasis
		Multiple lung abscesses
		Massive hemoptysis
		Bronchopleural fistula
Lobectomy	Resection of one or more lobes of lung	Lesions confined to a single lobe
		Pulmonary tuberculosis
		Bronchiectasis
		Lung abscesses or cysts
		Trauma
Segmental resection	Resection of bronchovascular segment of lung lobe	Small peripheral lesions
		Bronchiectasis
		Congenital cysts or blebs
Wedge resection	Removal of small wedge-shaped section of lung tissue	Small peripheral lesions (without lymph node involvement)
		Peripheral granulomas
		Pulmonary blebs
Bronchoplastic reconstruction (also called sleeve resection)	Resection of lung tissue and bronchus with end-to-end reanastomosis of bronchus	Small lesions involving the carina or major bronchus without evidence of metastasis
		May be combined with lobectomy

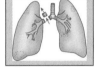

FIGURE 4-13

Images of thoracic surgeries: pneumonectomy, lobectomy, segmental resection, wedge resection, bronchoplastic resection (AKA sleeve). (From Urden L, Stacy K, Lough M, editors: Critical care nursing: diagnosis and management, ed 6, St Louis, 2010, Mosby.)

- *Thoracoscopy* (video-assisted thoracoscopic surgery): Examination, through the chest wall with a *thoracoscope,* of the pleura or lung parenchyma for pleural fluid biopsy or pulmonary resection
- *Tracheal resection and reconstruction:* Resection and reanastomosis (reconnection) of the trachea, main stem bronchi, or both; most commonly performed for tracheal carcinoma, trauma, stricture, or tracheomalacia
- *Tracheostomy:* Incision of the second or third tracheal rings or the creation of a stoma or opening for a tracheostomy tube; preferred for airway protection and prolonged ventilatory support or after laryngectomy, tracheal resection, or other head and neck surgery
- *Wedge resection:* Removal of lung parenchyma without regard to segment divisions (a portion of more than one segment but not a full lobe); most commonly performed for peripheral parenchymal carcinoma

Physical Therapy Intervention

Goals

The primary physical therapy goals in the treatment of patients with primary lung pathology include promoting independence in functional mobility; maximizing gas exchange (by improving ventilation and airway clearance); and increasing aerobic capacity, respiratory muscle endurance, and the patient's knowledge of his or her condition. General intervention techniques to accomplish these goals are breathing retraining exercises, secretion clearance techniques, positioning, functional activity and exercise with vital sign monitoring, and patient education.

A physiologically based treatment hierarchy for patients with impaired oxygen transport, developed by Elizabeth Dean, is a helpful tool in treating patients with cardiopulmonary impairments. The hierarchy is based on the principle that physiologic function is best when an individual is upright and moving.[42] Dean's hierarchy is shown in Table 4-12.

Management Concepts for Patients with Respiratory Impairments

Bronchopulmonary Hygiene. The following are basic concepts for implementing a bronchopulmonary hygiene, also known as airway clearance techniques (ACT), program for patients with respiratory dysfunction:

- A basic understanding of respiratory pathophysiology is necessary because bronchopulmonary hygiene is not indicated for certain conditions, such as a pleural effusion or pulmonary edema.
- To develop a proper plan of care, the physical therapist also must understand whether the respiratory pathology is acute or chronic, reversible or irreversible, or stable or progressive,

TABLE 4-12 Dean's Hierarchy for Treatment of Patients with Impaired Oxygen Transport

PREMISE: The Position of Optimal Physiologic Function is Being Upright and Moving		
I. Mobilization and exercise	Goal: To elicit an exercise stimulus that addresses one of the three effects on the various steps in the oxygen transport pathway, or some combination thereof	A. Acute effects B. Long-term effect C. Preventive effects
II. Body positioning	Goal: To elicit a gravitational stimulus that simulates being upright and moving as much as possible: active, active-assisted, or passive	A. Hemodynamic effects related to fluid shifts B. Cardiopulmonary effects on ventilation and its distribution, perfusion, ventilation, and perfusion matching and gas exchange
III. Breathing control maneuvers	Goal: To augment alveolar ventilation, to facilitate mucociliary transport, and to stimulate coughing	A. Coordinated breathing with activity and exercise B. Spontaneous eucapnic hyperventilation C. Maximal tidal breaths and movement in three dimensions D. Sustained maximal inspiration E. Pursed-lip breathing to end-tidal expiration F. Incentive spirometry
IV. Coughing maneuvers	Goal: To facilitate mucociliary clearance with the least effect on dynamic airway compression and the fewest adverse cardiovascular effects	A. Active and spontaneous cough with closed glottis B. Active-assisted (self-supported or supported by other) C. Modified coughing interventions with open glottis (e.g., forced expiratory technique, huff)
V. Relaxation and energy-conservation interventions	Goal: To minimize the work of breathing and of the heart and to minimize undue oxygen demand	A. Relaxation procedures at rest and during activity B. Energy conservation, (i.e., balance of activity and rest, performing activities in an energy-efficient manner, improved movement economy during activity) C. Pain-control interventions
VI. ROM exercises (cardiopulmonary indications)	Goal: To stimulate alveolar ventilation and alter its distribution	A. Active B. Assisted-active C. Passive
VII. Postural drainage positioning	Goal: To facilitate airway clearance using gravitational effects	A. Bronchopulmonary segmental drainage positions
VIII. Manual techniques	Goal: To facilitate airway clearance in conjunction with specific body positioning	A. Autogenic drainage B. Manual percussion C. Shaking and vibration D. Deep breathing and coughing
IX. Suctioning	Goal: To facilitate the removal of airway secretions collected centrally	A. Open suction system B. Closed suction system C. Tracheal tickle D. Instillation with saline E. Use of manual hyperinflation bag (bagging)

From Frownfelter D, Dean E: Cardiovascular and pulmonary physical therapy: evidence and practice, ed 4, St Louis, 2006, Mosby.

in addition to the potential for alterations in other body systems.

- The bronchopulmonary hygiene treatment plan will vary in direct correlation to the patient's respiratory or medical status. The physical therapist must be cognizant of the potential for rapid decline in patient status and modify treatment accordingly.
- Bronchopulmonary hygiene requires constant reassessment before, during, and after physical therapy intervention and on a daily basis.
- Bronchopulmonary hygiene may be enhanced by the use of supplemental O_2 and medication such as bronchodilators. Both O_2 and bronchodilators are medications that require a physician's order. Additionally, a combination of ACT may produce a more effective intervention (e.g., breathing assist techniques with inhaled hypertonic saline).
- Tolerance to bronchopulmonary hygiene can be monitored by pulse oximetry and can help determine the need for supplemental O_2 during therapy sessions.
- Cough effectiveness can be enhanced with pain medication before therapy, splinting (in cases of incision or rib fracture), positioning, and proper hydration.
- Patients with an ineffective cough for secretion removal may require nasotracheal suctioning. This technique should be performed only by well-trained therapists.
- Devices that provide oscillatory positive expiratory pressure, such as the Flutter device, can be a good adjunct to manual vibration/shaking in patients with large amounts of secretions (e.g., CF, bronchiectasis).[19,63,64]
- Patients with chronic respiratory diseases, such as CF or bronchiectasis, usually have an established routine for their bronchopulmonary hygiene. Although this routine may require modification in the hospital, maintaining this routine as much as possible optimizes the continuity of care. Be aware of the usual order of postural drainage positions and whether certain positions are uncomfortable.
- Document baseline sputum production, including certain times of the day when the patient is most productive.
- Patients with an obstructive pulmonary disorder generally do well with slow, prolonged exhalations, such as in pursed lip breathing. A patient may perform this maneuver naturally. Frequent rest breaks between coughs are also helpful to prevent air trapping and improve secretion clearance.
- Patients with a restrictive pulmonary disorder generally do well with therapeutic activities to improve inspiration, such

as diaphragmatic breathing, breathing assist techniques,[65] and chest wall stretching.
- Many hospitals (especially in the ICU setting) have incorporated rotational beds to facilitate frequent changes in patient positioning. Some beds also have modules for percussion/vibration. Although the use of these beds has shown positive outcomes,[66] they should not replace standard bronchopulmonary hygiene by physical therapists; they should supplement it.

✎ **CLINICAL TIP**

For persons with copious and chronic sputum production, education on independent forms of ACT, such as autogenic drainage and active cycle of breathing, improve adherence and therefore efficacy.[67,68]

Activity Progression. The following concepts should be considered when progressing activity in patients with respiratory dysfunction:

- Rating of perceived exertion or the dyspnea scale (see Table 4-3) are better indicators of exercise intensity than heart rate because a patient's respiratory limitations, such as dyspnea, generally supersede cardiac limitations. Monitoring O_2 saturation also can assist in determining the intensity of the activity.
- Shorter, more frequent sessions of activity are often better tolerated than are longer treatment sessions. Patient education regarding energy conservation and paced breathing contributes to increased activity tolerance.
- A treatment session may be scheduled according to the patient's other hospital activities to ensure that the patient is not overfatigued for therapy.
- Document the need and duration of seated or standing rest periods during a treatment session to help measure functional activity progression or regression.
- Although O_2 may not be needed at rest, supplemental O_2 with exercise may decrease dyspnea and prolong exercise duration and intensity.
- Bronchopulmonary hygiene before an exercise session may optimize activity tolerance.
- Table 4-13 provides some suggested treatment interventions based on common respiratory assessment findings.

TABLE 4-13 Respiratory Evaluation Findings and Suggested Physical Therapy Interventions

Evaluation	Finding	Suggested PT Intervention
Inspection	Dyspnea or tachypnea at rest or with exertion Asymmetric respiratory pattern Abnormal sitting or standing posture	Repositioning for comfort or more upright posture Relaxation techniques Energy conservation techniques Diaphragmatic or lateral costal expansion exercise Incentive spirometry Postural exercises Stretching of trunk and shoulder musculature Administer or request supplemental O_2
Palpation	Asymmetric respiratory pattern Palpable fremitus as a result of retained pulmonary secretions	Diaphragmatic or lateral costal expansion exercise Incentive spirometry Coughing exercises Upper extremity exercise Functional activity Manual techniques Postural drainage positions (see Chapter 22) Flutter valve, if applicable
Percussion	Increased dullness as a result of retained pulmonary secretions	See Palpation, above
Auscultation	Diminished or adventitious breath sounds as a result of retained pulmonary secretions	See Palpation, above
Cough effectiveness	Ineffective cough	Positioning for comfort or to maximize expiratory force Incisional splinting, if applicable Huffing and coughing techniques Functional activity or exercise External tracheal stimulation (tracheal tickle) Naso/endotracheal suctioning Requesting bronchodilator or mucolytic treatment

References

1. Thomas CL, editor: Taber's cyclopedic medical dictionary, ed 17, Philadelphia, 1989, FA Davis, pp 701, 635, 2121.
2. Urden L, Stacy K, Lough M, editors: Thelan's critical care nursing: diagnosis and management, ed 5, St Louis, 2006, Mosby.
3. Caruana-Montaldo B, Gleeson K, Zwillich CW: The control of breathing in clinical practice, Chest 117:205, 2000.
4. Ganong WF, editor: Review of medical physiology, ed 18, Norwalk, Conn, 1997, Appleton & Lange, pp 626-630.
5. Scanlon VC, Sanders T, editors: Essentials of anatomy and physiology, ed 3, Philadelphia, 1999, FA Davis, pp 342-343.
6. Vander AJ, Sherman JH, Luciano DS, editors: Human physiology, the mechanisms of body function, ed 4, New York, 1985, McGraw-Hill, p 379.
7. Kelsen SG, Borberly BR: The muscles of respiration. In Dantzker DR, Scharf SM, editors: Cardiopulmonary critical care, ed 3, Philadelphia, 1998, Saunders, pp 115-120.
8. Des Jardins T, editor: Clinical manifestations of respiratory disease, ed 3, St Louis, 1995, Mosby.
9. Scanlan CL, Wilkins RL: Gas exchange and transport. In Wilkins RL, Stoller JK, Scanlan CL, editors: Egan's fundamentals of respiratory care, ed 8, St Louis, 2003, Mosby.
10. Guyton AC, Hall JE, editors: Textbook of medical physiology, ed 11, Philadelphia, 2006, Saunders, pp 505, 510.
11. Hillegass EA, Sadowsky HS, editors: Essentials of cardiopulmonary physical therapy, ed 2, Philadelphia, 2001, Saunders.
12. Butler SM: Clinical assessment of the cardiopulmonary system. In Frownfelter DL, Dean E, editors: Cardiovascular and pulmonary physical therapy: evidence and practice, ed 4, St Louis, 2006, Mosby, pp 211-227.
13. Humberstone N, Tecklin JS: Respiratory evaluation. In Irwin S, Tecklin JS, editors: Cardiopulmonary physical therapy, ed 3, St Louis, 1995, Mosby, pp 334-335.
14. Boyars MC: Chest auscultation: how to maximize its diagnostic value in lung disease, Consultant 37(2):415-417, 1997.
15. American College of CP & ATS Joint Committee on Pulmonary Nomenclature: Pulmonary terms and symbols, Chest 67:583, 1975.
16. Flume PA, Mogayzel PJ, Robinson KA et al: Clinical practice guidelines for pulmonary therapies committee. Cystic fibrosis pulmonary guidelines, pulmonary complications: hemoptysis and pneumothorax, Am J Respir Crit Care Med 182(3):298-306, 2010.
17. Gutierrez G, Arfeen QV: Oxygent and utilization. In Dantzker DR, Scharf SM, editors: Cardiopulmonary critical care, ed 3, Philadelphia, 1998, Saunders, pp 195-196.
18. Ciesla ND, Murdock KR: Lines, tubes, catheters, and physiologic monitoring in the ICU, Cardiopulmonary Phys Ther J 11(1):18-19, 2000.
19. Sole ML, Byers JF: Ventilatory assistance. In Hartshorn JC, Sole ML, Lamborn ML, editors: Introduction to critical care nursing, ed 2, Saunders, 1997, Philadelphia, p 139.
20. Nettina SM, Mills EJ, editors: Lippincott manual of nursing practice, ed 8, Philadelphia, 2006, Lippincott, Williams & Wilkins.
21. Forrest JV, Feigin DS, editors: Essentials of chest radiology, Philadelphia, 1982, Saunders.
22. George RB, Matthay MA, Light RW et al, editors: Chest medicine: essentials of pulmonary and critical care medicine, ed 3, Baltimore, 1995, Williams & Wilkins, p 110.
23. Hetzed MR, editor: Minimally invasive techniques in thoracic medicine and surgery, London, 1995, Chapman & Hall Medical, p 4.

24. Rippe JM, Irwin RS, Fink MP et al, editors: Procedures and techniques in intensive care medicine, Boston, 1994, Little, Brown.

25. Lilington GA, editor: A diagnostic approach to chest diseases, ed 3, Baltimore, 1987, Williams & Wilkins, p 23.

26. Weiss CF, Scatarige JC et al: CT pulmonary angiography is the first-line imaging test for acute pulmonary embolism: a survey of US clinicians, Acad Radiol 13(4):434-446, 2006.

27. Bozlar U, Gaughen JR et al: Imaging diagnosis of acute pulmonary embolism, Expert Rev Cardiovasc Ther 5(3):519-529, 2007.

28. American Thoracic Society: The diagnostic approach to acute venous thromboembolism, Am J Respir Crit Care Med 160:1043-1066, 1999.

29. British Thoracic Society: British Thoracic Society guidelines for the management of suspected acute pulmonary embolism, Thorax 58:470-484, 2003.

30. Stein PD, Woodard PK et al: Diagnostic pathways in acute pulmonary embolism: recommendations of the PIOPED II investigators, Am J Med 119:1048-1055, 2006.

31. Ruppel GL, editor: Manual of pulmonary function testing, ed 7, St Louis, 1998, Mosby.

32. Thompson JM, Hirsch JE, MacFarland GK et al, editors: Clinical nursing practice, St Louis, 1986, Mosby, p 136.

33. Wilson AF, editor: Pulmonary function testing, indications and interpretations, Orlando, 1985, Orvine & Stratton.

34. Pauwels RA, Buist AS, Calverley PM et al: The GOLD Scientific Committee: global strategy for the diagnosis, management and prevention of chronic obstructive pulmonary disease. NHLBI/WHO Global Initiative for Chronic Obstructive Lung Disease (GOLD) workshop summary, Am J Respir Crit Care Med 163:1256-1276, 2001.

35. Anthonisen N: Chronic obstructive pulmonary disease. In Goldman L, Ausiello D, editors: Cecil textbook of medicine, ed 22, Philadelphia, 2004, Saunders.

36. Drazen MJ: Bronchial asthma. In Baum GL, Crapo JD, Celli BR et al, editors: Textbook of pulmonary diseases, ed 6, Philadelphia, 1998, Lippincott-Raven, pp 791-805.

37. Staton GW, Ingram RH: Asthma. In Dale DC, Federman DD, editors: Scientific American medicine 3, New York, 1998, Scientific American, pp 579-594.

38. Corbridge T, Hall JB: Status asthmaticus. In Hall JB, Schmidt GA, editors: Principles of critical care, ed 2, New York, 1998, McGraw-Hill, pp 579-594.

39. Fraser KL, Chapman KR: Chronic obstructive pulmonary disease: prevention, early detection, and aggressive treatment can make a difference, Postgrad Med 108:103, 2000.

40. Celli BR: Clinical aspects of chronic obstructive pulmonary disease. In Baum GL, Crapo JD, Celli BR et al, editors: Textbook of pulmonary diseases, ed 6, Philadelphia, 1998, Lippincott-Raven, pp 843-863.

41. Vaughan P, Waller DA: Surgical treatment of pulmonary emphysema, Surgery 23(12):435-438, 2005.

42. Frownfelter DL, Dean E, editors: Cardiovascular and pulmonary physical therapy: evidence and practice, ed 4, St Louis, 2006, Mosby.

43. Wood RE, Schafer IA, Karlinsky JB: Genetic diseases of the lung. In Baum GL, Crapo JD, Celli BR et al, editors: Textbook of pulmonary diseases, ed 6, Philadelphia, 1998, Lippincott-Raven, pp 1451-1468.

44. Selvaduari HC, Blimkie CJ, Meyers N et al: Randomized controlled study of in-hospital exercise training programs in children with cystic fibrosis, Ped Pulmonol 33:194-200, 2002.

45. Van Doorn N: Exercise programs for children with cystic fibrosis: a systematic review of randomized controlled trials, Disabil Rehabil 32(1):41-49, 2010.

46. O'Riordan T, Adam W: Bronchiectasis. In Baum GL, Crapo JD, Celli BR et al, editors: Textbook of pulmonary diseases, ed 6, Philadelphia, 1998, Lippincott-Raven, pp 807-822.

47. Chesnutt MS, Prendergast TJ, Stauffer JL: Lung. In Tierney LM, McPhess SJ, Papadakis MA, editors: Currents: medical diagnosis and treatment, ed 38, Stamford, Conn, 1999, Appleton & Lange, pp 225-337.

48. Donowitz GR, Mandell GL: Acute pneumonia. In Mandell GL, Bennett JE, Dolin R, editors: Principles and practice of infectious diseases, ed 6, Philadelphia, 2005, Churchill Livingstone.

49. Fraser RS, Muller NL, Colman N et al, editors: Pulmonary hypertension and edema. In Fraser RS, Muller NL, Colman NC et al: Fraser and Pare's diagnosis of diseases of the chest, vol 3, ed 4, Philadelphia, 1999, Saunders, p 1978.

50. O'Connor MF, Hall JB, Schmidt GA et al: Acute hypoxemic respiratory failure. In Hall JB, Schmidt GA, Wood LDH, editors: Principles of critical care, ed 2, New York, 1998, McGraw-Hill, pp 537-564.

51. Vollman KM: Prone positioning in the patient who has acute respiratory distress syndrome: the art and science, Crit Care Nurs Clin North Am 16(3):319-336, 2004.

52. Lynch JE, Cheek JM et al: Adjuncts to mechanical ventilation in ARDS, Semin Thorac Cardiovasc Surg 18(1):20-27, 2006.

53. Palevsky HI, Kelley MA, Fishman AP: Pulmonary thromboembolic disease. In Fishman AP 3rd, editor: Fishman's pulmonary diseases and disorders vol 1, New York, 1998, McGraw-Hill, pp 1297-1329.

54. Lazzara D: Respiratory distress, Nursing 31:58-63, 2001.

55. Toews GB: Interstitial lung disease. In Goldman L, Ausiello D, editors: Cecil textbook of medicine, ed 22, Philadelphia, 2004, Saunders.

56. Ragho G: Interstitial lung disease: a clinical overview and general approach. In Fishman AP 3rd, editor: Fishman's pulmonary diseases and disorders, vol 1, New York, 1998, McGraw-Hill, pp 1037-1053.

57. Vukich DJ, Markovick V: Thoracic trauma. In Rosen P, editor: Emergency medicine: concepts and clinical practice, St Louis, 1998, Mosby, pp 514-527.

58. Ruth-Sahd LA: Pulmonary contusions: management and implications for trauma nurses , J Trauma Nurs 90-98, 1997.

59. Hayes DD: Stemming the tide of pleural effusions, Nursing 31:49-52, 2001.

60. Goldman L, Ausiello D, editors: Cecil textbook of medicine, ed 22, Philadelphia, 2004, Saunders.

61. Baue AE, Geha AS et al, editors: Glenn's thoracic and cardiovascular surgery, vol 1, ed 6, Stamford, Conn, 1996, Appleton & Lange.

62. Sabiston DC, Spencer FC: In Surgery of the chest, ed 6, Philadelphia, 1995, Saunders.

63. Langenderfer B: Alternatives to percussion and postural drainage: a review of mucus clearance therapies: percussion and postural drainage, autogenic drainage, positive expiratory pressure, flutter valve, intrapulmonary percussive ventilation, and high-frequency chest compression with the ThAIRapy Vest, J Cardiopulm Rehabil 18(4):283-289, 1998.

64. Brooks D, Newbold E, Kozar L et al: The flutter device and expiratory pressures, J Cardiopulm Rehabil 22:53-57, 2002.

65. Nakano T, Ochi T, Ito N et al: Breathing assist techniques from Japan, Cardiopulm Phys Ther J 14(2):19-23, 2003.

66. Raoof S, Chowdhrey N et al: Effect of combined kinetic therapy and percussion therapy on the resolution of atelectasis in critically ill patients, Chest 115:1658-1666, 1658, 1999.

67. McIlwaine M, Wong LT, Chilvers M et al: Long-term comparative trial of two different physiotherapy techniques; postural drainage with percussion and autogenic drainage, in the treatment of cystic fibrosis, Pediatr Pulmonol 45: 1064-1069, 2010.

68. Robinson KA, McKoy N, Saldanha I et al: Active cycle of breathing techniques for cystic fibrosis (review), Cochrane Libr 11, 2010.

CHAPTER 5

Musculoskeletal System

Cathy S. Elrod

CHAPTER OBJECTIVES

The objectives of this chapter are the following:

1. Provide a brief overview of the structure and function of the musculoskeletal system
2. Describe the physical therapist's examination and management of the patient with musculoskeletal impairments in the acute care setting
3. Give an overview of fracture management and common orthopedic surgeries seen in the acute care setting
4. Describe the equipment commonly used by patients with musculoskeletal impairments in the acute care setting

PREFERRED PRACTICE PATTERNS

The most relevant practice patterns for the diagnoses discussed in this chapter, based on the American Physical Therapy Association's *Guide to Physical Therapist Practice*, second edition, are as follows:

- Fractures: 4G, 4H
- Dislocations: 4D
- Arthroplasty, Joint Resurfacing: 4H
- Limb Salvage Surgery: 4I
- Hip Disarticulation: 4I
- Hemipelvectomy: 4J
- Osteotomy: 4I
- Surgeries of the Spine: 4F

Please refer to Appendix A for a complete list of the preferred practice patterns, as individual patient conditions are highly variable and other practice patterns may be applicable.

An understanding of musculoskeletal health conditions, medical-surgical interventions, and use of orthotic and assistive devices in conjunction with weight-bearing restrictions is often the basis of physical therapy evaluation and treatment planning for patients with acute musculoskeletal impairments. Because a primary goal of the physical therapist working with a patient in the acute care setting is to initiate rehabilitative techniques that foster early restoration of maximum functional mobility and reduce the risk of secondary complications, the physical therapist is an integral member of the multidisciplinary health care team.

Structure and Function of the Musculoskeletal System

The musculoskeletal system is made up of the bony skeleton and contractile and noncontractile soft tissues, including muscles, tendons, ligaments, joint capsules, articular cartilage, and nonarticular cartilage. This matrix of soft tissue and bone provides the dynamic ability of movement, giving individuals the capacity to move through space, absorb shock, convert reactive forces, generate kinetic energy, and perform fine-motor tasks. The musculoskeletal system also provides housing and protection for vital organs and the central nervous system. As a result of its location and function, the musculoskeletal system commonly sustains traumatic injuries and degenerative changes. The impairments that develop from injury or disease can significantly affect an individual's ability to remain functional without further pathologic compromise.

Examination

Common orthopedic diagnoses seen by physical therapists in the acute care setting include degenerative joint disease, spinal disorders, and fractures associated with trauma. Because many patients with these conditions have undergone surgical interventions, physical therapists must be familiar with physician-dictated precautions such as weight-bearing limitations and range-of-motion (ROM) restrictions.

Patients with orthopedic impairments often experience pain, frustration, and anxiety while maneuvering in an environment that frequently includes peripheral lines, catheters, casts, and drains. A challenge for physical therapists in the acute care setting is to accurately interpret the reasons for the patient's presentation and then effectively achieve optimal outcomes in a very short time frame. To do this, the therapist must incorporate the judicious use of examination findings into the decision-making process. Various factors influence clinical reasoning. These factors include the therapist's knowledge, expertise, goals, values, beliefs, and use of evidence; the patient's age, diagnosis, and medical history, as well as his or her own goals, values, and beliefs; available resources; clinical practice environment; level of financial and social support; and the intended use of the collected information.[1,2]

Patient History

Information about the patient's history can be obtained from the medical record, the patient, and/or the patient's caregivers. According to the *Guide to Physical Therapist Practice*, the different types of data that can be generated from the patient history include general demographics, social history, employment/work, growth and development, general health status, social/health habits, family history, medical/surgical history, current condition(s)/chief complaint(s), functional status and activity level, medications, and other clinical tests.[3]

Medical Record Review

In addition to a standard medical review (see Chapter 2), information pertaining to the patient's musculoskeletal history should include the following:
- Medical diagnosis
- Cause and mechanism of injury
- Medical treatment and/or surgical procedures
- Physician-dictated orders
  - Weight-bearing status, limitations on ROM, positioning of extremities
  - Equipment such as braces, orthotics, assistive device use
  - Activity status
- Comorbidities and medical history
- Diagnostic test and laboratory results
- Medications (see Chapter 19)

Because many patients with musculoskeletal impairments have undergone some type of surgical procedure in which blood loss could have occurred, the physical therapist should review and monitor the patient's hematocrit and hemoglobin levels. If they are low, the patient is experiencing a reduction in the oxygen-carrying capacity of the blood. Thus the patient may have decreased exercise tolerance and complain of fatigue, weakness, and dyspnea on exertion.

Diagnostic test results should be reviewed by the physical therapist because they may indicate that certain activity limitations are warranted. The most commonly used diagnostic tests for the musculoskeletal system are listed in the following section. These tests may be repeated during or after a hospital stay to assess bone and soft-tissue healing and disease progression or whether there is a sudden change in vascular or neurologic status postoperatively.

Diagnostic Tests Review

Radiography. More commonly known as x-rays or plain films, radiographic photographs are the mainstay in the detection of fracture, dislocation, bone loss, and foreign bodies or air in tissue. Sequential x-rays are standard intraoperatively or postoperatively to evaluate component position with joint arthroplasty, placement of orthopedic hardware, or fracture reduction.

Computed Tomography. Computed tomography (CT) incorporates the use of radiography with a computer in order to provide images that have greater sensitivity than plain films alone. CT is the diagnostic test of choice for the evaluation of subtle and complex fractures; degenerative changes; trauma in which both soft-tissue and bone injuries are suspected; and loose bodies in a joint.[4]

Magnetic Resonance Imaging. Magnetic resonance imaging (MRI) is superior to x-ray or CT for the evaluation of soft tissue. MRI is the imaging modality of choice for the detection of partial or complete tendon, ligament, or meniscal tears; bony and soft-tissue tumors; and disc hernations.[4]

Bone Scan. A bone scan is the radiographic picture of the uptake in bone of a radionuclide tracer. Bone scans reflect the metabolic status of the skeleton at the time of the scan. They can provide an early indication of increased bone activity and are therefore used to detect skeletal tumors, subtle fractures, infections, and avascular necrosis.[4]

Myelography. A myelogram is a radiograph or CT of the spinal cord, nerve root, and dura mater with dye contrast. A myelogram can demonstrate spinal stenosis, spinal cord compression, intervertebral disc rupture, and nerve root injury.[4] As with any test that includes contrast media, contrast-related reactions postarthrogram or myelogram may occur.

Physical Therapy Implications
- X-rays may be ordered after any new event, such as an in-hospital fall, abnormal angulation of an extremity, or possible loss of fixation or reduction, or for a dramatic increase in pain. Regardless of the situation, defer physical therapy intervention until results are reported or the situation is managed.
- Physical therapy intervention is typically deferred for the patient post myelography secondary to specific postprocedure positioning and bed-rest restrictions. If physical therapy

is scheduled immediately following the completion of this test, the physical therapist should verify with the nurse that the patient is able to participate in rehabilitation.

Medication Review

Physical therapists should also be aware of the patient's medications. If the patient is being seen shortly after surgery, the residual effects of general anesthesia may be present. Specifically, the patient could be woozy, confused, delirious, and/or weak.[5] If a local anesthetic such as an epidural or spinal neural blockade is being used, the patient may have insufficient analgesia or diminished sensation or motor function.[5] Refer to Chapter 20 for more detailed information on anesthesia.

Pain medications, specifically opioid analgesics, are commonly used by this patient population. The physical therapist needs to be aware of the type of pain medication, its side effects, and dosing schedule in order to enhance the patient's participation in rehabilitation. Refer to Chapter 21 for more information on pain management.

Most patients status post orthopedic surgery are on an anticoagulant, specifically a low-molecular-weight heparin (LMWH). Other options include synthetic pentasaccharides that inhibit factor Xa indirectly by binding to antithrombin (e.g., Fondaparinux) and vitamin K antagonists (e.g., warfarin). Other venous thromboembolism deterrents include antiembolism stockings (e.g., TED hose) and pneumatic compression devices.

> ✎ **CLINICAL TIP**
> The coagulation profile of patients on a LMWH is not typically monitored via laboratory testing, whereas unfractionated heparin is monitored via the activated partial thromboplastin time (aPTT) test and warfarin via the prothrombin time (PT) test.

Coordination with Other Providers

After reviewing the medical record and before interacting with the patient, the physical therapist must have a conversation with the patient's nurse. The physical therapist needs to determine if there is any reason why further examination of the patient at that time is not warranted. The therapist should inquire about the following information:

- Most recent lab values
- Type and last dose of pain medication
- Whether or not the patient has been out of bed since admission to the hospital

Patient Interview

The physical therapist should also collect information from the patient about his or her:

- Functional level before admission
- Previous use of assistive device(s)
- Recreation or exercise level and frequency
- Need for adaptive equipment or footwear on a regular basis (e.g., a shoe lift)

- Any additional medical problems that limit use of assistive devices, participation in physical therapy
- History of falls
- History of chronic pain
- Support system
- Anticipated discharge location to determine the presence of stairs, railings, and so forth
- Goals

Tests and Measures

Based on the data from the patient history, the physical therapist determines the specific tests and measures necessary to confirm his or her working hypothesis as to the main reasons for the patient's presentation. These tests can also be used as outcome measurement tools to show patient improvement. The following tests and measures should be considered when examining patients with musculoskeletal impairments.

Mental Status

The screening of the patient's mental status begins once the physical therapist asks questions of the patient during the patient interview/history. Based on the patient's ability to effectively communicate, the physical therapist is able to determine if further specific testing is required. If a cognitive impairment is present, the therapist must determine whether onset occurred before or after the patient was hospitalized. The therapist should also screen the patient's hearing status to ensure that the apparent impairment in mental status is not because the patient cannot hear the questions that are being asked.

> ✎ **CLINICAL TIP**
> Because the adverse effects of certain pain medications include an altered mental status, the physical therapist needs to know the medication schedule of the patient.

Observation

A wealth of information can be gathered by simple observation of the patient. The physical therapist should note the presence of any equipment and if it is being used correctly by the patient. The therapist should also observe the patient's:

- General appearance
- Level of anxiety or stress
- Position of extremities
- Willingness to move or muscle guarding

The resting limb position of the involved extremity is important to observe. The therapist should note if the limb is resting in its natural anatomic position or if it is supported with a pillow, roll, or wedge. If the limb is being supported, the therapist needs to determine if the pillows are being used correctly. Some extremities must be elevated for edema management. In other situations, the patient might use pillows for comfort, but their use predisposes the limb to contracture development (i.e., pillows under the knee in a patient who has undergone total knee arthroplasty) and is contraindicated.

> ✎ **CLINICAL TIP**
>
> Joints should be placed in a neutral resting position to preserve motion and maintain soft-tissue length. A limb in a dependent position is at risk for edema formation, even if it is dependent for only a short period.

Cardiovascular and Pulmonary. The cardiovascular and pulmonary systems should be assessed for any signs or symptoms that indicate that the patient might not tolerate aerobic activities. As the energy expenditure (i.e., cardiopulmonary demand) required for use of an assistive device is greater than the demand imposed during ambulation without a device, it is important for the physical therapist to examine the aerobic capacity of the individual.[6,7] Heart rate and rhythm, blood pressure, respiratory rate, and oxygen saturation (if applicable) must be assessed at rest, before the initiation of further tests and measures, as well as during and at the completion of aerobic activities (e.g., walking).

> ✎ **CLINICAL TIP**
>
> Because orthostatic hypotension is a side effect of opioid use, the physical therapist needs to ensure that the patient's cardiovascular system has accommodated to positional changes before progressing with upright activities.

The physical therapist should also examine the circulatory status of the patient. With decreased mobility, the risk for the development of deep venous thrombosis (DVT) increases. The lower extremities should be observed for signs of a DVT. Deficits in skin temperature, capillary refill, and peripheral pulses at the level of or distal to the injury or surgical site should also be noted. Refer to Chapter 7 for a further discussion on vascular examination.

Integumentary. The patient's skin should be screened for the presence and location of edema, bruising, lacerations, or surgical incisions. Skin integrity and color should be examined, especially around and distal to injuries and incisions. Pressure sores from prolonged or increased bed rest after trauma or orthopedic surgery can develop in anyone, regardless of age or previous functional abilities. The therapist should be aware of signs and symptoms of infection, circulatory compromise, or pressure ulcer development that would warrant further testing. Refer to Chapter 12 for a further discussion of skin integrity.

Sensation. The neuromuscular system should be assessed for impairments in sensation, especially in the involved extremity. Physical therapists should be aware of signs and symptoms of sensory deficits in patients with diabetes, compartment syndrome, and peripheral nerve injury (e.g., after THA, acute foot drop may be present because of injury to the sciatic nerve). Patients should be asked if they are experiencing any changes in sensation. Light touch awareness should be performed by lightly brushing different areas (distal and proximal, medial and lateral) on the extremity. The patient with eyes closed must

recognize that a stimulus has been applied for the system to be intact. If deficits are noted, more formal testing is required. Refer to Chapter 6 for more detailed information on the nervous system.

Pain. Musculoskeletal pain quality and location should be determined subjectively and objectively. Pain scales appropriate for the patient's age, mental status, and vision should be used. The physical therapist should understand the dosing schedule of the patient's pain medication if the patient is not using a patient-controlled analgesia (PCA) pump in order to ensure that the patient can optimally participate in rehabilitation.

The physical therapist should observe the patient throughout the examination process (as well as during interventions) to determine if the patient is expressing or experiencing pain. The patient might present nonverbal indicators of pain such as behavior changes, facial expressions, and body language. The physical therapist should determine if pain is constant or variable and if movement or positioning increases or decreases the pain. Refer to Chapter 21 for more detailed information on pain assessment and management.

> ✎ **CLINICAL TIP**
>
> The patient's experience of pain might be masked by medications, and thus the patient can be "overworked" if the intensity of the intervention is too high.

Range of Motion and Strength. The musculoskeletal system, including the uninvolved extremities, should be assessed for impairments in ROM and muscle strength that might preclude the patient from successfully performing mobility activities. For example, a patient with a fracture of the femur who will require the use of an assistive device when ambulating should have both upper extremities examined to ensure that the patient can safely maintain the limited weight-bearing status.

It is optimal to determine if any deficits exist in the patient's ability to move his or her extremities before the performance of higher-level functional activities. A gross screen of upper extremity ROM can be performed by having the patient lift his or her arms over head through the full ROM (i.e., shoulder flexion/abduction, external rotation, and elbow extension). The patient can then be asked to touch his or her shoulders (i.e., elbow flexion), flex and extend the wrists, and make a fist. A gross screen of the lower extremities can include having the patient bring one knee at a time up to the chest and then return it to the surface of the bed (i.e., hip flexion and extension, knee flexion and extension). The patient can then bring the leg to the edge of the bed and back to midline (hip abduction and adduction). Finally, the patient can do dorsiflexion and plantarflexion of the ankle.

The ability to move through the full ROM gives the therapist a gross estimate of minimal strength capabilities as well.

If the patient is unable to move through the full available ROM, the therapist will then need to move the limb passively through the remaining range to determine if it is a strength deficit or loss of ROM. Further assessment of the magnitude of

TABLE 5-1 Normal Range-of-Motion Values*

	Joint	Normal Range of Motion (Degrees)
Shoulder	Flexion	0-180
	Extension	0-60
	Abduction	0-180
	Internal rotation	0-70
	External rotation	0-90†
Elbow	Flexion	0-150
Forearm	Pronation	0-80
	Supination	0-80
Wrist	Flexion	0-80
	Extension	0-70
Hip	Flexion	0-120
	Extension	0-30
	Abduction	0-45
	Adduction	0-30
	Internal rotation	0-45
	External rotation	0-45
Knee	Flexion	0-135
Ankle	Dorsiflexion	0-20
	Plantar flexion	0-50

*Values are from the American Academy of Orthopedic Surgeons (AAOS) as reported in Appendix B of Reese NB, Bandy WD: Joint range of motion and muscle length testing, ed 2, St Louis, 2010, Saunders.

†As the AAOS does not report a value for external rotation of the shoulder, the value is from the American Medical Association (AMA) as reported in Appendix B of Reese NB, Bandy WD: Joint range of motion and muscle length testing, ed 2, St Louis, 2010, Saunders.

the ROM impairment can be examined both passively and actively via the use of a goniometer (e.g., after total knee arthroplasty). Table 5-1 outlines normal ROM values.

If the patient is able to move through the full available ROM, the therapist should provide some manual resistance to the major muscle groups to determine if there are any strength deficits that would affect the patient's ability to successfully perform functional mobility activities and ADLs. If there are no contraindications, the therapist can do formal manual muscle testing (MMT).

If manual muscle testing is not possible secondary to conditions such as altered mental status and pain or if putting force across a fracture or surgical site is required when providing resistance, then strength should be described in functional terms such as how much movement occurred within the available ROM (e.g., active hip flexion is one-third range in supine) or during the performance of a functional activity (e.g., heel slide, ability to lift leg off and/or onto the bed).

Posture. The patient's resting posture should be observed in supine, sitting, and standing positions. An inspection of the head, trunk, and extremities for alignment, symmetry, and deformity is warranted.

> ### ✎ CLINICAL TIP
>
> A leg length discrepancy that could affect standing posture and gait may be present after some surgical procedures (e.g., total hip arthroplasty [THA]).

Functional Mobility and Balance. Functional mobility, including bed mobility, transfers, and ambulation on level surfaces and stairs, should be evaluated according to activity level, medical-surgical stability, and prior functional level. Safety is a key component of function. The patient's willingness to follow precautions with consistency, as well as his or her ability to maintain weight bearing and comply with proper equipment use, must be evaluated. The patient's self-awareness of risk for falls, speed of movement, onset of fatigue, and body mechanics should be monitored.

> ### ✎ CLINICAL TIP
>
> Safety awareness, or lack thereof, can be difficult to document. The physical therapist should try to describe a patient's level of safety awareness as objectively as possible (e.g., patient leaned on rolling tray table, unaware that it could move).

The therapist should be prepared for the patient to experience symptoms associated with decreased mobility and pain medications: the patient may complain of dizziness, nausea, and lightheadedness. Patients should be taught to slowly transition from sitting to standing activities, and standing to ambulatory activities. Orthostatic hypotension and syncope may be avoided by waiting several minutes after each transition and encouraging the patient to perform ankle pumps and two or three deep breaths.

Nearly all patients will fear or be anxious about moving out of bed for the first time, especially if a fall or traumatic event led to the hospital admission. Before mobilization, the physical therapist should use strategies such as clearly explaining what will be occurring and the sensations the patient may feel (e.g., "Your foot will throb a little when you lower it to the floor") to decrease the patient's apprehension.

The therapist should also consider the patient's aerobic capacity. The physical therapist needs to determine if the patient is only ambulating a certain distance because of pain, weakness, or fatigue. The patient's cardiopulmonary response to the functional task must be assessed through the taking of vital signs at rest, during, and immediately at the completion of the activity.

Because orthopedic injuries can often be the final result of other medical problems (e.g., balance disorders or visual or sensory impairments), it is important that the physical therapist take a thorough history, perform a physical examination, and critically observe the patient's functional mobility. Medical problems may be subtle in presentation but may dramatically influence the patient's capabilities, especially with new variables, such as pain or the presence of a cast. Collectively, these factors lead to a decreased functional level.

> ### ✎ CLINICAL TIP
>
> It may be the physical therapist who first appreciates an additional fracture, neurologic deficit, or pertinent piece of medical or social history. Any and all abnormal findings should be reported to the nurse or physician.

Evaluation and Prognosis

On completion of the examination, the physical therapist must evaluate the data and use his or her clinical judgment to identify possible problems that require the skilled interventions provided by physical therapists and/or referral to other health care professionals. The therapist then determines the patient's impairments and activity limitations, which will be the focus of the patient-related instruction and direct interventions.

Most patients with musculoskeletal impairments in the acute care setting do well and return to living at home. Medical complications or an inability to manage pain or achieve independent living in an environment of no social support may increase the length of hospital admission or lead to a transfer to another facility for continued nursing care or rehabilitation.

Interventions

Physical therapy interventions are provided either once or twice a day in the acute care setting and should be individualized to each patient according to the patient's goals and clinical presentation. General physical therapy goals for the patient with musculoskeletal impairments include:

- Decrease pain and/or muscle guarding
- Prevent circulatory and pulmonary complications
- Prevent ROM and strength deficits
- Improve functional mobility while protecting the involved structures

When providing interventions to the patient, the physical therapist must take into consideration the medical and/or surgical management of the musculoskeletal impairment, physician orders, and need for equipment use during mobilization activities. The patient's medical status, social support system, and ability to abide by all safety precautions will help guide the therapist in his or her decision making about prioritizing interventions.

Decrease Pain and/or Muscle Guarding

The physical therapist may choose to use relaxation and active assisted ROM exercises within the patient's tolerance to decrease the patient's experience of pain and muscle guarding. Cold, heat, and transcutaneous electrical nerve stimulation (TENS) are also options available in the acute care setting.

Prevent Circulatory and Pulmonary Complications

If edema is present, the limb can be elevated on pillows while the patient is resting. Active muscle-pumping exercises such as ankle pumps should be provided to all patients who have decreased mobility in order to minimize the potential for the development of a deep venous thromboembolism. The therapist should encourage the patient to take two or three deep breaths several times a day, especially on upright sitting, to minimize the development of pulmonary complications and discourage shallow breathing that can occur when a patient becomes anxious. Ultimately, having the patient perform functional activities, especially ambulatory tasks, will combat circulatory stasis and pulmonary impairments.

Prevent Range of Motion and Strength Deficits

The physical therapist should consider the use of isometrics to minimize muscle atrophy around an immobilized joint. Active ROM exercises can be used to maintain range of mobile joints. If strength deficits are present or loss of strength is expected and there are no contraindications to increasing the tension/force production of the muscle, initiating a strengthening program through progressive resistance exercises or the performance of functional activities is warranted.

Improve Functional Mobility While Protecting the Involved Structures

While ensuring that the patient has donned all prescribed equipment (e.g., braces, orthotics), the physical therapist must train the patient to perform all functional activities in a manner that maximizes the patient's capabilities and ensures that the patient abides by all precautions (e.g., weight-bearing status). If the injury is to the pelvis or lower extremity, use of an assistive device will be required to maintain any limited weight-bearing status. Gait training must be provided to minimize any inefficient gait deviations. Balance training during static and dynamic activities must occur to ensure that in different positions the patient is still able to abide by all precautions. The patient must be educated on proper and safe positioning and limb movements during the performance of functional activities.

Health Conditions

Traumatic Fracture

Traumatic Fracture Classification

The analysis and classification of fractures reveal the amount of energy imparted to bone, the extent of soft-tissue injury, and optimal fracture management. Traumatic fractures can be classified according to well-recognized classification systems such as the one established by the Orthopedic Trauma Association (OTA).[8] They can also be described according to the following[9,10]:

1. **The maintenance of skin integrity:**
   a. A closed fracture is a fracture without disruption of the skin.
   b. An open fracture is a fracture with an open laceration of the skin or protrusion of the bone through the skin.
2. **The site of the fracture:**
   a. An articular fracture involves a joint.
   b. An epiphyseal fracture involves the growth plate.
   c. A diaphyseal fracture involves the shaft of a long bone.
3. **The classification of the fracture:**
   a. A linear fracture lies parallel to the long axis of the bone.
   b. An oblique fracture lies on a diagonal to the long axis of the bone.

  c. A spiral fracture encircles the bone.
  d. A transverse fracture lies horizontal to the long axis of the bone.
  e. A comminuted fracture has two or more fragments; a butterfly (wedge-shaped) fragment may or may not be present.
  f. A segmental fracture has two or more fracture lines at different levels of the bone.
  g. A compression fracture occurs when the bone is crushed; it is common in the vertebrae.

4. The extent of the fracture:
  a. An incomplete fracture has only one portion of the cortex interrupted, and the bone is still in one piece.
  b. A complete fracture has all cortices of bone interrupted, and the bone is no longer in one piece.

5. The relative position of the fragments:
  a. A nondisplaced fracture is characterized by anatomic alignment of fracture fragments.
  b. A displaced fracture is characterized by abnormal anatomic alignment of fracture fragments.

Clinical Goal of Fracture Management

The goal of fracture management is bony union of the fracture without further bone or soft-tissue damage that enables early restoration of maximal function.[11] Early restoration of function minimizes cardiopulmonary compromise, muscle atrophy, and the loss of functional ROM. It also minimizes impairments associated with limited skeletal weight bearing (e.g., osteoporosis).

Fractures are managed either nonoperatively or operatively on an elective, urgent, or emergent basis depending on the location and type of fracture, presence of secondary injuries, and hemodynamic stability. Elective or nonurgent management (days to weeks) applies to stable fractures with an intact neurovascular system or fracture previously managed with conservative measures that have failed. Urgent management (24 to 72 hours) applies to closed, unstable fractures, dislocations, or long bone stabilization with an intact neurovascular system. Emergent management applies to open fractures, fractures/dislocations with an impaired neurovascular system or compartment syndrome, and spinal injuries with increasing neurologic deficits.[11]

Fracture reduction is the process of aligning and approximating fracture fragments. Reduction may be achieved by either closed or open methods. Closed reduction is noninvasive and is achieved by manual manipulation or traction. Open reduction with internal fixation (ORIF) techniques require surgery and fixation devices commonly referred to as hardware. ORIF is the treatment of choice when closed methods cannot maintain adequate fixation throughout the healing phase. In order to decrease the extent of soft-tissue disruption that occurs when direct reduction is required, minimally invasive surgical techniques for fracture fixation have been developed. In minimal access surgery or minimally invasive surgery (MIS), the surgeon uses the least invasive access portal and mainly indirect reduction techniques to fixate the fracture.[12]

Immobilization of the fracture is required to maintain reduction and viability of the fracture site. Immobilization is accomplished through noninvasive (casts or splints) or invasive (screws, plates, rods, pins, and external fixators) techniques (Figure 5-1). Regardless of the method of immobilization, the goal is to promote bone healing.

Fracture healing is complex and proceeds through two different processes. Primary cortical or direct healing occurs when bone fragments are anatomically aligned via rigid internal fixation, encounter minimal strain, and are stable.[13] More commonly, fracture healing occurs through endochondral or secondary bone healing (Figure 5-2).[14] The first stage (inflammatory stage) of this process involves the formation of a hematoma with a subsequent inflammatory response. The reparative phase follows and includes the influx of fibroblasts, chondroblasts, and osteoblasts that results in formation of a soft calcified cartilage callus. The remodeling phase begins with the transition of the soft callus to a permanent hard callus consisting of lamellar bone. In children, the healing of bone can take less than 2 months, whereas in adults it typically takes 2 or more months.[15] Box 5-1 lists the multitude of factors that contribute to fracture healing.

Complications of Fracture

Complications of fracture may be immediate (within days), delayed (weeks to months), or late (months to years). The immediate or early medical-surgical complications of special interest in the acute care setting include[16]:

- Loss of fixation or reduction
- Deep vein thrombosis, pulmonary or fat emboli
- Nerve damage, such as paresthesia or paralysis
- Arterial damage, such as blood vessel laceration
- Compartment syndrome
- Infection

BOX 5-1 Factors Contributing to Bone Healing

Favorable	Unfavorable
Early mobilization	Tobacco smoking
Early weight bearing	Presence of disease, such as
Maintenance of fracture reduction	diabetes, anemia, neuropathy, or malignancy
Younger age	Vitamin deficiency
Good nutrition	Osteoporosis
Minimal soft-tissue damage	Infection
Patient compliance	Irradiated bone
Presence of growth hormone	Severe soft-tissue damage
	Distraction of fracture fragments
	Bone loss
	Multiple fracture fragments
	Disruption of vascular supply to bone
	Corticosteroid use

Data from Wood GW II: General principles of fracture treatment. In Canale ST, Beaty JH, editors: Campbell's operative orthopaedics, vol 3, ed 11, Philadelphia, 2008, Mosby, pp 3040-3041; Buckwalter JA et al: Bone and joint healing. In Bucholz RW et al, editors: Rockwood and Green's fractures in adults, vol 1, ed 7, Philadelphia, 2010, Lippincott Williams & Wilkins, pp 90-97.

Type of Fixation: Compression Plate and Screws	
Biomechanics	Stress shielding
Type of bone healing	Primary
Speed of recovery	Slow
Advantages	Allows perfect alignment of the fracture Holds bone in compression allowing for primary healing
Disadvantanges	Stress shielding at the site of the plate Some periosteal stripping inevitable
Other information	May initially need secondary support such as a splint or cast
Applications	Tibial plateau fracture Displaced distal radial fracture

A

Type of Fixation: External Fixator Devices	
Biomechanics	Stress sharing
Type of bone healing	Secondary
Speed of recovery	Fast
Advantages	Allows access to soft tissue if wounds are open
Disadvantanges	Pin tract infections Cumbersome
Other information	Mainly used if patients have associated soft tissue injuries that prevent ORIF or if patient is too sick to undergo lengthy surgery
Applications	Open tibial fractures Severely comminuted distal radial fractures

B

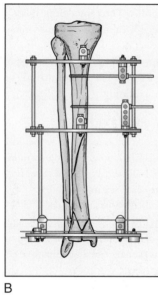

Type of Fixation: Screws, Pins, or Wires	
Biomechanics	Stress sharing
Type of bone healing	Secondary
Speed of recovery	Fast
Advantages	Minimal incision size often needed Less chance of growth plate damage with the use of smooth wires (Kirschner wires/ K-wires)
Disadvantanges	Difficult to get perfect alignment Hardware may need to be removed after healing is achieved
Other information	Often needs secondary support such as a splint or cast
Applications	Displaced patellar fractures Pediatric displaced supracondylar humeral fractures

C

FIGURE 5-1

Fracture fixation methods. **A,** Compression plate and screws; **B,** external fixator devices; **C,** screws, pins, or wires.

Type of Fixation: Rods/Nails	
Biomechanics	Stress sharing
Type of bone healing	Secondary
Speed of recovery	Fast
Advantages	Smaller incision than plates so often less soft tissue damage caused by surgery Early weight bearing possible
Disadvantanges	Disruption of endosteal blood supply Reaming may cause fat emboli
Other information	Reamed rods are most commonly used
Applications	Midshaft tibial and femoral fractures

D

Type of Fixation: Short or Long Cast of Plaster or Fiberglass; Brace	
Biomechanics	Stress sharing
Type of bone healing	Secondary
Speed of recovery	Fast
Advantages	Noninvasive Easy to apply Inexpensive
Disadvantanges	Skin breakdown or maceration Reduction of fracture may be lost if cast becomes loose Potential for harmful pressure on nerve/blood vessels
Other information	Most commonly used means of fracture support
Applications	Torus fracture of the wrist Nondisplaced lateral malleolar fracture

E

FIGURE 5-1, cont'd
D, Rods/nails; E, short or long cast of plaster or fiberglass; brace. *ORIF,* Open reduction with internal fixation.
(From Cameron MH, Monroe LG: Physical rehabilitation, St Louis, 2007, Saunders.)

- Orthostatic hypotension
Delayed and late complications are as follows[16]:
- Loss of fixation or reduction
- Delayed union (fracture fails to unite in a normal time frame in the presence of unfavorable healing factors)
- Nonunion (failure of fracture to unite)
- Malunion (fracture healed with an angular or rotary deformity)
- Pseudarthrosis (formation of a false joint at the fracture site)
- Posttraumatic arthritis
- Osteomyelitis
- Avascular necrosis
- Complex regional pain syndrome

Fracture Management According to Body Region
Pelvis and Lower Extremity

Pelvic Fractures. The pelvis is formed by the paired innominate bones, sacrum, sacroiliac joints, and the symphysis pubis. Stability of the pelvis is provided by the posterior sacroiliac ligamentous complex.[17] Pelvic fractures are classified, according to the Orthopedic Trauma Association (OTA) classification system, based on the mechanism of injury and the resultant stability of the pelvic ring (Figure 5-3).

Stable pelvic fractures (*Type A* injuries), due to low-impact direct blows or falls, do not disrupt the integrity of the pelvic ring.[8] Stable pelvic fractures include avulsion and localized nondisplaced iliac wing, pubic rami, or sacral fractures. When a pelvic fracture is described as stable, it is typically treated nonsurgically. Mobilization of the patient can occur in 1 to 2 days after a brief period of bed rest.[18,19] Ambulation with an assistive device that allows for limited weight bearing on the affected side is often prescribed.

Disruption of the pelvic ring is commonly the result of high-energy injuries that result in concurrent damage to the urinary, reproductive, and bowel systems as well as soft tissues, blood vessels, and nerves.[19] When two or more components of the

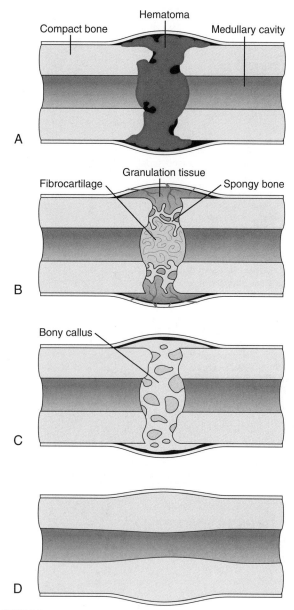

FIGURE 5-2
Fracture healing occurs in four stages. **A,** Hematoma; **B,** granulation tissue; **C,** bony callus; **D,** remodeling. (From Damjanov I: Pathology for the health professions, ed 4, St Louis, 2011, Saunders.)

FIGURE 5-3
Classification of pelvic fractures. Type *A*, Lesions sparing (or with no displacement of) the posterior pelvic arch. Type *B*, Incomplete disruption of the posterior arch (partially stable). Type *C*, Complete disruption of the posterior arch (unstable). (Courtesy of the Orthopedic Trauma Association.)

pelvic ring are injured, leading to rotational instability, but the pelvis remains stable vertically because the posterior osteoligamentous complex has been only partially disrupted, the pelvic fracture is considered to be partially stable (*Type B*).[8,17]

If the posterior osteoligamentous complex is completely disrupted, the pelvis becomes unstable both vertically and rotationally (*Type C*).[8,17] Type B and C injuries are treated with external fixation or internal fixation using plates and screws.[18] Based on the stability of the fracture and type of fixation, the physician will determine the patient's weight-bearing status, which could range from non–weight bearing (NWB) to weight bearing as tolerated (WBAT) on either one or both extremities. Functional mobility training, with the use of an assistive device, and active and active assisted ROM exercises for both lower

extremities are encouraged as soon as the patient is physiologically stable.[18]

Acetabulum Fractures. Acetabulum fractures occur when a high-impact blunt force is transmitted through the femoral head into the acetabulum. Depending on the direction of the force, different components of the acetabulum may be injured (Figure 5-4). If the hip is flexed and a force is transmitted through the femur posteriorly, as commonly occurs in a motor vehicle accident, the posterior wall will fracture.[20] An acetabulum fracture is a complex injury and is associated with retroperitoneal hematomas, injury to the lungs, shock, dislocation or fracture of the femoral head, and sciatic nerve palsy.[20,21] Acetabulum fractures are by nature intra-articular; hence, medical management focuses on the restoration of a functional

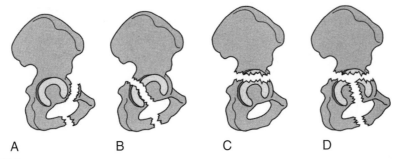

FIGURE 5-4
The innominate bone and the acetabulum are divided into anterior and posterior columns to reference the location of the trauma. Classification of acetabular fractures: **A**, anterior column; **B**, posterior column; **C**, transverse, involving both columns; **D**, complex or T-shaped, involving both columns. (From McKinnis LM: Fundamentals of musculoskeletal imaging, Philadelphia, 2010, FA Davis, p 348.)

and pain-free weight-bearing joint.[22] Closed reduction via skeletal traction with bed rest for the initial 6 to 8 weeks may be used if the patient is unable to undergo surgery.[22] Surgical management includes percutaneous pinning, open reduction with internal fixation, and hip arthroplasty.

On stabilization of the fracture, functional mobility activities should be initiated. Gait training with the appropriate assistive is required because the patient will have limited weight bearing, typically touchdown weight bearing (TDWB) or partial weight bearing (PWB), through the involved lower extremity. Active assisted exercises to the involved hip should be prescribed bearing in mind any hip precautions dictated by the physician (e.g., following THA).

Proximal Femur Fractures. Fractures of the proximal femur include proximal trochanteric, neck, and head fractures.[8] Collectively they are often referred to as hip fractures. They can be classified as intracapsular or extracapsular. In the older adult, a femoral neck fracture can occur with surprisingly little force owing to osteoporosis of the proximal femur. Femoral neck fractures in younger adults are almost always the result of high-impact forces, such as motor vehicle accidents.

Femoral head fractures are associated with a posterior hip dislocation and acetabular fracture, although the fracture can occur in the absence of either of these conditions.[23] Hip dislocations require urgent reduction because the vascular supply to the femoral head may be compromised.[23] Management of hip dislocation without fracture includes closed reduction under conscious sedation and muscle relaxation followed by traction or open reduction if closed reduction fails. Rehabilitation includes functional mobility activities with weight-bearing limitations, exercise, and positioning per physician order based on hip joint stability and associated neurovascular injury. Hip dislocation with fracture warrants surgical repair.

✎ CLINICAL TIP

After posterior hip dislocation, precautions typically include limiting hip flexion to 90 degrees, internal rotation to 0 degrees, and adduction to 0 degrees. For a confused or noncompliant patient who sustained a posterior hip dislocation, indirect restriction of hip movement during rest or functional activity can be achieved with the use of a knee immobilizer or hip abduction brace.

Intracapsular fractures are located within the hip joint capsule and include the femoral head, subcapital, and femoral neck regions. The four-stage Garden scale (Figure 5-5) is used to classify femoral neck fractures and is based on the amount of displacement and the degree of angulation.

- Garden stage I fractures are impacted and incomplete.
- Garden stage II fractures are complete and nondisplaced.
- Garden stage III fractures are complete and partially displaced.
- Garden stage IV fractures are completely displaced.

Femoral neck fractures require reduction and internal fixation, often through the use of cannulated screws.[23,24] In the older adult who has a displaced femoral neck fracture, some surgeons may elect to use a prosthetic replacement of the femoral head (hemiarthroplasty) in order to minimize the development of osteonecrosis or nonunion.[23,24]

Extracapsular fractures occur outside of the hip joint capsule. They can be further classified as intertrochanteric or subtrochanteric. *Intertrochanteric fractures* occur between the greater and lesser trochanters. *Subtrochanteric fractures* occur below the lesser trochanter and end at a point 5 cm distally.[25] Intertrochanteric and subtrochanteric fractures are shown in Figure 5-6. Extracapsular fractures are typically stabilized via open reduction and internal fixation through the use of a sliding hip screw or intramedullary nail.[26] Mobility and gait training focuses on ensuring protected weight bearing. Active or assisted hip ROM and strengthening exercises should be initiated to foster an early restoration of function.

Femoral Shaft Fractures. Fractures of the femoral shaft typically result from high-energy trauma and are associated with concurrent injuries to the pelvis and ipsilateral lower extremity.[27] Femoral shaft fractures can be accompanied by life-threatening systemic complications, such as hypovolemia, shock, or fat emboli. There also can be significant bleeding into the thigh with hematoma formation. Femoral shaft fractures can be classified based on their location (e.g., proximal, middle, and distal third) and through descriptive terms (Figure 5-7). In the presence of contamination or hemodynamic instability, external fixation or skeletal traction may be applied temporarily.[28] For most surgeons, the treatment of choice is the use of an intramedullary nail.[27] After intramedullary nailing, the patient should avoid rotation of and pivoting on the lower extremity, because microrotation of the intramedullary rod can occur and

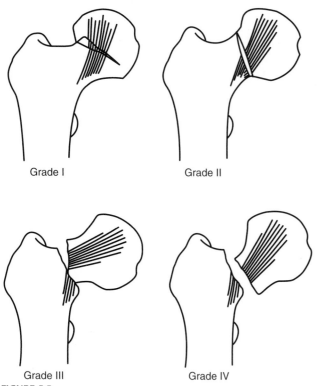

Grade I Grade II

Grade III Grade IV

FIGURE 5-5

The Garden classification of femoral neck fractures. *Grade I* is an incomplete, impacted fracture in valgus malalignment (generally stable). *Grade II* is a nondisplaced fracture. *Grade III* is an incompletely displaced fracture in varus malalignment. *Grade IV* is a completely displaced fracture with no engagement of the two fragments. The compression trabeculae in the femoral head line up with the trabeculae on the acetabular side. Displacement is generally more evident on the lateral view in grade IV. For prognostic purposes, these groupings can be lumped into nondisplaced/impacted (grades I and II) and displaced (grades III and IV) because the risk of nonunion and aseptic necrosis is similar within these grouped stages. (From Browner BD, Jupiter JB, Levine AM et al: Skeletal trauma: basic science, management, and reconstruction, ed 4, Philadelphia, 2009, Saunders.)

place stress on the fixation device. Initially, weight bearing is limited to touchdown weight bearing. Active and assisted ROM of the hip, quadriceps setting, straight-leg raises, and hip abduction exercises should be initiated.

> ✎ **CLINICAL TIP**
>
> The uninvolved leg or a single crutch can be used to assist the involved lower leg in and out of bed.

Distal Femur Fractures. Fractures of the distal femur are classified by the OTA classification system as extra-articular (*type A*), partial articular (*type B*), or complete articular (*type C*).[8] Involvement of the articular surface of the knee joint complicates the fracture. Typically, this type of fracture is caused by high-energy impact to the femur, especially in younger patients, or a direct force that drives the tibia cranially into the intercondylar fossa. Distal femur fractures may be accompanied by

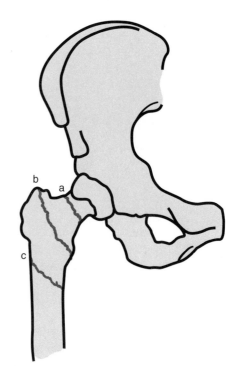

FIGURE 5-6

Fractures of the proximal femur: Neck (*a*); intertrochanteric (*b*); subtrochanteric (*c*). (From Pfenninger JL, Fowler GC, editors: Procedures for primary care, ed 3, Philadelphia, 2011, Mosby.)

injury to localized skin, muscle, and joint ligaments and cartilage with the potential for decreased knee joint mechanics.[29]

Postoperative rehabilitation will depend on the severity of the fracture and surgical techniques used for reduction and fixation. Early mobility and gentle active assisted knee ROM exercises are encouraged for the majority of these patients. Depending on the type of surgery, the physician will dictate weight-bearing limitations—typically NWB, TDWB, or PWB—and the need for any bracing (e.g., knee immobilizer or locked hinged brace).

Patella Fractures. A patella fracture results from direct trauma to the patella from a fall, blow, or motor vehicle accident (e.g., dashboard injury) or indirect mechanisms from a forceful contraction of the quadriceps with the knee flexed.[30] Injury to the patella may lead to alterations in the articular surface of the patellofemoral joint and abnormal extensor mechanism mechanics. Late complications include patellofemoral or hardware pain, osteoarthritis, decreased terminal extension, quadriceps weakness, or adhesions.[30] Nonsurgical management through immobilizing the knee in extension via a cast or brace may be chosen for nondisplaced fractures or patients with significant medical comorbidities.[31] Surgical treatment includes reduction and internal fixation, with a partial or total patellectomy reserved for highly comminuted fractures. Postoperatively, the knee is immobilized, and quadriceps setting exercises are initiated. Strong, forceful quadriceps contractions and straight-leg raises should be avoided. Protected weight bearing should ensue, abiding by the weight-bearing limitations prescribed by the physician.

Tibial Plateau Fractures. Tibial plateau fractures typically result from direct force on the proximal tibia (e.g., when a

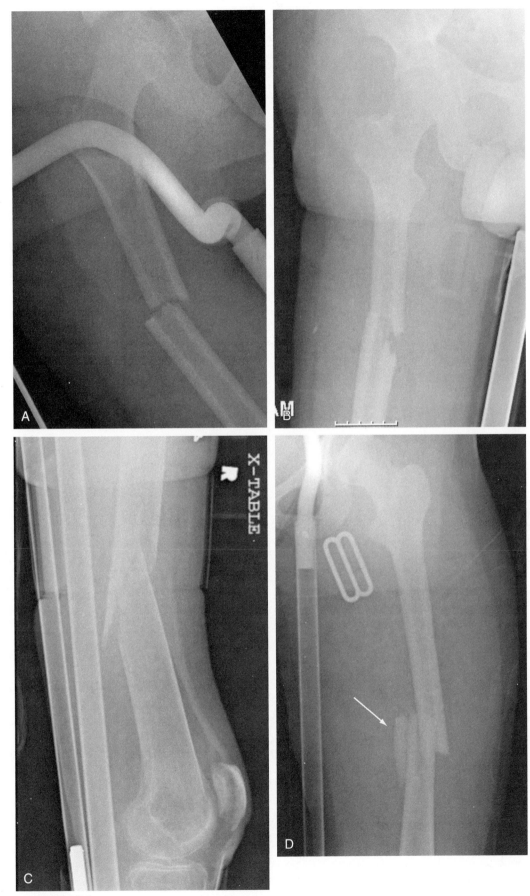

FIGURE 5-7
Femur fracture patterns. **A**, Transverse. **B**, Oblique. **C**, Spiral. **D**, Butterfly fragment *(arrow)*.

Continued

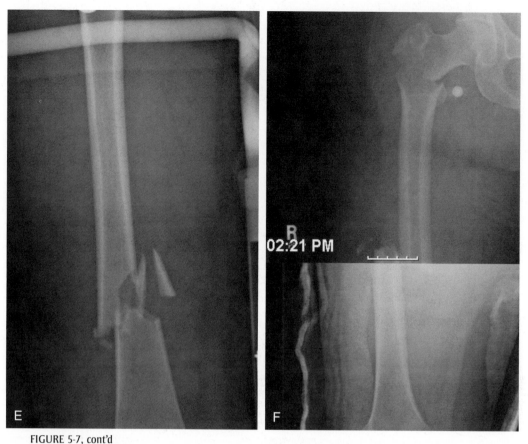

FIGURE 5-7, cont'd
E, Comminuted. **F,** Segmental. (From Townsend CM, Beauchamp D, Evers M, Mattox KL: Sabiston textbook of surgery, ed 19, Philadelphia, 2012, Saunders.)

pedestrian is hit by an automobile) and are considered extra-articular, partial articular, or complete articular.[8] The Schatzker classification system is commonly used with displaced fractures (Figure 5-8). This high-force injury often presents with open wounds and soft-tissue injuries, including capsular, ligamentous, and meniscal disruption. Immediate or early complications of tibial plateau fractures include popliteal or peroneal nerve compression, compartment syndrome, infection, and DVT.[27] Late complications include abnormal patellofemoral mechanics, lack of ROM or stability, and posttraumatic arthritis of the articular surface. Surgical management via internal or external fixation is used for fractures that are unstable or associated with ligamentous and articular disruption.[27] The complexity of the tibial plateau fracture will dictate the precautions for movement and mobility after surgery. In most situations, no weight bearing will be allowed during the initial healing phases, and gentle active or active assisted knee ROM exercises may be delayed for several days postoperatively.

Tibial Shaft and Fibula Fractures. Tibial shaft and fibula fractures typically result from high-energy trauma such as motor vehicle and skiing accidents. The higher the energy on impact, the more soft-tissue and bone damage occurs, including concomitant damage to the ankle (e.g., trimalleolar fracture, syndesmotic disruption, or talar dome fracture). Complications associated with tibial shaft fractures include anterior tibial artery and peroneal nerve injury and compartment syndrome.

Tibial shaft fractures can be classified based on their location (e.g., proximal, middle, and distal third) and through descriptive terms (e.g., simple, wedge, and complex) from the Orthopedic Trauma Association classification system.[8]

Nonsurgical management through the use of casts or braces may be provided for stable nondisplaced tibial and fibular fractures associated with low-energy trauma.[27] Surgical treatment typically includes reduction followed by plate and screw fixation, intramedullary nail insertion, or external fixation. Early mobility with restricted weight bearing is encouraged. Knee and ankle (unless the foot is involved) ROM and quadriceps strengthening exercises should also be initiated.

Distal Tibia and Ankle Fractures. Fractures of the distal tibia, distal fibula, and talus are described together because of their frequent simultaneous injury. Malleolar ankle fractures result from rotational mechanisms, whereas distal tibial fractures (i.e., pilon fractures) are the result of high vertical loading forces, such as falls from heights and motor vehicle accidents.[32] Often, long-axis compression throughout the proximal lower extremity can cause associated tibial plateau fracture, hip dislocation, or acetabular fracture. Ankle fractures commonly result from torque caused by abnormal loading of the talocrural joint with body weight. Fractures may be simple, involving avulsion of a portion of the distal fibula, or complex, involving the entire mortise (trimalleolar fracture) with disruption of the syndesmosis. Stability of the ankle depends on joint congruity and

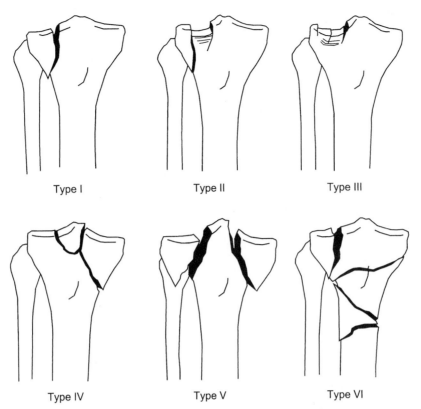

Type I   Type II   Type III

Type IV   Type V   Type VI

FIGURE 5-8
Tibial plateau fractures: Schatzker classification system. In this system, the treatment is more difficult and the prognosis poorer with higher fracture types. Types I, II, and III fractures are low-energy injuries that often occur in older persons and involve the lateral tibial plateau. Types IV, V, and VI fractures are higher-energy injuries and are associated with fracture comminution and involvement of the medial aspect of the tibia or medial tibial plateau. Type I injuries may also occur in young persons and are characterized by a split or wedge fracture line, although the size of the wedge is variable. These fractures are commonly associated with lateral meniscal tears or entrapment. Type II fractures are characterized by a lateral split fragment with or without articular depression just medial to the split. Type III fractures are characterized by pure articular depression. Type IV fractures involve the medial tibial plateau and may be further subdivided into those that are split fractures (type IVA) and those that are depression injuries (type IVB). These fractures may extend to the lateral aspect of the midline. Type V fractures involve both tibial plateaus and are often designated bicondylar fractures. Type VI fractures extend inferiorly to involve the metaphysis and diaphysis of the tibia. (From Langford JR, Jacofsky DJ, Haidukewych: Tibial plateau fractures. In Insall JN, Scott WN, editors: Surgery of the knee, ed 5, New York, 2012, Churchill Livingstone, p 775.)

ligamentous integrity. The majority of distal tibial and ankle fractures are managed through open reduction and internal fixation techniques. Surgical management for distal tibial and ankle fractures typically includes reduction and internal fixation with screws and plates. After fixation, the ankle may be immobilized in a neutral position a short leg cast, posterior plaster splint, removable splint, or fracture boot. Weight bearing will be limited. Knee ROM and proximal joint strengthening should be prescribed.

Calcaneal Fractures. The most commonly fractured bone of the foot is the calcaneus, with fractures caused by axial loading or a direct blow, such as a fall from a height or motor vehicle accident. Calcaneal fractures, usually bilateral, are associated with disruption of the subtalar joint. Nondisplaced fractures are managed nonsurgically, whereas reduction and internal fixation with plates and screws is used for displaced but reconstructable articular fractures.[33] Gait training with the appropriate assistive

is required, because the patient will be allowed no weight bearing through the ankle joint. Depending on the type of immobilization device, the physician may dictate specific ankle/forefoot motions.

Spine. Fractures to the vertebral column occur less frequently than fractures to the extremities. Approximately half of the individuals with spinal trauma sustain spinal cord or peripheral nerve root injury as well (refer to the Spinal Cord Injury section in Chapter 6).[34] Preservation of neurologic function is the primary goal of medical treatment. Thus, mechanical stability must be provided to unstable segments. The standard of treatment for most spinal injuries is closed reduction and stabilization through the use of external braces and orthoses.[34] The primary indication for surgical management is unstable ligamentous injury or disruption of the vertebral column with concomitant neurologic injury.[34] If surgical reduction and fixation is required, it is performed as soon as the patient is medically stable. Secondary management of spinal fracture may also include the following:

- Examination and treatment of associated extremity fracture, or head or internal injuries
- Very frequent (every 15 to 30 minutes) neurovascular assessment by nursing

Physical therapy management after spinal fracture without neurologic injury focuses on protecting the fracture and surgical site during all functional mobility activities. Before initiating physical therapy in a patient with suspected spinal trauma, the therapist must ensure that the spine has been "cleared" for mobility. Reviewing the results of diagnostic imaging as well as discussion with the nurse and/or physician will allow the therapist to verify the stability of the spine and the appropriateness of initiating mobilization activities. Also, temporary immobilization devices (such as a cervical collar) should not be removed until removal is ordered by the physician.

Once the spine has been "cleared," instructing the patient on proper "logroll" techniques is essential. These precautions include having the patient roll with the head, torso, and hips as one unit (i.e., no rotation). Patient education includes instruction on proper posture and body mechanics and use of any physician-ordered braces or orthotics. Therapeutic exercises including strengthening and ROM exercises will depend on the patient's clinical presentation. Refer to the Physical Therapy after Spinal Surgery section for additional tips on mobilizing a patient after spinal stabilization.

Upper Extremity

Shoulder Girdle Fractures. Fractures of the scapula typically occur during high-injury collisions; associated injuries include rib fracture, pneumothorax, spinal injuries, and ipsilateral upper extremity fracture.[35] They are classified as extra-articular (not glenoid), partial articular (glenoid), or total articular (glenoid).[8] Fractures that do not involve the articular surface often require minimal treatment (other than pain management) because the surrounding musculature serves to protect and immobilize the fracture site. Surgical reduction and fixation is necessary for intra-articular fractures and fractures of the coracoid with acromioclavicular separation.[36]

Fractures of the distal, middle, or medial third of the clavicle result from direct impact, such as falls or blows on the point of the shoulder. Management is conservative (sling immobilization for comfort) for nondisplaced fractures without ligamentous injury. ORIF is required acutely if the clavicle fracture is associated with nonunion, neurovascular compromise, coracoclavicular ligament tear, or floating shoulder (fracture of both the clavicle and surgical neck of the scapula), as well as for separation of fracture fragments by the deltoid or trapezius muscle.[36] Short-term immobilization in a sling is typical after ORIF.

Proximal Humerus and Humeral Shaft Fractures. Proximal humerus fractures occur when the humerus is subjected to direct or indirect trauma and are associated with rotator cuff injuries, and brachial plexus or peripheral nerve damage.[37] These fractures are typically defined as *minimally displaced* or *displaced* and may be classified according to the OTA classification system as an extra-articular, unifocal fracture (*type A*); extra-articular, bifocal fracture (*type B*); or articular fracture (*type C*).[8] Minimally

displaced fractures are managed nonsurgically. A sling is provided for comfort, and pendulum exercises initiated through physical therapy begin approximately 1 week after injury.[36] Displaced proximal fractures may be treated with closed reduction and percutaneous pinning, intramedullary nailing, or screw and plate fixation. Rehabilitation focuses on active assisted ROM exercises of the shoulder and functional mobility training while maintaining no weight bearing through the shoulder.

> ### ✎ CLINICAL TIP
> When the patient is lying supine, placing a thin pillow or folded sheet under the upper arm will help maintain neutral alignment and reduce pain.

Humeral shaft fractures are often the result of high-energy trauma such as a fall from a height or motor vehicle accident in the younger patient or a simple fall in the older adult.[38] Humeral shaft fractures may be associated with radial nerve or brachial plexus injury. Most humeral shaft fractures are managed nonsurgically with closed reduction and immobilization in a splint or brace. Functional mobility training while protecting the shoulder is encouraged. Typically, no weight bearing will be allowed through the involved upper extremity. The extent of assisted ROM exercises of the shoulder and elbow, if any, will be dictated by the physician.

> ### ✎ CLINICAL TIP
> Getting in and out of bed on the opposite side of an upper arm fracture is usually more comfortable for the patient.

Distal Humeral and Proximal Forearm Fractures. Distal humeral fractures are rare but complex fractures to manage because of the bony configuration of the elbow joint, adjacent neurovascular structures, and limited access to the articular surface.[37] Nonsurgical management is reserved for nondisplaced, stable fractures. All other fractures typically require surgical treatment, which consists of open reduction and internal fixation; total elbow arthroplasty (TEA) is an option for severely comminuted intra-articular fractures.

Proximal forearm fractures involve the olecranon, the head or neck of the radius, and the proximal third of the ulna. Olecranon fractures result from direct trauma to a flexed elbow or a fall on a partially flexed outstretched hand. If the fragments are displaced, surgical treatment will include open reduction and internal fixation. A fall onto an outstretched hand with a pronated forearm can cause a radial head or neck fracture. The majority of radial head fractures have good outcomes with nonsurgical management.[36] Severely comminuted fractures, loose bone fragments in the joint, and involvement of more than one third of the articular surface require surgical fixation.[36] Any displaced fracture of the radial neck and proximal ulna will also be managed with surgical fixation.

Rehabilitation management of distal humerus and proximal forearm fractures are similar. Initially the elbow is splinted, and early active assisted elbow ROM exercises may be initiated several days after surgery (physician dictated), although aggressive passive ROM should be avoided. No weight bearing should occur through the involved arm during any functional mobility activities.

Fractures of the Shaft of the Radius and Ulna. Fractures of the shaft or distal portion of the radius or ulna occur from a wide variety of direct trauma including falls, sports injuries, or motor vehicle accidents. Owing to the high-energy impact, the fracture is usually displaced and is associated with neurovascular injuries and compartment syndrome.[39] A distal radial fracture is often referred to as a Colles fracture if there is dorsal displacement of the radius. Treatment options include closed reduction and casting or percutaneous pinning, and open reduction with internal fixation. Immobilization with braces or splints may be ordered by the physician following surgical treatment. The physical therapist should note if there are any orders to initiate elbow, wrist, and hand active ROM exercises during the patient's hospitalization. Functional mobility training should occur while ensuring that no weight is applied through the involved arm.

> ✎ **CLINICAL TIP**
> Edema management should be initiated by elevating the forearm, wrist, and hand on pillows.

Carpal, Metacarpal, and Phalangeal Fractures. Carpal, metacarpal, and phalangeal fractures are typically associated with direct trauma from higher risk recreational, occupational, and sports activities.[40] Many of these fractures are accompanied by soft-tissue injuries that can result in treatment delay of several days to allow for a decrease in edema. Fractures are typically managed either by closed reduction and immobilization via casts or splints or by surgical fixation followed by immobilization with a splint or cast. Patients with isolated carpal, metacarpal, or phalangeal fracture are usually treated in the ambulatory care setting.

> ✎ **CLINICAL TIP**
> For patients who have concurrent lower- and upper-extremity injuries and require the use of a walker or crutches, a platform attachment placed on the assistive device will allow weight bearing to occur through the upper extremity proximal to the wrist.

Joint Arthroplasty

Joint arthroplasty is the surgical reconstruction of articular surfaces with prosthetic components. It is reserved for the individual with pain that is no longer responsive to conservative measures, such as antiinflammatory medication, restriction or modification of activity, exercise, weight loss, or the use of an assistive device. Its purpose is to restore function and motion to the involved joint. This surgery is elective and can be unilateral or bilateral. In recent years, the incidence of bilateral total joint arthroplasties, simultaneous or staged, being performed in the acute care setting has increased.

Joint arthroplasty provides patients and caregivers with a predictable postoperative course in the acute orthopedic care setting. For this reason, there are high expectations for these patients to achieve specific short- and long-term functional outcomes. Physical therapists must consider various factors when designing the treatment plan for these patients. Specifically, the therapist needs to understand the patient's preoperative history, including medical and rehabilitation management, impairments and activity limitations, surgical technique, prosthesis type, fixation method, soft-tissue disruption and repair, and type of anesthesia, as all of these will dictate any postoperative precautions or guidelines.

The following sections provide basic surgical information and acute rehabilitation management strategies for the acute care physical therapist.

Hip Arthroplasty

Hip arthroplasty involves the replacement of the femoral head, the acetabulum, or both with prosthetic components. A hip arthroplasty is most commonly performed on patients with severe hip arthritis (degenerative or rheumatoid), avascular necrosis (AVN), hip infection, or congenital disorders. The most common type of hip arthroplasty, a total hip arthroplasty or THA, is the replacement of both the femoral head and the acetabulum with a combination of metal (titanium or cobalt alloys), ceramic, and/or polyethylene components (Figure 5-9).

Fixation for the acetabular and femoral components may be cemented, cementless with porous surface for bony ingrowth, or cementless press-fit. With cementless components, weight bearing may be limited by surgeon protocol, although WBAT is becoming more prevalent. Weight bearing promotes bony ingrowth with the uncemented prosthetic components by allowing physiologic strain in the bone, thus increasing the activity of remodeling. With uncemented THA, the emphasis for the patient should be the prevention of torque or twisting on the operated leg while weight bearing. A cemented

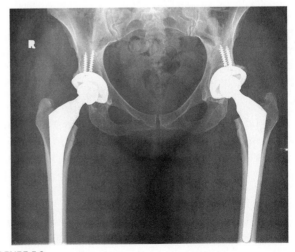

FIGURE 5-9
Bilateral total hip arthroplasty.

prosthesis allows for early weight bearing to tolerance in the recovery phase.

Surgical approaches for hip arthroplasty can be defined by how the hip joint is accessed in relation to the greater trochanter (i.e., posterior or posterolateral, anterior or anterolateral, transtrochanter or direct lateral), leg position for dislocating the femur (i.e., flexion=posterior dislocation, extension=anterior dislocation), and status of the surrounding musculature (i.e., need for detachment and repair of external rotators and abductors).[41] Recent studies suggest that there is no significant difference in clinical benefit in regard to pain, function, and gait mechanics between anterior and posterior approaches.[42,43] For all approaches, patients tend to walk faster and have an increased step length and stride length postoperatively as compared to preoperatively.[42]

A good understanding of the surgical approach taken to expose the hip joint is necessary to determine movement precautions that prevent dislocation postoperatively. Posterior dislocations usually occur in the presence of excessive flexion, adduction, and internal rotation, especially in a patient who has had a posterolateral approach that has weakened the posterior capsule and soft-tissue structures. Anterior dislocation usually occurs during excessive extension, adduction, and external rotation. In the acute care setting, the risk of dislocation is significant because of the incision made in the muscle mass and joint capsule for exposure of the hip during surgery. Consequently, the hip remains at risk for dislocation until these structures are well healed, edema is reduced, and the surrounding musculature is strengthened. Scientific evidence is lacking to support the benefit of incorporating hip dislocation precautions into the immediate postoperative management of all patients who have undergone a THA.[44,45] Despite these findings, the therapist should be aware of common hip dislocation precautions following THA (Table 5-2).

✎ CLINICAL TIP

If a physical therapist suspects the patient has dislocated his or her hip, the therapist should immediately contact the patient's nurse and physician so further testing and appropriate medical management can be initiated. Signs and symptoms of hip dislocation include excessive pain with motion, abnormal internal or external rotation of the limb with limited active and passive motion, inability to bear weight through the limb, and shortening of the limb.

Complications that may occur during or after THA include fracture, aseptic loosening, hematoma formation, heterotopic ossification, infection, dislocation, nerve injury, vascular damage, thromboembolism that can cause pulmonary embolism, myocardial infarction, cerebral vascular accident, and limb-length discrepancy.[46]

Physical Therapy after Hip Arthroplasty. Ideally, physical therapy should begin before the surgery. Preoperative physical therapy should focus on educating the patient and caregivers on the expected course of rehabilitation after surgery and

---

TABLE 5-2 Surgical Approaches and Common Hip Dislocation Precautions for Total Hip Arthroplasty

Surgical Approach	Dislocation Precautions
Posterolateral or posterior	No hip flexion beyond 90 degrees No internal rotation past neutral No hip adduction past neutral
Anterolateral or anterior	No hip extension and external rotation

Hip surgery performed in conjunction with a trochanteric osteotomy (removal and reattachment of the greater trochanter) will require an additional movement restriction of no active abduction or passive adduction. Weight bearing of the surgical limb may be limited further.

BOX 5-2 Common Activity Restrictions after Total Hip Arthroplasty

- Avoid hip motion into prohibited ranges based on dislocation precautions dictated by the surgeon
- No sitting on low surfaces
- No sleeping on operative side

Data from Harkess JW, Crockarell JR, Arthroplasty of the hip. In Canale ST, Beaty JH, editors: Campbell's operative orthopaedics, vol 1, ed 11, Philadelphia, 2007, Mosby, pp 312-481.

---

any postoperative precautions, and training on proper transfer techniques, appropriate assistive device use, and postoperative exercises.

Early postoperative physical therapy intervention is focused on functional mobility training, patient education about movement precautions during activities of daily living (ADLs), and strengthening of hip musculature.[47-49] Physical therapy may assist in preventing complications, such as atelectasis, blockage of the intestines because of decreased peristalsis secondary to anesthesia (postoperative ileus), and DVT. Early mobilization improves respiration, digestion, and venous return from the lower extremities. Patients should be educated about these risks to help prevent secondary complications. In addition, the potential for perioperative nerve compression exists; thus all peripheral innervations should be examined postoperatively, with emphasis on the femoral nerve that innervates the quadriceps and the sciatic nerve that innervates the peroneals. Neurapraxia of the femoral nerve can impact knee extension, and if the peroneals are affected, then footdrop may also occur on the affected side. In such a situation, a custom-fit ankle-foot orthosis may be indicated for the patient to optimize gait.

The priority of treatment is to achieve safe functional mobility (i.e., bed mobility, transfers, and ambulation with assistive devices) to maximize independence and functional outcomes. Because the stability of the hip is affected by the surgical approach, the physical therapist must confirm the presence of any activity restrictions with the patient's surgeon (Box 5-2). The physical therapist should educate the patient about hip dislocation precautions and activity restrictions while encouraging use of the operated limb with functional activities.

Verbal and tactile cueing may assist a patient in precaution maintenance; failure to do so may result in hip dislocation. As noted earlier in the chapter, the use of a knee immobilizer reduces hip flexion by maintaining knee extension. This technique can be helpful in preventing dislocation in patients who are unable to maintain posterior hip dislocation precautions independently. A knee immobilizer may also be necessary to provide stability if the quadriceps lacks adequate strength and stability for ambulation. The therapist should also educate the patient that movement of the operated hip can decrease postoperative pain and stiffness.

Physical therapy should be initiated the day of or the first day after surgery. The patient should be premedicated for pain control before the treatment session. Any surgical drains should be noted. Patients commonly are prescribed antiembolism stockings and external compression devices to reduce the risk of a thromboembolic event.

Patient education should include:
- Proper positioning for comfort and maintenance of the integrity of the surgical procedure
  - When supine, operative leg should be positioned with patella and toes pointing toward ceiling. Most patients are typically in a reclined position or sitting in a chair postoperatively, which allows for hip flexor tightness.

Lying flat in bed will allow the hip joint and surrounding areas to adjust more comfortably to a neutral position.
  - Use of abduction splint (Figure 5-10), if ordered
- Hip dislocation precautions and activity restrictions, as dictated by the surgeon (see Figure 5-10)
- Weight-bearing limitations
- Avoidance of low chairs
- Therapeutic exercise program

Muscle spasm often occurs in the musculature surrounding the hip postoperatively. Instructing the patient in exercises to gain control of the musculature around the hip can help to reduce muscle spasms and can also improve control of the limb during functional activities. Patients should be encouraged to perform all exercises several times a day. The patient should be educated in and perform strengthening exercises on the nonoperative extremities, as the patient will be using them more to maintain any weight-bearing limitations through the use of an assistive device.

Isometric exercises for quadriceps and gluteal muscles can be performed immediately post surgery, progressing to active-assisted and active exercises as tolerated. As maximal gluteal isometrics have been shown to generate greater acetabular contact pressures than weight-bearing activities themselves, a submaximal effort should be encouraged.[50-52] Straight-leg raises

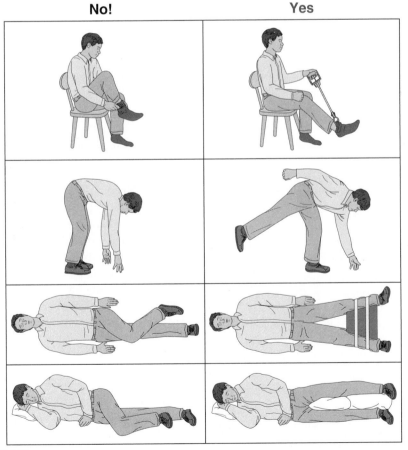

FIGURE 5-10
Total hip arthroplasty: positions to be avoided and recommended alternatives. (From Cameron MH, Monroe LG: Physical rehabilitation, St Louis, 2007, Saunders.)

should also be avoided as they put rotational stresses on the femoral component.[46]

Before establishing an advanced strengthening program consisting of progressive resistive exercises or weight training, the surgeon should be consulted to determine the appropriate time frame for initiation of these exercises because excessive strain can hinder healing of surgically involved structures.

Therapeutic exercises during the immediate postoperative phase should include:

- Deep breathing and antiembolism exercises (e.g., ankle pumps)
- Passive, active assisted, and active ROM within the parameters of any hip movement precautions in supine
  - Hip flexion and abduction
- Submaximal isometrics for gluteal muscles in supine
- Isometrics for quadriceps muscles in supine, progressing to active-assisted and active as tolerated in supine and sitting
- As out-of-bed activities increase, initiate active, gravity-only hip flexion, abduction, and extension within the parameters of any hip movement or activity restriction guidelines

Transfer and gait training with the appropriate assistive device based on the patient's weight-bearing restrictions should begin as soon as possible. Elevation of the height of the bed can facilitate sit-to-stand transfers by reducing the degree of hip flexion and the work of the hip abductors and extensors. This elevated position is especially helpful for patients with bilateral THA. If available, a hip chair (or other elevated seating surface) and commode chair should be used to facilitate transfers while maintaining hip movement precautions after a posterior or posterolateral approach. Preoperative and postoperative education in the use of furniture of the appropriate height in the home should be initiated by the physical therapist.

During gait training, the patient should be instructed to avoid pivoting on the operated extremity when ambulating by taking small steps and turning away from the operated leg to maintain movement precautions. Patients should also be trained how to safely ascend and descend stairs before discharge. Additionally, based on the patient's presentation, an aerobic exercise program may be added to the therapeutic exercise regimen because the patient's limitations in functional performance

could be attributed to deconditioning and a decreased aerobic capacity. Patients should be provided with printed instructions on their therapeutic exercise program, dislocation precautions and activity restrictions, and signs and symptoms of dislocation as well as what they should do if it occurs.

Trochanteric Osteotomy

A trochanteric osteotomy is a procedure that may be used during hip arthroplasty to allow for easier dislocation of the hip and exposure of the articular surfaces, especially in the presence of distorted anatomy.[46] If abductor muscle laxity has resulted in hip instability, a trochanteric osteotomy can change the length of the abductors and improve stability. In this procedure, the greater trochanter is excised from the femur, leaving the vastus lateralis, gluteus medius, and gluteus minimus attached to the osteotomized bone. After the fixation is complete, the trochanter is reattached to the femur with wires (Figure 5-11).

Physical Therapy after Trochanteric Osteotomy. As most trochanteric osteotomies occur during hip arthroplasty, physical therapy management follows the same general guidelines for patients who have undergone a THA. Because a portion of the greater trochanter with the abductor muscles attached was resected and then reattached to the femur, activity restrictions will be present. Specifically, no active or active assistive abduction is allowed. Procedures differ based on surgeon preference, so the physical therapist should verify these and any other weight bearing or activity restrictions. Patients should be educated in how to perform all therapeutic exercises and functional mobility activities while maintaining these precautions.

> ✎ **CLINICAL TIP**
>
> The patient can be instructed in using a leg lifter to support the surgical extremity and assist with positioning and getting the limb in and out of bed to avoid active abduction of the hip.

Hip Resurfacing Arthroplasty

Hip resurfacing arthroplasty (HRA) has evolved over time as an alternative to THA in young, active patients with end-stage osteoarthritis. It is desirable because of its femoral bone conserving properties and its ability to better preserve the biomechanics of the hip, resulting in higher postsurgery activity levels when compared to conventional THA.[53-55] Modern implants use metal-on-metal components with a cemented femoral stem and cementless press-fit acetabular cup (Figure 5-12). Complications include infection, femoral neck fracture or notching, avascular necrosis of the femoral head, component loosening, hypersensitivity to metal ions, and higher incidence rates of revision than for THA.[53,55,56]

Physical Therapy after Hip Joint Resurfacing. Specific precautions and therapeutic exercise restrictions should be confirmed with the surgeon because they are dependent on the surgical approach and procedure performed. If the hip was approached posterolaterally, hip dislocation precautions may be warranted. Full weight bearing (FWB) immediately

> ✎ **CLINICAL TIP**
>
> As the initial healing stages begin, the patient may feel as though one leg is longer while ambulating. This condition is referred to as "apparent leg length discrepancy" and is associated with the newly restored joint space that was preoperatively lessened by cartilage wearing. Patients are usually concerned because it is a sudden noticeable increase in height, whereas the progressive decrease in joint space preoperatively was over time and less noticeable. It is important to educate the patient on this subject and assure him or her that this discrepancy most typically resolves in 4 to 6 weeks. In the interim, instructing the patient to wear a shoe on the nonoperative leg and a slipper on the operative leg may help to facilitate a more "even" sensation during ambulation.

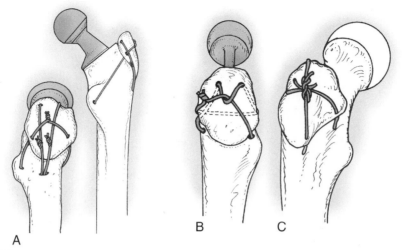

A   B   C

FIGURE 5-11
Wire fixation of trochanter. **A,** Two vertical wires are inserted in hole drilled in lateral cortex below abductor tubercle; they emerge from cut surface of neck, and one is inserted in hole in osteotomized trochanter. Two vertical wires are tightened and twisted, and transverse wire that was inserted in hole drilled in lesser trochanter and two holes in osteotomized trochanter is tightened and twisted. **B,** One-wire technique of Coventry. After component has been cemented in femur, two anteroposterior holes are drilled in femur beneath osteotomized surface, and two holes are drilled in osteotomized trochanter. One end of wire is inserted through lateral loop before being tightened and twisted. **C,** Oblique interlocking wire technique of Amstutz for surface replacement. (**A** modified from Smith & Nephew, Memphis, Tenn; **B** and **C** redrawn from Markolf KL, Hirschowitz DL, Amstutz HC: Mechanical stability of the greater trochanter following osteotomy and reattachment by wiring, Clin Orthop Relat Res 141:111, 1979.)

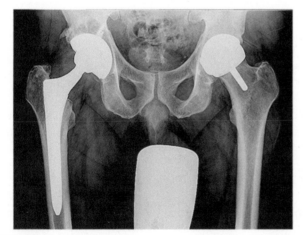

FIGURE 5-12
Radiograph of a patient with a right total hip replacement and a left hip resurfacing. The total hip replacement consists of a longer stem placed in the medullary canal of the femur. The hip resurfacing implant preserves the proximal femoral bone. (From Schafer AI, Goldman L: Goldman's Cecil medicine, ed 24, Philadelphia, 2012, Saunders.)

postsurgery is commonly prescribed, although an initial period of restricted weight bearing has been recommended when the surgeon is concerned about bone healing at the femoral neck implant interface.[57-59]

Physical therapy should focus on bed mobility, transfer training, and gait training reflecting specific weight-bearing restrictions. Immediately postoperative functional outcomes should be consistent with those of a THA, with emphasis on increasing hip ROM and strength and maximizing independence with functional activities and ambulation.

Knee Arthroplasty

Knee arthroplasty involves the replacement of the articular surfaces of the knee with prosthetic implants. It is indicated for patients with end-stage arthritis. Pain reduction, gaining intrinsic joint stability, and restoration of function are the primary goals associated with knee arthroplasty and should only be considered when conservative measures have failed.

A unicompartmental (unicondylar) knee arthroplasty is the replacement of the worn femoral and tibial articulating surfaces in either the medial or lateral compartment of the joint. This surgery is indicated for individuals who have osteoarthritis or osteonecrosis confined to one compartment with intact cruciate and collateral ligaments. In unicompartmental knee arthroplasty (UKA), the goal is to maximize the preservation of the articular cartilage of the healthier compartment and spare bone that may in turn delay a total knee arthroplasty. More of the joint is preserved, including the opposite tibiofemoral compartment and the patellofemoral joint. Preservation of the joint helps to maintain the normal kinematics of the knee joint, allowing for a quicker rehabilitation process because the patient can typically tolerate more aggressive mobility training in the immediate postoperative stage. Associated valgus deformities may also be corrected by a tibial osteotomy and release of soft tissue during the unicompartmental knee replacement.

The tricompartmental or total knee arthroplasty (TKA) is the replacement of the femoral condyles, the tibial articulating surface, and the dorsal surface of the patella. This type of

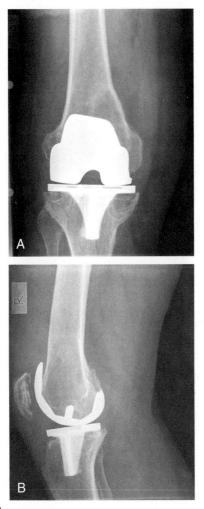

FIGURE 5-13
A, Anterior view of a right total knee arthroplasty. **B,** Lateral view of a right total knee arthroplasty.

knee arthroplasty involves the medial and lateral compartments of the joint, as well as resurfacing the patellofemoral articulation with prosthetic components (Figure 5-13, *A*). The femoral condyles are replaced with a metal-bearing surface that articulates with a polyethylene tray implanted on the proximal tibia. The dorsal aspect of the patella is often resurfaced if excessive erosion of the cartilage has occurred; however, some surgeons refrain from the patellar implant if the articular cartilage of the patella seems reasonably intact, as shown in Figure 5-13, *B*.[60]

Prosthesis systems used in knee arthroplasty vary depending on the extent of tissue damage, varus or valgus deformity, and joint laxity. Prostheses options include posterior cruciate ligament (PCL)-retaining (mild deformity) or PCL-substituting (more severe deformity), and fixed-bearing or mobile-bearing. The more recent mobile-bearing prosthesis has a congruent rotating platform between the tibial and femoral components and was designed to lower contact pressures and decrease long-term wear found in fixed-bearing devices.[61,62]

The methods of fixation in TKA are similar to those of hip arthroplasty. Cementing techniques can be used to fix the components, or the prosthetic design can allow for either porous ingrowth or press-fit fixation. Weight bearing is typically limited initially with cementless fixation techniques, whereas early WBAT as tolerated is encouraged when cement is used.

The most common surgical technique for accessing the knee joint is an anterior midline incision and medial parapatellar retinacular approach.[60] Because of some concern over the extent of quadriceps weakness with this technique, other methods for accessing the knee have been developed, such as the subvastus approach, which uses a more medial incision (Figure 5-14, *A*), and the midvastus approach, which splits the vastus medialis oblique fibers (Figure 5-14, *B*).[60,63-65]

Patients who undergo knee arthroplasty may also have associated preoperative soft-tissue contractures. A lateral retinacular release can be performed to centralize patellar tracking. If performed, there may be an increased risk of patellar subluxation with flexion. Following this technique, the surgeon may impose restrictions to ROM and weight bearing. Any additional soft-tissue balance procedures may prolong healing time secondary to increased edema and pain, which limits the patient's functional mobility and tolerance to exercise. Complications after TKA include thromboembolism, infection, joint instability, fractures, patellar tendon rupture, patellofemoral instability, component failure or loosening, and peroneal nerve injury.[60]

Physical Therapy after Knee Arthroplasty. As with all patients who are scheduled to have joint arthroplasty, physical therapy should begin before the surgery. Preoperative physical therapy should focus on educating the patient and caregivers on the expected course of rehabilitation after surgery and any postoperative activity restrictions, and training on proper transfer techniques, appropriate assistive device use, and postoperative exercises.

Postoperative physical therapy after knee arthroplasty is focused on improving knee ROM and strength as well as maximizing independence and safety with all mobility activities (i.e., bed mobility, transfers, and ambulation with assistive devices).[66-68] The physical therapist should confirm with the surgeon if there are restrictions on weight bearing or any activity/movement precautions.

Physical therapy should be initiated the day of or the first day after surgery. The patient should be premedicated for pain control before the treatment session. Any surgical drains should be noted. Patients commonly are prescribed antiembolism stockings and external compression devices to reduce the risk of a thromboembolic event.

Knee immobilizers may be prescribed to protect the knee from twisting and buckling secondary to decreased quadriceps strength. With a lateral release, there may be increased pain and edema that might hinder quadriceps functioning; therefore, a knee immobilizer or brace may be required for a longer period of time. Proper fit of the brace or knee immobilizer should be checked in order to maintain appropriate knee extension. The nursing staff may need to be educated about proper donning and doffing of the brace.

Positioning and edema control should be initiated immediately to help reduce pain and increase ROM. The patient should be educated to elevate the operated extremity with pillows or towel rolls under the calf to promote edema reduction and knee

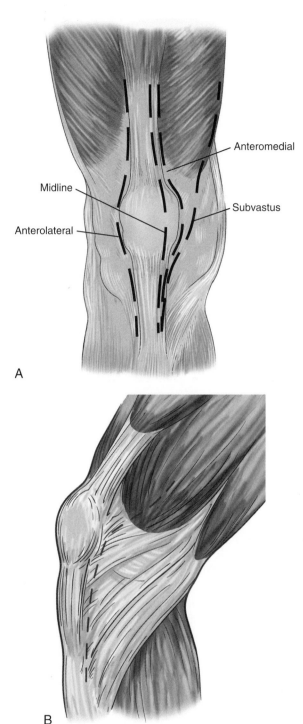

FIGURE 5-14

A, Preferred anterior approaches to the knee. **B,** Midvastus approach. (**A,** Redrawn from Scott WN: The knee, vol 1, St Louis, 1994, Mosby-Year Book, in Scott WN: Insall & Scott surgery of the knee, ed 5, Philadelphia, 2012, Churchill Livingstone. **B,** From Scott WN: Insall & Scott surgery of the knee, ed 5, Philadelphia, 2012, Churchill Livingstone.)

extension. Ice should be applied after exercise or whenever needed for patient comfort. The therapist can also place a towel roll or blanket along the lateral aspect of the femur, near the greater trochanter, to maintain the operated extremity in a neutral position. Any external rotation at the hip can result in slight flexion at the knee.

Patient education should include:
- Proper positioning for comfort and maintenance of the integrity of the surgical procedure
  - Avoid the use of pillows directly under the knee to minimize the development of knee flexion contractures
  - Use of continuous passive motion (CPM), if ordered
  - Use of knee immobilizer, if ordered
- Any activity restrictions and weight-bearing limitations, as dictated by the surgeon
- Therapeutic exercise program

ROM and strengthening exercises should begin immediately after TKA. ROM must be gained early in the rehabilitation process and is initially accomplished by passive, active-assisted, or active exercises, progressing to passive and active stretching. A CPM machine may be used to assist in achieving knee flexion ROM.[69] The limitations to ROM are often attributed to pain, swelling, muscle guarding, and apprehension, all of which can be addressed through physical therapy interventions and patient education.

The focus of strengthening exercises is typically the operated limb, although addressing any deficits in the uninvolved limb should be incorporated into the strengthening program.[70] Isometric progressing to active-assisted and active quadriceps and hamstring exercises through the full available ROM should be performed to increase stability around the operated knee and enhance performance of functional activities.[71,72] Quadriceps retraining may be accomplished with overflow from the uninvolved limb or distal limb. The patient should be encouraged to perform exercises independently, within the limits of comfort.

Therapeutic exercises during the immediate postoperative phase should include:
- Deep breathing and antiembolism exercises (e.g., ankle pumps)
- Passive, active-assisted, and active ROM
  - Knee extension and flexion (e.g., heel slides)
- Gentle stretching at end ranges of knee flexion and extension within limits of pain in supine and sitting
  - Minimize tension on incision site to ensure that integrity of surgical closure is not compromised
- Isometrics for gluteal, quadriceps, and hamstring muscles in supine, progressing to active-assisted and active exercises in supine, sitting, and standing (e.g., seated long arc quads)
- While performing isometric quadriceps exercises, the therapist should place a small towel roll under the knee. This position will produce a stronger quadriceps contraction by reducing passive stretch on joint receptors and pain receptors. It will also provide posterior support to the knee, providing increased tactile feedback for the patient.
- When performing active-assisted ROM, the use of hold/relax techniques to the hamstrings assists in decreasing muscle guarding and increases knee flexion through reciprocal inhibition of the quadriceps muscle. This technique also provides a dorsal glide to the tibia, preparing the posterior capsule for flexion.
- Active-assisted progressing to active exercises for hip flexion with knee extension in supine

- Straight-leg raises with isometric quad setting to ensure full knee-extension ROM should be achieved before lifting of leg off bed (i.e., no quad lag)
- Active exercises for hip abduction and hip adduction in supine or standing to assist in controlling limb when getting into and out of bed

Transfer, gait, and stair training with the appropriate assistive device should begin as soon as possible. Based on the patient's presentation, an aerobic exercise program may be added to the therapeutic exercise regimen because the patient's limitations in functional performance could be attributed to deconditioning and a decreased aerobic capacity. As the patient progresses through rehabilitation, balance retraining should also be considered, especially if significant soft-tissue trauma occurred during surgery; mechanoreceptor functioning around the knee joint may be disrupted, leading to balance deficits.[73]

Minimally Invasive Hip and Knee Arthroplasty

Minimally invasive surgery (MIS) refers to a variety of procedures and techniques that are used to decrease the amount of soft-tissue injury during surgery. Surgeons use special instrumentation and smaller incision sites (Figure 5-15) to access the hip

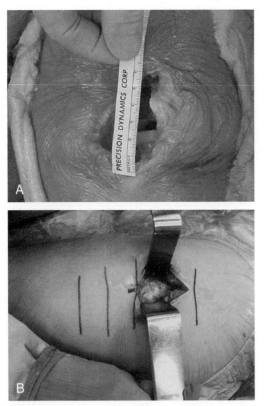

FIGURE 5-15
A, Minimally invasive knee: intraoperative measurement of incision line during MIS-TKA. **B,** Minimally invasive hip: a typical length mini-incision. (**A** from Bonutti PM: Minimally invasive total knee arthroplasty: a 10-feature evolutionary approach, Orthop Clin North Am 35(2):217-226, 2004; **B** from Sculco TP, Jordan LC, Walter WL: Minimally invasive total hip arthroplasty: the Hospital for Special Surgery experience, Orthop Clin North Am 35(2):137-142, 2004.)

or knee joint. The indications for MIS are very similar to those for traditional arthroplasty; however, this technique is not commonly used for complex joint replacements or joint revisions. Physical therapy follows the same guidelines as presented for a patient who has had a THA or TKA.

Proponents of minimally invasive techniques state that these surgical methods have the potential to decrease postoperative pain, perioperative blood loss, and hospital length of stay as well as increase healing times and speed of postoperative rehabilitation.[46] A significant clinical advantage of MIS over conventional surgery has not been supported in the literature. Contrasting literature reports improved pain relief and early functional mobility, whereas others suggest no clinical improvement.[74-77]

Shoulder Arthroplasty

Shoulder arthroplasty is indicated for patients with severe pain and limited ROM that has not responded to conservative treatment. Surgical options include replacing both the humeral and glenoid surfaces (i.e., total shoulder arthroplasty [TSA]) or replacing only the humeral head (i.e., hemiarthroplasty) with prosthetic components. The surgeon takes many factors into consideration when determining which surgical procedure to perform. Several systematic reviews suggest superior outcomes with respect to pain, ROM, function and revision rates after TSA as compared to hemiarthroplasty.[78,79]

TSA involves the use of cemented or press-fit modular prosthetic designs that are unconstrained, semiconstrained, or constrained (Figure 5-16). The most commonly used prosthesis is the unconstrained type that relies on the soft-tissue integrity of the rotator cuff and deltoid muscles. If these structures are insufficient or damaged, soft-tissue repair may take place during shoulder arthroplasty surgery and may prolong rehabilitation.

The shoulder is typically accessed anteriorly via the deltopectoral approach. Surgeons may choose to access the humeral head via a subscapularis tenotomy or a lesser tubercle osteotomy (LTO). Recently the LTO approach has gained popularity because some evidence suggests it decreases the extent of diminished subscapularis function after TSA.[80,81] The success of TSA is associated with accurate surgical placement of the prosthesis and the ability of the surgeon to reconstruct the anatomic congruency of the joint. Proper orientation of the prosthetic components and preservation of structural length and muscular integrity are key aspects of the surgery that predispose favorable outcomes. Peri- and postoperative complications include rotator cuff tearing, glenohumeral instability, and humeral fracture.

A proximal humeral hemiarthroplasty can be performed when arthritic changes have affected only the humeral head. The humeral head is replaced with a prosthetic component through a technique similar to that used in TSA. Results are dependent on the integrity of the rotator cuff and deltoid, the precision of the surgeon, and the willingness of the patient to commit to a continual rehabilitation program. With hemiarthroplasty, there is less risk for shoulder instability than with TSA, but there is also less consistent pain relief.[82]

Physical Therapy after Shoulder Arthroplasty. Initial postoperative rehabilitation after TSA or shoulder

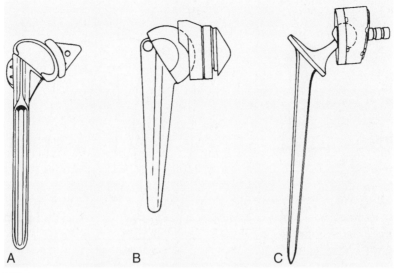

FIGURE 5-16

A variable amount of constraint is incorporated in the various designs of total shoulder replacement. **A,** Many implants have their articular surfaces shaped much like a normal joint surface. The system may be partially constrained by virtue of a hooded or more cup-shaped socket (**B**), or the components may be secured to one another as in a ball-in-socket prosthesis (**C**). (From Cofield RH: The shoulder and prosthetic arthroplasty. In Evarts CM, editor: Surgery of the musculoskeletal system, New York, 1983, Churchill Livingstone, pp 125-143.)

BOX 5-3 Common Precautions after Total Shoulder Arthroplasty

- Avoid shoulder active range of motion
- No lifting, pushing, or pulling objects with involved upper extremity
- No excessive shoulder motion behind back, especially into internal rotation
- No excessive stretching, especially into external rotation
- No supporting body weight by hand on involved side
- No driving for 3 weeks

Data from Wilcox RB 3rd, Arslanian LE, Millett PJ: Rehabilitation following total shoulder arthroplasty, J Orthop Sports Phys Ther 35(12):836, 2005.

---

hemiarthroplasty should emphasize functional mobility training to ensure independence with all ADLs, transfers, and ambulation and patient education on therapeutic exercises to minimize adhesion formation. Because the stability of the shoulder is dependent on the rotator cuff and deltoid muscles, the rehabilitation program will be dictated by their integrity. Thus, the physical therapist must confirm the presence of any precautions with the patient's surgeon (Box 5-3). Although some publications provide suggested guidelines for rehabilitation after TSA,[83-87] few studies have examined the effectiveness of specific interventions. It is imperative that the physical therapist have a collegial relationship with the patient's surgeon to ensure that the patient's unique needs after surgery are considered during the development of the therapy plan.

Physical therapy should be initiated the day of or the first day after surgery. The patient should be premedicated for pain control before the treatment session. Any surgical drains or postoperative slings or immobilizers should be noted. Instruction should be given to the patient and family/care providers on donning and doffing any supportive braces. Typically, patients are allowed to remove the sling or brace for exercise, dressing, and hygiene.

Patient education should include:

- Use of ice for the management of pain and inflammation
- Proper positioning for comfort and maintenance of the integrity of the surgical procedure
  - Avoid lying on the involved shoulder
  - Use a towel roll under the elbow when supine
- Bringing the hand to the mouth with the elbow held at the side of the trunk
- Therapeutic exercise program

To decrease distal edema, hand, wrist, and elbow active range-of-motion (AROM) exercises and ice packs may be used. Having the patient squeeze a ball or sponge will help maintain grip strength.

Therapeutic exercises during the immediate postoperative phase should include[82-84,86]:

- Supine passive forward flexion with elbow flexed; patient may passively move involved arm by using opposite hand to guide the movement (Figure 5-17, *A*)
- Supine passive external rotation with arm at side and elbow flexed to no more than 30 degrees; patient may passively move involved arm by using a wand or cane
- Pendulum exercises, clockwise and counterclockwise (see Figure 5-17, *B*)

Based on the patient's surgical procedure, other therapeutic exercises might be encouraged by the surgeon; some of the listed exercises might also be postponed until later in the rehabilitation process. Outpatient physical therapy during which further

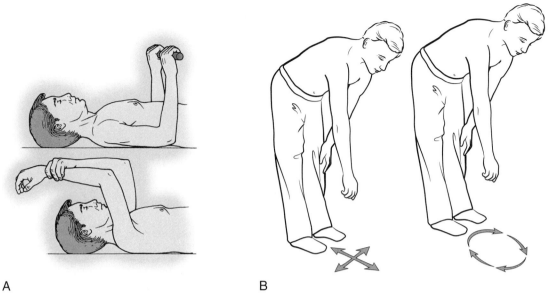

A   B

FIGURE 5-17
A, *Top*, Assisted external rotation exercise (supine). Elbows are flexed and held close to body, and movement is assisted with stick. Position aids pain-free excursion of motion soon after surgery. *Bottom*, Assisted flexion exercise (supine). Lifting power is provided by good arm. Early range of motion without stressing deltoid and subscapularis repair is possible with this exercise. **B**, Pendulum. (**A** redrawn from Hughes M, Neer CS 2nd: Glenohumeral joint replacement and postoperative rehabilitation, Phys Ther 55:850, 1975, in Campbell's operative orthopedics. **B** from Gartsman GM: Shoulder arthroscopy, ed 2, Philadelphia, 2009, Saunders.)

ROM and strengthening exercises will be initiated and progressed should begin shortly after the follow-up visit with the surgeon.

Reverse Total Shoulder Arthroplasty

A reverse total shoulder arthroplasty (rTSA) is usually chosen when the patient presents with rotator cuff arthropathy, failed shoulder arthroplasty, multiple failed rotator cuff repairs with poor function and anterosuperior instability, or malunion of the tuberosity after fracture.[82] The success of this technique is primarily due to positioning the center of rotation of the shoulder more inferior and medial, which causes shoulder stability and function to rely heavily on the deltoid muscle.[88] The new position of the deltoid allows it to elevate the arm in the presence of rotator cuff deficiency. The great advantage to this semiconstrained technique is that it is found to exhibit movement patterns similar to those of the normal shoulder.[89]

Physical Therapy after Reverse Total Shoulder Arthroplasty. The physical therapy protocol and precautions for an rTSA is similar to that of a TSA as described previously. However because of the significance of the deltoid muscle resection in this procedure, patients are typically immobilized in slight abduction and neutral rotation. The physical therapist must consult with the surgeon to determine the surgical approach to the shoulder because the extent of soft-tissue injury and reconstruction can vary and influences the aggressiveness of the immediate postoperative rehabilitation. For example, if the standard deltopectoral approach was used, active ROM exercises can be initiated the first day after surgery, whereas if a deltoid-splitting approach was used, only gentle passive forward elevation and external rotation is started immediately postoperatively; active assisted exercises are held for 2 to 3 weeks.[90]

Total Joint Arthroplasty Infection and Resection

The percentage of total joint arthroplasties that become infected (septic) is relatively small. However, a patient may present at any time after a joint arthroplasty with fever, wound drainage, persistent pain, or erythema. Infection is often diagnosed by aspirating the joint, culturing joint fluid specimens, and examining laboratory results from the aspirate. Once the type of organism is identified, there are several different avenues to follow for treatment of the infection. Treatment choices include antibiotic therapy, debridement with prosthesis retention or removal, one- or two-stage reimplantation, arthrodesis, or, in life-threatening instances, amputation.[46,60]

Resection arthroplasty involves the removal of the infected hardware and cement. The greatest potential for a functional joint occurs with a reimplantation arthroplasty.[60] The two-step process includes the removal of the infected material followed by a period of intravenous antibiotics. Once the joint is cleared of infection, new prostheses are implanted. During the interim, antibiotic spacers are typically placed between the joint surfaces.

Patients who had an infected THA, but for whom reimplementation is not an option, commonly experience instability at the hip and limited hip ROM and require the use of an assistive device during ambulatory activities.[46] If reimplantation is not an option for the knee, the limb may be braced for 6 months to maximize stability, although long-term function tends to be poor because of instability and limited ROM.[60] Because of these results, arthrodesis with an intramedullary nail may be chosen to provide stability at the knee.

Physical Therapy after Hip or Knee Resection Arthroplasty. Physical therapy after a resection arthroplasty without reimplantation or a two-staged reimplantation is dependent on the extent of joint or bone destruction caused by the infection and the removal of the prosthetic components and cement and debridement of soft tissue. Weight-bearing restrictions depend on use of cement spacers and vary from NWB to WBAT, as established by the surgeon. Physical therapy sessions focus on functional mobility, safety, proper assistive device use, and maintenance of muscle strength and endurance in anticipation of reimplantation of the joint.

Patients who have an infection and joint resection arthroplasty may be compromised by general malaise and decreased endurance secondary to the infection, as well as possibly from increased blood loss during surgery. These conditions may lead to decreased pain tolerance. The physical therapist should take these factors into account when mobilizing the patient. Functional mobility training should begin when the patient is stable, and physical therapy sessions should be modified to patient tolerance.

A hip resection arthroplasty, otherwise known as a Girdlestone procedure, may leave a patient with a significant leg-length discrepancy. With decreased leg length, the musculature surrounding the hip shortens. Shortened muscles may spasm; isometric exercises should be encouraged to gain control of these muscles to reduce spasm. For patients who are NWB, a shoe on the unaffected side and a slipper sock on the affected side can assist with toe clearance when advancing the affected leg during the swing phase of gait. Conversely, with a patient who has a significant leg-length discrepancy, a slipper sock on the unaffected side and a shoe on the affected side can assist with ambulation until a shoe lift is obtained.

> ### ✎ CLINICAL TIP
> A patient's shoes should be adapted with a lift to correct gait and increase weight bearing on the affected extremity. However, this intervention is not typically advised until the healing stages are complete because the significance of the discrepancy may change from the acute to chronic stages of healing.

THA precautions often do not apply after removal of the prosthesis. The physical therapist should verify any other precautions, such as trochanteric osteotomy precautions and weight-bearing status, with the surgeon. Without movement precautions, most isometric, active, and active-assisted exercises are appropriate. Progress the patient as tolerated to maximize function, strength, and endurance in preparation for eventual reimplantation of the prosthesis.

For knee resection surgery, strengthening exercises for the quadriceps muscle can be initiated as long as the extensor mechanism is intact. Isometrics, active-assisted exercises, and active straight-leg raises as well as active hip abduction and adduction exercises can be initiated according to patient comfort.

Edema should be controlled with ice and elevation. Positioning of the limb is important to decrease discomfort from muscle spasm and the potential for deformities caused by muscle contractures around the hip and knee.

Musculoskeletal Tumor Resection

Limb Salvage Surgery

Musculoskeletal tumors can originate in bone or soft tissues such as muscle and cartilage. If they are malignant, they are considered sarcomas (e.g., osteosarcoma, chondrosarcoma). Although tumors of the musculoskeletal system are uncommon, a major concern with bone tumors is the development of pathologic fractures. In many instances, when the tumor is in an extremity, complete tumor resection is necessary via either limb salvaging (limb-sparing) techniques or amputation.[91]

Limb-sparing procedures typically have three phases: tumor resection, bone reconstruction, and soft-tissue reconstruction for wound closure.[92] One example of a limb salvage procedure is the total femur replacement. Patients undergoing this procedure achieve good long-term prosthetic survival; 90% have limb survival.[93] A major determining factor in outcome is the oncologic diagnosis and associated complications. Confounding factors affecting patient outcomes include the presence of metastases, chemotherapy, and radiation therapy. Refer to Chapter 11 for suggestions on physical therapy management of the patient with cancer.

Early postoperative rehabilitation is essential to minimize the risks associated with immobility and to promote independence with functional activities. Transfer and gait training in the presence of restricted weight bearing, ROM and strengthening exercises for the involved and uninvolved extremities, positioning for comfort, edema management, contracture prevention, and aerobic conditioning should be components of the physical therapy plan of care.

Hip Disarticulation and Hemipelvectomy

Malignant soft-tissue or bone tumors of the hip and pelvis are treated in multiple ways. If the tumor is located on the femur or thigh and cannot be managed with limb-salvaging techniques, a hip disarticulation may be performed. This procedure involves releasing key pelvic/hip musculature, dislocating the hip joint, dividing the ligamentum teres, and removing the lower limb.[94]

In contrast, an external hemipelvectomy is indicated when the tumor involves the hip joint or a large portion of the ilium. A hemipelvectomy is very similar to a hip disarticulation but is more extensive, because the resection encompasses more of the pelvis. It typically begins at the posterior sacroiliac spine and extends along the iliac crest to the pubic symphysis and requires an osteotomy through the sacroiliac joint after the soft-tissue and neurovascular structures have been divided.[94]

In specific cases where the tumor has not interrupted the neuromuscular system and obtains only a small portion of the pelvis, an internal hemipelvectomy (Figure 5-18) is a more favorable option because the lower extremity is typically spared with this procedure.[94] The internal hemipelvectomy is similar

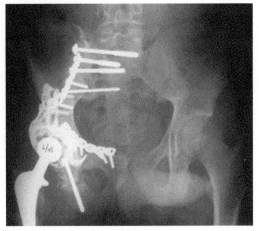

FIGURE 5-18
Internal hemipelvectomy. Anterior-posterior radiograph of pelvis demonstrating reconstruction, after modified internal hemipelvectomy, using hemipelvic allograft-prosthetic composite and total hip arthroplasty. Compression plate internal fixation of reconstructed sacroiliac joint and superior pubic ramus. Cemented total hip arthroplasty with acetabular metallic cage. (From Cheng EY: Surgical management of sarcomas, Hematol Oncol Clin North Am 19(3):451-470, 2005.)

to the external hemipelvectomy described previously, as a large portion of the pelvis and soft tissue is resected. The critical difference is the sparing of the extremity. There are many different approaches for this surgical procedure that may or may not involve internal fixation and/or THA.

These procedures are invasive and complex. It is important to consider the entire patient in these situations because such patients typically have multiple medical complications. Often they are in the process of chemotherapy and/or radiation. In addition, the emotional component involved with this type of amputation and the expected decrease in functional performance should not be disregarded.[95]

There are also many postoperative complications to consider, including infection, poor wound healing, blood loss, orthostatic hypotension, and, when the lower limb is amputated, phantom pain. In regard to the expected blood loss and anemia during surgery and postoperatively, the patient will most likely have a drain placed to remove excess blood from the surgical site. These drains should be left intact and carefully monitored when performing mobility activities. The physician should be notified immediately if they become dislodged because the patient is then at increased risk of infection and/or bleeding.

Physical Therapy after Hip Disarticulation or Hemipelvectomy. Physical therapy after a hip disarticulation or hemipelvectomy is focused on increasing functional independence. Compared to patients who have undergone joint arthroplasty, these patients typically have a more difficult time initiating mobility because they have more medical complications and limited activity tolerance at first. Extensive rehabilitation typically results in the patient ambulating independently with forearm or Lofstrand crutches. Because the amputation involves such a large portion of limb, many patients choose not to use prosthetics, which can be awkward and cumbersome, but instead live an independent life on crutches.

Rehabilitation should begin immediately postoperatively, as soon as the patient is hemodynamically stable. Bed mobility, transfer training, gait and balance training, and overall functional strength and endurance training make up the primary goals of rehabilitation.

Because mobility is encouraged from day 1, the patient should begin to build sitting tolerance, as this is usually the biggest challenge. Patients are typically unable to tolerate increased sitting as a result of pain and orthostatic hypotension. The patient should be educated on the importance of mobility, but the concept of gradual and slow progression should also be stressed and carefully monitored. Not uncommonly, it takes months before a patient can tolerate prolonged sitting without pain.

To alleviate pressure and pain during sitting, it is helpful to have the patient transfer to a reclining wheelchair. When the patient is no longer able to sit in an upright position, the wheelchair can be reclined for comfort and to disperse pressure. Using this type of wheelchair is an easy way to allow the patient to quickly lie down without having to transfer him or her back to bed. Custom seating cushions are essential for these patients to avoid any excess skin breakdown on the incision and also for added comfort. A seating consult should be initiated while the patient is in the acute care setting.

Crutch and/or walker training is essential for the patient to obtain functional independence. Progression of these activities should include increasing distance gradually and eventually incorporating stair training.

The patient should be instructed on ROM and strengthening exercises for the nonoperative extremities, especially the upper extremities, because they will become a greater contributor to weight bearing.

> ✎ **CLINICAL TIP**
> The patient should be educated on proper scooting techniques so he or she can avoid shearing or irritation to the incision while moving about in bed.

Spinal Pathology

The vertebral column forms the central axial support of the body and consists of bony segments and fibrocartilaginous discs connected by ligamentous structures and supportive musculature. Degenerative, traumatic, or congenital changes can cause compensation in the vertebral bodies, intervertebral discs, facets, and intervertebral foramen. Any changes in these structures can result in dysfunction that in turn causes pain. Some common dysfunctions of the spine and associated structures are ligamentous sprain, muscle strain, herniated nucleus pulposus, rupture of the intervertebral disc, spinal stenosis with nerve root compression, spondylolisthesis, and degenerative disease of the disc, vertebral body, or facet joints. Any dysfunction can present itself in the cervical, thoracic, and lumbar spine.

Back pain is the major indication for spinal surgery. Pain can be disabling to a patient, limiting the ability to work or complete ADLs. Any acute injury, such as muscle spasm, herniated nucleus pulposus, or chronic low back pain exacerbations, should be managed conservatively before surgical treatment is recommended. Surgery may be indicated when these measures fail to relieve a patient's symptoms or if his or her neurologic status declines.

Surgeries of the Spine

Advances have been made in all areas of spinal surgery; however, there is still no cure for low back pain. Low back pain and leg pain can arise from degenerative disc disease and herniation or rupture of the intervertebral disc. Surgical procedures can be performed to relieve the symptoms associated with degenerative disc disease when conservative measures have failed. Spinal surgeries are also indicated for the management of fractures, hypermobile spinal segments (e.g., subluxation), deformities (e.g., scoliosis), and spinal tumors.

The spinal column can be approached anteriorly (Figure 5-19, A and B) and posteriorly (Figure 5-19, C). A variety of surgical procedures have been developed over time to meet the challenges of working on and around the spine (Table 5-3). The extent of soft-tissue trauma has diminished with the advent of minimally invasive techniques. Minimally invasive procedures

have evolved as a favorable approach to posterior lumbar spinal surgery intervention. Because the dorsal muscles of the lower back are large and deep, spinal incisions can often cause more discomfort than the compromised vertebral column. Given the significant muscle soreness postoperatively, it is advantageous to the patient to use a smaller incision. Techniques include a percutaneous approach with fluoroscopic imaging and the use of microendoscopes with tubular retraction systems for lumbar discectomies and fusion.[96,97]

A discectomy removes disc fragments and herniated disc material that compress the adjacent nerve root. Microdiscectomy is a minimally invasive procedure that uses magnification to view the surgical area, allowing for decreased surgical exposure.[98] Most microdiscectomy surgeries can be done on an outpatient basis, and early return to activity is possible. If additional exposure of the nerve root is needed, associated procedures, such as a laminectomy, may be performed in conjunction with the discectomy.

Spinal instability is commonly treated surgically with spinal fusion. If neural structures are being compromised, a laminectomy or decompression in which elements of the vertebral column are removed can also be performed. Stability is achieved

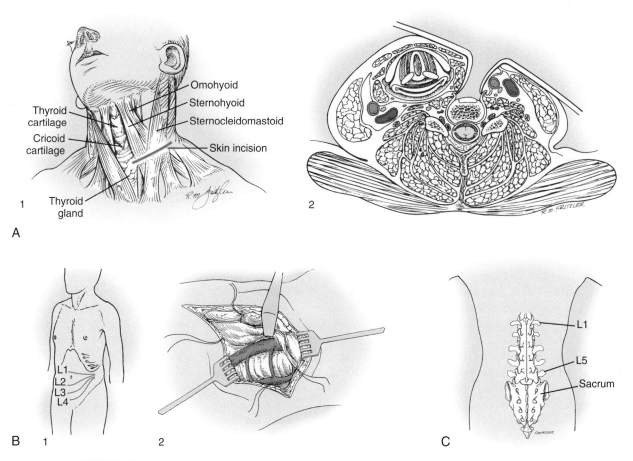

FIGURE 5-19
Surgical approaches to the spine. **A,** Anterior approach to C3-7. *1,* Incision. *2,* Thyroid gland, trachea, and esophagus have been retracted medially, and carotid sheath and its contents have been retracted laterally in opposite direction. **B,** Anterior retroperitoneal approach. *1,* Skin incisions for lumbar vertebrae. *2,* Exposure of spine before ligation of segmental vessels. **C,** Posterior approach to lumbar spine. (From Canale ST, Beaty JH, editors: Campbell's operative orthopedics, ed 11, Philadelphia, 2007, Mosby.)

TABLE 5-3 Common Spinal Surgeries

Surgery	Purpose	Procedure
Fusion	Stabilization of hypermobile or unstable joints	Use of internal fixation (e.g., Harrington rods, plates, pedicle screws, wires, interbody cages) and/or bone grafts
Laminectomy	Relieve pressure on neural structures	Removal of the lamina
Decompression	Relieve pressure on neural structures	Removal of elements of the vertebral column
Discectomy	Excision of protruding or herniated interdiscal material	Removal of a portion of or the entire intervertebral disc. Can be combined with laminectomy, decompression, and/or fusion
Corpectomy	Removal of part of the vertebral body	Use of special instruments to remove fragments or components of the vertebral body

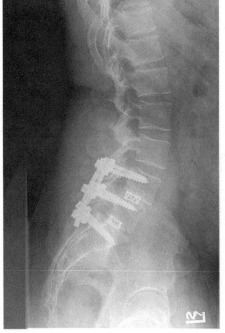

FIGURE 5-20
Lateral view of a posterior interbody fusion with pedicle screws.

through implantation of various types of instrumentation and/or bone struts. Spinal segments can be fixed using different types of rods, plates, pedicle screws, and interbody fusion cages that are packed with bone graft harvested from the iliac crest (autograft) or from a bone bank (Figure 5-20).

Total disc replacement for the lumbar spine has been developed as an alternative to spinal fusion. It is designed to reconstruct the disc, maintain disc height, and preserve segmental motion of the spine.[99] Although there is a trend toward improved outcomes compared to spinal fusion surgeries, few high-quality clinical trials have evaluated its effectiveness and efficacy.[100-102]

Complications that can occur perioperatively from spinal surgery are neurologic injury, infection, cauda equina syndrome, dural tear with cerebrospinal fluid leak, and nonunion, as well as general surgical complications noted in previous sections.

Physical Therapy after Spinal Surgery. In the acute care setting, physical therapy should emphasize early functional mobilization, education on proper body mechanics, and gait training. Patients should be educated on movement precautions if applicable to their surgical procedure. Typically patients who have undergone a decompression procedure without fusion, including microdiscectomy or laminectomy, only need to follow a 10-lb lifting precaution recommended by the surgeon. The patient should be encouraged to mobilize as tolerated and avoid any excessively painful motions., Decompression combined with a fusion or any type of instrumentation requires patients to follow specific precautions that include minimizing bending and twisting with activity, lifting restrictions per the surgeon, and use of braces or corsets if prescribed. For surgical procedures with an anterior approach, the patient should be given a splinting pillow and be educated in its use to promote deep breathing and coughing. A corset may be prescribed to aid patient comfort with activity.

Treatment should be coordinated with the administration of pain medication. Patients should be educated in relaxation techniques or breathing exercises to help manage their pain. They should be encouraged to limit the amount of time in sitting to 30 minutes.

Functional mobility training should begin the first postoperative day. The physical therapist should always check orders to determine if a brace has been prescribed by the surgeon and if there are any restrictions on activity. Braces are worn when the patient is out of bed but must be applied while the patient is supine. The patient needs to be instructed in proper donning and doffing techniques before mobilization.

Patients should be taught to logroll to get out of bed by having the body roll as a unit, minimizing any trunk rotation.

A walking program should be stressed as the only formal exercise immediately after spinal surgery to promote healing of all tissues. The patient must be informed of the need to discontinue any previous exercises he or she was performing before surgery. If an assistive device is necessary for safety, balance, and/or pain reduction during ambulatory activities, a rolling walker is useful to promote a step-through gait pattern and decrease stress on the spine caused by lifting a standard walker. Patients should quickly progress to a cane or no assistive device to promote upright posture. After several weeks of soft-tissue healing, initiating a progressive exercise program has been shown to be beneficial in improving functional performance.[103-106]

Symptoms, such as radiating pain and sensory changes present before surgery, may persist for a significant period postoperatively because of edema surrounding the surgical site. Patients should be informed of this fact and should be told to notify the nurse, surgeon, or both immediately if any significant increase in pain or change in bladder and bowel function occurs.

> ### ✎ CLINICAL TIP
>
> If an iliac crest bone graft is harvested through a second incision, a patient may complain of increased pain at the surgical site. Ice can decrease swelling at the donor site. With this type of graft, a patient will likely need an assistive device to increase safety with ambulation and decrease pain.

Kyphoplasty and Vertebroplasty

Vertebral augmentation is a surgical intervention used for progressive symptomatic osteoporotic vertebral compression fractures. These minimally invasive procedures are most commonly referred to as vertebroplasty or kyphoplasty and have been shown to be effective in restoring function and relieving acute pain associated with compression fractures.[107] Conflicting literature, however, shows that long-term outcomes following vertebral augmentation are no different from conservative management (e.g., bed rest, analgesics, and braces).[108,109]

A vertebroplasty is a procedure that consists of injecting a polymethylmethacrylate (PMMA) cement into the vertebral space to stabilize the compression fracture (Figure 5-21, A).[110] The cement is injected percutaneously in a fluid state and is intended to permeate into the cancellous bone. There are several benefits to this procedure, including stabilization of the fracture and immediate pain relief; however, the lack of height restoration and deformity restoration may lead to more chronic pathologies.[111]

A kyphoplasty differs in that it creates a space by percutaneously inserting an inflatable balloon to allow accurate placement of the PMMA cement and restores the height of the collapsed vertebral body and deformities of the spine (Figure 5-21, B).[110] Advantages of this procedure compared to a vertebroplasty are the restoration of vertebral height and alignment of the spine.[111]

Physical Therapy after Vertebroplasty or Kyphoplasty. Although there are limited evidence-based practice guidelines for physical therapy after vertebral augmentation procedures, the primary goal immediately postoperatively is to increase functional mobility.[112,113] As in most spinal protocols, a walking program is the primary source of exercise immediately postoperatively. However, the physical therapist should consult with the surgeon to determine if there are any activity restrictions, especially given a medical diagnosis of osteoporosis.

The patient should also be encouraged and instructed to use a logroll technique when getting in and out of bed to avoid any additional pain or stress on the spinal regions. Instructing the patient in good body mechanics is essential in the acute and chronic rehabilitation stages to help prevent any further injury.

Soft-Tissue Surgeries

Soft-tissue surgeries are primarily aimed at improving joint stability by repairing the functional length of muscles, tendons, and ligaments. Common soft-tissue surgeries of the lower extremity include tendon transfers, muscle repairs, fasciotomies,

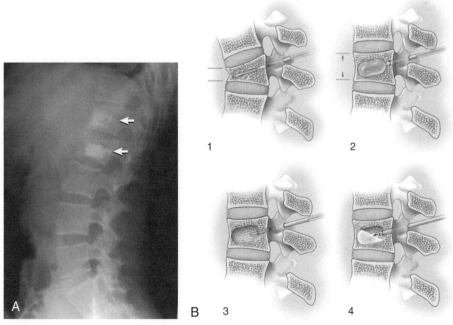

FIGURE 5-21

A, Vertebroplasty. At two levels, insertion via needle of radiopaque cement (*arrows*) has been used to arrest compression fractures. **B,** Kyphoplasty. Balloon kyphoplasty. (**A** from Mettler FA Jr: Essentials of radiology, ed 2, Philadelphia, 2005, Saunders; **B** redrawn from Garfin S: What the experts say: treatment options for VCF, including balloon kyphoplasty, Daly City, Calif, Kyphon, Inc. In Canale TS, Beaty JH, editors: Campbell's operative orthopaedics, vol 2, ed 11, Philadelphia, 2007, Mosby.)

TABLE 5-4 Soft-Tissue Repair and Reconstruction Surgeries of the Knee and Physical Therapy Intervention

Type of Repair and Reconstruction	Procedure
Meniscectomy	Removal of all or part of the medial or lateral meniscus secondary to an irreparable tear
Meniscal repair	Repair of a torn meniscus in the vascular portion of the meniscus, where the likelihood of healing is greatest
Lateral retinacular release	Release of the synovium, capsular, and retinacular structures lateral to the patella, and proximal muscle fibers of the vastus lateralis
Anterior cruciate ligament (ACL) reconstruction	Reconstruction of the ligament using autograft or allograft of the patellar tendon or hamstring tendon
Posterior cruciate ligament (PCL) reconstruction	Reconstruction of the ligament with autograft or allograft using the central third of the patellar tendon or Achilles tendon

Data from Canale ST, Beaty JH, editors: Campbell's operative orthopaedics, vol 3, ed 11, Philadelphia, 2007, Mosby.

cartilage resections or repairs, and ligament reconstructions (Table 5-4). Many of these surgeries are performed arthroscopically in an ambulatory surgery setting. However, in some cases, discharge may be delayed because of complications such as disruption of articular cartilage, menisci, and fat pads; damage to blood vessels, nerves, ligaments, and tendons; temporary paresis after tourniquet use; surgical instrument breakage; hemarthrosis; thrombophlebitis; and infection.[114] At this point, physical therapy may be involved with functional activity progression and patient education before discharge.

Equipment Used in the Management of Musculoskeletal Pathologies

Casts

A cast is a circumferential rigid external dressing used to maintain optimal skeletal alignment of a stable fracture. It is typically applied after closed reduction and encapsulates the joints above and below the fracture site. Casts can be made of plaster, fiberglass, or synthetic material and can be used on almost any body part. Table 5-5 lists common types of casts. Some casts may be split into two pieces (bivalved cast) to allow periodic visualization of the involved area or to relieve pressure or be hinged at joints (hybrid cast braces). Casts can also be used to provide low-load, prolonged, passive stretch to soft tissue to improve ROM. This application is known as serial casting.

Complications associated with casts include nerve compression of a peripheral nerve over a bony prominence by the cast,

skin breakdown, and compartment syndrome.[115] Compartment syndrome occurs when elevated interstitial pressures within a closed fascial compartment lead to tissue hypoxia; the pressure gradient becomes so high that perfusion to distal structures diminishes.[116] If compartment syndrome is left untreated, tissue necrosis will occur. It may be caused by excessive swelling or the improper fit of a cast. The classic signs and symptoms of compartment syndrome are pain (out of proportion to the injury, unrelieved by pain medicine, and increased by passive stretching of muscle groups), pressure, paresthesia, pallor, weakness (paralysis), and decreased peripheral pulses (pulselessness).[117]

> ✎ **CLINICAL TIP**
>
> The therapist should instruct the patient to contact the physician if any of the following develops: symptoms of burning or warmth, numbness, or tingling; movement of the limb within the cast; increased edema; a discolored and cool hand or foot; or a strong odor from within the cast.

Physical Therapy Implications

- The physical therapist should notify the nurse and physician immediately for any signs and symptoms of compartment syndrome, nerve compression, suspected skin breakdown, or new drainage from within the cast.
- The therapist should elevate all distal extremities 4 to 5 inches above the heart to allow gravity to assist venous return. Elevation of more than 5 inches can increase venous pressure, causing increased cardiovascular workload, and may be contraindicated for patients with congestive heart failure.
- Casts, especially plaster casts, should not get wet. The therapist should instruct the patient to wrap the cast in a waterproof bag during bathing or showering. Exposing casting materials to water weakens the structure and traps moisture against the skin.
- The therapist should discourage patients from sliding objects into the cast to scratch itchy skin. Such objects can be lost in the cast or displace the stockinet beneath the cast and cause a wound or increase the risk of pressure sore formation. Because the cast provides a moist and warm environment, bacterial growth can develop at an accelerated rate and progress into a gangrenous lesion.
- Because most casts are not rigid enough to withstand the forces of weight bearing, the physical therapist must verify any weight-bearing parameters with the physician.
- A nonslip cast shoe should be provided for patients who have casts encompassing the foot and are allowed to weight bear during transfers and ambulation.
- It is important to reinforce that the patient should move all joints proximal and distal to the cast to maintain functional ROM.

External Fixators

An external fixator is a device consisting of aluminum or titanium percutaneous pins or wires inserted into the long axis of

TABLE 5-5 Common Types of Casts

Type of Cast	Description
Short leg cast (SLC)	Extends from metatarsal heads to tibial tubercle. For distal tibia/fibula, ankle, and rear or midfoot fractures. Immobilizes foot and ankle, usually 90 degrees neutral or slight dorsiflexion. Plantar flexion immobilization is used for Achilles tendon rupture.
Patellar tendon–bearing cast (PTB)	Extends from metatarsal heads to mid- or suprapatella. Used for weight-bearing activity. A patellar tendon bar dissipates some limb loading force to the external cast shell. Knee position is 90 degrees flexion, neutral ankle, or slight dorsiflexion.
Long leg cast (LLC)	Extends from metatarsal heads to the proximal/mid femur (to stabilize the tibia) or to the greater trochanter (to stabilize the distal femur). For proximal tibia and distal femur fractures. Knee immobilized in 5 degrees flexion.
Hip spica cast	Extends from lower trunk/pelvis to the involved distal thigh (single hip spica) or to the involved entire lower extremity and thigh of the uninvolved side (1½ hip spica). For proximal femur and hip joint fractures, or hip dislocation. Hip is immobilized approximately 30 degrees of hip flexion and abduction with 30 degrees knee flexion.
Forearm cast (Colles cast)	Extends from metacarpal phalangeal (MCP) joint to proximal forearm. For radius and ulna fractures. Wrist immobilized in best position for fracture reduction or slight extension. Allows elbow flexion/extension and thumb/finger movement.
Long arm cast (LAC)	Extends from MCP joint to proximal upper arm, or just below the axilla. For distal humerus, elbow, and forearm fractures. Elbow flexion typically immobilized at 90 degrees.
Spinal cast	Extends from above sternal notch to pubic symphysis, enclosing the chest and abdomen. For stable thoracolumbar spine injuries, such as burst fractures. Immobilizes the thoracic and lumbar spine.

Data from Lusardi MM, Barringer WJ, Stills ML: Orthotics in the rehabilitation of congenital, developmental, and trauma-related musculoskeletal impairment of the lower extremities, In Lusardi MM, Nielsen CC, editors: Orthotics and prosthetics in rehabilitation, ed 2, St Louis, 2007, Saunders, pp 357-395; and Court-Brown CM: Principles of nonoperative fracture treatment. In Bucholz R, Heckman J, Court-Brown CM et al, editors: Rockwood and Green's fractures in adults, vol 1, ed 7, Philadelphia, 2010, Lippincott Williams & Wilkins, pp 125-161.

a bone that connect externally to a frame. The frame provides the alignment forces to fracture fragments and maintains reduction while healing occurs.[118] The pins and wires can be connected to longitudinal connecting bars (monolateral external fixation) or metal rings (circular external fixation).[119] External fixation devices are often the treatment of choice for severely comminuted or open long-bone fractures; unstable pelvic fractures; fractures with severe soft-tissue or vascular injuries; or when significant bone loss has occurred.[119] An advantage of external fixation is the ability to manage associated injuries, such as skin grafts and areas of debridement. It also allows for early functional mobilization.

Complications of external fixation devices include pin site infection; nerve, blood vessel, or tendon damage; loss of fracture reduction or new fractures; nonunion or malunion; joint and muscle stiffness; and compartment syndrome.[118]

Physical Therapy Implications

- It is important to maintain full ROM of all joints proximal and distal to the external fixator. A footplate can be attached to the lower leg fixator to maintain neutral ankle dorsiflexion.
- The metal rods of the external fixator should not be used to assist with movement of the extremity.
- Extra care should be taken to prevent the inadvertent tapping or banging of the external fixator against objects such as a walker or footstool because the force (vibration) is transferred to the bone and can be painful.

Braces and Splints

Orthotic devices such as braces and splints are used in conjunction with medical and surgical intervention techniques for management of musculoskeletal impairments. Functional bracing is based on the concept that continued function during the fracture healing phase promotes osteogenesis (bone growth) and enhances soft-tissue healing while preventing joint hypomobility and disuse atrophy. Bracing and splinting can be used to maintain fracture and joint alignment during healing and to unload weight-bearing forces. They can be applied immediately at the time of injury or used as part of a progressive treatment course after conventional casting or traction. They may be prefabricated or custom made.

> ✎ **CLINICAL TIP**
>
> Often, a manufacturer's brand name is used to identify its most popular brace or splint. Therefore, it is important to clarify and understand the specific function of the brace or splint, not just the style or popular name.

Patient education is vital for every patient receiving a brace, splint, or orthosis. The patient or caregiver should have a good working knowledge of the function and purpose of the device, as well as the ability to don and doff the device.

Table 5-6 lists some of the most commonly used orthoses.

TABLE 5-6 Braces and Splints Commonly Used in the Acute Care Setting

Type of Orthosis	Description
Spine	
Soft cervical collar	Foam cylinder with a cloth cover that secures with Velcro around the neck.
	Used as a kinesthetic reminder to limit neck movement for injuries that do not require rigid cervical fixation.
Reinforced cervical collar (e.g., Philadelphia, Miami J, Aspen)	Bivalved total-contact soft inner padding reinforced within a semirigid plastic frame that secures with Velcro.
	Used to control motion of the cervical spine.
Cervicothoracic orthoses	Reinforced cervical collars are connected via occipital and mandibular struts to thoracic shells.
	Used to control motion of the lower cervical and upper thoracic spine.
Halo vest	Percutaneous pins to the skull connect at the level of the forehead to a circumferential frame, which is attached via vertical rods to a vest lined with sheepskin.
	Used for strict immobilization of the cervical or high thoracic spine.
Hyperextension orthosis (e.g., Jewett, CASH)	Anterolateral aluminum frame with pads at the sternum, lateral midline of the trunk, pubis, and lumbar spine; three-point pressure system.
	Used to limit flexion and encourage hyperextension of low thoracic and upper lumbar vertebrae.
Molded thoracolumbosacral orthosis (TLSO)	Custom-fabricated, total-contact thermoplastic shell (single unit or bivalved) secured with Velcro.
	Used to limit flexion/extension, side bending, and rotation of the thoracic and upper lumbar spine.
Corset	Fabric bands with or without stays sewn into the corset that encircle the thoracolumbar and/or sacral region.
	Used for pain management; reduction of spinal and abdominal muscle activity.
Lower Extremity	
Short leg walking boot	Prefabricated, bivalved, hard, plastic outer shell with foam-filled air cells that encloses the foot and lower leg below the knee; plantar surface has a nonslip rubber grip.
	Used for conditions that allow weight bearing but require immobilization (e.g., stable ankle fracture) or cushioning (e.g., bruised calcaneus).
Ankle-foot orthosis (AFO) with anterior shell	Thermoplastic shell encompasses lower leg, ankle, and foot.
	Worn with standard lace-up shoes if weight bearing allowed.
	Used to control ankle and distal tibial motion for patients with distal tibial or fibular fractures.
Knee immobilizer	Cylinder-shaped foam secured with Velcro with either posterior or medial/lateral aluminum stays; extends from the upper thigh to the lower calf.
	Used to promote extension when rigid immobilization is not required.
Drop-lock brace (Bledsoe)	Lateral and medial metal struts adhered to foam at the thigh and lower leg connect to a hinge mechanism at the knee; hinge has a dial to select the desired degree of flexion or extension at the knee.
	Used for knee injuries requiring intermittent rigid immobilization.
Hip abduction orthosis	A padded pelvic band with a lateral extension toward the greater trochanter connects to a thigh cuff by a metal upright, including an adjustable hip joint; thigh cuff extends medially across the knee joint; may be used with a spine orthosis or knee ankle foot orthosis (KAFO).
	Used to keep hip in slight abduction while limiting hip flexion/extension.
Upper Extremity	
Simple arm sling	Fabric sling with a strap around the neck positions the elbow in approximately 90-degree flexion across the chest with the shoulder internally rotated.
	Used for comfort and gentle support of the shoulder and upper extremity.

Data from Lusardi MM, Nielsen CC: Orthotics and prosthetics in rehabilitation, ed 2, St Louis, 2007, Saunders.

Traction

Traction involves the use of a distractive force on an extremity to stabilize a fracture. For skeletal traction, a system of weights and pulleys restores the alignment of bone and muscle. It is most commonly used for fractures of the femur, although internal or external fixation has become the preferred method of stabilization.[120] The traction apparatus connects to the patient (positioned in supine) either directly into the bone via pins through the proximal tibial metaphysis or indirectly via the skin through boots, slings, or belts.[121] It is maintained continuously; therefore, the patient is on strict bed rest.

Spinal traction can be used for the initial management of cervical fractures and dislocations, allowing for decompression of neural elements and stabilization of the spine. Frequently, the patient will be transitioned to halo rings (halo vest) or undergo internal fixation.[121] Cranial tongs are made up of a metal ring with pins that are placed into the skull and a weighted pulley system. Similar to skeletal traction, the patient is supine and on strict bed rest while the cranial tongs are in place. Halo rings allow the patient to have more mobility because the rings can be incorporated into a brace or vest. They typically include two anterior and two posterior pins that are inserted into the skull and are then stabilized by metal struts attached to a plastic body brace.[121]

Complications associated with traction include generalized muscle atrophy of the immobilized limb, deconditioning of the cardiovascular system and the general side effects of prolonged bed rest, skin breakdown or pressure ulcer formation of the immobilized limb over high-pressure areas, pin tract infection, and pin loosening.[121]

Physical Therapy Implications

- If loosening or any other complication or alteration of the traction apparatus is suspected, the patient's nurse and physician should be notified immediately. The physical therapist should not adjust, remove, or reapply traction.

- The patient's body alignment or the position of the bed is specifically selected for proper countertraction; therefore, the therapist must not change the positioning of the head or foot of the bed or the placement of blanket rolls or sandbags.
- The weight should be hanging free when the patient is in traction. The head of the bed should not be lowered to a level at which the weight inadvertently rests on the floor.
- It is important to monitor the patient's skin integrity, pain report, and lower-extremity position when in skeletal traction because abnormal traction or extremity position can cause discomfort or nerve palsy (e.g., external hip rotation can compress the peroneal nerve against a suspension device).
- Isometric or active exercise of both the involved and uninvolved extremities should be initiated as appropriate to minimize strength loss, joint stiffness, and restlessness associated with prolonged bed rest.

References

1. O'Sullivan S, Schmitz T, editors: Physical rehabilitation, ed 5, Philadelphia, 2007, FA Davis.
2. McGinnis PQ, Hack LM, Nixon-Cave K et al: Factors that influence the clinical decision making of physical therapists in choosing a balance assessment approach, Phys Ther 89(3):233-247, 2009.
3. American Physical Therapy Association: Guide to physical therapist practice, ed 2, Alexandria, VA, 2001, American Physical Therapy Association.
4. McKinnis L: Fundamentals of musculoskeletal imaging, ed 3, Philadelphia, 2010, FA Davis.
5. Ciccone C: Pharmacology in rehabilitation, ed 4, Philadelphia, 2007, FA Davis.
6. Foley M, Prax B, Crowell R et al: Effects of assistive devices on cardiorespiratory demands in older adults, Phys Ther 76(12):1313-1319, 1996.
7. Westerman RW, Hull P, Hendry RG et al: The physiological cost of restricted weight bearing, Injury 39:725-727, 2008.
8. Marsh JL, Slongo TF, Agel JN et al: Fracture and dislocation classification compendium—2007: Orthopaedic Trauma Association Classification, Database and Outcomes Committee, J Orthop Trauma 21(10):S1-S163, 2007.
9. Lundon K: Injury, regeneration, and repair in bone. In Lundon K, editor: Orthopedic rehabilitation science. Boston, 2000, Butterworth-Heinemann, pp 93-113.
10. McCance K, Huether S. Pathophysiology: the biologic basis for disease in adults and children, ed 6, St Louis, 2010, Mosby.
11. Wood G: General principles of fracture treatment. In Canale ST, Beaty J, editors: Campbell's operative orthopaedics, vol 3, ed 11, Philadelphia, 2007, Mosby, pp 3017-3084.
12. Jones C, Babst R, Anders M: Minimally invasive fracture care. In Schmidt A, Teague D, editors: Orthopaedic knowledge update: trauma, ed 4, Rosemont, IL, 2010, American Academy of Orthopaedic Surgeons, pp 41-49.
13. Donovan S, Brechter J, Sueki D: Tissue injury and healing. In Orthopedic rehabilitation clinical advisor, Maryland Heights, MO, 2010, Mosby, pp 3-16.
14. Kakar S, Einhorn T: Biology and enhancement of skeletal repair. In Browner B, Jupiter J, Levine A et al, editors: Skeletal trauma: basic science, management, and reconstruction, vol 1, ed 4, Philadelphia, 2008, Saunders, pp 33-50.
15. Gould B, Dyer R: Pathophysiology for the health professions, ed 4, St Louis, 2011, Saunders.
16. Roberts D, Lappe J: Management of clients with musculoskeletal trauma or overuse. In Black J, Hawks J, editors: Medical-surgical nursing: clinical management for positive outcomes, ed 8, St Louis, 2009, Saunders, pp 470-543.
17. Smith W, Suzuki T, Tornetta III P: Pelvic fractures: evaluation and acute management. In Schmidt A, Teague D, editors: Orthopaedic knowledge update: trauma, ed 4, Rosemont, IL, 2010, American Academy of Orthopaedic Surgeons, pp 279-292.
18. Sagi HC, Jimenez M: Pelvic fractures: definitive treatment and expected outcomes. In Schmidt A, Teague D, editors: Orthopaedic knowledge update: trauma, ed 4, Rosemont, IL, 2010, American Academy of Orthopaedic Surgeons, pp 293-307.
19. McKinnis L. Radiologic evaluation of the pelvis and hip. In McKinnis L, editor: Fundamentals of musculoskeletal imaging, ed 3, Philadelphia, 2010, FA Davis, pp 333-369.
20. Ahn J, Reilly M, Lorich D et al: Acetabular fractures: acute evaluation. In Schmidt A, Teague D, editors: Orthopaedic knowledge update: trauma, ed 4, Rosemont, IL, 2010, American Academy of Orthopaedic Surgeons, pp 309-321.
21. Porter SE, Schroeder AC, Dzugan SS et al: Acetabular fracture patterns and their associated injuries, J Orthop Trauma 22(3):165-170, 2008.
22. Routt M, Agarwal A: Acetabular fractures: definitive treatment and expected outcomes. In Schmidt A, Teague D, editors: Orthopaedic knowledge update: trauma, ed 4, Rosemont, IL, 2010, American Academy of Orthopaedic Surgeons, pp 323-335.
23. Egol K, Leighton R, Evans A et al: Hip dislocations and femoral head and neck fractures. In Schmidt A, Teague D, editors: Orthopaedic knowledge update: trauma, ed 4, Rosemont, IL, 2010, American Academy of Orthopaedic Surgeons, pp 399-416.
24. LaVelle D: Fractures and dislocations of the hip. In Canale ST, Beaty J, editors: Campbell's operative orthopaedics, vol 3, ed 11, Philadelphia, 2007, Mosby, pp 3237-3308.
25. Nork S, Reilly M: Subtrochanteric fractures of the femur. In Browner B, Jupiter J, Levine A et al, editors: Skeletal trauma: basic science, management, and reconstruction, vol 1, ed 4, Philadelphia, 2008, Saunders, pp 1977-2034.

26. Lee M, Harvey E: Fractures of the proximal femur. In Schmidt A, Teague D, editors: Orthopaedic knowledge update: trauma, ed 4, Rosemont, IL, 2010, American Academy of Orthopaedic Surgeons, pp 417-430.

27. Whittle AP: Fractures of the lower extremity. In Canale ST, Beaty J, editors: Campbell's operative orthopaedics, vol 3, ed 11, Philadelphia, 2007, Mosby, pp 3085-3236.

28. Ricci W, Gruen G, Summers H et al: Fractures of the femoral diaphysis. In Schmidt A, Teague D, editors: Orthopaedic knowledge update: trauma, ed 4, Rosemont, IL, 2010, American Academy of Orthopaedic Surgeons, pp 431-444.

29. Collinge C, Smith J: Fractures of the distal femur. In Schmidt A, Teague D, editors: Orthopaedic knowledge update: trauma, ed 4, Rosemont, IL, 2010, American Academy of Orthopaedic Surgeons, pp 445-459.

30. Bedi A, Karunakar M: Patella fractures and extensor mechanism injuries. In Bucholz R, Heckman J, Court-Brown C et al, editors: Rockwood and Green's fractures in adults, vol 2, ed 7, Philadelphia, 2010, Lippincott Williams & Wilkins, pp 1752-1779.

31. Levy B, Stuart M, Kottmeier S: Knee injuries. In Schmidt A, Teague D, editors: Orthopaedic knowledge update: trauma, ed 4, Rosemont, IL, 2010, American Academy of Orthopaedic Surgeons, pp 461-474.

32. Barei D, Crist B: Fractures of the ankle and distal tibial pilon. In: Schmidt A, Teague D, editors: Orthopaedic knowledge update: trauma, ed 4, Rosemont, IL, 2010, American Academy of Orthopaedic Surgeons, pp 499-518.

33. Tejwani N, Pugh K: Foot injuries. In Schmidt A, Teague D, editors: Orthopaedic knowledge update: trauma, ed 4, Rosemont, IL, 2010, American Academy of Orthopaedic Surgeons, pp 519-531.

34. Oleson C, Simmons N, Mirza S: Principles of spine trauma care. In Bucholz R, Heckman J, Court-Brown C et al, editors: Rockwood and Green's fractures in adults, vol 2, ed 7, Philadelphia, 2010, Lippincott Williams & Wilkins, pp 1279-1311.

35. Krieg J, Green A, Cole P: Shoulder trauma. In Schmidt A, Teague D, editors: Orthopaedic knowledge update: trauma, ed 4, Rosemont, IL, 2010, American Academy of Orthopaedic Surgeons, pp 181-200.

36. Crenshaw A, Perez E: Fractures of the shoulder, arm, and forearm. In Canale ST, Beaty J, editors: Campbell's operative orthopaedics, vol 3, ed 11, Philadelphia, 2007, Mosby, pp 3371-3460.

37. Graves M, Nork S: Fractures of the humerus. In Schmidt A, Teague D, editors: Orthopaedic knowledge update: trauma, ed 4, Rosemont, IL, 2010, American Academy of Orthopaedic Surgeons, pp 201-224.

38. McKee M, Larsson S: Humeral shaft fractures. In Bucholz R, Heckman J, Court-Brown C et al, editors: Rockwood and Green's fractures in adults, vol 1, ed 7, Philadelphia, 2010, Lippincott Williams & Wilkins, pp 999-1038.

39. Schwartz A, Rosenwasser M, White N et al: Fractures of the forearm and distal radius. In Schmidt A, Teague D, editors: Orthopaedic knowledge update: trauma, ed 4, Rosemont, IL, 2010, American Academy of Orthopaedic Surgeons, pp 241-262.

40. Fuller D, Capo J: Injuries of the hand and carpus. In Schmidt A, Teague D, editors: Orthopaedic knowledge update: trauma, ed 4, Rosemont, IL, 2010, American Academy of Orthopaedic Surgeons, pp 263-275.

41. Hansen B, Hallows R, Kelley S: The Rottinger approach for total hip arthroplasty: technique and review of literature, Curr Rev Musculoskelet Med 4:132-138, 2011.

42. Queen R, Butler R, Watters T et al: The effect of total hip arthroplasty surgical approach on postoperative gait mechanics, J Arthroplasty 26(6):66-71, 2011.

43. Palan J, Beard DJ, Murray DW et al: Which approach for total hip arthroplasty: anterolateral or posterior? Clin Orthop Rel Res 467(2):473-477, 2009.

44. Restrepo C, Mortazavi SMJ, Brothers J et al: Hip dislocation: are hip precautions necessary in anterior approaches? Clin Orthop Rel Res 469(2):417-422, 2011.

45. Tejwani NC, Immerman I: Myths and legends in orthopaedic practice: are we all guilty? Clin Orthop Rel Res 466(11): 2861-2872, 2008.

46. Harkess J, Crockarell J: Arthroplasty of the hip. In Canale ST, Beaty J, editors: Operative orthopaedics, vol 1, ed 11, Philadelphia, 2007, Mosby.

47. Husby VS, Helgerud J, Bjørgen S et al: Early postoperative maximal strength training improves work efficiency 6-12 months after osteoarthritis-induced total hip arthroplasty in patients younger than 60 years, Am J Phys Med Rehabil 89(4):304-314, 2010.

48. Robbins C, Bierbaum B, Ward D: Total hip arthroplasty: day of surgery physical therapy intervention, Curr Orthop Pract 20(2):157-160, 2009.

49. Di Monaco M, Vallero F, Tappero R et al: Rehabilitation after total hip arthroplasty: a systematic review of controlled trials on physical exercise programs, Eur J Phys Rehabil Med 45(3):303-317, 2009.

50. Strickland EM, Fares M, Krebs DE et al: In vivo acetabular contact pressures during rehabilitation, part I: acute phase, Phys Ther 72(10):691-699, 1992.

51. Givens-Heiss DL, Krebs DE, Riley PO et al: In vivo acetabular contact pressures during rehabilitation, part II: postacute phase, Phys Ther 72(10):700-705, 1992.

52. Krebs DE, Elbaum L, Riley PO et al: Exercise and gait effects on in vivo hip contact pressures, Phys Ther 71(4):301-309, 1991.

53. Bow JK, Rudan JF, Grant HJ et al: Are hip resurfacing arthroplasties meeting the needs of our patients? A 2-year follow-up study, J Arthroplasty 27(6):984-989, 2012.

54. Corten K, Ganz R, Simon J-P et al: Hip resurfacing arthroplasty: current status and future perspectives, Eur Cell Mater 21:243-258, 2011.

55. Jiang Y, Zhang K, Die J et al: A systematic review of modern metal-on-metal total hip resurfacing vs standard total hip arthroplasty in active young patients, J Arthroplasty 26(3):419-426, 2011.

56. Kohan L, Field CJ, Kerr DR: Early complications of hip resurfacing, J Arthroplasty 27(6):997-1002, 2012.

57. Jensen C, Aagaard P, Overgaard S: Recovery in mechanical muscle strength following resurfacing vs standard total hip arthroplasty—a randomised clinical trial, Osteoarthritis Cartilage 19(9):1108-1116, 2011.

58. Amanatullah D, Cheung Y, Di Cesare P: Hip resurfacing arthroplasty: a review of the evidence for surgical technique, outcome, and complications, Orthop Clin North Am 41: 263-272, 2010.

59. Muirhead-Allwood S, Sandiford N, Kabir C: Total hip resurfacing as an alternative to total hip arthroplasty: indications and precautions, Semin Arthroplasty 19(4):274-282, 2008.

60. Crockarell J, Guyton J: Arthroplasty of the knee. In Canale ST, Beaty J, editors: Campbell's operative orthopaedics, vol 1, ed 11, Philadelphia, 2007, Mosby, pp 241-311.

61. Oh KJ, Pandher DS, Lee SH et al: Meta-analysis comparing outcomes of fixed-bearing and mobile-bearing prostheses in total knee arthroplasty, J Arthroplasty 24(6):873-884, 2009.

62. Post ZD, Matar WY, van de Leur T et al: Mobile-bearing total knee arthroplasty: better than a fixed-bearing? J Arthroplasty 25(6):998-1003, 2010.

63. Sastre S, Sanchez M-D, Lozano L et al: Total knee arthroplasty: better short-term results after subvastus approach. A

randomized, controlled study, Knee Surg Sports Traumatol Arthrosc 17(10):1184-1188, 2009.

64. van Hemert WL, Senden R, Grimm B et al: Early functional outcome after subvastus or parapatellar approach in knee arthroplasty is comparable, Knee Surg Sports Traumatol Arthrosc 19(6):943-951, 2011.

65. Bathis H, Perlick L, Blum C et al: Midvastus approach in total knee arthroplasty: a randomized, double-blinded study on early rehabilitation, Knee Surg Sports Traumatol Arthrosc 13: 545-550, 2005.

66. Bade MJ: Outcomes before and after total knee arthroplasty compared to healthy adults, J Orthop Sports Phys Ther 40(9):559-567, 2010.

67. Lenssen A, Crijns Y, Waltje E et al: Efficiency of immediate postoperative inpatient physical therapy following total knee arthroplasty: an RCT, BMC Musculoskelet Disord 7:71-79, 2006.

68. Meier W: Total knee arthroplasty: muscle impairments, functional limitations and recommended rehabilitation approaches, J Orthop Sports Phys Ther 38(5):246-256, 2008.

69. Denis M, Moffet H, Caron F et al: Effectiveness of continuous passive motion and conventional physical therapy after total knee arthroplasty: a randomized clinical trial, Phys Ther 86(2):174-185, 2006.

70. Zeni JA, Snyder-Mackler L: Early postoperative measures predict 1- and 2-year outcomes after unilateral total knee arthroplasty: importance of contralateral limb strength, Phys Ther 90(1):43-54, 2010.

71. Judd DL, Eckhoff DG, Stevens-Lapsley JE: Muscle strength loss in the lower limb after total knee arthroplasty, Am J Phys Med Rehabil 91(3):220-230, 2012.

72. Stevens-Lapsley J, Balter JE, Kohrt WM et al: Quadriceps and hamstrings muscle dysfunction after total knee arthroplasty, Clin Orthop Rel Res 468:2460-2468, 2010.

73. Piva SR, Gil AB, Almeida GJM et al: A balance exercise program appears to improve function for patients with total knee arthroplasty: a randomized clinical trial, Phys Ther 90(6):880-894, 2010.

74. Liu Z, Yang H: Comparison of the minimally invasive and standard medial parapatellar approaches for total knee arthroplasty: systematic review and meta-analysis, J Int Med Res 39(5):1607-1617, 2011.

75. Reininga IHF, Zijlstra W, Wagenmakers R et al: Minimally invasive and computer-navigated total hip arthroplasty: a qualitative and systematic review of the literature, BMC Musculoskelet Disord 11:92-104, 2010.

76. Stevens-Lapsley JE, Bade MJ, Shulman BC et al: Minimally invasive total knee arthroplasty improves early knee strength but not functional performance: a randomized controlled trial, J Arthroplasty 27(10):1812-1819, 2012. http://www.sciencedirect.com/science/article/pii/S088354031200126X. Accessed May 1, 2012.

77. Smith T, Blake V, Hing C: Minimally invasive versus conventional exposure for total hip arthroplasty: a systematic review and meta-analysis of clinical and radiological outcomes, Int Orthop 35:173-184, 2011.

78. Radnay CS, Setter KJ, Chambers L et al: Total shoulder replacement compared with humeral head replacement for the treatment of primary glenohumeral osteoarthritis: a systematic review, J Shoulder Elbow Surg 16(4):396-402, 2007.

79. Bryant D, Litchfield R, Sandow M et al: A comparison of pain, strength, range of motion, and functional outcomes after hemiarthroplasty and total shoulder arthroplasty in patients with osteoarthritis of the shoulder, J Bone Joint Surg Am 87(9):1947-1956, 2005.

80. Qureshi S, Hsiao A, Klug RA et al: Subscapularis function after total shoulder replacement: Results with lesser tuberosity osteotomy, J Shoulder Elbow Surg 17(1):68-72, 2008.

81. Jandhyala S, Unnithan A, Hughes S et al: Subscapularis tenotomy versus lesser tuberosity osteotomy during total shoulder replacement: a comparison of patient outcomes, J Shoulder Elbow Surg 20(7):1102-1107, 2011.

82. Azar F, Calandruccio J: Arthroplasty of the shoulder and elbow. In Canale ST, Beaty J, editors: Campbell's operative orthopaedics, vol 1, ed 11, Philadelphia, 2007, Mosby, pp 483-557.

83. Wilcox R 3rd, Arslanian L, Millett P: Rehabilitation following total shoulder arthroplasty, J Orthop Sports Phys Ther 35(12):821-836, 2005.

84. Brems JJ: Rehabilitation after total shoulder arthroplasty: current concepts, Semin Arthroplasty 18(1):55-65, 2007.

85. Watson JD, Murthi AM: Conventional shoulder arthroplasty in the athlete, Oper Tech Sports Med 16(1):37-42, 2008.

86. Kelley M, Leggin B: Rehabilitation. In Williams G, Yamaguchi K, Ramsey M et al, editors: Shoulder and elbow arthroplasty, Philadelphia, 2005, Lippincott Williams & Wilkins, pp 255-268.

87. Sebelski C, Guanche C: Total shoulder arthroplasty. In Maxey L, Magnusson J, editors: Rehabilitation for the postsurgical orthopedic patient, ed 2, St Louis, 2007, Mosby, pp 113-137.

88. Hatzidakis A, Norris T, Boileau P: Reverse shoulder arthroplasty indications, technique, and results, Tech Shoulder Elbow Surg 6(3):135-149, 2005.

89. Mahfouz M, Nicholson G, Komistek R et al: In vivo determination of the dynamics of normal, rotator cuff-deficient, total, and reverse replacement shoulders, J Bone Joint Surg Am 87(Suppl 2):107-113, 2005.

90. Ekelund A, Seebauer L: Advanced evaluation and management of glenohumeral arthritis in the cuff-deficient shoulder. In Rockwood C Jr, Matsen III F, Wirth M et al, editors: The shoulder, vol 1, ed 4, Philadelphia, 2009, Saunders, pp 1247-1276.

91. Heck R Jr: General principles of tumors. In Canale ST, Beaty J, editors: Campbell's operative orthopaedics, vol 1, ed 11, Philadelphia, 2007, Mosby, pp 775-854.

92. Goodman C: Musculoskeletal neoplasms. In Pathology: implications for the physical therapist, ed 3, St Louis, 2009, Saunders, pp 1201-1234.

93. Karla S, Abuda A, Murata H et al: Total femur replacement: primary procedure for treatment of malignant tumours of the femur, Eur J Surg Oncol 36:378-383, 2010.

94. Parrish W: Hip disarticulation and hemi-pelvectomy, Oper Tech Gen Surg 7(2):96-101, 2005.

95. Griesser MJ, Gillette B, Crist M et al: Internal and external hemipelvectomy or flail hip in patients with sarcomas, Am J Phys Med Rehabil 91(1):24-32, 2012.

96. Anderson DG, Samartzis D, Shen F et al: Percutaneous instrumentation of the thoracic and lumbar spine, Orthop Clin North Am 38:401-408, 2007.

97. Marcus J, James A, Hartl R: Minimally invasive surgical treatment options for lumbar disc herniations and stenosis, Semin Spine Surg 23:20-26, 2011.

98. Williams K, Park A: Low back pain and disorders of intervertebral discs. In Canale ST, Beaty J, editors: Campbell's operative orthopaedics, vol 2, ed 11, Philadelphia, 2007, Mosby, pp 2159-2236.

99. Mayer HM: Total lumbar disc replacement, J Bone Joint Surg Brit Vol 87-B(8):1029-1037, 2005.

100. van den Eerenbeemt KD, Ostelo RW, van Royen BJ et al: Total disc replacement surgery for symptomatic degenerative lumbar disc disease: a systematic review of the literature, Eur Spine J 19(8):1262-1280, 2010.

101. Yu L, Song Y, Yang X et al: Systematic review and meta-analysis of randomized controlled trials: comparison of total disc replacement with anterior cervical decompression and fusion, Orthopedics 34(10):e651-658, 2011.

102. Berg S, Tullberg T, Branth B et al: Total disc replacement compared to lumbar fusion: a randomised controlled trial with 2-year follow-up, Eur Spine J 18(10):1512-1519, 2009.

103. Canbulat N, Sasani M, Ataker Y et al: A rehabilitation protocol for patients with lumbar degenerative disc disease treated with lumbar total disc replacement, Arch Phys Med Rehabil 92(4):670-676, 2011.

104. Ostelo RWJG, Pena Costa LO, Maher CG et al: Rehabilitation after lumbar disc surgery, Spine 34(17):1839-1848, 2009.

105. Kulig K, Beneck GJ, Selkowitz DM et al: An intensive, progressive exercise program reduces disability and improves functional performance in patients after single-level lumbar microdiscectomy, Phys Ther 89(11):1145-1157, 2009.

106. Hebert J, Marcus R, Koppenhaver S et al: Postoperative rehabilitation following lumbar discectomy with quantification of trunk muscle morphology and function: a case report and review of the literature, J Orthop Sports Phys Ther 40(7): 402-412, 2010.

107. Klazen CA, Lohle PN, de Vries J et al: Vertebroplasty versus conservative treatment in acute osteoporotic vertebral compression fractures (Vertos II): an open-label randomised trial, Lancet 376(9746):1085-1092, 2010.

108. Voormolen MHJ, Mali WPTM, Lohle PNM et al: Percutaneous vertebroplasty compared with optimal pain medication treatment: short-term clinical outcome of patients with subacute or chronic painful osteoporotic vertebral compression fractures. The VERTOS Study, Am J Neuroradiol 28(3):555-560, 2007.

109. Rousing R, Hansen KL, Andersen MO et al: Twelve-months follow-up in forty-nine patients with acute/semiacute osteoporotic vertebral fractures treated conservatively or with percutaneous vertebroplasty, Spine 35(5):478-482, 2010.

110. Wood G 2nd: Fracture, dislocations, and fracture-dislocations of the spine. In Canale ST, Beaty J, editors: Campbell's operative orthopaedics, vol 2, ed 11, Philadelphia, 2007, Mosby, pp 1761-1850.

111. Pateder D, Khanna AJ, Lieberman I: Vertebroplasty and kyphoplasty for the management of osteoporotic vertebral compression fractures, Orthop Clin North Am 38:409-418, 2007.

112. Cahoj P, Cook J, Robinson B: Efficacy of percutaneous vertebral augmentation and use of physical therapy intervention following vertebral compression fractures in older adults: a systematic review, J Geriatr Phys Ther 30(1):31-40, 2007.

113. Boonen S, Van Meirhaeghe J, Bastian L et al: Balloon kyphoplasty for the treatment of acute vertebral compression fractures: 2-year results from a randomized trial, J Bone Mineral Res 26(7):1627-1637, 2011.

114. Azar F: General principles of arthroscopy. In Canale ST, Beaty J, editors: Campbell's operative orthopedics, vol 3, ed 11, Philadelphia, 2007, Mosby, pp 2789-2810.

115. Halanski M, Noonan KJ: Cast and splint immobilization: complications, J Am Acad Orthop Surg 16(1):30-40, 2008.

116. Prasarn ML, Ouellette EA: Acute compartment syndrome of the upper extremity, J Am Acad Orthop Surg 19(1):49-58, 2011.

117. Olson SA, Glasgow RR: Acute compartment syndrome in lower extremity musculoskeletal trauma, J Am Acad Orthop Surg 13(7):436-444, 2005.

118. Lavini F, Dall'Oca C, Renzi Brivio L: Principles of monolateral external fixation. In Bulstrode C, editor: Oxford textbook of trauma and orthopaedics, ed 2, Oxford, England, 2011, Oxford University Press, pp 952-967.

119. Watson JT: Principles of external fixation. In Bucholz R, Heckman J, Court-Brown C et al, editors: Rockwood and Green's fractures in adults, vol 1, ed 7, Philadelphia, 2010, Lippincott Williams & Wilkins, pp 191-243.

120. DeCoster TA, Xing Z: Femur shaft fractures. In Bulstrode C, editor: Oxford textbook of trauma and orthopaedics, ed 2, Oxford, England, 2011, Oxford University Press, pp 1328-1337.

121. Court-Brown C: Principles of nonoperative fracture treatment. In Bucholz R, Heckman J, Court-Brown C et al, editors: Rockwood and Green's fractures in adults, vol 1, ed 7, Philadelphia, 2010, Lippincott Williams & Wilkins, pp 124-161.

CHAPTER 6

Nervous System

Hillary A. Reinhold
Michele P. West

CHAPTER OBJECTIVES

The objectives of this chapter are to provide the following:

1. Provide a brief review of the structure and function of the nervous system
2. Give an overview of neurologic evaluation, including the physical examination and diagnostic tests
3. Describe common neurologic diseases and disorders, including clinical findings, medical and surgical management, and physical therapy interventions

PREFERRED PRACTICE PATTERNS

The most relevant practice patterns for the diagnoses discussed in this chapter, based on the American Physical Therapy Association's *Guide to Physical Therapist Practice*, second edition, are as follows:

- Common Degenerative Central Nervous System Diseases (Amyotrophic Lateral Sclerosis, Guillain-Barré Syndrome, Multiple Sclerosis, Parkinson's Disease, Huntington's Disease): 5A, 5E, 5G, 6B, 6E, 7A
- Vestibular Dysfunction (Bilateral Vestibular Hypofunction, Ménière's Disease, Acute Vestibular Neuronitis, Benign Positional Paroxysmal Vertigo, Vertigo, Lightheadedness, Dysequilibrium): 5A
- Neuroinfectious diseases (Encephalitis, Meningitis, and Poliomyelitis [more information in Chapter 13]): 4A, 5C, 5D, 5G, 5H, 6E, 7A
- Syncope: 5A
- Seizure (Status Epilepticus, Epilepsy, Simple Partial Seizures, Complex Partial Seizures, Tonic-Clonic Seizures): 5A, 5C, 5D, 5E
- Ventricular Dysfunction (Cerebrospinal Fluid Leak and Hydrocephalus): 5C, 5D
- Spinal Cord Injury: 5H, 7A, 7C
- Traumatic Brain Injury: 5C, 5D, 5I
- Cerebrovascular Disease and Disorders (Transient Ischemic Attack, Cerebrovascular Accident, Dementia, Subarachnoid Hemorrhage, Arteriovenous Malformation and Cerebral Aneurysm): 5C, 5D, 5I, 6E, 6F, 7A

Please refer to Appendix A for a complete list of the preferred practice patterns, as individual patient conditions are highly variable and other practice patterns may be applicable.

The nervous system is linked to every system of the body and is responsible for the integration and regulation of homeostasis. It is also involved in the action, communication, and higher cortical function of the body. A neurologic insult and its manifestations therefore have the potential to affect multiple body systems. To safely and effectively prevent or improve the neuromuscular, systemic, and functional sequelae of altered neurologic status in the acute care setting, the physical therapist requires an understanding of the neurologic system and the principles of neuropathology.

Body Structure and Function of the Nervous System

The nervous system is divided as follows:
- The central nervous system (CNS), consisting of the brain and spinal cord
- The peripheral nervous system, consisting of efferent and afferent nerves outside the CNS

The peripheral nervous system is divided into:
- The autonomic (involuntary) nervous system, consisting of the sympathetic and parasympathetic systems innervating the viscera, smooth muscles, and glands
- The somatic (voluntary) nervous system, consisting of efferent and afferent nerves to all parts of the body except the viscera, smooth muscles, and glands

Central Nervous System

Brain

The brain is anatomically divided into the cerebral hemispheres, diencephalon, brain stem, and cerebellum. A midsagittal view of the brain is shown in Figure 6-1, *A*. Figure 6-1, *B* shows the basal ganglia and the internal capsule. Although each portion of the brain has its own function, it is linked to other portions via tracts and rarely works in isolation. When lesions occur, disruption of these functions can be predicted. Tables 6-1 and 6-2 describe the basic structure, function, and dysfunction

of the cerebral hemispheres, diencephalon, brain stem, and cerebellum.

Protective Mechanisms. The brain is protected by the cranium, meninges, ventricular system, and blood-brain barrier.

Cranium. The cranium encloses the brain. It is composed of eight cranial and 14 facial bones connected by sutures and contains approximately 85 foramina for the passage of the spinal cord, cranial nerves (CNs), and blood vessels.[1] The cranium is divided into the cranial vault, or calvaria (the superolateral and posterior aspects), and the cranial floor, which is composed of fossae (the anterior fossa supports the frontal lobes; the middle fossa supports the temporal lobes; and the posterior fossa supports the cerebellum, pons, and medulla).[2]

Meninges. The meninges are three layers of connective tissue that cover the brain and spinal cord. The dura mater, the outermost layer, lines the skull (periosteum) and has four major folds (Table 6-3). The arachnoid, the middle layer, loosely encloses the brain. The pia mater, the inner layer, covers the convolutions of the brain and forms a portion of the choroid plexus in the ventricular system. The three layers create very

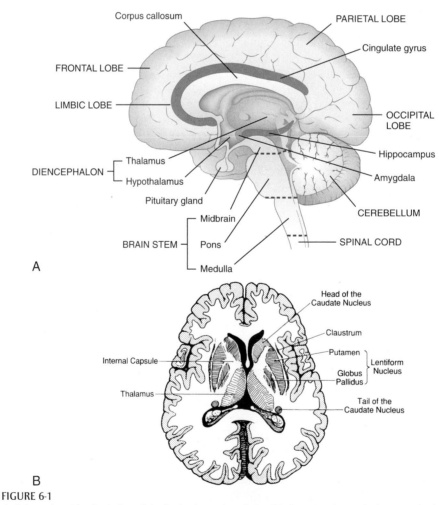

FIGURE 6-1

A, Schematic midsagittal view of the brain shows the relationship between the cerebral cortex, cerebellum, spinal cord, and brainstem and the subcortical structures important to functional movement. **B,** Horizontal section of the cerebrum showing the basal ganglia. (**A,** From Cech DJ, Martin ST: Functional movement development across the life span, ed 3, St Louis, 2012, Saunders. **B,** From Love RJ, Webb WG, editors: Neurology for the speech-language pathologist, ed 4, Boston, 2001, Butterworth-Heinemann, p 38.)

TABLE 6-1 Structure, Function, and Dysfunction of the Cerebral Hemispheres

Lobe of Cerebrum	Structure	Function	Dysfunction
Frontal lobe	Precentral gyrus	Voluntary motor cortex of contralateral face, arm, trunk, and leg	Contralateral mono- or hemiparesis or hemiplegia
	Supplementary motor area	Advanced motor planning	Contralateral head and eye paralysis
		Contralateral head and eye turning (connections to cranial nerves III, IV, VI, IX, X, and XII nuclei)	Akinesia or inability to perform complex tasks
	Prefrontal pole	Personality center, including abstract ideas, concern for others, conscience, initiative, judgment, persistence, and planning	Loss of inhibition and demonstration of antisocial behaviors
			Ataxia, primitive reflexes, and hypertonicity
	Paracentral lobule	Bladder and bowel inhibition	Urinary and bowel incontinence
	Broca's area	D: Motor speech center	Broca's (expressive) aphasia
		ND: Appreciation of intonation and gestures with vocalization	
Parietal lobe	Postcentral gyrus	Somatosensory cortex of contralateral pain; posture; proprioception; touch of arm, trunk, and leg	Contralateral sensation loss
	Parietal pole	D: Ability to perform calculations	D: Acalculia, agraphia, finger agnosia
		ND: Ability to construct shapes, awareness of external environment, and body image	ND: Constructional apraxia, geographic agnosia, dressing apraxia, anosognosia
	Wernicke's area	D: Sensory speech (auditory and written) comprehension center	Wernicke's (receptive) aphasia
		ND: Appreciation of content of emotional language (e.g., tone of voice)	
	Optic radiation	Visual tract	Lower homonymous quadrantanopia
	Gustatory cortex	Perception of taste	Dysfunction is very uncommon
Temporal lobe	Superior temporal gyrus (auditory cortex)	D: Appreciation of language	D: Decreased ability to hear
		ND: Appreciation of music, rhythm, and sound	ND: Decreased ability to appreciate music
	Middle and inferior temporal gyri	Learning and memory centers	Learning and memory deficits
	Limbic lobe and olfactory cortex	Affective and emotion center, including mood, primitive behavior, self-preservation, short-term memory, visceral emotion processes, and interpretation of smell	Aggressive or antisocial behaviors Inability to establish new memories
	Wernicke's area	See Parietal lobe, above	Wernicke's (receptive) aphasia
	Optic radiation	Visual tract	Upper homonymous quadrantanopia
Occipital lobe	Striate and parastriate cortices	Perception of vision (visual cortex)	Homonymous hemianopsia with or without macular involvement

Data from Gilman S, Newman SW, editors: Manter and Gatz's essentials of clinical neuroanatomy and neurophysiology, ed 7, Philadelphia, 1989, FA Davis; Kiernan JA, editor: Introduction to human neuroscience, Philadelphia, 1987, Lippincott; Marieb EN, editor: Human anatomy and physiology, ed 5, San Francisco, 2001, Benjamin-Cummings; Thelan L, Davie J, Lough M, editors: Critical care nursing: diagnosis and management, ed 2, St Louis, 1994, Mosby; Mancell EL, editor: Gray's clinical neuroanatomy: the anatomic basis for clinical neuroscience, Philadelphia, 2011, Elsevier Saunders; O'Sullivan SB, Schmitz TJ, editors: Physical rehabilitation, ed 5, Philadelphia, 2007, FA Davis.

D, Dominant; *ND,* nondominant.

important anatomic and potential spaces in the brain, as shown in Figure 6-2 and described in Table 6-4.

Ventricular System. The ventricular system nourishes the brain and acts as a cushion by increasing the buoyancy of the brain. It consists of four ventricles and a series of foramina, through which cerebrospinal fluid (CSF) passes to surround the CNS. CSF is a colorless, odorless solution produced by the choroid plexus of all ventricles at a rate of 400 to 500 ml per day.[2] CSF circulates in a pulse-like fashion through the

ventricles and around the spinal cord with the beating of ependymal cilia that line the ventricles and intracranial blood volume changes that occur with breathing and cardiac systole.[3] The flow of CSF under normal conditions, as shown in Figure 6-3, is as follows[4]:

- From the lateral ventricles via the interventricular foramen to the third ventricle
- From the third ventricle to the fourth ventricle via the cerebral aqueduct

TABLE 6-2 Structure, Function, and Dysfunction of the Diencephalon, Brain Stem, and Cerebellum

Brain Structure	Substructure	Function	Dysfunction
Diencephalon			
Thalamus	Specific and association nuclei	Cortical arousal Integrative relay station for all ascending and descending motor stimuli and all ascending sensory stimuli except smell Memory	Altered consciousness Signs and symptoms of increased ICP Contralateral hemiplegia, hemiparesis, or hemianesthesia Altered eye movement Thalamic pain syndrome
Hypothalamus	Mamillary bodies Optic chiasm Infundibulum (stalk) connects to the pituitary gland Forms inferolateral wall of third ventricle	Autonomic center for sympathetic and parasympathetic responses Visceral center for regulation of body temperature, food intake, thirst, sleep and wake cycle, water balance Produces ADH and oxytocin Regulates anterior pituitary gland Association with limbic system	Altered autonomic function and vital signs Headache Visual deficits Vomiting with signs and symptoms of increased ICP See Chapter 10 for more information on hormones and endocrine disorders
Epithalamus	Pineal body Posterior commissure, striae medullares, habenular nuclei and commissure	Association with limbic system	Dysfunction unknown
Subthalamus	Substantia nigra Red nuclei	Association with thalamus for motor control	Dyskinesia and decreased motor control
Pituitary	Anterior and posterior lobes	Production, storage, and secretion of reproductive hormones Secretion of ADH and oxytocin	See Chapter 10 for more information on hormones and endocrine disorders
Internal capsule	Fiber tracts connecting thalamus to the cortex	Conduction pathway between the cortex and spinal cord	Contralateral hemiparesis or hemiplegia and hemianesthesia
Brain Stem			
Midbrain	Superior cerebellar peduncles Superior and inferior colliculi Medial and lateral lemniscus CNs III and IV nuclei Reticular formation Cerebral aqueduct in its center	Conduction pathway between higher and lower brain centers Visual reflex Auditory reflex	Contralateral hemiparesis or hemiplegia and hemianesthesia, altered consciousness and respiratory pattern, cranial nerve palsy
Pons	Middle cerebellar peduncles Respiratory center CNs V-VIII nuclei Forms anterior wall of fourth ventricle	Conduction pathway between higher and lower brain centers	See Midbrain, above
Medulla	Decussation of pyramidal tracts Inferior cerebellar peduncles Inferior olivary nuclei Nucleus cuneatus and gracilis CNs IX-XII nuclei	Homeostatic center for cardiac, respiratory, vasomotor functions	See Midbrain, above
Cerebellum			
Anterior lobe	Medial portion Lateral portion	Sensory and motor input of trunk Sensory and motor input of extremities for coordination of gait	Ipsilateral ataxia and discoordination or tremor of extremities
Posterior lobe	Medial and lateral portions	Sensory and motor input for coordination of motor skills and postural tone	Ipsilateral ataxia and discoordination of the trunk
Flocculonodular	Flocculus nodule	Sensory input from ears Sensory and motor input from eyes and head for coordination of balance and eye and head movement	Ipsilateral facial sensory loss and Horner's syndrome, nystagmus, visual overshooting Loss of balance

Data from Gilman S, Newman SW, editors: Manter and Gatz's essentials of clinical neuroanatomy and neurophysiology, ed 7, Philadelphia, 1989, FA Davis; Kiernan JA, editor: Introduction to human neuroscience, Philadelphia, 1987, Lippincott; Marieb EN, editor: Human anatomy and physiology, ed 5, San Francisco, 2001, Benjamin-Cummings; Thelan L, Davie J, Lough M, editors: Critical care nursing: diagnosis and management, ed 2, St Louis, 1994, Mosby; Mancell EL, editor: Gray's clinical neuroanatomy: the anatomic basis for clinical neuroscience, Philadelphia, 2011, Elsevier Saunders; O'Sullivan SB, Schmitz TJ, editors: Physical rehabilitation, ed 5, Philadelphia, 2007, FA Davis.
ADH, Antidiuretic hormone; *CN*, cranial nerve; *ICP*, intracranial pressure.

TABLE 6-3 Dural Folds

Falx cerebri	Vertical fold that separates the two cerebral hemispheres to prevent horizontal displacement of these structures
Falx cerebelli	Vertical fold that separates the two cerebellar hemispheres to prevent horizontal displacement of these structures
Tentorium cerebelli	Horizontal fold that separates occipital lobes from the cerebellum to prevent vertical displacement of these structures
Diaphragm sellae	Horizontal fold that separates the subarachnoid space from the sella turcica and is perforated by the stalk of the pituitary gland

Data from Wilkinson JL, editor: Neuroanatomy for medical students, ed 3, Oxford, UK, 1998, Butterworth-Heinemann.

TABLE 6-4 Dural Spaces

Epidural (extradural) space	Potential space between the skull and outer dura mater
Subdural space	Potential space between the dura and the arachnoid mater; a split in the dura contains the venous sinus
Subarachnoid space	Anatomic space between the arachnoid and pia mater containing cerebrospinal fluid and the vascular supply of the cortex

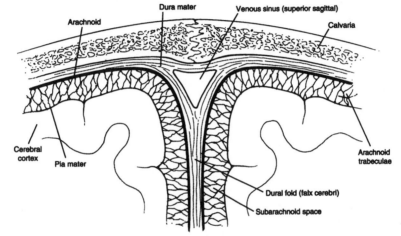

FIGURE 6-2
Coronal section of cranial meninges showing a venous sinus and dural fold. (From Young PA, Young PH: Basic clinical neuroanatomy, Philadelphia, 1997, Williams & Wilkins, p 8.)

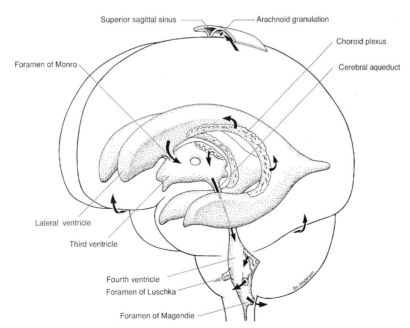

FIGURE 6-3
The ventricular system of the brain. Arrows indicate the circulation of cerebrospinal fluid from the site of formation in the choroid plexus to the site of absorption in the villi of the sagittal sinus. (From Bogousslavsky J, Fisher M, editors: Textbook of neurology, Boston, 1998, Butterworth-Heinemann, p 656.)

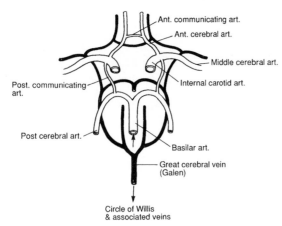

FIGURE 6-4
Schematic representation of the arterial circle of Willis and accompanying veins. *Ant.,* Anterior; *art.,* artery; *Post.,* posterior. (From Gonzalez EG, Meyers SJ, editors: Downey and Darling's physiological basis of rehabilitation medicine, ed 3, Boston, 2001, Butterworth-Heinemann, p 22.)

- From the fourth ventricle to the cisterns, subarachnoid space, and spinal cord via the median and lateral apertures

When ventricular pressure is greater than venous pressure, CSF is absorbed into the venous system via the arachnoid villi, capillary walls of the pia mater, and lymphatics of the subarachnoid space near the optic nerve.[2]

Blood-Brain Barrier. The blood-brain barrier is the physiologic mechanism responsible for keeping toxins, such as amino acids, hormones, ions, and urea, from altering neuronal firing of the brain. It readily allows water, oxygen, carbon dioxide, glucose, some amino acids, and substances that are highly soluble in fat (e.g., alcohol, nicotine, and anesthetic agents) to pass across the barrier.[5,6] The barrier consists of fused endothelial cells on a basement membrane that is surrounded by astrocytic foot extensions.[6] Substances must therefore pass through, rather than around, these cells. The blood-brain barrier is absent near the hypothalamus, pineal region, anterior third ventricle, and floor of the fourth ventricle.[3]

Central Brain Systems. The central brain systems are the reticular activating system and the limbic system. The reticular activating system (RAS) is composed of an ascending tract and a descending tract. The ascending RAS is responsible for human consciousness level and integrates the functions of the brain stem with cortical, cerebellar, thalamic, hypothalamic, and sensory receptor functions.[5] The descending RAS promotes spinal cord antigravity reflexes or extensor tone needed to maintain standing.[7]

The limbic system is a complex interactive system, with primary connections between the cortex, hypothalamus, amygdala, and sensory receptors. The limbic system plays a major role in memory, emotion, and visceral and motor responses involved in defense and reproduction by mediating cortical autonomic function of internal and external stimuli.[8,9]

Circulation. The brain receives blood from the internal carotid and vertebral arteries, which are linked together by the circle of Willis, as shown in Figure 6-4. Each vessel supplies blood to a certain part of the brain (Table 6-5). The circulation of the brain is discussed in terms of a single vessel or by region

TABLE 6-5 Blood Supply of the Major Areas of the Brain

Artery	Area of Perfusion
Anterior Circulation	
Internal carotid artery (ICA)	The dura, optic tract, basal ganglia, midbrain, uncus, lateral geniculate body, pituitary gland, trigeminal ganglion, and tympanic cavity. Ophthalmic branch supplies the eyes and orbits
External carotid artery (ECA)	All structures external to the skull, the larynx, and the thyroid
Anterior cerebral artery (ACA)	Medial and superior surface of frontal and parietal lobes. Medial striate branch supplies anterior portion of the internal capsule, optic chiasm and nerve, portions of the hypothalamus, and basal ganglia
Middle cerebral artery (MCA)	Lateral surface of the frontal, parietal, and occipital lobes, including the superior and lateral surfaces of temporal lobes, posterior portion of the internal capsule, and portions of the basal ganglia
Posterior Circulation	
Vertebral artery	Medulla, dura of the posterior fossa, including the falx cerebri and tentorium cerebelli
Basilar artery	Pons, midbrain, internal ear, cerebellum
Posterior inferior cerebellar artery (PICA)	Posterior and inferior surface of the cerebellum, choroid plexus of the fourth ventricle
Anterior inferior cerebellar artery (AICA)	Anterior surface of the cerebellum, flocculus, and inferior vermis
Superior cerebellar artery (SCA)	Superior surface of the cerebellum and vermis
Posterior cerebral artery (PCA)	Occipital lobe and medial and lateral surfaces of the temporal lobes, thalamus, lateral geniculate bodies, hippocampus, and choroid plexus of the third and lateral ventricles

Data from Rumbaugh CL, Wang A, Tsai FY, editors: Cerebrovascular disease imaging and interventional treatment options, New York, 1995, Igaku-Shoin Medical Publishers; Moore KI, Dalley AF, editors: Clinically oriented anatomy, ed 4, Baltimore, 1999, Lippincott Williams & Wilkins; O'Sullivan SB, Schmitz TJ, editors: Physical rehabilitation, ed 5, Philadelphia, 2007, FA Davis.

(usually as the anterior or posterior circulation). There are several anastomotic systems of the cerebral vasculature that provide essential blood flow to the brain. Blood is drained from the brain through a series of venous sinuses. The superior sagittal sinus, with its associated lacunae and villi, is the primary drainage site. The superior sagittal sinus and sinuses located in the dura and scalp then drain blood into the internal jugular vein for return to the heart.

Spinal Cord

The spinal cord lies within the spinal column and extends from the foramen magnum to the first lumbar vertebra, where it

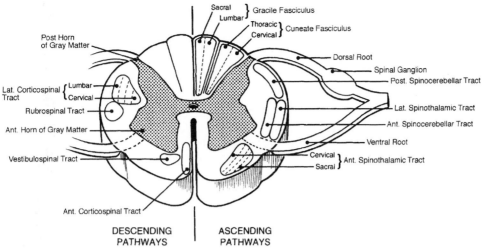

FIGURE 6-5

Cross-section of the spinal cord. *Ant.*, Anterior; *Lat.*, lateral; *Post.*, posterior. (From Love RJ, Webb WG, editors: Neurology for the speech-language pathologist, ed 4, Boston, 2001, Butterworth-Heinemann, p 44.)

forms the conus medullaris and the cauda equina and attaches to the coccyx via the filum terminale. Divided into the cervical, thoracic, and lumbar portions, it is protected by mechanisms similar to those supporting the brain. The spinal cord is composed of gray and white matter and provides the pathway for the ascending and descending tracts, as shown in cross-section in Figure 6-5 and outlined in Table 6-6.

Peripheral Nervous System

The peripheral nervous system consists of the cranial and spinal nerves and the reflex system. The primary structures include peripheral nerves, associated ganglia, and sensory receptors. There are 12 pairs of CNs, each with a unique pathway and function (sensory, motor, mixed, or autonomic). Thirty-one pairs of spinal nerves (all mixed) exit the spinal cord to form distinct plexuses (except T2 to T12). The peripheral nerves of the trunk and the upper and lower extremities are listed in Table 6-7, and the dermatomal system is shown in Figure 6-6. The reflex system includes spinal, deep tendon, stretch, and superficial reflexes and protective responses.

Autonomic Nervous System

The portion of the peripheral nervous system that innervates glands and cardiac and smooth muscle is the autonomic nervous system. The parasympathetic division is activated in times of rest, whereas the sympathetic division is activated in times of work or "fight or flight" situations. The two divisions work closely together, with dual innervation of most organs, to ensure homeostasis.

Neurologic Examination

The neurologic examination is initiated on hospital admission or in the field and is reassessed continuously, hourly, or daily, as necessary. The neurologic examination consists of patient

TABLE 6-6 Major Ascending and Descending White Matter Tracts*

Tract	Function
Fasciculus gracilis	Sensory pathway for lower-extremity and lower-trunk joint proprioception, vibration, two-point discrimination, graphesthesia, and double simultaneous stimulation
Fasciculus cuneatus	Sensory pathway for upper-extremity, upper-trunk, and neck joint proprioception, vibration, two-point discrimination, graphesthesia, and double simultaneous stimulation
Lateral spinothalamic	Sensory pathway for pain, temperature, and light touch
Ventral spinocerebellar	Sensory pathway for ipsilateral subconscious proprioception
Dorsal spinocerebellar	Sensory pathway for ipsilateral and contralateral subconscious proprioception
Lateral corticospinal (pyramidal)	Motor pathway for contralateral voluntary fine-muscle movement
Anterior corticospinal (pyramidal)	Motor pathway for ipsilateral voluntary movement
Rubrospinal (extrapyramidal)	Motor pathway for gross postural tone
Tectospinal (extrapyramidal)	Motor pathway for contralateral gross postural muscle tone associated with auditory and visual stimuli
Vestibulospinal (extrapyramidal)	Motor pathway for ipsilateral gross postural adjustments associated with head movements

Data from Gilman S, Newman SW, editors: Manter and Gatz's essentials of clinical neuroanatomy and neurophysiology, ed 7, Philadelphia, 1989, FA Davis; Marieb EN, editor: Human anatomy and physiology, ed 5, San Francisco, 2001, Benjamin-Cummings.

*Sensory tracts ascend from the spinal cord; motor tracts descend from the brain to the spinal cord.

TABLE 6-7 Major Peripheral Nerves of the Trunk, Upper Extremity, and Lower Extremity

Nerve	Spinal Root	Innervation
Trunk		
Spinal accessory	C3 and C4	Trapezius
Phrenic	C3, C4, and C5	Diaphragm
Long thoracic	C5, C6, and C7	Serratus anterior
Medial pectoral	C6, C7, and C8	Pectoralis minor and major
Lateral pectoral	C7, C8, and T1	Pectoralis major
Thoracodorsal	C7 and C8	Latissimus dorsi
Intercostal	Corresponds to nerve root level	External intercostals, internal intercostals, levatores costarum longi and brevis
Iliohypogastric and ilioinguinal	L1	Transversus abdominis, internal abdominal oblique
Upper Extremity		
Dorsal scapular	C5	Levator scapulae, rhomboid major and minor
Suprascapular	C5 and C6	Supraspinatus, infraspinatus, and glenohumeral joint
Lower subscapular	C5 and C6	Teres major and inferior portion of subscapularis
Upper subscapular	C5 and C6	Superior portion of subscapularis
Axillary	C5 and C6	Teres minor, deltoid, and glenohumeral joint
Radial	C5, C6, C7, C8, and T1	Triceps, brachioradialis, anconeus, extensor carpi radialis longus and brevis, supinator, extensor carpi ulnaris, extensor digitorum, extensor digiti minimi, extensor indicis, extensor pollicis longus and brevis, abductor pollicis brevis
Ulnar	C8 and T1	Flexor digitorum profundus, flexor carpi ulnaris, palmaris brevis, abductor digiti minimi, flexor digiti minimi brevis, opponens digiti minimi, palmar and dorsal interossei, third and fourth lumbricals
Median	C6, C7, C8, and T1	Pronator teres, flexor carpi radialis, palmaris longus, flexor digitorum superficialis and profundus, flexor pollicis longus, pronator quadratus, abductor pollicis brevis, opponens pollicis, flexor pollicis brevis, first and second lumbricals
Musculocutaneous	C5, C6, and C7	Coracobrachialis, brachialis, biceps
Lower Extremity		
Femoral	L2, L3, and L4	Iliacus, psoas major, sartorius, pectinous, rectus femoris, vastus lateralis, intermedius, and medialis, articularis genu
Obturator	L2, L3, and L4	Obturator externus, adductor brevis, longus, and magnus, gracilis, pectineus
Superior gluteal	L4, L5, and S1	Gluteus medius and minimus, tensor fasciae latae
Inferior gluteal	L5, S1, and S2	Gluteus maximus
Sciatic	L4, L5, S1, S2, and S3	Biceps femoris, adductor magnus, semitendinosus, semimembranosus
Tibial	L4, L5, S1, S2, and S3	Gastrocnemius, soleus, flexor digitorum longus, tibialis posterior, flexor hallucis longus
Common peroneal	L4, L5, S1, and S2	Peroneus longus and brevis, tibialis anterior, extensor digitorum longus, extensor hallucis longus, extensor hallucis brevis, extensor digitorum brevis

Data from Netter FH, editor: Atlas of human anatomy, Summit City, NJ, 1989, Ciba-Geigy; Moore KL, Dalley AF, editors: Clinically oriented anatomy, ed 4, Baltimore, 1999, Lippincott Williams & Wilkins.

history; observation; mental status examination; vital sign measurement; vision, motor, sensory, and coordination testing; and diagnostic testing.

Patient History

A detailed history, initially taken by the physician, is often the most helpful information used to delineate whether a patient presents with a true neurologic event or another process (usually cardiac or metabolic in nature). The history may be presented by the patient or, more commonly, by a family member or person witnessing the acute or progressive event(s) responsible for hospital admission. One common framework for organizing questions regarding each neurologic complaint, sign, or symptom is as follows[10,11]:

- What is the patient feeling?
- When did the problem initially occur, and has it progressed?
- What relieves or exacerbates the problem?
- What are the onset, frequency, and duration of signs or symptoms?

In addition to the general medical record review (see Chapter 2), questions relevant to a complete neurologic history include:

- Does the problem involve loss of consciousness?
- Did a fall precede or follow the problem?
- Is there headache, dizziness, or visual disturbance?
- What are the functional deficits associated with the problem?
- Is there an alteration of speech?

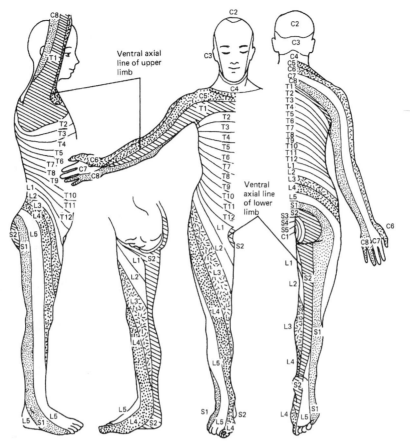

FIGURE 6-6
Dermatome chart based on embryologic segments. (From Maitland GD, editor: Vertebral manipulation, ed 5, Oxford, UK, 1986, Butterworth-Heinemann, p 46.)

- Does the patient demonstrate memory loss or altered cognition?
- Does the patient have an altered sleep pattern?
- What is the handedness of the patient? (Handedness is a predictor of brain [language] dominance.)

Observation

Data that can be gathered from close or distant observation of the patient include the following:
- Level of alertness, arousal, distress, or the need for restraint
- Body position
- Head, trunk, and extremity posture, including movement patterns
- Amount and quality of active movement
- Amount and quality of interaction with the environment or family members
- Degree of ease or difficulty with activities of daily living
- Presence of involuntary movements, such as tremor
- Eye movement(s)
- Presence of hemibody or hemispace neglect
- Presence of muscle atrophy
- Respiratory rate and pattern
- Facial expression and symmetry

The therapist should correlate these observations with other information from the chart review and other health care team members to determine:

1. If the diagnosis is consistent with the physical presentation,
2. What types of commands or tone of voice to use,
3. How much assistance is needed, and
4. How to prioritize the portions of the physical therapy evaluation.

Mental Status Examination

The mental status examination includes assessment of level of consciousness, cognition, emotional state, memory, and speech and language ability.

Level of Consciousness

Consciousness consists of arousal and the awareness of self and environment, including the ability to interact appropriately in response to any normal stimulus.[12] Coma is often considered the opposite of consciousness. Table 6-8 describes the different states of consciousness. Evaluating a patient's level of consciousness is important because it serves as a baseline to monitor stability, improvement, or decline in the patient's condition. It also helps to determine the severity and prognosis of neurologic insult or disease state, thus directing the medical plan of care.

Physical Therapy Implications. Time of day, fatigue, and side effects of medication are factors that can cause variable levels of alertness or participation in physical therapy. The documentation of these factors is important for communication

TABLE 6-8 Normal and Abnormal States of Consciousness

Alert	Completely awake Attentive to normal levels of stimulation Able to interact meaningfully with clinician
Lethargic or somnolent	Arousal with stimuli Falls asleep when not stimulated Decreased awareness Loss of train of thought
Obtunded	Difficult to arouse Requires constant stimulation to maintain consciousness Confused when awake Interactions with clinicians may be largely unproductive
Stupor (semicoma)	Arousal only with strong, generally noxious stimuli and returns to unconscious state when stimulation is stopped Patient is unable to interact with clinician
Coma (deep coma)	Unarousable to any type of stimulus Reflex motor responses may or may not be seen
Delirium	State of disorientation marked by irritability or agitation, paranoia, and hallucinations Patient demonstrates offensive, loud, and talkative behaviors
Dementia	Alteration in mental processes secondary to organic disease that is not accompanied by a change in arousal

TABLE 6-9 Glasgow Coma Scale

Response		Score
Eye opening (E)	Spontaneous: eyes open without stimulation	4
	To speech: eyes open to voice	3
	To pain: eyes open to noxious stimulus	2
	Nil: eyes do not open despite variety of stimuli	1
Motor response (M)	Obeys: follows commands	6
	Localizes: purposeful attempts to move limb to stimulus	5
	Withdraws: flexor withdrawal without localizing	4
	Abnormal flexion: decorticate posturing to stimulus	3
	Extensor response: decerebrate posturing to stimulus	2
	Nil: no motor movement	1
Verbal response (V)	Oriented: normal conversation	5
	Confused conversation: vocalizes in sentences, incorrect context	4
	Inappropriate words: vocalizes with comprehensible words	3
	Incomprehensible words: vocalizes with sounds	2
	Nil: no vocalization	1

Data from Teasdale G, Jennett B: Assessment of coma and impaired consciousness: a practical scale, Lancet 2:81, 1974.

among the health care team and for the rehabilitation screening process. A progressive intensity of stimuli should be used to arouse a patient with decreased alertness or level of consciousness. For example, call the patient's name in a normal tone of voice before using a loud tone of voice, or tap the patient's shoulder before rubbing the shoulder. Changes in body position, especially the transition from a recumbent position to sitting upright, can also be used to stimulate increased alertness. Other stimuli to increase alertness include daylight, radio or television sound, or a cold cloth on the forehead.

Glasgow Coma Scale. The Glasgow Coma Scale (GCS) is a widely accepted measure of level of consciousness and responsiveness and is described in Table 6-9. The GCS evaluates best eye opening (E), motor response (M), and verbal response (V). To determine a patient's overall GCS, add each score (i.e., E + M + V). Scores range from 3 to 15. A score of 8 or less signifies coma.[13]

Calculation of the GCS usually occurs at regular intervals. The GCS should be used to confirm the type and amount of cueing needed to communicate with a patient, determine what time of day a patient is most capable of participating in physical therapy, and delineate physical therapy goals.

Cognition

Cognitive testing includes the assessment of attention, orientation, memory, abstract thought, and the ability to perform calculations or construct figures. General intelligence and vocabulary are estimated with questions regarding history, geography, or current events. Table 6-10 lists typical methods of testing the components of cognition.

> ✎ **CLINICAL TIP**
>
> A & O × 3 is a common abbreviation for alert and oriented to person, place, and time. The number may be modified to reflect the patient's orientation (e.g., A & O × 1 [self]). A & O × 4 may also be used to identify that the patient is oriented to the situation.

Emotional State

Emotional state assessment entails observation and direct questioning to ascertain a patient's mood, affect, perception, and thought process, as well as to evaluate for behavioral changes. Evaluation of emotion is not meant to be a full psychiatric examination; however, it provides insight as to how a patient may complete the cognitive portion of the mental status examination.[14]

It is important to note that a patient's culture may affect particular emotional responses. Patients who recently have had a stroke or have a history of stroke, for example, can be emotionally labile depending on the site of the lesion. This can be quite

TABLE 6-10 Tests of Cognitive Function

Cognitive Function	Definition	Task
Attention	Ability to attend to a specific stimulus or task	Repetition of a series of numbers or letters Spelling words forward and backward
Orientation	Ability to orient to person, place, and time	Identify name, age, current date and season, birth date, present location, town, etc.
Memory	Immediate recall Short-term memory Long-term memory	Recount three words after a few seconds Recount words (after a few minutes) or recent events Recount past events
Calculation	Ability to perform verbal or written mathematical problems	Add, subtract, multiply, or divide whole numbers
Construction	Ability to construct a two- or three-dimensional figure or shape	Draw a figure after a verbal command or reproduce a figure from a picture
Abstraction	Ability to reason in an abstract rather than a literal or concrete fashion	Interpret proverbs Discuss how two objects are similar or different
Judgment	Ability to reason (according to age and lifestyle)	Demonstrate common sense and safety

Data from Bickley LS, Hoekelman RA, editors: Bates' guide to physical examination and history taking, ed 7, Philadelphia, 1999, Lippincott Williams & Wilkins.

stressful for patients because they feel that they have little control over their emotions.

Speech and Language Ability

The physician should perform a speech and language assessment as soon as possible according to the patient's level of consciousness. The main goals of this assessment are to evaluate the patient's ability to articulate and produce voice and the presence, extent, and severity of aphasia.[15] These goals are achieved by testing comprehension and repetition of spoken speech, naming, quality and quantity of conversational speech, and reading and writing abilities.[15]

A speech-language pathologist is often consulted to perform a longer, more in-depth examination of cognition, speech, and swallow using standardized tests and skilled evaluation of articulation, phonation, hearing, and orofacial muscle strength testing. The physical therapist should be aware of, and use, as appropriate, the speech-language pathologist's suggestions for types of commands, activity modification, and positioning as related to risk of aspiration.

> ✎ **CLINICAL TIP**
>
> Be sure to allow the patient ample time to respond to a command or a question. Slowed response time can be mistaken for aphasia.

Vital Signs

The brain is the homeostatic center of the body; therefore, vital signs are an indirect measure of neurologic status and the body's ability to perform basic functions, such as respiration and temperature control.

Blood pressure, heart rate, respiratory rate and pattern (see Table 4-3), temperature, and other vital signs from invasive monitoring (see Table 18-4) are assessed continuously or hourly to determine neurologic and hemodynamic stability.

Physical Therapy Implications

The therapist should be aware of blood pressure parameters determined by the physician for the patient with neurologic dysfunction. These parameters may be set greater than normal to maintain adequate perfusion to the brain or lower than normal to prevent further injury to the brain.

It is important for the therapist to be aware of vital sign trends (especially blood pressure) in the neurologic patient over the course of the day(s). An increase or decrease in blood pressure over time may be intentional and related to medication changes, or it may be unrelated to medication changes. A change unrelated to medication (or intravenous fluid administration) may be related to neurologic decline due to increased intracranial pressure (ICP). Trends in vital signs should be used by the clinician to determine the safety of physical therapy intervention.

Cranial Nerves

Cranial nerve (CN) testing provides information about the general neurologic status of the patient and the function of the special senses. The results assist in the differential diagnosis of neurologic dysfunction and may help in determining the location of a lesion. CNs I through XII are tested on admission, daily in the hospital, or when there is a suspected change in neurologic function (Table 6-11).

Vision

Vision testing is an important portion of the neurologic examination because alterations in vision can indicate neurologic lesions, as illustrated in Figure 6-7. In addition to the visual field, acuity, reflexive, and ophthalmoscopic testing performed by the physician during CN assessment, the pupils are further examined for size and equality, shape, and reactivity. PERRLA is an acronym that describes pupil function: *p*upils *e*qual, *r*ound, and *r*eactive to *l*ight and *a*ccommodation.

Note any baseline pupil changes, such as those associated with cataract repair (keyhole shape). If the patient's vision or

TABLE 6-11 Origin, Purpose, and Testing of the Cranial Nerves

Nerve/Origin	Purpose	How to Test	Signs/Symptoms of Impairment
Olfactory (CN I)/ cerebral cortex	Sense of smell	Have the patient close one nostril, and ask the patient to sniff a mild-smelling substance and identify it.	Anosmia
Optic (CN II)/ thalamus	Central and peripheral vision	Acuity: Have the patient cover one eye, and ask the patient to read a visual chart. Fields: Have the patient cover one eye, and hold an object (e.g., pen cap) at arm's length from the patient in his or her peripheral field. Hold the patient's head steady. Slowly move the object centrally, and ask the patient to state when he or she first sees the object. Repeat the process in all quadrants.	Blindness, myopia, presbyopia Homonymous hemianopsia
Oculomotor (CN III)/midbrain	Upward, inward, and inferomedial eye movement Eyelid elevation Pupil constriction Visual focusing	CNs III, IV, and VI are tested together. Saccadic (patient is asked to look in each direction) and pursuit (patient follows moving finger) eye movements should both be tested. Ask the patient to open eyes wide. Pupil reaction to light: Shine a flashlight into one eye and observe bilateral pupil reaction. Gaze: Hold object (e.g., pen) at arm's length from the patient, and hold the patient's head steady. Ask the patient to follow the object with a full horizontal, vertical, and diagonal gaze.	Ophthalmoplegia with eye deviation downward and outward Strabismus causing diplopia Ptosis Loss of ipsilateral pupillary light and accommodation reflexes
Trochlear (CN IV)/midbrain	Inferolateral eye movement	See Oculomotor (CN III), above.	Diplopia Head tilt to unaffected side Weakness in depression of ipsilateral adducted eye
Trigeminal (CN V)/pons	Sensation of face Mastication Corneal reflex Jaw jerk*	Conduct touch, pain, and temperature sensory testing over the patient's face. Observe for deviation of jaw. Wisp of cotton on the patient's cornea. Palpate masseter as the patient clamps his or her jaw.	Loss of facial sensation Ipsilateral deviation of opened jaw Loss of ipsilateral corneal reflex Muscle wasting When opened, deviation of jaw to ipsilateral side
Abducens (CN VI)/pons	Lateral eye movement and proprioception	See Oculomotor (CN III), above.	Diplopia Convergent strabismus Ipsilateral abductor paralysis
Facial (CN VII)/ pons	Facial expression Taste (anterior two thirds of tongue)* Autonomic innervation of lacrimal and salivary glands*	Ask the patient to smile, wrinkle brow, purse lips, and close eyes tightly. Inspect closely for symmetry. Ask patient to differentiate between saline and sugar solutions applied to the tongue with a cotton swab. Introduce a stimulus to produce tears such as exposing patient to a cut onion.	Paralysis of ipsilateral upper and lower facial muscles, resulting in inability to close eye, facial droop, and/or difficulty with speech articulation Loss of taste on ipsilateral two thirds of tongue Loss of lacrimation, dry mouth
Vestibulocochlear (CN VIII)/ pons	Vestibular branch: sense of equilibrium Cochlear branch: sense of hearing	Oculocephalic reflex (doll's eyes): Rotate the patient's head and watch for eye movement. (Normal: Eyes will move in the opposite direction of the head before return to midline.) Test balance: Vestibulospinal function. Test auditory acuity. Weber test: Vibrate a tuning fork, place it on the mid forehead, and ask the patient if sound is heard louder in one ear. Rinne test: Vibrate a tuning fork on the mastoid bone, then close to ear canal; sound heard longer through air than bone.	Vertigo, nystagmus, dysequilibrium Deafness, impaired hearing, tinnitus Unilateral conductive loss: Sound lateralized to impaired ear Sensorineural loss: Sound heard in good ear Conductive loss: Sound heard through bone is equal to or longer than air. Sensorineural loss: Sound heard through air is longer

TABLE 6-11　Origin, Purpose, and Testing of the Cranial Nerves—cont'd

Nerve/Origin	Purpose	How to Test	Signs/Symptoms of Impairment
Glossopharyngeal (CN IX)/ medulla	Gag reflex Motor and proprioception of superior pharyngeal muscle Autonomic innervation of salivary gland Taste (posterior one third of tongue)* Sensation from the external auditory meatus and skin of posterior ear Blood pressure regulation	Test CNs IX and X together. Induce gag with tongue depressor (one side at a time). Patient phonates a prolonged vowel sound or talks for an extended period of time. Listen for voice quality and pitch. Ask patient to differentiate between saline and sugar solutions applied to the tongue with a cotton swab. Test sensation in posterior ear.	Loss of gag reflex Dysphagia Dry mouth Loss of taste to ipsilateral one third of tongue Impaired sensation to ipsilateral ear
Vagus (CN X)/ medulla	Swallowing Palatal pharynx control Parasympathetic innervation of heart, lungs, and abdominal viscera	See Glossopharyngeal (CN IX), above. Have patient say "ah"; observe motion of soft palate (elevates) and position of uvula (remains midline).	Dysphagia Soft palate paralysis, contralateral deviation of uvula, hoarseness
Spinal accessory (CN XI)/ C1-C5	Motor control of the trapezius and sternocleidomastoid muscles	Ask patient to rotate the head or shrug the shoulders. Offer gentle resistance to movement.	LMN: Weakness with head turning to contralateral side and ipsilateral shoulder shrug UMN: Weakness with head turning to ipsilateral side and contralateral shoulder shrug
Hypoglossal (CN XII)/medulla	Movement and proprioception of tongue for chewing and speech	Ask the patient to stick out his or her tongue, observe for midline, and ask patient to move side-to-side. Listen for articulation problems.	Ipsilateral deviation of tongue during protrusion Dysarthria

Data from Lindsay KW, Bone I, Callander R, editors: Neurology and neurosurgery illustrated, ed 2, Edinburgh, UK, 1991, Churchill Livingstone; Marieb EN, editor: Human anatomy and physiology, ed 5, San Francisco, 2001, Benjamin-Cummings; McNeill ME, editor: Neuroanatomy primer, Baltimore, 1997, Lippincott Williams & Wilkins; O'Sullivan SB, Schmitz TJ, editors: Physical rehabilitation, ed 5, Philadelphia, 2007, FA Davis.

CN, Cranial nerve; *LMN,* lower motor neuron; *UMN,* upper motor neuron.

*Rarely tested.

pupil size or shape changes during physical therapy intervention, discontinue the treatment and notify the nurse or physician immediately.

- Size and equality: Pupil size is normally 2 to 4 mm or 4 to 8 mm in diameter in the light and dark, respectively.[16] The pupils should be of equal size, although up to a 1-mm difference in diameter can normally occur between the left and right pupils.[17]
- Shape: Pupils are normally round but may become oval or irregularly shaped with neurologic dysfunction.
- Reactivity: Pupils normally constrict in response to light, as a consensual response to light shone in the opposite eye or when fixed on a near object. Conversely, pupils normally dilate in the dark. Constriction and dilation occur briskly under normal circumstances. A variety of deviations of pupil characteristics can occur. Pupil reactivity can be tested by shining a light directly into the patient's eye. Dilated, nonreactive (fixed), malpositioned, or disconjugate pupils can signify very serious neurologic conditions (especially oculomotor compression, increased ICP, or brain herniation).[17]

> ✎ **CLINICAL TIP**
>
> For a patient with diplopia (double vision), a cotton or gauze eye patch can be worn temporarily over one eye to improve participation during physical therapy sessions.

The presence of nystagmus during the visual exam should also be noted. Nystagmus is an involuntary rhythmic movement of the eyes that may be present at rest or occur with eye or head movements.[18] Nystagmus can be the result of vestibular dysfunction, a cerebellar lesion, or an imbalance in the reflex activity coordinating the two. While observing nystagmus, it is important to note the orientation (vertical versus horizontal), direction (right versus left), and head motions that increase the nystagmus. This will aid the clinician in determining the cause. Nystagmus involving the tracts/reflexes between the vestibular system and cerebellum is usually horizontal in nature and more pronounced when looking to the side of the lesion.[18] Vertical nystagmus is usually present with lesions involving the anterior vermis of the cerebellum or medulla and indicates a poor

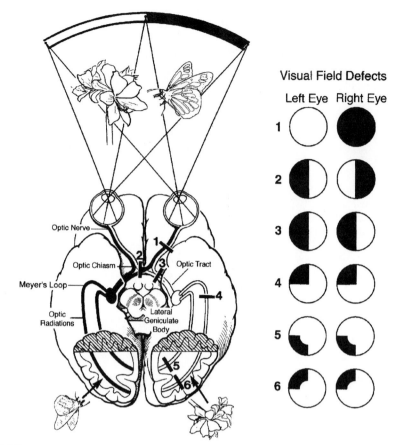

FIGURE 6-7

Visual pathway with lesion sites and resulting visual field defects. The occipital lobe has been cut away to show the medial aspect and the calcarine sulci. (From Love RJ, Webb WG, editors: Neurology for the speech-language pathologist, ed 4, Boston, 2001, Butterworth-Heinemann, p 103.)

prognosis for recovery. Spontaneous (at rest) nystagmus is most often observed after an acute unilateral insult to the vestibular system.[7]

Motor Function

The evaluation of motor function consists of strength, tone, and reflex testing.

Strength Testing

Strength is the force output of a contracting muscle directly related to the amount of tension that it can produce.[19] Strength can be graded in the following ways in the acute care setting:

- Graded 0-5/0-N (normal) with manual muscle testing
- Graded as strong or weak with resisted isometrics
- Graded by the portion of a range of motion in which movement occurs (e.g., hip flexion through one fourth of available range)
- Graded functionally

The manner in which muscle strength is tested depends on the patient's ability to follow commands, arousal, cooperation, and activity tolerance, as well as on constraints on the patient, such as positioning, sedation, and medical equipment. If it is not possible to grade strength in any of the described ways, then only the presence, frequency, and location of spontaneous movements are noted instead.

Muscle Tone

Muscle tone has been described in a multitude of ways; however, neither a precise definition nor a quantitative measure has been determined.[20] It is beyond the scope of this book to discuss the various definitions of tone, including variants such as clonus and tremor. For simplicity, muscle tone is discussed in terms of hypertonicity, hypotonicity, or dystonia. Hypertonicity, an increase in muscle contractility, includes spasticity (velocity-dependent increase in resistance to passive stretch) and rigidity (increased uniform resistance that is present throughout the whole range of motion and is independent of velocity) secondary to a neurologic lesion of the CNS or upper motor neuron system.[7] Hypotonicity, a decrease in muscle contractility, includes flaccidity (diminished resistance to passive stretching and tendon reflexes)[21] from a neurologic lesion of the lower motor neuron system (or as in the early stage of spinal cord injury [SCI] known as spinal shock). Dystonia, a hyperkinetic

TABLE 6-12 Modified Ashworth Scale for Grading Abnormal Tone

Grade	Description
0	No increase in muscle tone.
1	Slight increase in muscle tone, manifested by a slight catch and release or by minimal resistance at the end of the range of motion when the affected part(s) is moved in flexion or extension.
1+	Slight increase in muscle tone, manifested by a catch, followed by minimal resistance throughout the remainder (less than half) of the range of motion.
2	More marked increased in muscle tone through most of the range of motion, but affected part(s) easily moved.
3	Considerable increase in muscle tone; passive movement difficult.
4	Affected part(s) rigid in flexion and extension.

From Bohannon RW, Smith MB: Interrater reliability of a Modified Ashworth Scale of Muscle Spasticity, Phys Ther 67:206, 1987.

TABLE 6-13 Tardieu Scale for Grading Spasticity

Grade	Description
0	No resistance throughout the course of movement.
1	Slight resistance throughout the course of movement, but no clear catch.
2	Clear catch at a precise angle, interrupting the movement, followed by release.
3	Fatigable clonus with less than 10 seconds when maintaining the pressure and appearing at a precise angle.
4	Unfatigable clonus with more than 10 seconds when maintaining the pressure and appearing at a precise angle.
5	Joint is immovable.

Measurements are taken at three different velocities: V1: As slow as possible (slower than the natural drop of the limb segment under gravity); V2: Speed of limb segment falling under gravity; V3: As fast as possible (faster than the natural drop of the limb segment under gravity).

Responses are recorded at each velocity as X/Y, with X indicating the 0 to 5 rating, and Y indicating the degree of angle at which the muscle reaction occurs. Refer to Appendix 6-A for an example of a scoring sheet for this particular scale.

From Tardieu G, Shentoub S, Delarue R: A la recherché d'une technique de mesure de la spasticite. Revue Neurologique. Research on a technic for measurement of spasticity, Rev Neurol (Paris) 91:143-144, 1954.

movement disorder, is characterized by disordered tone and involuntary movements involving large portions of the body resulting from a lesion in the basal ganglia (as in Parkinson's disease with excessive L-dopa therapy).[7] Regardless of the specific definition of muscle tone, clinicians agree that muscle tone may change according to a variety of factors, including stress, febrile state, pain, body position, medical status, medication, CNS arousal, and degree of volitional movement.[7]

Muscle tone can be evaluated qualitatively in the following ways:

- Passively as mild (i.e., mild resistance to movement with quick stretch), moderate (i.e., moderate resistance to movement, even without quick stretch), or severe (i.e., resistance great enough to prevent movement of a joint)[22]
- Passively or actively as the ability or inability to achieve full joint range of motion
- Actively as the ability to complete functional mobility and volitional movement
- As abnormal decorticate (flexion) or decerebrate (extension) posturing. (Decortication is the result of a hemispheric or internal capsule lesion that results in a disruption of the corticospinal tract.[17] Decerebration is the result of a brain stem lesion and is thus considered a sign of deteriorating neurologic status.[17] A patient may demonstrate one or both of these postures.)

Muscle tone and spasticity can also be evaluated objectively using the following scales:

- Modified Ashworth Scale as described in Table 6-12. This scale has been considered the "gold standard" of measuring muscle tone due to initial studies showing high interrater (0.84) and intrarater (0.83) reliability.[23] However, more recent studies have had less favorable results, showing moderate reliability.[24-26]
- Modified Tardieu Scale as described in Table 6-13. The Tardieu Scale was developed by Tardieu in 1954[26a] (the

TABLE 6-14 Deep Tendon Reflexes of the Upper and Lower Extremities

Reflex	Spinal Level	Normal Response
Biceps	C5	Elbow flexion
Brachioradialis	C6	Elbow flexion
Triceps	C7	Elbow extension
Patellar	L4	Knee extension
Posterior tibialis	L5	Plantar flexion and inversion
Achilles	S1	Plantar flexion

patient is in the supine position) and modified by Boyd and Graham in 1999[26b] (the patient is in supine, sitting, or standing, depending on the joint tested). This scale measures the quality of muscle reaction to passive stretch at three different velocities. Not only is the muscle reaction quantified (as in the Modified Ashworth Scale), but it also controls for the velocity of the stretch and measures the angle at which the catch, or clonus, occurs.[26b] This scale has been shown in recent studies to be a more accurate measure of spasticity than the Modified Ashworth Scale.[27,28]

Reflexes

A reflex is a motor response to a sensory stimulus and is used to assess the integrity of the motor system in the conscious or unconscious patient. The reflexes most commonly tested are deep tendon reflexes (DTRs). A DTR should elicit a muscle contraction of the tendon stimulated. Table 6-14 describes DTRs according to spinal level and expected response. DTR testing should proceed in the following manner:

TABLE 6-15 Deep Tendon Reflex Grades and Interpretation

Grade	Response	Interpretation
0	No response	Abnormal
1+	Diminished or sluggish response	Low normal
2+	Active response	Normal
3+	Brisk response	High normal
4+	Very brisk response, with or without clonus	Abnormal

Data from Bickley LS, Hoekelman RA: Bates' guide to physical examination and history taking, ed 7, Philadelphia, 1999, Lippincott Williams & Wilkins.

1. The patient should be sitting or supine and as relaxed as possible.
2. The joint to be tested should be in midposition to stretch the tendon.
3. The tendon is then directly tapped with a reflex hammer. Both sides should be compared.

Reflexes are typically graded as present (normal, exaggerated, or depressed) or absent. Reflexes can also be graded on a scale of 0 to 4, as described in Table 6-15. Depressed reflexes signify lower motor neuron disease or neuropathy. Exaggerated reflexes signify upper motor neuron disease, or they may be due to hyperthyroidism, electrolyte imbalance, or other metabolic abnormalities.[29]

> ✎ **CLINICAL TIP**
>
> The numeric results of DTR testing may appear in a stick figure drawing in the medical record. The DTR grades are placed next to each of the main DTR sites. An arrow may appear next to the stick figure as well. Arrows pointing upward signify hyperreflexia; conversely, arrows pointing downward signify hyporeflexia.

A superficial reflex should elicit a muscle contraction from the cornea, mucous membrane, or area of the skin that is stimulated. The most frequently tested superficial reflexes are the corneal (which involve CNs V and VII), gag and swallowing (which involve CNs IX and X), and perianal reflexes (which involve S3 to S5). These reflexes are evaluated by physicians and are graded as present or absent. Superficial reflexes may also be recurrent primitive reflexes that are graded as present or absent.

The most commonly tested cutaneous reflex is the Babinski sign. A positive (abnormal) Babinski sign is great-toe extension with splaying of the toes in response to stroking the lateral plantar surface of the foot with the opposite end of a reflex hammer. It indicates corticospinal tract damage, as seen in spinal cord injury, stroke, and multiple sclerosis.[30]

> ✎ **CLINICAL TIP**
>
> A positive Babinski sign may be noted in a patient's chart as "upgoing toe(s) on the right (or left)."

Other primitive reflexes that can be tested are flexor withdrawal and plantar or palmar grasp. These are all reflexes normally seen in infants that become integrated at an early age. The presence of any of these three reflexes in an adult is abnormal and usually indicates significant upper motor neuron lesion or brain injury. If the patient does squeeze the clinician's hand while the clinician is testing for the palmar grasp reflex, then the clinician should also ask the patient to release his or her hand: if the patient releases the hand it will be a better indicator as to whether the patient is truly following commands.

Sensation

Sensation testing evaluates the ability to sense light touch, proprioception, pressure, temperature, vibration sense, and pain. For each modality, the face, neck, trunk, and extremities are tested bilaterally, proceeding in a dermatomal pattern (see Figure 6-6). For more reliable sensation testing results, the patient should be asked to close his or her eyes or look away from the area being tested. Table 6-16 outlines the method of sensation testing by stimulus.

Before performing the sensory examination, the physical therapist should be sure that the patient can correctly identify stimuli (e.g., that a pinprick feels like a pinprick). If more primitive sensation (such as light touch) is not intact, then it may not be advisable to proceed with the more complex sensation testing, such as graphesthesia or two-point discrimination.

Coordination

Although each lobe of the cerebellum has its own function, coordination tests cannot truly differentiate among them. Coordination tests evaluate the presence of ataxia (general incoordination), dysmetria (overshooting), and dysdiadochokinesia (inability to perform rapid alternating movements) with arm, leg, and trunk movements, as well as with gait.[11] The results of each test (Table 6-17) are described in terms of the patient's ability to complete the test, accuracy, regularity of rhythm, and presence of tremor.[31]

Testing for pronator drift in the acute care setting is important because it can be an early indication of evolving hemiparesis or supratentorial mass lesion.[32] While the patient is sitting or standing, he or she flexes both shoulders and extends the elbows with the palms upward. The patient is then asked to close his or her eyes. The forearm is observed for 10 to 20 seconds for (1) pronation or downward drift, which suggests a contralateral corticospinal lesion, or (2) an upward or sideward drift, which suggests loss of position sense.[33]

Diagnostic Procedures

A multitude of diagnostic tests and procedures is used to evaluate, differentiate, and monitor neurologic dysfunction. Each has its own cost, accuracy, advantages, and disadvantages. For the purposes of this text, only the procedures most commonly used in the acute care setting are described.

TABLE 6-16 Sensation Testing

Sensation	Modality and Method
Light touch	Apply light touch with the finger, a cotton ball, or washcloth over the extremities or trunk. The patient is asked to identify if there is a stimulus present and the location of the stimulus.
Pain	Touch a pin or pen cap over the extremities or trunk. Ask the patient to distinguish between dull (pen cap) and sharp (the pin) stimuli.
Pressure	Using the therapist's fingertip, apply pressure on the skin surface that is firm enough to indent the skin and stimulate the deep receptors. The patient is asked to identify if there is a stimulus present.
Proprioception	Lightly grasp the distal interphalangeal joint of the patient's finger or great toe, and move the joint slowly up and down. Ask the patient to state in which direction the joint is moved. Test distal to proximal (e.g., toe to ankle to knee).
Vibration	Activate a tuning fork and place on a bony prominence. Ask the patient to state when the vibration slows and stops. Proceed distal to proximal.
Temperature	Place test tubes filled with warm or cold water on the area of the patient's body to be tested. Ask the patient to state the temperature. (Rarely done in the acute care setting.)
Stereognosis	Place a familiar object in the patient's hand and ask the patient to identify it.
Two-point discrimination	Place two-point caliper or drafting compass on area to be tested. Ask the patient to distinguish whether it has one or two points.
Graphesthesia	Trace a letter or number in the patient's open palm and ask the patient to state what was drawn.
Double simultaneous stimulation	Simultaneously touch two areas on the same side of the patient's body. Ask patient to locate and distinguish both points.

Data from Lindsay KW, Bone I, Callander R, editors: Neurology and neurosurgery illustrated, ed 2, Edinburgh, UK, 1991, Churchill Livingstone; Gilman S, Newman SW, editors: Manter and Gatz's essentials of clinical neuroanatomy and neurophysiology, ed 7, Philadelphia, 1989, FA Davis; Hickey JV, editor: The clinical practice of neurological and neurosurgical nursing ed 4, Philadelphia, 1997, Lippincott.

TABLE 6-17 Coordination Tests

Test	Method	Impairment
Upper Extremity		
Finger to nose	Ask the patient to touch his or her nose. Then, ask patient to touch his or her nose and then touch your finger (which should be held an arm's length away). Ask the patient to repeat this rapidly.	Dysmetria Intention tremor
Finger opposition	Ask the patient to touch the thumb to each finger in sequence, gradually increasing the speed.	Dysmetria Intention tremor
Supination and pronation	Ask the patient to rapidly and alternately supinate and pronate his or her forearms.	Dysdiadochokinesia
Tapping	Ask the patient to rapidly tap his or her hands on a surface simultaneously, alternately, or both.	Dysdiadochokinesia
Arm bounce	Have the patient flex his or her shoulder to 90 degrees with elbow fully extended and wrist in the neutral position; then apply a brief downward pressure on the arm. (Excessive swinging of the arm indicates a positive test.)	Cerebellar dysfunction—impaired postural stability
Rebound phenomenon	Ask the patient to flex his or her elbow to approximately 45 degrees. Apply resistance to elbow flexion; then suddenly release the resistance. Normally the triceps would contract and keep the elbow/arm in position. Be careful that the patient does not strike his/her face in the case of a positive test.	Cerebellar dysfunction—impaired postural stability Triceps weakness
Lower Extremity		
Heel to shin	Ask the patient to move his or her heel up and down the opposite shin and repeat rapidly.	Dysmetria
Tapping	Ask the patient to rapidly tap his or her feet on the floor simultaneously, alternately, or both.	Dysdiadochokinesia
Romberg test	Ask the patient to stand (heels together) with eyes open. Observe for swaying or loss of balance. Repeat with eyes closed.	Inability to maintain balance when the eyes are closed is a positive test indicating a loss of proprioception, vestibular dysfunction, or both.
Gait	Ask the patient to walk. Observe gait pattern, posture, and balance. Repeat with tandem walking to exaggerate deficits.	Ataxia

Data from Gilroy J, editor: Basic neurology, ed 3, New York, 2000, McGraw-Hill; and O'Sullivan SB, Schmitz TJ, editors: Physical rehabilitation, ed 5, Philadelphia, 2007, FA Davis.

X-Ray

X-rays can provide anterior, posterior, lateral, and base views of the skull that are used to assess the presence of calcification, bone erosion, or fracture, especially after head or facial trauma or if a tumor is suspected.[34] Anterior, lateral, posterior, and oblique views of the cervical, thoracic, lumbar, and sacral spine are used to assess the presence of bone erosion, fracture, dislocation, spondylosis, spur, or stenosis, especially after trauma or if there are motor or sensory deficits.[17,35] X-rays are a quick way to screen for serious injury in the trauma victim, but this method of imaging is quickly being replaced by computed tomography and/or magnetic resonance imaging.

Computed Tomography and Angiography

Computed tomography (CT) is a series of successive x-ray films put together and analyzed by a computer to provide a three-dimensional view of the body part being imaged. The CT image of the brain is taken in the sagittal or coronal planes, with or without contrast, and is used to identify such abnormalities as neoplasm, cortical atrophy, cerebral aneurysm, intracranial hemorrhage, arteriovenous malformation (AVM), cerebral infarction, and ventricular displacement or enlargement.[36] Head CT is the preferred neuroimaging test in the ER, to rule out subarachnoid hemorrhage (SAH) and for the evaluation of acute cerebrovascular accident (CVA), as it can readily distinguish a primary ischemic from a primary hemorrhagic process and thus determine the appropriate use of tissue plasminogen activator (tPA) (see Table 19-7).[7] CT of the spine and orbits is also available to evaluate for fractures, neoplasm, spinal cord compromise, or sinusitis. Xenon CT can be used to evaluate cerebral blood flow (CBF). The patient inhales xenon gas while in the CT scanner. Xenon is diffused almost immediately into the bloodstream and into the brain. The concentration of the gas is calculated by the computer and converted into CBF. Abnormalities identified using this scan include cerebrovascular occlusive disease, increased ICP, intracranial bleeding, and "brain death" where CBF would equal zero.[36,37]

Computed tomography angiography (CTA) is a noninvasive method used to visualize blood vessels throughout the body. It is faster, is less expensive, and exposes the patient to less radiation than traditional invasive angiography. CTA can be used to screen for SAH, aneurysm, and stenosis.

Magnetic Resonance Imaging and Angiography

Views in any plane of the head, with or without contrast, taken with magnetic resonance imaging (MRI) are used to assess intracranial neoplasm, degenerative disease, cerebral and spinal cord edema, ischemia, hemorrhage, AVM, cerebral atrophy, and congenital anomalies.[17,35] MRI has several advantages over CT scans, including providing better contrast between normal and pathologic tissues allowing for quicker identification of areas of ischemia, improved visualization of blood vessels, less obscuring bone artifact, and the ability to image in any plane.[36] However, MRI is not as sensitive as CT in detecting and evaluating SAH, calcification, or bony abnormalities, and it cannot be performed in patients with pacemakers, metallic implants, or pain stimulator implants, or in patients with severe claustrophobia.[38] Magnetic resonance angiography (MRA) is a noninvasive method used to assess the intracranial vasculature for CVA, transient ischemic attack (TIA), venous sinus thrombosis, AVM, and vascular tumors or extracranially for carotid bifurcation stenosis.[39]

Doppler Flowmetry

Doppler flowmetry is the use of ultrasound to assess blood flow.

Transcranial Doppler Sonography

Transcranial Doppler sonography (TCD) involves the passage of low-frequency ultrasound waves over thin cranial bones (temporal) or over gaps in bones to determine the velocity and direction of blood flow in the anterior, middle, or posterior cerebral and basilar arteries. It is used to assess arteriosclerotic disease, collateral circulation, vasospasm, and brain death and to identify AVMs and their supply arteries.[17,35]

Carotid Noninvasive Studies

Carotid noninvasive studies use the passage of high-frequency ultrasound waves over the common, internal, and external carotid arteries to determine the velocity of blood flow in these vessels. It is used to assess location, presence, and severity of carotid occlusion and stenosis.[17,35] Carotid ultrasound is now often done in color and is referred to as a *carotid duplex ultrasound.*

Digital-Subtraction Angiography

Digital-subtraction angiography (DSA) is the computer-assisted radiographic visualization of the carotids and cerebral vessels with a minimal view of background tissues. An image is taken before and after the injection of a contrast medium. The first picture is "subtracted" from the second, a process that creates a highlight of the vessels. DSA is used to assess aneurysm, AVM, fistula, occlusion, or stenosis. It is considered the "gold standard" in assessment for carotid stenosis; however, it is less cost efficient and carries a small but significant risk of stroke or death due to the invasive nature of the test compared with MRA or carotid ultrasound.[40] It is also used in the operating room (i.e., television display) to examine the integrity of anastomoses or cerebrovascular repairs.[17,35]

Cerebral Angiography

Cerebral angiography remains the gold standard for imaging the cervicocerebral vasculature and related flow because of its ability to identify very small lesions that may be missed by noninvasive studies such as CTA and MRA.[41] It involves the radiographic visualization (angiography) of the displacement, patency, stenosis, or vasospasm of intracranial or extracranial arteries after the injection of a radiopaque contrast medium via a catheter (usually in the femoral artery). It is used to assess aneurysm, AVMs, occlusions, or stenosis as a single procedure or in the operating room to examine blood flow after surgical procedures (e.g., after an aneurysm clipping).[17]

Lumbar Puncture

A lumbar puncture (LP) is the collection of CSF from a needle placed into the subarachnoid space below the L1 vertebra, usually between L3 and L4. The patient is placed in a side-lying position with the neck and hips flexed as much as possible (to open the laminae for the best access to the subarachnoid space). Multiple vials of CSF are collected and tested for color, cytology, chlorine, glucose, protein, and pH. The opening and closing pressures are noted. LP is used to assist in the diagnosis of primary or metastatic brain or spinal cord neoplasm, cerebral hemorrhage, meningitis, encephalitis, degenerative brain disease, autoimmune diseases involving the central nervous system, neurosyphilis, and demyelinating disorders (such as multiple sclerosis [MS] and acute demyelinating polyneuropathy). This procedure may also be performed to inject therapeutic or diagnostic agents, to administer spinal anesthetics, or to reduce/drain the volume of CSF to a normal level in normal pressure hydrocephalus or in patients with pseudotumor cerebri.

Positron Emission Tomography

In positron emission tomography (PET), radioactive chemicals that mimic the normal metabolic process of the brain are administered to the patient (most commonly fluorodeoxyglucose or FDG). The positrons emitted from the radioactive chemicals are sensed by a series of detectors placed around the patient, and in combination with CT the emissions are recorded into a high-resolution two- or three-dimensional image.[36] Areas in the brain that are more metabolically active will take up more of the FDG than normal areas of the brain, indicating pathology such as cancer. Areas with less uptake would indicate hypometabolism such as that seen in Alzheimer's disease. PET scanning is most commonly used to assist in the diagnosis of brain tumor, cerebrovascular disease or trauma, dementia including Alzheimer's disease, seizure disorders, Parkinson's disease, and psychiatric disorders.[42,43]

Electroencephalography

Electroencephalography (EEG) is the recording of electrical brain activity, using electrodes affixed to the scalp at rest or sleep, after sleep deprivation, after hyperventilation, or after photic stimulation.[43] Brain waves may show abnormalities of activity, amplitude, pattern, or speed. Electroencephalography is used in conjunction with other neurodiagnostic tests to assess seizure focus, sleep and metabolic disorders, dementia, and brain death. In epileptic states, seizure activity is characterized by rapid, spiking waves on the graph, whereas cerebral lesions such as tumors or infarctions show abnormally slow EEG waves, depending on the size and location of the lesion. EEG can also be used during surgery when a carotid vessel is temporarily occluded to evaluate for tissue ischemia in the brain, indicating the need for temporary shunting of blood to avoid CVA.[36]

Evoked Potentials

Evoked potentials (EPs) are electrical responses generated by the stimulation of a sensory organ. EP studies allow clinicians to measure and assess the entire sensory pathway from the peripheral sensory organ to the brain cortex. Conduction delays indicate damage or disease anywhere along the pathway to the cortex.[36] A visual evoked potential (VEP) or visual evoked response (VER) is measured using electrodes that are placed over the occipital lobe to record occipital cortex activity after a patient is shown flashing lights or a checkerboard pattern. Visual evoked potentials are used to assess optic neuropathies and optic nerve lesions. Ninety percent of patients with MS show abnormal latencies of VERs.[36] A brain stem auditory evoked response is measured using electrodes that are placed over the cortex to record CN VIII, pons, and midbrain activity after a patient listens to a series of clicking noises through headphones. Brain stem auditory evoked responses are used to assess acoustic tumors, brain stem lesions in MS, or brain stem function (in comatose patients). A somatosensory evoked potential is measured using electrodes over the contralateral sensory cortex after the median or posterior tibial nerve is electrically stimulated. Somatosensory evoked potentials are used to assess SCI, cervical disc disease, sensory dysfunction associated with MS, or parietal cortex tumor.[17,35]

Electromyography and Nerve Conduction Velocity Studies

Electromyography (EMG) is the recording of muscle activity at rest, with voluntary movement, and with electrical stimulation with needle electrodes. Nerve conduction velocity studies are the measurement of the conduction time and amplitude of an electrical stimulus along a peripheral nerve(s). EMG and nerve conduction velocity studies are used to assess and differentiate myopathy and peripheral nerve injury, respectively.[17]

Myelography

Myelography uses x-ray to show how a contrast medium flows through the subarachnoid space and around the vertebral column after the removal of a small amount of CSF and the injection of dye via LP. It is used to assess bone displacement, disc herniation, cord compression, or tumor.[17,35]

After myelography, typical orders include restricting activity for 24 hours to no heavy lifting or bending, vigorous rehydration, elevation of the head to limit contrast flowing intracranially, and resumption of restricted medications after 24 hours. Other side effects are similar to with LP, including spinal headache.[38]

Transesophageal Echocardiography

Transesophageal echocardiography (TEE) and the less invasive transthoracic echocardiography (TTE) are useful imaging techniques in patients who have had or suspected to have had an ischemic stroke or TIA. These images can help to identify cardiac sources of arterial embolism and can guide treatments to avoid a recurrence of CVA or TIA.[36] Please refer to Chapter 3 for more specific details of these tests.

Health Conditions

Traumatic Brain Injury

The medical-surgical treatment of traumatic brain injury (TBI) is a complex and challenging task. Direct or indirect trauma to the skull, brain, or both typically results in altered consciousness and systemic homeostasis. TBI can be described by location, extent, severity, and mechanism of injury.[44]

Location

TBI may involve damage to the cranium only, the cranium and brain structures, or brain structures only. Frequently, head trauma is categorized in the following manner:
- Closed: Protective mechanisms are maintained
- Open: Protective mechanisms are altered
- Coup: The lesion is deep to the site of impact
- Contrecoup: The lesion is opposite the site of impact
- Coup-contrecoup: A combination of coup and contrecoup

Extent

TBI may be classified as primary (in reference to the direct biomechanical changes in the brain) or secondary (in reference to the latent intracranial or systemic complications that exacerbate the original injury). The terms *focal* and *diffuse* are often used to describe a specific or gross lesion, respectively.

Severity

In addition to diagnostic tests, TBI may be classified according to cognitive skill deficit and GCS as mild (13 to 15), moderate (9 to 12), or severe (3 to 8).

Mechanism of injury

The most common mechanisms responsible for primary TBI are acceleration-deceleration, rotation forces, and direct impact. These forces may be of low or high velocity and result in the compression, traction, or shearing of brain structures.

Secondary brain injury occurs within minutes to hours of the traumatic primary injury and is characterized by inflammatory, vascular, and biomolecular abnormalities. These changes include the release of cytokines and a disruption of the blood-brain barrier, which causes the development of vasogenic (extracellular) brain edema; impaired cerebral autoregulation and

ischemia in the setting of hypoxia and hypotension; tissue acidosis and an influx of electrolytes, which causes cytotoxic (intracellular) brain edema; and the loss of neurons, glial cells, and presynaptic terminals from neurochemical and oxygen–free radical reactions.[45,46]

Table 6-18 defines the most common types of TBI and describes the clinical findings. The management of these conditions is discussed later in the General Management section.

> ✎ **CLINICAL TIP**
>
> The therapist should be aware of the most recent activity orders and blood pressure and heart rate parameters to minimize secondary brain injury during treatment.

Spinal Cord Injury

In the United States, there are approximately 12,000 new cases of SCI per year, costing, on average $1 million to $4.3 million per lifetime, depending on age and level of injury.[47] SCI can be identified as traumatic (most common) or nontraumatic. The two most common causes of traumatic SCI are motor vehicle accidents (40%) and falls (27%). Causes of nontraumatic injury include impingement from abscess or tumor; disruption of vasculature due to thrombosis, AVM, or hemorrhage; transverse myelitis; or disease process such as MS. SCI is classified broadly as:

1. Paraplegia or tetraplegia and
2. Complete or incomplete

It is very important to determine the appropriate level of injury, with respect to both sensation and motor function (Table 6-19). The American Spinal Injury Association (ASIA) Impairment Scale is used to determine the appropriate level of injury and has helped to standardize classification across the country.[48,49] Table 6-20 describes the anticipated return of function for each spinal cord level of injury.

As with TBI, the key to optimizing recovery is to monitor for and treat secondary SCI in the acute phase of injury. Secondary SCI is a complex series of pathologic vascular and inflammatory responses to primary SCI, which further compound the original injury over the course of several days. A summary of secondary SCI includes (1) vasospasm of superficial spinal vessels, intraparenchymal hemorrhage and disruption of the blood-brain and spinal cord barrier, complicated by neurogenic shock and loss of autoregulation, and (2) increased calcium levels, which stimulate free radical production to cause further ischemia, the release of catecholamines and opioids, and the accumulation of activated microglia and macrophages.[50,51]

The most common types of incomplete SCI syndromes are described in Table 6-21. The immediate physiologic effect of SCI is spinal shock; the triad of hypotension, bradycardia, and hypothermia is secondary to altered sympathetic reflex activity.[50] It is beyond the scope of this book to discuss in detail the physiologic sequelae of SCI. However, other major physiologic effects of SCI include autonomic dysreflexia; orthostatic hypotension; impaired respiratory function; bladder, bowel, and sexual dysfunction; malnutrition; pressure ulcer; diabetes insipidus (DI); syndrome of inappropriate secretion of antidiuretic

TABLE 6-18 Classifications and Clinical Findings of Traumatic Brain Injuries

Injury	Definition	Clinical Findings
Cerebral concussion	Shaking of the brain secondary to acceleration-deceleration forces, usually as a result of a fall or during sports activity. Can be classified as mild or classic. Signs and symptoms of cerebral concussion are reversible in most cases.	Brief loss of consciousness or "dazed" presentation, headache, dizziness, irritability, inappropriate laughter, nausea, decreased concentration and memory, retrograde or antegrade amnesia, altered gait
Postconcussive syndrome (PCS)	Clinical findings after a concussion that last for weeks to months. (Patients who initially presented with headache, nausea, and dizziness are at higher risk for PCS.)	Headache, nausea, dizziness, sensory sensitivity, memory or concentration difficulties, irritability, sleep disturbances, and depression
Cerebral contusion	Bruise (small hemorrhage) secondary to acceleration-deceleration forces or beneath a depressed skull fracture, most commonly in the frontal or temporal areas.	See Cerebral concussion, above. (Patients with a contusion are often delayed in their clinical presentation.)
Cerebral laceration	Tear of the cortical surface secondary to acceleration-deceleration forces, commonly in occurrence with cerebral contusion over the anterior and middle fossa where there are sharp bony surfaces.	S/S dependent on area involved, ICP, and degree of mass effect.
Diffuse axonal injury (DAI)	Occurs with widespread white matter shearing secondary to high-speed acceleration-deceleration forces, usually as a result of a motor vehicle accident. Can be classified as mild (6-24 hours of coma), moderate (>24 hours of coma), or severe (days to weeks of coma).	Coma, abnormal posturing (if severe), other S/S dependent on area involved, ICP, and degree of mass effect.
Epidural hematoma (EDH)	Blood accumulation in the epidural space secondary to tearing of meningeal arteries that compresses deep brain structures. Associated with cranial fractures, particularly the thin temporal bone and frontal and middle meningeal tears.	Headache, altered consciousness, abnormal posture, contralateral hemiparesis, and other S/S dependent on specific location of the lesion, ICP, and degree of mass effect. Can present with a "lucid" interval before loss of consciousness for a second time.
Subdural hematoma (SDH)	Blood accumulation in the subdural space that compresses brain structures as a result of traumatic rupture or tear of cerebral veins, increased intracranial hemorrhage, or continued bleeding of a cerebral contusion. The onset of symptoms may be acute (up to 24 hours), subacute (2 days to 3 weeks), or chronic (3 weeks to 3-4 months).	See Epidural hematoma, above.
Intracerebral hematoma (ICH)	Blood accumulation in the brain parenchyma secondary to acceleration-deceleration forces, the shearing of cortical blood vessels, or beneath a fracture. May also arise as a complication of hypertension or delayed bleeding with progression of blood into the dural, arachnoid, or ventricular spaces.	See Epidural hematoma, above.

Data from Marx JA, editor: Rosen's emergency medicine: concepts and clinical practice, ed 6, Philadelphia, 2006, Mosby.

ICP, Intracranial pressure, *S/S,* signs and symptoms.

hormone (SIADH); edema; and increased risk of deep venous thrombosis.

The management of SCI typically includes medical stabilization with ventilatory support (if indicated); immobilization of the spine with a collar, orthosis, traction, halo vest, or surgical repair; methylprednisolone or other pharmacologic therapies; treatment of secondary injuries; pain management; and psychosocial support.

> ✎ **CLINICAL TIP**
>
> The key to successful recovery for patients with SCI are early mobilization with thigh-high elastic stockings and abdominal binder to prevent orthostatic hypotension; aggressive chest physical therapy including assisted cough as indicated; multidisciplinary positioning schedule; range of motion; and early splinting to prevent contractures.

TABLE 6-19 American Spinal Injury Association Impairment Scale

A	Complete	No sensory function or motor function is preserved in S4-S5.
B	Incomplete	The preservation of sensory function without motor function below the neurologic level and includes S4-S5.
C	Incomplete	The preservation of motor function below the neurologic level. Muscle function of more than half of key muscles below this level is less than 3/5.
D	Incomplete	The preservation of motor function below the neurologic level. Muscle function of at least half of key muscles below this level is equal to or greater than 3/5.
E	Normal	Motor function and sensory function are intact.

From American Spinal Injury Association: http://asia-spinalinjury.org/publications/59544_sc_Exam_Sheet_r4.pdf. Accessed October 18, 2012.

TABLE 6-20 Level of Spinal Cord Injury with Expected Return of Function

Level of Lesion	Expected Return of Function
C4	Spontaneous breathing
C5	Elbow flexion
C6	Wrist extension
C7	Elbow extension*
C8-T1	Finger flexion
T1-T12	Intercostal and abdominal muscles—trunk control
L1-L2	Hip flexion
L3	Knee extension
L4	Ankle dorsiflexion
L5	Toe extension
S1-S2	Ankle plantarflexion
S2-S4	Rectal sphincter tone

* Key muscle group for reaching goal of independent transfers.

TABLE 6-21 Incomplete Spinal Cord Injury Syndromes

Syndrome	Mechanism of Injury	Description
Central cord	Most commonly a hyperextension injury to the cervical spine, often with preexisting spondylosis; less often resulting from tumor	Lesion of the central cord exerts pressure on anterior horn cells. Typically presents with bilateral motor paralysis/paresis of upper extremities greater than lower extremities, variable sensory deficits, and possible bowel/bladder dysfunction. Majority of patients have residual deficits in hand function.
Anterior cord	Hyperflexion injury, acute large disc herniation, or as a result of anterior spinal artery injury	Lesion of the anterior cord damages the anterolateral spinothalamic tract, corticospinal tract, and anterior horn (gray matter). Typically presents with bilateral loss of pain and temperature sensation and motor function below the level of the lesion, with retained light touch, proprioception, and vibration sense. Worse prognosis than other cord syndromes.
Brown-Séquard	Most frequently caused by penetrating spinal trauma (e.g., stab wound); rarely from epidural hematoma, spinal AVM, cervical spondylosis, or unilateral articular process fracture or dislocation	Lesion of one half of the spinal cord; typically presents with contralateral loss of pain and temperature sensation several levels below the lesion; ipsilateral loss of touch, proprioception, and vibration sense; ipsilateral motor paresis or paralysis; and ipsilateral decrease in reflexes with positive Babinski. Typically patients maintain bowel and bladder function. Most become ambulatory.
Cauda equina	Burst fracture or herniated disc	Lower motor neuron injury. Absent deep tendon reflexes, flaccid bladder, and hypotonicity of lower extremities. Has the same potential to regenerate as peripheral nerves. Regeneration usually stops about 1 year from injury.

Data from Daroff RB, Fenichel GM, Jankovic J et al, editors: Bradley's neurology in clinical practice, ed 6, Philadelphia, 2012, Saunders; O'Sullivan SB, Schmitz TJ, editors: Physical rehabilitation, ed 5, Philadelphia, 2007, FA Davis.

Cerebrovascular Disease and Disorders

Patent cerebral vasculature is imperative for the delivery of oxygen to the brain. Alterations of the vascular supply or vascular structures can cause neurologic dysfunction from cerebral ischemia or infarction.

Transient Ischemic Attack

A TIA is characterized by a brief episode of neurologic dysfunction caused by a focal disturbance of brain or retinal ischemia, with clinical symptoms typically lasting less than 1 hour, and without evidence of infarction.[52] TIA is often a strong prognostic indicator of stroke and is commonly caused by carotid or vertebrobasilar disease. About 10% to 15% of patients with TIA will go on to have a stroke within 90 days; 5% will have a stroke within 2 days.[53] The management of TIAs involves observation, treatment of causative factor (if possible), anticoagulation, and carotid endarterectomy.

Cerebrovascular Accident

A CVA, otherwise known as a stroke or brain attack, is characterized by the sudden onset of focal neurologic deficits of more than 24 hours' duration or imaging of an acute, clinically relevant lesion in patients with rapidly resolving symptoms secondary to insufficient oxygen delivery to the brain.[54]

The most prominent risk factors for CVA include older age, African-American race, hypertension, coronary artery disease, hyperlipidemia, atrial fibrillation, hypercoagulable state, diabetes mellitus, obesity, smoking, alcohol abuse, and physical inactivity.[54,55] There are several types of cerebrovascular accident, including ischemic, hemorrhagic, and lacunar:

• Ischemic cerebrovascular accident: Ischemic CVA is the result of cerebral hypoperfusion. An ischemic CVA due to thrombotic disease, such as carotid artery stenosis or arteriosclerotic intracranial arteries, usually has a slow onset. Symptoms of an ischemic stroke caused by embolus from the heart in the setting of atrial fibrillation, meningitis, prosthetic valves, patent foramen ovale, or endocarditis will have a sudden onset. Refer to Figure 6-8 for the most frequent sites of arterial and cardiac abnormalities causing ischemic stroke. The management of ischemic CVA involves blood pressure control (normal to elevated range), treatment of causative factors (if possible), anticoagulation, recombinant tPA,[56-58] cerebral edema control, prophylactic anticonvulsant therapy, blood glucose control,[58] and carotid endarterectomy (if indicated).

• Hemorrhagic cerebrovascular accident: Hemorrhagic CVA involves cerebral hypoperfusion, which is abrupt in onset and is secondary to intraparenchymal hemorrhage associated with hypertension, AVM, trauma, or aneurysm rupture. Patients usually present with sudden onset of headache, vomiting, severely elevated blood pressure, altered mental status, and focal neurologic deficits that progress over minutes.[59] The management of hemorrhagic CVA involves blood pressure control (low to normal range), treatment of causative factors (if possible), blood glucose control, close monitoring of ICP and treatment of elevated ICP, prophylactic anticonvulsant therapy, and surgical hematoma evacuation (if appropriate).[60] Patients with hemorrhagic CVA have a poorer prognosis than those with ischemic stroke, with a 30-day mortality rate of 35% to 50%.[59,60]

• Lacunar cerebrovascular accident: Lacunar or small-vessel strokes are common in patients with diabetes and hypertension and are caused by small-vessel disease deep in cerebral white matter. Infarctions range in size from a few millimeters to 2 cm and occur most commonly in the basal ganglia, thalamus, pons, and internal capsule.[59] Several syndromes have been identified dependent on the site of infarcts, most commonly with pure motor symptoms, pure sensory symptoms, or ataxic hemiparesis. Lacunar strokes do not cause cognitive impairment, aphasia, or visual deficits because the higher cortical areas are preserved.[7]

Experimental treatment options for CVA include:

• Cytoprotective drugs such as antioxidants, calcium channel blockers, and glutamate receptor antagonists
• Catheter-based fibrinolysis, extending the current therapeutic window beyond 3 hours[61]
• Mild to moderate hypothermia as a neuroprotective strategy
• A variety of mechanical clot retrieval devices[57,59]

> **⬗ CLINICAL TIP**
> A patient who has received tPA is at risk for intracranial hemorrhage or bleeding from other sites and requires strict blood pressure control during the first 24 hours of infusion.[62] Physical therapy is usually not initiated during this time frame. Be aware that the window of time for administration of tPA has expanded from 3 to 4.5 hours from the onset of symptoms. Patients more than 80 years of age may also be included under certain circumstances.[62a]

The signs and symptoms of CVA depend on the location (anterior versus posterior, and cortical versus subcortical) and the extent of the cerebral ischemia or infarction. General signs and symptoms include contralateral motor and sensory loss, speech and perceptual deficits, altered vision, abnormal muscle tone, headache, nausea, vomiting, and altered affect. Refer to Table 6-22 for presentation of symptoms dependent on the specific area of infarction.

Other terms commonly used to describe CVA include the following:

• Completed stroke: A CVA in which the neurologic impairments have fully evolved
• Stroke-in-evolution: A CVA in which the neurologic impairments continue to evolve or fluctuate over hours or days[63]

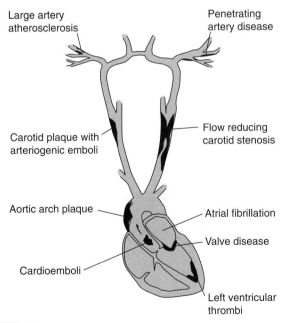

FIGURE 6-8
The most frequent sites of arterial and cardiac abnormalities causing ischemic stroke. (From Albers GW, Amarenco P, Easton JD, et al: Antithrombotic and thrombolytic therapy for ischemic stroke: The Seventh ACCP Conference on Antithrombotic and Thrombolytic Therapy, Chest 126[3 Suppl]:483S-512S, 2004.)

TABLE 6-22 Neurologic Signs Associated with CVA by Location

Artery Affected	Neurologic Signs
Internal carotid artery supplies the diencephalon and the cerebral hemispheres via the middle cerebral artery and the anterior cerebral artery	Unilateral blindness Severe contralateral hemiplegia and hemianesthesia Profound aphasia
Middle cerebral artery supplies the frontal lobe, parietal lobe, and cortical surfaces of temporal lobe (affecting structures of higher cerebral processes of communication; language interpretation; and perception and interpretation of space, sensation, form, and voluntary movement).	Alterations in communication, cognition, mobility, and sensation Contralateral homonymous hemianopsia Contralateral hemiplegia or hemiparesis, motor and sensory loss, greater in the face and arm than in the leg
Anterior cerebral artery supplies superior surfaces of frontal and parietal lobes and medial surface of cerebral hemispheres (includes motor and somesthetic cortex serving the legs), basal ganglia, and corpus callosum.	Emotional lability Confusion, amnesia, personality changes Urinary incontinence Contralateral hemiplegia or hemiparesis, greater in the leg than in the arm
Posterior cerebral artery supplies medial and inferior temporal lobes, medial occipital lobe, thalamus, posterior hypothalamus, and visual receptive area	Hemianesthesia Contralateral hemiplegia, greater in the face and arm than in the leg Cerebellar ataxia, tremor Homonymous hemianopsia, cortical blindness Receptive aphasia Memory deficits Weber's syndrome

Vertebral or basilar arteries supply the brain stem and cerebellum
   Incomplete occlusion
 	
   Anterior portion of the pons
 	
   Complete occlusion or hemorrhage
	
	Unilateral and bilateral weakness of extremities; upper motor neuron weakness involving face, tongue, and throat; loss of vibratory sense, two-point discrimination, and position sense
	Diplopia, homonymous hemianopsia
	Nausea, vertigo, tinnitus, and syncope
	Dysphagia, dysarthria
	Sometimes confusion and drowsiness
	"Locked-in" syndrome—no movement except eyelids; sensation and consciousness preserved
	Coma or death
	Miotic pupils
	Decerebrate rigidity
	Respiratory and circulatory abnormalities

Posterior inferior cerebellar artery supplies the lateral and posterior portion of the medulla	Wallenberg syndrome Dysphagia, dysphonia Nystagmus, vertigo, nausea, and vomiting Ipsilateral anesthesia of face and cornea for pain and temperature (touch preserved) Contralateral anesthesia of trunk and extremities for pain and temperature Ipsilateral Horner syndrome Ipsilateral decompensation of movement
Anterior inferior and superior cerebellar arteries supply the cerebellum	Difficulty with articulation, gross movements of limbs—ipsilateral ataxia Nystagmus, vertigo, nausea, and vomiting Ipsilateral Horner syndrome

Data from Hunt WE, Hess RM: Surgical risk as related to time of intervention in the repair of intracranial aneurysms, J Neurosurg 28(1):14-20, 1968; Hunt WE, Meagher JN, Hess RM: Intracranial aneurysm: a nine-year study, Ohio State Med J 62(11):1168-1171, 1966.

- Watershed stroke: A cerebral infarct between the terminal areas of perfusion of two different arteries, typically between the anterior and middle cerebral arteries[17]

Arteriovenous Malformation

AVM is a malformation in which blood from the arterial system is shunted to the venous system (thereby bypassing the capillaries) through abnormally thin and dilated vessels, making them prone to ruptures causing intracerebral hemorrhage. An AVM can occur in a variety of locations, shapes, and sizes. The result of the bypass of blood is degeneration of brain parenchyma around the site of the AVM, which creates a chronic ischemic state. Signs and symptoms of AVM include headache, dizziness, fainting, seizure, aphasia, bruit, and motor and sensory deficits.[64] Management of AVM includes cerebral angiogram to evaluate the precise location of the AVM, followed by

TABLE 6-23 Focal Signs in Patients with Aneurysms at Various Sites

Site of Aneurysms	Clinical Findings
Internal carotid—post communicating	Cranial nerve III palsy
Middle cerebral artery	Contralateral face or hand paresis Aphasia (left side) Contralateral visual neglect (right side)
Anterior communicating	Bilateral leg paresis Bilateral Babinski sign
Basilar artery apex	Vertical gaze paresis Coma
Intracranial vertebral artery/posterior inferior cerebellar artery	Vertigo Elements of lateral medullary syndrome

From Goetz CG, editor: Textbook of clinical neurology, ed 2, Philadelphia, 2003, Saunders.

TABLE 6-24 Hunt and Hess Scale for Measuring Subarachnoid Hemorrhage

I	Asymptomatic, mild headache and mild nuchal rigidity, no neurologic deficit
II	Moderate to severe headache, nuchal rigidity, without neurologic deficit other than cranial nerve palsy
III	Drowsiness, confusion, with mild focal neurologic deficit
IV	Stupor, moderate to severe focal deficits, such as hemiplegia
V	Comatose, decerebrate posturing

Adapted from Daroff RB, Fenichel GM, Jankovic J et al, editors: Bradley's neurology in clinical practice, ed 6, Philadelphia, 2012, Saunders, p 1078.

surgical AVM repair, embolization, radiosurgery (stereotactic), photon beam therapy, or medical management alone with close monitoring in some cases.[43]

Cerebral Aneurysm

Cerebral aneurysm is the dilation of a cerebral blood vessel wall owing to a smooth muscle defect through which the endothelial layer penetrates. Cerebral aneurysms most commonly occur at arterial bifurcations and in the larger vessels of the anterior circulation. Signs and symptoms of unruptured cerebral aneurysm are determined by size and location, detailed in Table 6-23. When an aneurysm ruptures, blood is released under arterial pressure into the subarachnoid space and quickly spreads through the CSF around the brain and spinal cord.[43] Signs and symptoms of ruptured aneurysm include violent headache, stiff neck, photophobia, vomiting, hemiplegia, aphasia, seizure, and CN (III, IV, VI) palsy.[17] Management of cerebral aneurysm involves CT scan or angiogram to closely evaluate the aneurysm, followed by aneurysm clipping, embolization, coiling, or balloon occlusion.

Subarachnoid Hemorrhage

Subarachnoid hemorrhage, the accumulation of blood in the subarachnoid space, is most commonly the result of aneurysm rupture, or less commonly a complication of AVM, tumor, infection, or trauma. It is graded from I to V according to the Hunt and Hess scale (Table 6-24).[17,65]

SAH is diagnosed by history, clinical examination, noncontrast CT scan, LP, or angiogram. The management of SAH depends on its severity and may include surgical aneurysm repair with blood evacuation; ventriculostomy; and supportive measures to maximize neurologic, cardiac, and respiratory status, rehydration, and fluid-electrolyte balance.

Complications of SAH include rebleeding, hyponatremia, hydrocephalus, seizure, and vasospasm. Vasospasm is the spasm (constriction) of one or more cerebral arteries that occurs 4 to 12 days after SAH.[66] The etiology is unknown and is diagnosed by either transcranial Doppler, cerebral angiography, or CT. Vasospasm results in cerebral ischemia distal to the area of spasm if untreated. The signs and symptoms of vasospasm are worsening level of consciousness, agitation, decreased strength, altered speech, pupil changes, headache, and vomiting, and they may wax and wane with the degree of vasospasm. There is currently a vast amount of research concerning treatment of vasospasm. HHH therapy (hypertension, hypervolemia, and hemodilution) has traditionally been the treatment of choice for vasospasm[66]; however, recent studies have questioned the validity of hemodilution as an effective strategy.[67,68] Additional treatment options being studied include angioplasty[69,70] and administration of intra-arterial medicines such as calcium channel blockers[71] or inotropes, specifically milrinone.[72]

Dementia

Dementia is a syndrome of acquired persistent dysfunction in several domains of intellectual function including memory, language, visuospatial ability, and cognition (abstraction, mathematics, judgment, and problem solving).[73] There are numerous conditions that can cause or contribute to dementia, including:

- Alzheimer's disease
- Acquired immunodeficiency syndrome
- Alcoholism
- Lewy body dementia
- Metabolic disorders
- Multi-infarct dementia
- Multiple sclerosis
- Neoplasms
- Parkinson's disease
- Vascular dementia

It is beyond the scope of this book to discuss each type in depth. The following are some of the most common dementias encountered in the acute care setting.

Alzheimer's disease (AD) is the most common cause of dementia.[73] Patients with AD usually experience a gradual onset of cognitive deficits caused by amyloid plaques in the brain that replace healthy white matter. There is no specific test for diagnosis. A detailed medical history, mini–mental exam, neurologic exam, and MRI assist in diagnosing AD. In the acute care setting, patients with AD are often admitted with a sudden decline in function including decreased interactions with caregivers, decrease in initiation, apraxia, or combative behavior. Infections such as urinary tract infection can cause the decline in function, and symptoms usually improve with antibiotics.

Lewy body dementia (LBD) is characterized by marked fluctuations in cognition, visual and auditory hallucinations, clouding of consciousness, and mild spontaneous extrapyramidal symptoms caused by a pathologic accumulation of Lewy bodies in the brain stem and cortex.[73] These patients also display a pronounced sensitivity to antipsychotics, with a tendency to develop severe parkinsonism.[74] The diagnosis is made in a similar manner as Alzheimer's disease and is differentiated from AD by the day-to-day fluctuations and the sensitivity to antipsychotics. The disease process is progressive with an average mortality of 12 to 13 years after diagnosis.[74]

Vascular dementia is usually abrupt in onset and may be a consequence of multiple cortical infarctions, multiple subcortical infarctions (lacunar state), ischemic injury to the deep hemispheric white matter, or a combination of these.[73] Diagnosis is made through an accurate history that may include atherosclerosis with myocardial infarction, retinopathy, hypertension, or stroke; EEG; and MRI. The patient presents with relative preservation of personality with emotional lability, depression, somatic preoccupation, and nocturnal confusion.

The focus of physical therapy in the acute care setting for all of these patients is to maximize function while ensuring safety of the patient.

> ✎ **CLINICAL TIP**
>
> Patients with dementia have an elevated fear of falling, which can interfere with mobility. It is helpful to stand in front of the patient during transfers so that the patient cannot see the floor. Keep instructions functional and simple. Reduce stimuli and avoid distractions during treatment by closing the door or pulling the curtain.

Ventricular Dysfunction

Hydrocephalus

Hydrocephalus is the acute or gradual accumulation of CSF, causing excessive ventricular dilation and increased ICP. CSF permeates through the ventricular walls into brain tissue secondary to a pressure gradient.

There are two types of hydrocephalus:

1. Noncommunicating (obstructive) hydrocephalus, in which there is an obstruction of CSF flow within the ventricular system. There may be thickening of the arachnoid villi or an increased amount or viscosity of CSF. This condition may be congenital or acquired, often as the result of aqueduct stenosis, tumor obstruction, abscess, or cyst, or as a complication of neurosurgery.[4]

2. Communicating hydrocephalus, in which there is an obstruction in CSF flow as it interfaces with the subarachnoid space. This condition can occur with meningitis, after head injury, with SAH, or as a complication of neurosurgery.[2]

Hydrocephalus may be of acute onset characterized by headache, altered consciousness, decreased upward gaze, and papilledema.[11] Management includes treatment of the causative factor if possible, or placement of a ventriculoperitoneal (VP) or ventriculoatrial (VA) shunt.

Normal-pressure hydrocephalus (NPH) is a type of communicating hydrocephalus without an associated rise in ICP and occurs primarily in the elderly.[56] NPH is typically gradual and idiopathic but may be associated with previous meningitis, trauma, or SAH.[56] The hallmark triad of NPH is altered mental status (confusion), altered gait (usually wide-based and shuffling with difficulty initiating ambulation), and urinary incontinence. NPH is diagnosed by history, CT scan, or MRI to document ventriculomegaly, and lumbar puncture. LP is performed to remove excessive CSF (usually 40 to 50 ml).[56] A video recording is often made of the patient before and after the lumbar puncture to observe for improvements in gait and cognition. If symptoms are significantly improved, the decision may be made for VP shunt placement. Recent studies have shown up to a 90% success rate in shunt placement in patients who showed improvement after lumbar puncture.[75]

> ✎ **CLINICAL TIP**
>
> The clinician should be aware that patients with NPH often present with a similar gait pattern to patients with Parkinson's disease.

Cerebrospinal Fluid Leak

A CSF leak is the abnormal discharge of CSF from a scalp wound, the nose (rhinorrhea), or the ear (otorrhea) as a result of a meningeal tear. A CSF leak can occur with anterior fossa or petrous skull fractures or, less commonly, as a complication of neurosurgery. With a CSF leak, the patient becomes at risk for meningitis with the altered integrity of the dura. A CSF leak, which usually resolves spontaneously in 7 to 10 days,[17] is diagnosed by clinical history, CT cisternography, and testing of fluid from the leak site. If the fluid is CSF (and not another fluid [e.g., mucus]), it will test positive for glucose. The patient may also complain of a salty taste in the mouth. Management of CSF leak includes prophylactic antibiotics (controversial), lumbar drainage for leaks persisting more than 4 days, dural repair for leaks persisting more than 10 days, or VP or VA shunt placement.[64]

> ✎ **CLINICAL TIP**
>
> If it is known that a patient has a CSF leak, the therapist should be aware of vital sign or position restrictions before physical therapy intervention. If a CSF leak increases or a new leak occurs during physical therapy intervention, the therapist should stop the treatment, loosely cover the leaking area, and notify the nurse immediately.

Seizure

A seizure is defined as abnormal neurologic functioning caused by abnormally excessive activation of neurons, either in the cerebral cortex or in the deep limbic system.[59] The signs and symptoms of the seizure depend on the seizure locus on the cortex (e.g., visual hallucinations accompany an occipital cortex locus). Seizures can occur as a complication of CVA, head trauma, brain tumor, meningitis, or surgery. Febrile state, hypoxia, hyperglycemia or hypoglycemia, hyponatremia, severe uremic or hepatic encephalopathy, drug overdose, and drug or alcohol withdrawal are also associated with seizures.[76] Seizures are classified as partial (originating in a focal region of one hemisphere) or generalized (originating in both hemispheres or from a deep midline focus) (Table 6-25).

Seizures are of acute onset, with or without any of the following: aura, tremor, paresthesia, sensation of fear, gustatory hallucinations, lightheadedness, and visual changes. Seizure history, including prodrome or aura (if any), for the patient with a recent seizure or epilepsy should be established by either chart review or interview to be as prepared as possible to assist the patient if seizure activity should occur.

Seizure activity can be irrefutably identified only by EEG. Synchronized EEG with video recording may be required to differentiate pseudoseizures (also called *psychogenic* seizures) from seizures, and both may coexist in the same patient.[59] Medical management of seizures involves the treatment of causative factors (if possible) and antiepileptic drugs. Surgical management for seizure refractory to medical management may consist of the resection of the seizure focus or the implantation of a vagal nerve stimulator.[77]

Terms related to seizure include[17,76]:
- Prodrome: The signs and symptoms (e.g., smells, auditory hallucinations, a sense of déjà vu) that precede a seizure by hours
- Aura: The signs and symptoms (as just listed) that precede a seizure by seconds or minutes
- Epilepsy or seizure disorder: Refers to recurrent seizures
- Status epilepticus: More than 30 minutes of continuous seizure activity or two or more seizures without full recovery of consciousness between seizures. Generalized tonic-clonic status epilepticus is a medical emergency marked by the inability to sustain spontaneous ventilation with the potential for hypoxia requiring pharmacologic and life support. Often the result of tumor, CNS infection, or drug abuse in adults.
- Postictal state: The period of time immediately after a seizure characterized by lethargy, confusion, and, in some cases, paralysis. This state can last minutes to hours and even days.

Syncope

Syncope is the transient loss of consciousness and postural tone secondary to cerebral hypoperfusion, usually accompanied by bradycardia and hypotension.[77] Syncope can be any of the following[78]:
- Cardiogenic syncope, resulting from drug toxicity; dysrhythmias, such as atrioventricular block or supraventricular tachycardia; cardiac tamponade; atrial stenosis; aortic aneurysm; pulmonary hypertension; or pulmonary embolism
- Neurologic syncope, resulting from benign positional vertigo, carotid stenosis, cerebral atherosclerosis, seizure, spinal cord lesions, or peripheral neuropathy associated with diabetes mellitus or with degenerative diseases, such as Parkinson's disease
- Metabolic syncope, resulting from hypoglycemia, hyperventilation-induced alkalosis, or hypoadrenalism
- Reflexive syncope, resulting from carotid sinus syndrome, pain, emotions, or a vasovagal response after eating, coughing, or defecation
- Orthostatic syncope, resulting from the side effects of drugs, volume depletion, or prolonged bed rest

The cause of syncope is diagnosed by clinical history, blood work such as hematocrit and blood glucose, electrocardiogram, Holter or continuous-loop event recorder, echocardiogram, or tilt-table testing. CT and MRI are performed only if new neurologic deficits are found.[78] EEG may be performed to rule out seizure. The management of syncope, dependent on the etiology and frequency of the syncopal episode(s), may include treatment of the causative factor; pharmacologic agents, such as

TABLE 6-25   Seizure Classifications

Classification	Type	Characteristics
Partial seizures[76]	Simple partial	Partial seizures without loss of consciousness
	Complex partial	Brief loss of consciousness marked by motionless staring
	Partial evolving to secondary generalization	Progression to seizure activity in both hemispheres
Generalized seizures[76]	Tonic	Sudden flexor or extensor rigidity
	Tonic-clonic	Sudden extensor rigidity followed by flexor jerking. This type of seizure may be accompanied by incontinence or a crying noise owing to rigidity of the truncal muscles
	Clonic	Rhythmic jerking muscle movements without an initial tonic phase
	Atonic	Loss of muscle tone
	Absence	Very brief period (seconds) of unresponsiveness with blank staring and the inability to complete any activity at the time of the seizure
	Myoclonic	Local or gross rapid, nonrhythmic jerking movements

beta-adrenergic blockers; fluid repletion; or cardiac pacemaker placement. Compression stockings, an abdominal binder, slowly raising the head of the bed before sitting at the edge of the bed, and lower extremity exercises once sitting can help to reduce orthostatic hypotension.

Neuroinfectious Diseases

Refer to Chapter 13 for a description of encephalitis, meningitis, and poliomyelitis.

Vestibular Dysfunction

Dizziness is one of the leading complaints of patients seeking medical attention. It is up to the clinician to take a detailed history of the complaint to determine the primary etiology. Patients use the term *dizzy* to describe a multitude of symptoms:

- Vertigo: A sense that the environment is moving or spinning (usually caused by vestibular dysfunction)
- Lightheadedness: A feeling of faintness (usually caused by orthostatic hypotension, hypoglycemia, or cardiac in origin; refer to Chapters 3 and 7 for further details)
- Dysequilibrium: Sensation of being off balance (usually associated with lower extremity weakness or decreased proprioception caused by neuropathy)

Vertigo is the hallmark symptom of vestibular dysfunction. The vestibular system is complex and made up of a peripheral system and a central system. The peripheral system includes three semicircular canals and two otolith organs in the inner ear. The central system includes pathways between the inner ear, the vestibular nuclei in the brainstem, cerebellum, cerebral cortex, and the spinal cord. The vestibular system functions to:

- Stabilize visual images on the retina during head movement for clear vision
- Maintain postural stability during head movements
- Maintain spatial orientation

After the clinician has determined that there is a vestibular system pathology (Table 6-26), the next step is to determine if the pathology is peripheral or central (Table 6-27).

Peripheral vestibular system pathology includes benign positional paroxysmal vertigo (BPPV), acute vestibular neuronitis, Ménière's disease, and ototoxicity. These conditions are discussed next. Central vestibular pathology is caused by stroke affecting the cerebellar supply and/or vertebral artery; TIA; traumatic brain injury; migraine; tumor; and demyelinating diseases such as MS that affect the eighth cranial nerve.[7,79,80] The underlying cause of the pathology must be treated for optimal recovery. Physical therapy focuses on the primary diagnosis and compensatory strategies to help with nystagmus or unresolved vertigo.

Benign Positional Paroxysmal Vertigo

BPPV, the most common peripheral vestibular disorder,[79] is characterized by severe vertigo associated with specific changes in head position with or without nausea and vomiting. The impairments are directly caused by a misplaced otoconium in the semicircular canal from head trauma, whiplash injury, surgery, prolonged inactivity, or aging.[9] The otoconia are either

"free-floating" in the canal, giving rise to canalithiasis, or adhered to the cupola in the canal, called cupulolithiasis. Typically, symptoms of vertigo last less than 60 seconds[7] and are precipitated by specific head movements such as looking up to a high shelf, rolling over in bed to one direction, or lying on a specific side.

The Hallpike-Dix test (Figure 6-9) is the most common test for BPPV and is performed in the following manner[79]: The patient is positioned on an examination table such that when he or she is placed supine, the head extends over the edge. The patient is lowered quickly with the head supported and turned 45 degrees to one side or the other. The eyes are carefully observed. If no abnormal eye movements are seen in a 30-second time period, the patient is returned to the upright position. The maneuver is repeated with the head turned in the opposite direction. The direction, duration, and time of onset of the nystagmus is noted and is helpful in determining which semicircular canal is involved as well as differentiating between canalithiasis and cupulolithiasis. In canalithiasis, onset of symptoms will be delayed 2 to 20 seconds and will last less than 40

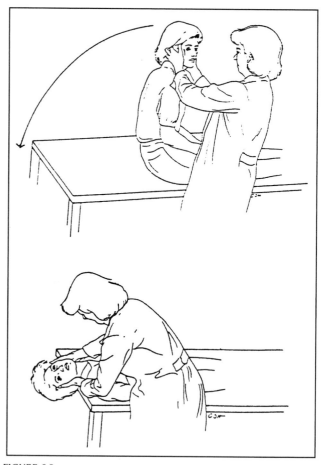

FIGURE 6-9

Hallpike-Dix maneuver for eliciting nystagmus and vertigo due to posterior or anterior canal BPPV. The patient's head is first turned 45 degrees to the right. The patient's neck and shoulders are then brought into the supine position with the neck extended below the level of the examination table. The patient is observed for nystagmus or complaints of vertigo. The patient is next returned to the upright position if the test is negative. (From Herdman S: Treatment of benign paroxysmal positional vertigo, *Phys Ther* 70:381-388,1990.)

TABLE 6-26 Tests and Measures for Vestibular Dysfunction*

Test	Test Procedure	Vestibular Pathology
Static ocular observation	The eyes are examined for the presence of nystagmus while the head is still. If nystagmus is present, the clinician observes for any change with gaze fixation.	Nystagmus is present when the head is still and improves with gaze fixation indicative of unilateral vestibular hypofunction.
Examination of saccades	Saccades are examined by asking the patient to alternately fixate (with the head still) the examiner's nose and then finger, held at different locations at approximately 15 degrees away from primary position. The velocity, accuracy, and initiation time are observed.	Slowed saccades or the inability to complete without also moving the head indicates vestibular pathology.
Head thrust test	The patient fixates on a close object (examiner's nose) while the head is manually rotated, by the examiner, in an unpredictable direction using a small-amplitude, high-acceleration angular thrust.	The eyes will not move as quickly as the head rotation, and the eyes move off the target with a corrective saccade to reposition the eyes on the target. This is indicative of vestibular hypofunction.
Head-shaking–induced nystagmus	The patient closes his or her eyes while the examiner flexes the head 30 degrees and oscillates the head horizontally for 20 cycles at a frequency of 2 reps per second. Once the oscillations are stopped, the patient opens his or her eyes and the examiner observes for nystagmus.	Horizontal nystagmus indicates a unilateral peripheral vestibular lesion, with the slow phase of nystagmus toward the side of the lesion. Vertical nystagmus suggests a central lesion.
Hallpike-Dix test	The patient's head is rotated 45 degrees to one side in sitting and moved into a supine position with the head extended 30 degrees over the end of the examination table with the head still rotated. The examiner observes for the presence of nystagmus.	The presence of nystagmus indicates BPPV.
Dynamic visual acuity (DVA) test	The patient attempts to read the lowest line of an eye chart while the clinician horizontally oscillates the patient's head at a frequency of 2 reps per second.	A decrement in visual acuity of three or more lines during the head movement indicates vestibular hypofunction.
Caloric testing	Air or water is infused into the external auditory canal. The change in temperature generates nystagmus within the horizontal SCC in intact vestibular systems.	The absence of or slowed nystagmus indicates pathology in the horizontal SCC.
Rotary chair test	Patients are rotated in a chair in the dark. Nystagmus is present in intact vestibular systems.	The absence of or slowed nystagmus indicates pathology in the horizontal SCC.
Rhomberg test	Patient stands with the feet together with eyes open and then with the eyes closed.	Increase in sway or loss of balance with the eyes closed may indicate vestibular dysfunction.
Sensory organization test	There are six parts to the test: In condition 1, the patient stands on a fixed platform with eyes open. In 2, the patient stands on a fixed platform with the eyes closed. In 3, the patient stands on a fixed platform with moving vision screen. In conditions 1-3, the patient is relying on somatosensory and vestibular input. The test is repeated with a moving platform to distort somatosensory input, and in condition 6 (moving platform and moving vision screen), the patient is relying on vestibular input alone. Sway is noted and recorded as minimal, mild or moderate, and fall.	The patient will be unable to maintain balance in condition 6 if vestibular dysfunction is present and vision and somatosensory input are intact. The examiner has to be aware that patients may also lose their balance in other conditions because of impaired vision or sensation that is seen normally in the aging process.

Data from O'Sullivan SB, Schmitz TJ, editors: Physical rehabilitation, ed 5, Philadelphia, 2007, FA Davis; Cummings CW, Flint PW et al, editors: Otolaryngology: head & neck surgery, ed 4, Philadelphia, 2005, Mosby.
BPPV, Benign positional paroxysmal vertigo; SCC, semicircular canal.
*Before performing these tests, ensure that the patient's cervical spine is intact and can tolerate neck/head rotation. Also ensure that the vertebral arteries are not compromised.

TABLE 6-27 Symptoms Associated with Peripheral versus Central Vestibular Pathology

Symptom	Peripheral	Central
Balance deficits	Mild to moderate	Severe, ataxia usually present
Hearing loss	Accompanied with fullness of the ears and tinnitus	Rare; if it does occur, often sudden and permanent
Nystagmus	Unidirectional in all gaze positions; decreases with visual fixation	Changes direction in different gaze positions; no change with visual fixation
Nausea	Can be severe	Variable, may be absent
Additional neurologic impairment	Usually not present	Can include diplopia, altered consciousness, lateropulsion

Data from Cummings CW et al, editors: Otolaryngology: head & neck surgery, ed 4, Philadelphia, 2005, Mosby; Schubert MC: Vestibular disorders. In O'Sullivan SB, Schmitz TJ, editors: Physical rehabilitation, ed 5, Philadelphia, 2007, FA Davis, p 1013.

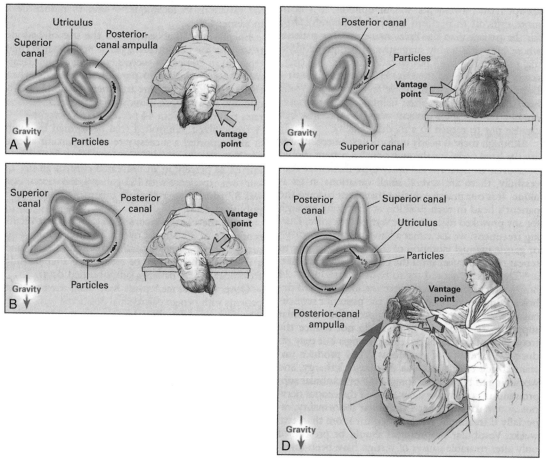

FIGURE 6-10

The Epley maneuver. (From Furman JM, Cass SP: Benign paroxysmal positional vertigo, N Engl J Med 341:1590-1596, 1999. Copyright 1999 Massachusetts Medical Society. All rights reserved.)

seconds.[81] In cupulolithiasis, onset of symptoms is immediate and continues for more than 60 seconds.

If the Hallpike-Dix test is positive for canalithiasis, the Epley maneuver (Figure 6-10) is utilized to reposition the otoconia by sequentially moving the head into four positions, staying in each position for roughly as long as the nystagmus lasted during the Hallpike-Dix test. For example, if the nystagmus lasted for 25 seconds during the Hallpike-Dix test, each position during the Epley maneuver is held for 25 seconds. Of cases of BPPV, 95% are posterior canalithiasis and can be treated with the Epley maneuver. Treatment of cupulolithiasis and horizontal canalithiasis are beyond the scope of this book. The reader is encouraged to refer to Susan Herdman's *Vestibular Rehabilitation*, ed 3, for more information. The recurrence rate for BPPV after these maneuvers is about 30% at 1 year, and in some instances a second treatment may be necessary.[81]

Physical Therapy Implications.

• Contraindications for the Hallpike-Dix test and Epley maneuver include vertebral artery stenosis, cervical spine dysfunction, or osteoporosis.

- Recommend discussing with the physician whether premedicating the patient with meclizine before performing the Epley or Hallpike-Dix maneuvers is appropriate. It may help to reduce or eliminate nausea/vomiting from the maneuvers.
- The clinician should direct the patient to keep his/her chin tucked to the shoulder (closest to the ground) when transitioning from the last position of the Epley maneuver to sitting, to avoid the otoconia dropping into the horizontal canal.

Acute Vestibular Neuronitis

Acute vestibular neuronitis (vestibular neuritis) is an inflammation of the vestibular nerve, usually caused by viral infection.[80] Symptoms include a dramatic, sudden onset of vertigo lasting days, with gradual improvement. Nystagmus may or may not be present, and hearing deficits are not noted. Treatment is usually supportive, and symptoms should resolve in 1 to 2 weeks. Treatment with antivirals has not been shown to be effective.[82]

Vestibular neuritis can be mistaken for BPPV. A detailed history can usually differentiate between these two disorders before the patient is examined. In cases of neuritis, the patient usually can tell the examiner in vivid detail what they were doing at the sudden onset of dizziness. Dizziness is constant and usually associated with nausea and vomiting. With BPPV, symptoms usually are provoked by a change in position or specific head movement and resolve with rest or gaze stabilization. In cases of neuritis, patients should be encouraged to keep well hydrated and to sit out of bed, in a supportive chair and well-lit room, to maximize somatosensory and visual input.

Ménière's Disease

Ménière's disease (idiopathic endolymphatic hydrops) is a disorder of the inner ear associated with spontaneous, episodic attacks of vertigo; sensorineural hearing loss that usually fluctuates; tinnitus; and often a sensation of aural fullness.[79] This is likely caused by an increase in endolymphatic fluid causing distention of the membranous labyrinth.[9] Ménière's disease is usually treated with a salt-restricted diet and the use of diuretics to control the fluid balance within the ear as well as vestibular suppressing medications such as meclizine. When conservative treatment has failed, an endolymphatic shunt can be placed; ablation of a portion of the labyrinth can be attempted; or vestibular neurectomy can be performed. Physical therapy focuses on patient education and compensatory strategies such as gaze and postural stabilization.

Bilateral Vestibular Hypofunction

Bilateral vestibular hypofunction (BVH) is most commonly caused by ototoxicity of aminoglycosides (gentamicin, streptomycin). The bilateral loss of vestibular function leads to oscillopsia (oscillating or swinging vision) and unsteady gait to varying degrees.[79] Impairments are usually permanent, although patients can return to high levels of function by learning to use visual and somatosensory information to make up for the loss of vestibular function. Other, less common causes of BVH include meningitis, autoimmune disorders, head trauma, tumors on each eighth cranial nerve, TIA of vessels supplying the vestibular system, and sequential unilateral vestibular neuronitis.[7]

Common Degenerative Central Nervous System Diseases

Amyotrophic Lateral Sclerosis

Amyotrophic lateral sclerosis (ALS), or Lou Gehrig's disease, is the progressive degeneration of upper and lower motor neurons, primarily the motor cells of the anterior horn and the corticospinal tract. The etiology of ALS is unknown except for familial cases. Signs and symptoms of ALS depend on the predominance of upper or lower motor neuron involvement and may include hyperreflexia, muscle atrophy, fasciculation, and weakness, which result in dysarthria, dysphagia, respiratory weakness, and immobility.[83] If more upper motor neurons are affected, the symptoms will be primarily clumsiness, stiffness, and fatigue, whereas lower motor neuron degeneration will present as weakness or atrophy and occasionally fasciculations. Bulbar symptoms include hoarseness, slurring of speech, choking on liquids, and difficulty initiating swallowing and are more predominant in cases of familial ALS.[43] ALS is diagnosed by clinical presentation, EMG, nerve conduction velocity (NCV) studies, muscle and nerve biopsies, and neuroimaging studies to rule out other diagnoses.[7] Owing to the progressive nature of ALS, management is typically supportive or palliative, depending on the disease state, and may include pharmacologic therapy (Rilutek [riluzole]), spasticity control, bronchopulmonary hygiene, and nutritional and psychosocial support.[64] Physical therapy and rehabilitation are important with patients with ALS to maximize compensatory strategies and to prescribe appropriate adaptive equipment to maintain the patient's independence for as long as possible.

Guillain-Barré Syndrome

Guillain-Barré syndrome (GBS), or acute inflammatory demyelinating polyradiculopathy, is caused by the breakdown of Schwann cells by antibodies.[64] There is an onset of paresthesia, pain (especially of the lumbar spine), symmetric weakness (commonly distal to proximal, including the facial and respiratory musculature), diminishing reflexes, and autonomic dysfunction approximately 1 to 3 weeks after a viral infection. GBS is diagnosed by history, clinical presentation, CSF sampling (increased protein level), and EMG studies (which show decreased motor and sensory velocities).[84] Once diagnosed, the patient with GBS is hospitalized because of the potential for rapid respiratory muscle paralysis.[84] Functional recovery varies from full independence to residual weakness that takes 12 to 24 months to resolve.[64,84] GBS is fatal in 5% to 10% of cases.[85] The management of GBS may consist of pharmacologic therapy (immunosuppressive agents), plasma exchange, intravenous immunoglobulin, respiratory support, physical therapy, and the supportive treatment of associated symptoms (e.g., pain management).

BOX 6-1   Definitions and Terminology Used to Describe Categories of Multiple Sclerosis

- Relapsing-remitting MS (RRMS): Characterized by relapses with either full recovery or some remaining neurologic signs/symptoms and residual deficit on recovery; the periods between relapses are characterized by lack of disease progression.
- Primary-progressive MS (PPMS): Characterized by disease progression from onset, without plateaus or remissions or with occasional plateaus and temporary minor improvements.
- Secondary-progressive MS (SPMS): Characterized by initial relapsing-remitting course, followed by progression at a variable rate that may also include occasional relapses and minor remissions.
- Progressive-relapsing MS (PRMS): Characterized by progressive disease from onset but without clear acute relapses that may or may not have some recovery or remission; commonly seen in patients who develop the disease after 40 years of age.
- Benign MS: Characterized by mild disease in which patients remain fully functional in all neurologic systems 15 years after disease onset.
- Malignant MS (Marburg's variant): Characterized by rapid progression leading to significant disability or death within a relatively short time after onset.

Multiple Sclerosis

MS is the demyelination of the white matter of the CNS and of the optic nerve, presumably an autoimmune reaction induced by a viral or other infectious agent.[7] Symptoms of MS are highly variable from person to person, and the specific type of MS is categorized by the progression of symptoms (Box 6-1).[7]

MS typically occurs in 20 to 40 year olds and in women more than in men. It is diagnosed by history (onset of symptoms must occur and resolve more than once), clinical presentation, CSF sampling (increased myelin protein and immunoglobulin G levels, called oligoclonal bands), evoked potential recording, and MRI (which shows the presence of two or more plaques of the CNS).[7,11] These plaques are located at areas of demyelination where lymphocytic and plasma infiltration and gliosis have occurred. Signs and symptoms of the early stages of MS may include focal weakness, fatigue, diplopia, blurred vision, equilibrium loss (vertigo), paresthesias, Lhermitte's sign, and urinary incontinence. Additional signs and symptoms of the later stages of MS may include ataxia, paresthesias, spasticity, sensory deficits, hyperreflexia, tremor, and nystagmus.[83] The management of MS may include pharmacologic therapy (corticosteroids for

---

✎ CLINICAL TIP

Patients with MS usually present with an adverse reaction to heat, triggering an exacerbation marked by decline in function and an increase in fatigue. Heat stressors are anything that can raise body temperature, including sun exposure, hot environment, or a hot bath or pool. This exacerbation usually resolves within 24 hours.

---

acute relapse/exacerbations; synthetic interferons such as interferon beta-1a [Avonex, Rebif]; or immunosuppressants such as mitoxantrone [Novantrone]), skeletal muscle relaxants (baclofen), physical therapy, and the treatment of associated disease manifestations (e.g., bladder dysfunction).

Parkinson's Disease

Parkinson's disease (PD) is a neurodegenerative disorder caused by a loss of dopaminergic neurons in the substantia nigra, as well as other dopaminergic and nondopaminergic areas of the brain.[86] PD is characterized by progressive onset of bradykinesia, altered posture and postural reflexes, resting tremor, and cogwheel rigidity. Other signs and symptoms may include shuffling gait characterized by the inability to start or stop, blank facial expression, drooling, decreased speech volume, an inability to perform fine-motor tasks, and dementia.[43,83] PD is diagnosed by history, clinical presentation, and MRI (which shows a light rather than dark substantia nigra).[11,65] The management of PD mainly includes pharmacologic therapy with antiparkinsonian agents and physical therapy. Levodopa is the most effective treatment for PD, but chronic use can cause hallucinations, dyskinesias, and motor fluctuations.[43] There are also several surgical options that have emerged including the placement of a deep brain stimulator (DBS) and, most recently, stem cell implants. The DBS has showed the most promise, with recent studies showing improvement in quality of life rating[87] and a decrease in tremors.[88] To date there have been limited studies completed to support the effectiveness of fetal graft transplantation in humans,[88] although multiple studies using rat models have showed improvements.[89,90]

✎ CLINICAL TIP

The clinician should be aware that patients with PD, especially those taking a beta blocker, have a higher incidence of orthostatic hypotension and have a tendency toward retropulsion (pushing posteriorly in sitting and standing) with mobility.

General Management

Intracranial and Cerebral Perfusion Pressure

The maintenance of normal ICP or the prompt recognition of elevated ICP is one of the primary goals of the team caring for the postcraniosurgical patient or the patient with cerebral trauma, neoplasm, or infection.

ICP is the pressure CSF exerts within the ventricles. This pressure (normally 4 to 15 mm Hg) fluctuates with any systemic condition, body position, or activity that increases cerebral blood flow, blood pressure, or intrathoracic or abdominal pressure; decreases venous return; or increases cerebral metabolism.

The three dynamic variables within the fixed skull are blood, CSF, and brain tissue. As ICP rises, these variables change in an attempt to lower ICP via the following mechanisms: cerebral vasoconstriction, compression of venous sinuses, decreased CSF production, or shift of CSF to the subarachnoid space. When

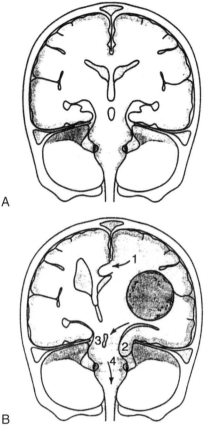

FIGURE 6-11

Herniation syndromes depicted. Intracranial shifts from supratentorial lesions. **A,** Normal location of structures. **B,** Various herniation syndromes are demonstrated: *1,* Cingulate gyrus herniating under falx cerebri. *2,* Temporal lobe herniating downward through the tentorial notch. *3,* Compression of contralateral cerebral peduncle. *4,* Downward displacement of brain stem through tentorial notch showing central herniation syndrome. (From Beare PG, Myers JL, editors: Adult health nursing, ed 3, Philadelphia, 1998, Saunders, p 919.)

these compensations fail, compression of brain structures occurs, and fatal brain herniation will develop if untreated (Figure 6-11). The signs and symptoms of increased ICP are listed in Table 6-28. The methods of controlling ICP, based on clinical neurologic examination and diagnostic tests, are outlined in Table 6-29. Table 18-5 describes the different types of ICP monitoring systems.

Cerebral perfusion pressure (CPP), or cerebral blood pressure, is mean arterial pressure minus ICP. It indicates oxygen delivery to the brain. Normal CPP is 70 to 100 mm Hg. CPPs at or less than 60 mm Hg for a prolonged length of time correlate with ischemia and anoxic brain injury.[91]

The following are terms related to ICP:

- Brain herniation: The displacement of brain parenchyma through an anatomic opening; named according to the location of the displaced structure (e.g., transtentorial herniation is the herniation of the cerebral hemispheres, diencephalon, or midbrain beneath the tentorium cerebelli).
- Mass effect: The combination of midline shift, third ventricle compression, and hydrocephalus.[11]

TABLE 6-28 Early and Late Signs of Increased Intracranial Pressure

Observation	Early	Late
Level of consciousness	Confusion, restlessness, lethargy	Coma
Pupil appearance	Ipsilateral pupil sluggish to light, ovoid in shape, with gradual dilatation	Papilledema, ipsilateral pupil dilated and fixed, or bilateral pupils dilated and fixed (if brain herniation has occurred)
Vision	Blurred vision, diplopia, and decreased visual acuity	Same as early signs but more exaggerated
Motor	Contralateral paresis	Abnormal posturing, bilateral flaccidity if herniation has occurred
Vital signs	Stable blood pressure and heart rate	Hypertension, bradycardia, and altered respiratory pattern (Cushing's triad); increased temperature
Additional findings	Headache, seizure, cranial nerve palsy	Headache, vomiting, altered brain stem reflexes

Data from Hickey JV: The clinical practice of neurological and neurosurgical nursing, ed 4, Philadelphia, 1997, Lippincott.

- Midline shift: The lateral displacement of the falx cerebri secondary to a space-occupying lesion.
- Space-occupying lesion: A mass lesion, such as a tumor or hematoma that displaces brain parenchyma and may result in the elevation of ICP and shifting of the brain.

Another primary goal of the team is to prevent further neurologic impairment. The main components of management of the patient with neurologic dysfunction in the acute care setting include pharmacologic therapy, surgical procedures, and physical therapy intervention.

Pharmacologic Therapy

A multitude of pharmacologic agents can be prescribed for the patient with neurologic dysfunction. These include antianxiety medications (see Chapter 19, Table 19-15), anticonvulsants (see Chapter 19, Table 19-16), antidepressants (see Chapter 19, Table 19-17), antipsychotics (see Chapter 19, Table 19-18), mood stabilizers (see Chapter 19, Table 19-19), Parkinson's medications (see Chapter 19, Table 19-21), diuretics (see Chapter 19, Table 19-3), and adrenocorticosteroids (see Chapter 19, Table 19-8).

Additional pharmacologic agents for medical needs include antibiotics (e.g., for infection or after neurosurgery), antihypertensives, thrombolytics, anticoagulants, chemotherapy and

TABLE 6-29 Treatment Options to Decrease Intracranial Pressure (ICP)

Variable	Treatment
Blood pressure	Inotropic drugs to maintain mean arterial pressure > 90 mm Hg to aid in cerebral perfusion, or antihypertensives
Osmotherapy	Osmotic diuretic to minimize cerebral edema
Mechanical ventilation	Normocapnia* to maximize cerebral oxygen delivery by limiting cerebral ischemia from the vasoconstrictive effects of decreased $PaCO_2$
Cerebrospinal fluid drainage	Ventriculostomy to remove cerebrospinal fluid
Sedation/paralysis	Barbiturates to decrease cerebral blood flow or other medication to decrease the stress of noxious activities
Positioning	Head of the bed positioned at 30-45 degrees to increase cerebral venous drainage. Promote neutral cervical spine and head position
Environment	Dim lights, decreased noise, frequent rest periods to decrease external stimulation
Seizure control	Prophylactic anticonvulsant medication
Temperature control	Normothermia or induced hypothermia to 32-35° C (e.g., cooling blanket or decreased room temperature) to decrease cerebral metabolism

Data from Wong F: Prevention of secondary brain injury, Crit Care Nurs 20:18-27, 2000.

*Routine aggressive hyperventilation is no longer used for the control of elevated ICP. Hyperventilation can contribute to secondary brain injury because of a rebound increase in cerebral blood flow and volume in response to a decreased cerebrospinal fluid pH.

TABLE 6-30 Common Neurosurgery Procedures

Aneurysm clipping	The obliteration of an aneurysm with a surgical clip placed at the stem of the aneurysm.
Burr hole	A small hole made in the skull with a drill for access to the brain for the placement of ICP monitoring systems, hematoma evacuation, or stereotactic procedures; a series of burr holes is made before a craniotomy.
Craniectomy	The removal of incised bone, usually for brain (bone flap) tissue decompression; the bone may be permanently removed or placed in the bone bank or temporarily placed in the subcutaneous tissue of the abdomen (to maintain blood supply) and replaced at a later date.
Cranioplasty	The reconstruction of the skull with a bone graft or acrylic material to restore the protective properties of the scalp and for cosmesis.
Craniotomy	An incision through the skull for access to the brain for extensive intracranial neurosurgery, such as aneurysm or AVM repair or tumor removal; craniotomy is named according to the area of the bone affected (e.g., frontal, bifrontal, frontotemporal [pterional], temporal, occipital).
Embolization	The use of arterial catheterization (entrance usually at the femoral artery) to place a material, such as a detachable coil, balloon, or sponge, to clot off an AVM or aneurysm.
Evacuation	The removal of an epidural, subdural, or intraparenchymal hematoma via burr hole or craniotomy.
Shunt placement	The insertion of a shunt system that connects the ventricular system with the right atrium (VA shunt) or peritoneal cavity (VP shunt) to allow the drainage of CSF when ICP rises.
Stereotaxis	The use of a stereotactic frame (a frame that temporarily attaches to the patient's head) in conjunction with head CT results to specifically localize a pretargeted site, as in tumor biopsy; a burr hole is then made for access to the brain.

AVM, Arteriovenous malformation; *CSF*, cerebrospinal fluid; *CT*, computed tomography; *ICP*, intracranial pressure; *VA*, ventriculoatrial; *VP*, ventriculoperitoneal.

radiation for CNS neoplasm, stress ulcer prophylaxis (e.g., after SCI), pain control, and neuromuscular blockade.

Neurosurgical Procedures

The most common surgical and nonsurgical neurologic procedures are described in Table 6-30. Refer to Table 5-3 for a description of surgical spine procedures and Table 18-5 for a description of ICP monitoring devices.

The clinician should pay close attention to head-of-bed positioning restrictions for the patient who has recently had neurosurgery. Often, the head of the bed is at 30 degrees, or it may be flat for an initial 24 hours and then gradually elevated 15 to 30 degrees per day depending on the location of surgery (supratentorial or infratentorial, respectively).[17]

> ### ✎ CLINICAL TIP
>
> The physical therapist should be aware of the location of a craniectomy because the patient should not have direct pressure applied to that area. Look for signs posted at the patient's bedside that communicate positioning restrictions.

Physical Therapy Intervention

Goals

The primary physical therapy goals in treating patients with primary neurologic pathology in the acute care setting include maximizing independence and promoting safety with gross functional activity. Another main goal is to assist in the prevention of the secondary manifestations of neurologic dysfunction and immobility, such as pressure sores, joint contracture, and the deleterious effects of bed rest (see Chapter 1, Table 1-1).

Management Concepts for Patients with Neurologic Dysfunction

- A basic understanding of neurologic pathophysiology is necessary to create appropriate functional goals for the patient. The therapist must appreciate the difference between reversible and irreversible and between nonprogressive and progressive disease states.

- There are a number of natural changes of the nervous system with aging, such as decreased coordination, reflexes, balance, and visual acuity. Be sure to accommodate for these normal changes in the examination of and interaction with the elderly patient.

- Take extra time to observe and assess the patient with neurologic dysfunction, as changes in neurologic status are often very subtle.

- A basic knowledge of the factors that affect ICP and the ability to modify treatment techniques or conditions during physical therapy intervention for the patient with head trauma, after intracranial surgery, or other pathology interfering with intracranial dynamics is necessary for patient safety.

- Patient and family or caregiver education is an important component of physical therapy. Incorporate information about risk factor reduction (e.g., stroke prevention) and reinforce health care team recommendations (e.g., swallowing strategies per the speech-language pathologist).

- There are a variety of therapeutic techniques and motor-control theories for the treatment of the patient with neurologic dysfunction. Do not hesitate to experiment with or combine techniques from different schools of thought.

- Be persistent with patients who do not readily respond to typical treatment techniques because these patients most likely present with perceptual impairments superimposed on motor and sensory deficits.

- Recognize that it is rarely possible to address all of the patient's impairments at once; therefore, prioritize the plan of care according to present physiologic status and future functional outcome.

References

1. Marieb EN, editor: Human anatomy and physiology, Redwood City, CA, 1989, Benjamin-Cummings, p 172.
2. Moore KL, Dalley AF: The head. In Moore KL, Dalley AF, editors: Clinically oriented anatomy, ed 4, Baltimore, 1999, Lippincott Williams & Wilkins, pp 832-891.
3. Westmoreland BF, Benarroch EE, Daube JR et al, editors: Medical neurosciences: an approach to anatomy, pathology, and physiology by systems and levels, ed 3, New York, 1986, Little, Brown, p 107.
4. Young PA, Young PH, editors: Basic clinical neuroanatomy, Baltimore, 1997, Williams & Wilkins, pp 251-258.
5. Marieb EN, editor: Human anatomy and physiology, Redwood City, CA, 1989, Benjamin-Cummings, p 375.
6. Wilkinson JL, editor: Neuroanatomy for medical students, ed 3, Oxford, UK, 1998, Butterworth-Heinemann, pp 189-200.
7. O'Sullivan SB, Schmitz TJ, editors: Physical rehabilitation, ed 5, Philadelphia, 2007, FA Davis.
8. Kiernan JA, editor: Barr's the human nervous system: an anatomical viewpoint, ed 7, Philadelphia, 1998, Lippincott-Raven, p 324.
9. Goodman CG, Boissonnault WG, editors: Pathology: implications for the physical therapist, Philadelphia, 1998, Saunders, p 685.
10. Goldberg S, editor: The four-minute neurological exam, Med-Master, 1992, Miami, p 20.
11. Lindsay KW, Bone I, Callander R, editors: Neurology and neurosurgery illustrated, ed 2, Edinburgh, UK, 1991, Churchill Livingstone, Edinburgh, UK.
12. Plum F, Posner J, Saper CB et al, editors: The diagnosis of stupor and coma, ed 4, New York, 2007, Oxford University Press, p 5.
13. Jennett B, Teasdale G, editors: Management of head injuries, Philadelphia, 1981, FA Davis, p 77.
14. Strub RL, Black FW, editors: Mental status examination in neurology, ed 2, Philadelphia, 1985, FA Davis, p 9.
15. Love RJ, Webb WG, editors: Neurology for the speech-language pathologist, ed 4, Boston, 2001, Butterworth-Heinemann, p 205.
16. Specter RM: The pupils. In Walker HK, Hall WD, Hurst JW, editors: Clinical methods: the history, physical, and laboratory examinations, ed 3, Boston, 1990, Butterworth, p 300.
17. Hickey JV, editor: The clinical practice of neurological and neurosurgical nursing, ed 4, Philadelphia, 1997, Lippincott.
18. Gilroy J: Neurological evaluation. In Gilroy J, editor: Basic neurology, ed 3, New York, 2000, McGraw-Hill, pp 29-30.
19. Kisner C, Colby LA: Therapeutic exercise foundations and techniques, ed 3, Philadelphia, 1996, FA Davis, p 57.
20. Katz RT, Dewald J, Schmit BD: Spasticity. In Braddon RL, editor: Physical medicine and rehabilitation, ed 2, Philadelphia, 2000, Saunders, p 592.
21. Victor M, Ropper AH: Motor paralysis. In Victor M, Ropper AH, editors: Adam and Victor's principles of neurology, New York, 2001, McGraw-Hill, pp 50-58.
22. Charness A: Gathering the pieces: evaluation. In Charness A, editor: Stroke/head injury: a guide to functional outcomes in physical therapy management, Rockville, MD, 1986, Aspen, p 1.
23. Bohannon RW, Smith MB: Interrater reliability of a Modified Ashworth Scale of Muscle Spasticity, Phys Ther 67:206, 1987.
24. Craven BC, Morris AR: Modified Ashworth Scale reliability for measurement of lower extremity spasticity among patients with SCI, Spinal Cord 48(3):207-213, 2010.

25. Ansari NN: The interrater and intrarater reliability of the Modified Ashworth Scale in the assessment of muscle spasticity: limb and muscle group effect. NeuroRehabilitation 23(3):231-237, 2008.

26. Fleuren JF: Stop using the Ashworth Scale for the assessment of spasticity, J Neurol Neurosurg Psychiatry 81(1):46-52, 2010.

26a. Tardieu G, Shentoub S, Delarue R: Research on a technic for measurement of spasticity [in French], Rev Neurol (Paris) 91:143-144, 1954.

26b. Boyd R, Graham H: Objective measurement of clinical findings in the use of botulinum toxin type A for the management of children with cerebral palsy, Eur J Neurol 6:S23-S35, 1999.

27. Singh P, Joshua AM, Ganeshan S et al: Intra-rater reliability of the Modified Tardieu Scale to quantify spasticity in elbow flexors and ankle plantar flexors in adult stroke subjects, Ann Indian Acad Neurol 14(1):23-26, 2011.

28. Merholz J, Wagner K, Meissner D et al: Reliability of the Modified Tardieu Scale and Modified Ashworth Scale in adult patients with severe brain injury: a comparison study, Clin Rehabil 19(7), 751-759, 2005.

29. Swartz MH: The nervous system. In Swartz MH, Schmitt W, editors: Textbook of physical diagnosis history and examination, ed 6, Philadelphia, 2009, Saunders, p 675.

30. O'Young BJ, Young MA, Stiens SA, editors: Physical medicine and rehabilitation secrets, ed 3, Philadelphia, 2008, Mosby, p 105.

31. Gelb DJ: The neurologic examination. In Gelb DJ, editor: Introduction to clinical neurology, ed 2, Boston, 2000, Butterworth-Heinemann, pp 43-90.

32. Kruse JA, Fink MP, Carlson RW, editors: Saunders manual of critical care, ed 1, Philadelphia, 2003, Saunders, p 498.

33. Bickley LS, Hoekelman RA: The nervous system. In Bickley LS, Bates B, Hoekelman RA, editors: Bates' guide to physical examination and history taking, ed 7, Philadelphia, 1999, Lippincott Williams & Wilkins, p 585.

34. Grainger RG, Allison D: In Grainger and Allison's diagnostic radiology: a textbook of medical imaging, ed 4, New York, 2001, Churchill Livingstone, p 1611.

35. Shpritz DW: Neurodiagnostic studies, Nurs Clin North Am 34(3):593-606, 1999.

36. Pagana KD, Pagana TJ, editors: Mosby's diagnostic and test reference, St Louis, 2007, Mosby.

37. Carlson AP, Brown AM, Zager E et al: Xenon-enhanced cerebral blood flow at 28% xenon provides uniquely safe access to quantitative, clinically useful cerebral blood flow information: a multicenter study, Am J Neuroradiol 32(7):1315-1320, 2011.

38. Yousem DM, Grossman RI, editors: Neuroradiology—the requisites, ed 3, Philadelphia, 2010, Mosby, pp 15-19.

39. Delapaz R, Chan S: Computed tomography and magnetic resonance imaging. In Rowland LP, editor: Merritt's neurology, ed 10, Philadelphia, 2000, Lippincott Williams & Wilkins, pp 55-63.

40. U-King-Im JM, Trivedi RA, Graves MJ et al: Contrast-enhanced MR angiography for carotid disease: diagnostic and potential clinical impact, Neurology 62(8):1282-1290, 2004.

41. Mohr JP, Wolf PA, Grotta JC et al, editors: Stroke—pathophysiology, diagnosis, and management, ed 5, Philadelphia, 2011, Saunders, p 910.

42. Chernecky CC, Berger BJ: Laboratory tests and diagnostic procedures, ed 4, Philadelphia, 2004, Saunders.

43. Goetz CG, editor: Textbook of clinical neurology, ed 2, Philadelphia, 2003, Saunders.

44. McNair ND: Traumatic brain injury, Nurs Clin North Am 34:637-659, 1999.

45. Wong F: Prevention of secondary brain injury, Crit Care Nurs 20:18-27, 2000.

46. Zink BJ: Traumatic brain injury outcome: concepts for emergency care, Ann Emerg Med 37:318-332, 2001.

47. National Spinal Cord Injury Statistical Center (NSISC). https://www.nscisc.uab.edu. [cited 2012 April 14].

48. Mitcho K, Yanko JR: Acute care management of spinal cord injuries, Crit Care Nurs Q 22:60-79, 1999.

49. Selzer ME, Tessler AR: Plasticity and regeneration in the injured spinal cord. In Gonzalez EG, Myers SJ, editors: Downey and Darling's physiological basis of rehabilitation medicine, ed 3, Boston, 2001, Butterworth-Heinemann, pp 629-632.

50. Dubendorf P: Spinal cord injury pathophysiology, Crit Care Nurs Q 22(2):31-35, 1999.

51. Mautes A, Weinzierl MR, Donovan F et al: Vascular events after spinal cord injury: contribution to secondary pathogenesis, Phys Ther 80:673-687, 2000.

52. Albers GW, Caplan LR, Easton JD et al for the TIA Working Group: Transient ischemic attack: proposal for a new definition, N Engl J Med 347:1713-1716, 2002.

53. Easton JD, Saver JL, Albers GW et al: Definition and evaluation of transient ischemic attack, Stroke 40:2276-2293, 2009.

54. Sacco RL, Adams R, Albers G et al: Guidelines for prevention of stroke in patients with ischemic stroke of transient ischemic attack: a statement for healthcare professionals from the American Heart Association/American Stroke Association Council on Stroke, Stroke 37:577-617, 2006.

55. Furie KL, Kasner SE, Adams RJ et al: Guidelines for the prevention of stroke in patients with stroke or transient ischemic attack. a guideline for healthcare professionals from the American Heart Association/American Stroke Association, Stroke 42(1):227-276, 2011.

56. Ferri FF: In Ferri's clinical advisor 2007: instant diagnosis and treatment, ed 9, Philadelphia, 2007, Mosby.

57. Lansberg MG, O'Donnel MJ, Khatri P et al: Antithrombotic and thrombolytic therapy for ischemic stroke, Chest 141(2 Suppl):e601S-636S, 2012.

58. Adams HP, del Zopp G, Alberts MJ et al: Guidelines for the early management of adults with ischemic stroke, Stroke 38:1655-1711, 2007.

59. Marx JA, editor: Rosen's emergency medicine: concepts and clinical practice, ed 6, Philadelphia, 2006, Mosby.

60. Broderick J, Connolly S, Feldmann E et al: Guidelines for the management of spontaneous intracerebral hemorrhage in adults, Stroke 38:2001-2023, 2007.

61. Furlan A, Higashida R, Wechsler L et al: Intra-arterial prourokinase for acute ischemic stroke: the PROACT II Study: a randomized control trial. Prolyse in Acute Cerebral Thromboembolism, JAMA 282(21):2003-2011, 1999.

62. Blank F, Keyes M: Thrombolytic therapy for patients with acute stroke in the ED setting, J Emerg Nurs 26:24-30, 2000.

62a. del Zoppo G, Saver J, Jauch EC et al: Expansion of the time window for treatment of acute ischemic stroke with intravenous tissue plasminogen activator: a science advisory from the American Heart Association/American Stroke Association, Stroke 40:2945, 2009.

63. Hock NH: Brain attack: the stroke continuum, Nurs Clin North Am 34:689-724, 1999.

64. Bradley WG, Daroff RB, Fenichel GM et al, editors: Pocket companion to neurology in clinical practice, ed 3, Boston, 2000, Butterworth-Heinemann.

65. Daroff RB, Fenichel GM, Jankovic J et al, editors: Bradley's neurology in clinical practice, ed 6, Philadelphia, 2012, Saunders, p 1078.

66. Mower-Wade D, Cavanaugh MC, Bush D: Protecting a patient with ruptured cerebral aneurysm, Nursing 31:52-57, 2001.

67. Chittboina P, Conrad S, McCarthy P et al: The evolving role of hemodilution in treatment of cerebral vasospasm: a historical perspective, World Neurosurg 75(5-6):660-664, 2011.

68. Robinson JS, Walid MS, Hyun S et al: Computational modeling of HHH therapy and impact on blood pressure and hematocrit, World Neurosurg 74(2-3):294-296, 2010.

69. Brisman JL, Eskridge JM, Newell DW: Neurointerventional treatment of vasospasm, Neurol Res 28(7):769-776, 2006.

70. Terry A, Zipfel G, Milner E et al: Safety and technical efficacy of over-the-wire balloons for the treatment of subarachnoid hemorrhage-induced cerebral vasospasm, Neurosurg Focus 21(3):E14, 2006.

71. Hui C, Lau KP: Efficacy of intra-arterial nimodipine in the treatment of cerebral vasospasm complicating subarachnoid hemorrhage, Clin Radiol 60(9):1030-1036, 2005.

72. Shankar JJ, dos Santos MP, Deus-Silva L et al: Angiographic evaluation of the effect of intra-arterial milrinone therapy in patients with vasospasm from aneurysmal subarachnoid hemorrhage, Neuroradiology 53(2):123-128, 2011.

73. Duthie EH, Katz PR, editors: Practice of geriatrics, ed 3, Philadelphia, 1998, Saunders.

74. Moore DP, Jefferson JW, editors: Handbook of medical psychiatry, ed 2, Philadelphia, 2004, Mosby.

75. Kilic K, Czorny A, Auque J et al: Predicting the outcome of shunt surgery in normal pressure hydrocephalus, J Clin Neurosci 14(8):729-736, 2007.

76. Drury IJ, Gelb DJ: Seizures. In Gelb DJ, editor: Introduction to clinical neurology, ed 2, Boston, 2000, Butterworth-Heinemann, pp 129-151.

77. Aminoff MJ: Nervous system. In Tierney LM, McPhee SJ, Papadakis MA, editors: Current medical diagnosis and treatment 2001, ed 40, New York, 2001, Lange Medical Books/McGraw-Hill, pp 979-980, 983-986.

78. Cox MM, Kaplan D: Uncovering the cause of syncope, Patient Care 34:39-48, 59, 2000.

79. Cummings CW, Flint PW et al, editors: Otolaryngology: head & neck surgery, ed 4, Philadelphia, 2005, Mosby.

80. Labuguen RH: Initial evaluation of vertigo, Am Fam Physician 73(2):244-251, 2006.

81. Luxon LM, Bamiou DE: Vestibular system disorders. In Schapira AHV, Byrne E, DiMauro S et al, editors: Neurology and clinical neuroscience, ed 1, Philadelphia, 2008, Mosby, pp 337-352.

82. Strupp M, Zingler VC, Arbusow V: Methylprednisolone, valacyclovir, or the combination for vestibular neuritis, N Engl J Med 351(4):354-361, 2004.

83. Fuller KS: Degenerative diseases of the central nervous system. In Goodman CC, Boissonnault WG, editors: Pathology: implications for the physical therapist, Philadelphia, 1998, Saunders, p 723.

84. Newswanger DL, Warren CR: Guillain-Barré syndrome, Am Fam Physician 69(10):2405-2410, 2004.

85. Aminoff MJ, editor: Neurology and general medicine, ed 4, Philadelphia, 2007, Churchill Livingstone, p 843.

86. Suchowersky O, Reich S, Perlmutter J et al: Practice parameters: diagnosis and prognosis of new onset Parkinson disease (an evidence-based review): report of the Quality Standards Subcommittee of the American Academy of Neurology, Neurology 66(7):976-982, 2006.

87. The Deep-Brain Stimulator for Parkinson's Disease Study Group: Deep-brain stimulation of the subthalamic nucleus or pars interna of the globus pallidus in Parkinson's disease, N Engl J Med 345:956-963, 2001.

88. Diamond A, Shahed J, Jankovic J: The effects of subthalamic nucleus deep brain stimulation on parkinsonian tremor, J Neurol Sci 260(1-2):199-203, 2007.

89. Anderson L, Caldwell MA: Human neural progenitor cell transplants into the subthalamic nucleus lead to functional recovery in a rat model of Parkinson's disease, Neurobiol Dis 27(2):133-140, 2007.

90. Wang XJ, Liu WG, Zhang YH et al: Effect of transplantation of c17.2 cells transfected with interleukin-10 gene on intracerebral immune response in rat model of Parkinson's disease, Neurosci Lett 423(2):95-99, 2007.

91. King BS, Gupta R, Narayan RJ: The early assessment and intensive care unit management of patients with severe traumatic brain and spinal cord injuries, Surg Clin North Am 80:855-870, 2000.

APPENDIX 6A MODIFIED TARDIEU SCALE SCORING SHEET

Date/Time	Joint/Muscle	Position of Patient	Velocity (V)	Muscle Response (X)	Angle of Catch (Y)

Example of a completed scoring sheet:

Date/Time	Joint/Muscle	Position of Patient	Velocity (V)	Muscle Response (X)	Angle of Catch (Y)
7/5/2012 8:15 am	Hamstring	Supine with the hip flexed to 90°	V1	0	N/A
			V2	2	−50° of extension
			V3	4	−60° of extension
7/7/2012 8:20 am (after Botox injection)	Hamstring	Supine with the hip flexed to 90°	V1	0	N/A
			V2	0	N/A
			V3	2	−30° of extension

As you can see, this is a more objective way of measuring spasticity, and trends can be more easily identified.

CHAPTER 7

Vascular System and Hematology

Falguni Vashi

CHAPTER OBJECTIVES

The objectives of this chapter are to provide the following:

1. Review the structure and function of blood and blood vessels
2. Review the vascular and hematologic evaluation, including physical examination and diagnostic and laboratory tests
3. Describe vascular, hematologic, and lymphatic health conditions, including clinical findings, medical and surgical management, and physical therapy intervention

PREFERRED PRACTICE PATTERNS

The most relevant practice patterns for the diagnoses discussed in this chapter, based on the American Physical Therapy Association's *Guide to Physical Therapist Practice*, second edition, are as follows:

- Arterial Disorders (Atherosclerosis, Aneurysm, Aortic Dissection, Hypertension, Raynaud's Disease), Chronic Regional Pain Syndrome, Compartment Syndrome: 4C, 4J, 6D, 7A
- Venous Disorders (Varicose Veins, Venous Thrombosis, Pulmonary Embolism, Chronic Venous Insufficiency): 4C, 6D, 7A
- Combined Arterial and Venous Disorders (Arteriovenous Malformations): 4C, 6D, 7A
- Hematologic Disorders (Erythrocytic Disorders [Anemia], Polycythemia), Thrombocytic Disorders: 4C, 6D
- Lymphatic Disorders (Lymphedema): 4C, 6D, 6H

Please refer to Appendix A for a complete list of the preferred practice patterns, as individual patient conditions are highly variable and other practice patterns may be applicable.

Alterations in the integrity of the vascular and hematologic systems can alter a patient's activity tolerance. The physical therapist must be aware of the potential impact that a change in blood composition or blood flow has on a multitude of body functions, including cardiac output, hemostasis, energy level, and healing.

Body Structure

The network of arteries, veins, and capillaries composes the vascular system. Living blood cells and plasma within the blood vessels are the structures that compose the hematologic system. The lymphatic system assists the vascular system by draining unabsorbed plasma from tissue spaces and returning this fluid (lymph) to the heart via the thoracic duct, which empties into the left jugular vein. The flow of lymph is regulated by intrinsic contractions of the lymph vessels, muscular contractions, respiratory movements, and gravity.[1]

Vascular System Structure

All blood vessels are composed of three similar layers (Figure 7-1 and Table 7-1). Blood vessel diameter, length, and wall thickness vary according to location and function (Table 7-2). Note

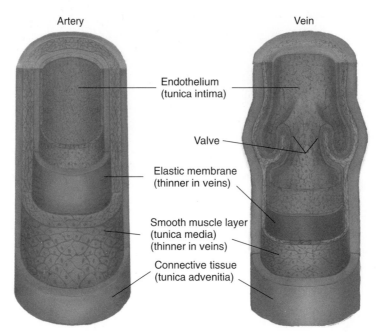

FIGURE 7-1
Structure of the arteries and veins. (From Lewis SL, Heitkepmer M, Dirksen S et al: Medical-surgical nursing: assessment and management of clinical problems, ed 7, St Louis, 2007, Mosby.)

TABLE 7-1 Blood Vessel Layers

Layer	Description	Function
Tunica intima	Innermost layer: Endothelial layer over a basement membrane	Provides a smooth surface for laminar blood flow
Tunica media	Middle layer: Smooth muscle cells and elastic connective tissue with sympathetic innervation	Constricts and dilates for blood pressure regulation
Tunica adventitia	Outermost layer: Composed of collagen fibers, lymph vessels, and the blood vessels that supply nutrients to the blood vessel	Protects and attaches blood vessels to nearby structures

Data from Marieb EN: Human anatomy and physiology, ed 3, Redwood City, CA, 1995, Benjamin-Cummings.

TABLE 7-2 Characteristics of Blood Vessels

Vessel	Description
Artery	Large or elastic arteries—aorta and its large branches and pulmonary artery. Medium or muscular arteries—composing other branches of aorta (i.e., coronary arteries). Small arteries and arterioles. Thick tunica media layer allows arteries to readily accommodate to pressure changes from the heart.
Vein	Small, medium, or large in diameter. Thin tunica media and thick tunica adventitia. Valves prevent backflow of blood to maintain venous return to the heart.
Capillary network	The interface of the arterial and venous systems where blood cells, fluids, and gases are exchanged. Capillary beds can be open or closed, depending on the circulatory requirements of the body.

Data from Marieb EN: Human anatomy and physiology, ed 3, Redwood City, CA, 1995, Benjamin-Cummings; Kumar V: Robbins and Cotran pathologic basis of disease, ed 7, Philadelphia, 2005, Saunders.

that the arteries are divided into three types, depending on their size and structural features.

Hematologic System Structure

Blood is composed of living cells (Table 7-3) in a nonliving plasma solution and accounts for 8% of total body weight, or 4 to 5 liters in women and 5 to 6 liters in men. Plasma is composed almost completely of water and contains more than 100 dissolved substances. The major solutes include albumin, fibrinogen, protein globules, nitrogenous substances, nutrients, electrolytes, and respiratory gases.[2]

Lymphatic System Structure

The lymphatic system includes lymph vessels, lymph fluid, and lymph tissues and organs (lymph nodes, tonsils, spleen, thymus, and the thoracic duct). The lymphatic system is parallel to and works in concert with the venous system. Lymphatics are fragile and are more likely to collapse under pressure than the veins. Lymphatics are located in all portions of the body except the central nervous system and cornea. Lymph moves throughout the body through a number of mechanisms, and the excess

TABLE 7-3 Blood Cell Types

Cell	Description
Erythrocyte (red blood cell; RBC)	Contains hemoglobin molecules responsible for oxygen transport to tissues. Composed of four protein chains (two alpha and two beta chains) bound to four iron pigment complexes. An oxygen molecule attaches to each iron atom to become oxyhemoglobin.
Leukocyte (white blood cell; WBC)	Five types of WBCs (neutrophils, basophils, eosinophils, lymphocytes, and monocytes) are responsible for launching immune defenses and fighting infection. WBCs leave the circulation to gain access to a site of infection.
Thrombocyte (platelet; Plt)	Cell fragment responsible for clot formation.

Data from Marieb EN: Human anatomy and physiology, ed 3, Redwood City, CA, 1995, Benjamin-Cummings.

TABLE 7-4 Functions of Blood

Function	Method
Oxygen and carbon dioxide transport	Binding to hemoglobin; dissolved in plasma
Nutrient and metabolite transport	Bound to plasma proteins; dissolved in plasma
Hormone transport	In plasma
Transport of waste products to kidneys and liver	In plasma
Transport of cells and substances involved in immune reactions	In plasma to site of infection or foreign body
Clotting at breaks in blood vessels	Hemostasis
Maintenance of fluid balance	Blood volume regulation
Body temperature regulation	Peripheral vasoconstriction or dilation
Maintenance of acid-base balance	Acid-base regulation

Data from Nettina S: The Lippincott manual of nursing practice, ed 8, Philadelphia, 2005, Lippincott Williams & Wilkins.

lymph is transported to the thoracic duct and emptied into the jugular vein trunks. Lymph fluid is first absorbed at the capillary level, then channeled through the small vessels and finally picked up by the larger valved vessels.[3]

Body Function

The function of the blood vessels is to carry blood throughout the body to and from the heart (Table 7-4). Normal alterations in the vessel diameter will occur, depending on circulating blood volume and the metabolic needs of the tissues.

The function of the lymphatic system is to (1) protect the body from infection and disease via the immune response and (2) to facilitate movement of fluid back and forth between the bloodstream and the interstitial spaces, removing excess fluid, blood waste, and protein molecules in the process of fluid exchange.[3]

The vascular and hematologic systems are intimately linked, and the examination of these systems is often similar. For the purpose of this chapter, however, the evaluations of the vascular and hematologic systems are discussed separately.

Physical Examination

Vascular Evaluation

History

In addition to the general chart review (see Chapter 2), it is important to gather the following information during examination of the patient with a suspected vascular disorder[4-8]:

- Relevant medical history that includes diabetes mellitus, hypertension, hyperlipidemia, syncope or vertigo, and non-healing ulcers.
- Relevant social history that includes exercise and dietary habits, as well as the use of tobacco or alcohol.
- History of recent prolonged bed rest and/or surgery or a long flight.
- Pain in arms and legs. (Visceral pain and arthritis pain may radiate to the extremities.)
- Presence of intermittent claudication (pain, ache, sense of fatigue, or other discomfort that occurs in the affected muscle group with exercise, particularly walking, and resolves with rest.) The speed, distance, and the site of the pain, including what relieves the pain, should be noted.
- Buttock, hip, or thigh claudication typically occurs in patients with obstruction of the aorta and iliac arteries. Calf claudication characterizes femoral and popliteal artery stenosis. The gastrocnemius muscle consumes more oxygen during walking than other muscle groups in the leg and hence causes the most frequent symptom reported by patients.
- Presence of nocturnal pain that can develop as the vascular occlusion worsens. This type of pain occurs when the patient is in bed and is caused by a combination of leg elevation and reduced cardiac output.
- Presence of rest pain refers to pain that occurs in the absence of activity and with legs in a dependent position. Rest pain signals advanced occlusive disease, typically greater than 90% occlusion.
- Presence or history of acute or chronic peripheral edema. If chronic, what is the patient's baseline level of edema?
- Precautions, such as weight bearing or blood pressure parameters after vascular surgery.

> ✎ **CLINICAL TIP**
>
> Intermittent claudication is often abbreviated in the clinical setting as IC.

Inspection

Observation of the following features can help delineate the location and severity of vascular disease and help determine whether these manifestations are arterial or venous in origin[1,4,5,9]:

- Skin color: Note the presence of any discoloration of the distal extremities/nail bed, which is indicative of decreased blood flow (e.g., mottled skin).
- Hair distribution: Patchy hair loss on the lower leg may indicate arterial insufficiency.
- Venous pattern: Dilation or varicosities—dilated, purplish, ropelike veins, particularly in the calf.
- Edema or atrophy: Peripheral edema from right-sided congestive heart failure occurs bilaterally in dependent areas; edema from trauma, lymphatic obstruction, or chronic venous insufficiency is generally unilateral. Refer to Table 3-5 for grading of pitting edema. Measurement of the extremities may help to identify the edema or atrophy. With a flexible tape, measure:
  - The forefoot
  - The smallest possible circumference above the ankle
  - The largest circumference at the calf
  - The mid-thigh, a measured distance above the patella with the knee extended

  A difference greater than 1 cm just above the ankle or 2 cm at the calf is suggestive of edema.
- Presence of cellulitis.
- Presence of petechiae: Small, purplish, hemorrhagic spots on the skin.
- Skin lesions: Ulcers, blisters, or scars.
- Digital clubbing: Could be indicative of poor arterial oxygenation or circulation.
- Gait abnormalities.

Palpation

During the palpation portion of the examination, the physical therapist can assess the presence of pain and tenderness, strength and rate of peripheral pulses, respiratory rate, blood pressure, skin temperature, and limb girth (if edematous). Changes in heart rate, blood pressure, and respiratory rate may correspond to changes in the fluid volume status of the patient. For example, a decrease in fluid volume may result in a decreased blood pressure that results in a compensatory increase in heart and respiratory rates. The decreased fluid volume and resultant increased heart rate in this situation may then result in a decreased strength of the peripheral pulses on palpation. A decreased or absent pulse provides insight into the location of arterial stenoses.[7] In patients with suspected or diagnosed peripheral vascular disease, monitoring distal pulses is more important than monitoring central pulses in the larger, more proximal vessels.[4]

The following system/scale is used to grade peripheral pulses[10]:

- 0: Absent, not palpable
- 1: Diminished, barely palpable
- 2: Brisk, expected
- 3: Full, increased
- 4: Bounding

Peripheral pulses can be assessed in the following arteries (see Chapter 3, Figure 3-6):

- Temporal
- Carotid
- Brachial
- Ulnar
- Radial
- Femoral
- Popliteal
- Posterior tibial
- Dorsalis pedis

> ### ✎ CLINICAL TIP
>
> A small percentage of the adult population may normally have absent peripheral pulses; 10% to 17% lack dorsalis pedis pulses.[1] Peripheral pulse grades are generally denoted in the medical record by physicians in the following manner: dorsalis pedis +1. The aorta can also be palpated in thin people.

Physical Therapy Considerations

- In patients who have disorders resulting in vascular compromise (e.g., diabetes mellitus, peripheral vascular disease, or hypertension), pulses should be monitored before, during, and after activity not only to determine any rate changes, but, more important, to determine any changes in the strength of the pulse.
- Notation should be made if the strength of pulses is correlated to complaints of pain, numbness, or tingling of the extremity.
- Compare the two extremities for color, temperature, and swelling. Bilateral coldness is most often due to cold environment and/or anxiety.[5]
- Carotid arteries should never be palpated simultaneously, as excessive carotid sinus massage can cause slowing of the pulse, cause a drop in blood pressure, and compromise blood flow to the brain. If the pulse is difficult to palpate, the patient's head should be rotated to the side being examined to relax the sternocleidomastoid.[10]

Auscultation

Systemic blood pressure and the presence of bruits (whooshing sound indicative of turbulent blood flow from obstructions) are assessed through auscultation.[4] Bruits are often indicative of accelerated blood flow velocity and flow disturbance at sites of stenosis.[7] Bruits are typically assessed by physicians and nurses (see Chapter 3 for further details on blood pressure measurement).

Vascular Tests

Various tests that can be performed clinically to evaluate vascular flow and integrity are described in Table 7-5. These tests can be performed easily at the patient's bedside without the use of diagnostic equipment. The Wells Clinical Decision Rule for Deep Venous Thrombosis is described in Table 7-6.

TABLE 7-5 Vascular Tests

Test	Indication	Description	Normal Results and Values
Capillary refill time*	To assess vascular perfusion and indirectly assess cardiac output.	Nail beds of fingers or toes are squeezed until blanching (whitening) occurs, and then they are released.	Blanching should resolve (capillary refill) in less than 2 seconds.
Elevation pallor	To assess arterial perfusion Normally color should not change. A gray (dark-skinned individuals) or pale/pallor (fair-skinned individuals) discoloration will result from arterial insufficiency or occlusion.	A limb is elevated 30-40 degrees for 15-60 seconds, and color changes are observed over 60 seconds.	Observe the amount of time it takes for pallor to appear: Pallor within 25 seconds indicates severe occlusive disease. Pallor within 25-40 seconds indicates moderate occlusive disease. Pallor within 40-60 seconds indicates mild occlusive disease.
Trendelenburg's test/ Retrograde filling test	To determine if superficial or deep veins and their valves are involved in causing varicosities.	To do Trendelenburg's test, mark the distended veins with a pen while the patient stands. Then have the patient lie on the examination table and elevate his or her leg for about a minute to drain the veins. Next, have the patient stand while you measure venous filling time. If the veins fill in less than 30 seconds, have the patient lie on the examination table again, and elevate his or her leg for 1 minute. Then apply a tourniquet around his or her upper thigh. Next, have the patient stand. Next, remove the tourniquet. To pinpoint incompetent valve location, repeat this procedure by applying the tourniquet just below the knee and then around the upper calf.	Competent valves take at least 30 seconds to fill. If leg veins still fill in less than 30 seconds, suspect incompetent perforating vein and deep vein valves (functioning valves block retrograde flow). If the veins fill again in less than 30 seconds, suspect incompetent superficial vein valves that allow backward blood flow.
Manual compression test	To detect competent valves in the veins.	Palpate the dilated veins with the fingertips of one hand. With the other hand, firmly compress the vein at a point at least 8 inches (20.3 cm) higher. Palpate the impulse under your finger.	With a competent valve, there will be no detectable impulse. A palpable impulse indicates incompetent valves in the vein segment between the two hands.
Allen's test	To assess the patency of the radial and ulnar arteries, to ensure the collateral circulation of the hand.	Flex the patient's arm with the hand above level of the elbow. Then compress the radial and ulnar arteries at the level of the wrist while the patient clenches his or her fist. The patient then opens his or her hand and either the radial or the ulnar artery is released. The process is repeated for the other artery.	When the patient opens the hand, the blanched area should flush within seconds if collateral circulation is adequate. If the blanched area does not flush quickly, then it may indicate that collateral circulation is inadequate to support circulation to the hand.
Homans' sign†	To detect the presence of deep vein thrombosis.	The calf muscle is gently squeezed, or the foot is quickly dorsiflexed.	Pain that is elicited with either squeezing or dorsiflexing may indicate a deep vein thrombosis.

Continued

TABLE 7-5 Vascular Tests—cont'd

Test	Indication	Description	Normal Results and Values
Ankle-brachial index (ABI)‡	To compare the perfusion pressures in the lower leg with the upper extremity using a blood pressure cuff and Doppler probe. This test is commonly used to screen patients for evidence of significant arterial insufficiency.	Place the patient in supine at least 10 minutes before the test. Obtain the brachial pressure in each arm, and record the highest pressure. Obtain the ankle pressure in each leg. Place the cuff around the lower leg 2.5 cm above the malleolus. Apply acoustic gel over the dorsalis pedis or posterior tibialis pulse location. Hold the Doppler probe lightly over the pedal pulse. Inflate the cuff to a level 20-30 mm Hg above the point at which the pulse is no longer audible. Slowly deflate the cuff while monitoring for the return of the pulse signal; the point at which the arterial signal returns is recorded as the ankle pressure. Calculate the ABI by dividing the higher of the two ankle systolic pressures by the higher of the brachial systolic pressures.	The diagnosis of peripheral arterial disease is based on the limb symptoms or an ABI. Interpretation of ABI ABI ≥ 1.0-1.3: normal range.§ ABI ≥ 0.7-0.8: borderline perfusion. ABI ≤ 0.5: severe ischemia, wound healing unlikely. ABI ≤ 0.4: critical limb ischemia.

Data from Seidel HM, Ball JW, Dains JE et al: Mosby's guide to physical examination, ed 7, St Louis, 2010, Mosby; Lanzer P, Rosch J, editors: Vascular diagnostics: noninvasive and invasive techniques, peri-interventional evaluations, Berlin, 1994, Springer Verlag; Springhouse: Handbook of medical-surgical nursing, ed 4, Philadelphia, 2005, Lippincott Williams & Wilkins; Newberry L, Sheehy S, editors: Sheehy's emergency nursing: principles and practice, ed 6, St Louis, 2009, Mosby; Dormandy JA, Rutherford RB: Management of peripheral arterial disease (PAD). TASC Working Group, J Vasc Surg 31:S1–S296, 2000; Hallet JW, Brewster DC, Darling RC, editors: Handbook of patient care in vascular surgery, ed 3, Boston, 1995, Little, Brown; Goodman CC: The hematologic system. In Goodman CC, Boisonnault WG, editors: Pathology: implications for the physical therapist, ed 3, Philadelphia, 2009, Saunders.

*Variability is found in defining the time by different individuals, so capillary refill time should not be considered an observation with exquisite sensitivity and specificity and should be used more to confirm clinical judgment.

†A 50% false-positive rate occurs with this test. Vascular laboratory studies are more sensitive.

‡ABI measurements may be of limited value in anyone with diabetes because calcification of the tibial and peroneal arteries may render them noncompressible.

§An ABI of less than 0.95 is considered abnormal and is 95% sensitive for the angiographically verified peripheral arterial stenosis.

Diagnostic Studies

Noninvasive Laboratory Studies. Various noninvasive procedures can examine vascular flow. The phrases *lower-extremity noninvasive studies* and *carotid noninvasive studies* are general descriptions that are inclusive of the noninvasive tests described in Table 7-7.

Invasive Vascular Studies. The most common invasive vascular study is arteriography, typically referred to as contrast angiography (Figure 7-2). This study is performed by injecting radiopaque dye into the femoral, lumbar, brachial, or axillary arteries, followed by radiographic viewing. Blood flow dynamics, abnormal blood vessels, vascular anomalies, normal and abnormal vascular anatomy, and tumors are easily seen during the radiographic viewing. With the use of digital-subtraction angiography (DSA), bony structures can be obliterated from the picture. DSA is useful when adjacent bone inhibits visualization of the blood vessel to be evaluated.[11] An angiogram is a picture produced by angiography. Angiography is generally performed before or during therapeutic interventions, such as percutaneous angioplasty, thrombolytic therapy, or surgical bypass grafting.

Postangiogram care includes the following[12]:

- Bed rest for 4 to 8 hours.
- Pressure dressings to the injection site with assessment for hematoma formation.
- Intravenous fluid administration to help with dye excretion. Blood urea nitrogen (BUN) and creatinine are monitored to ensure proper renal function (refer to Chapter 9 for more information on BUN and creatinine).
- Frequent vital sign monitoring with pulse assessments.
- If a patient has been on heparin before angiography, the drug is not resumed for a minimum of 4 hours.[12]

The complications of arteriography can be due to the catheterization or due to the contrast agent that is injected (Table 7-8).

Hematologic Evaluation

The medical workup of the patient with a suspected hematologic abnormality includes the patient's medical history and laboratory studies, in addition to the patient's clinical presentation.

History

In addition to the general chart review (see Chapter 2), the following questions are especially relevant in the evaluation of the patient with a suspected hematologic disorder[13-15]:

- What are the presenting symptoms?
- Was the onset of symptoms gradual, rapid, or associated with trauma or other disease?

TABLE 7-6 Wells Clinical Decision Rule (CDR) for Deep Venous Thrombosis

Clinical Characteristic	Score*
Active cancer (treatment ongoing within previous 6 mo or palliative)	1
Paralysis, paresis, or recent plaster immobilization of the lower extremities	1
Recently bedridden for more than 3 days or major surgery, within 4 weeks	1
Localized tenderness along the distribution of the deep venous system	1
Entire leg swollen	1
Calf swelling by more than 3 cm when compared with the asymptomatic leg (measured 10 cm below tibial tuberosity)	1
Pitting edema (greater in the symptomatic leg)	1
Collateral superficial veins (nonvaricose)	1
Alternative diagnosis as likely as or more likely than deep vein thrombosis	−2

From Wells PS, Anderson DR, Bormanis J et al: Value of assessment of pretest probability of deep-vein thrombosis in clinical management, Lancet 350(9094):1795-1798, 1997.

*−2 to 0: Low probability of DVT (3%); 1 to 2: Moderate probability of DVT (17%); 3 or more: High probability of DVT (75%). Medical consultation is advised in the presence of low probability; medical referral is required with moderate or high score.

TABLE 7-7 Noninvasive Vascular Studies

Test	Description
Doppler ultrasound	High-frequency and low-intensity (1-10 MHz) sound waves are applied to the skin with a Doppler probe (and acoustic gel) to detect the presence or absence of blood flow, direction of flow, and flow character over arteries and veins with an audible signal. Low-frequency waves generally indicate low-velocity blood flow. Ultrasound examination has a sensitivity and specificity of approximately 95%.
Color duplex scanning or imaging	Velocity patterns of blood flow along with visual images of vessel and plaque anatomy can be obtained by combing ultrasound with a pulsed Doppler detector. Distinctive color changes indicate blood flow through a stenotic area.
Plethysmography	Plethysmography is a noninvasive test that provides measurement of changes in the volume of the blood distal to the affected area indicating an occlusion and specifically for the amount of time required for the veins to refill after being emptied.
Exercise testing	Exercise testing is performed to assess the nature of claudication by measuring ankle pressures and pulse volume recordings (PVRs) after exercise. A drop in ankle pressures can occur with arterial disease. This type of testing provides a controlled method to document onset, severity, and location of claudication. Screening for cardiorespiratory disease can also be performed, as patients with peripheral vascular disease often have concurrent cardiac or pulmonary disorders (see Chapter 3).
Computed tomography (CT)	CT is used to provide visualization of the arterial wall and its structures. Indications for CT include diagnosis of abdominal aortic aneurysms and postoperative complications of graft infections, occlusions, hemorrhage, and abscess.
Magnetic resonance imaging (MRI)	MRI has multiple uses in evaluating the vascular system and is now more commonly used to visualize the arterial system than arteriograms. Specific uses for MRI include detection of deep venous thrombosis and evaluation of cerebral edema. (Serial MRIs can also be used to help determine the optimal operative time for patients with cerebrovascular accidents by monitoring their progression.)
Magnetic resonance angiography (MRA)	MRA uses blood as a physiologic contrast medium to examine the structure and location of major blood vessels and the flow of blood through these vessels. The direction and rate of flow can also be quantified. MRA minimizes complications that may be associated with contrast medium injection. Figure 7-2 illustrates the MRA of the aorta and lower extremity.

Data from Black JM, Matassarin-Jacobs E, editors: Luckmann and Sorensen's medical-surgical nursing: a psychophysiologic approach, ed 4, Philadelphia, 1993, Saunders, p 1286; Bryant RA, Nix DP: Acute and chronic wounds. Current management concepts, ed 4, St Louis, 2012, Mosby; Lanzer P, Rosch J, editors: Vascular diagnostics: noninvasive and invasive techniques, peri-interventional evaluations, Berlin, 1994, Springer Verlag; Kee JL, editor: Laboratory and diagnostic tests with nursing implications, ed 8, Stamford, CT, 2009, Appleton & Lange, p 606; Malarkey LM, Morrow ME, editors: Nurses manual of laboratory tests and diagnostic procedures, ed 2, Philadelphia, 2000, Saunders, p 359; Mettler FA: In Essentials of radiology, ed 2, Philadelphia, 2005, Saunders; Fahey VA, editor: Vascular nursing, ed 4, Philadelphia, 2003, Saunders; McCance KL, Huether SE, editors: Pathophysiology: the biologic basis for disease in adults and children, ed 6, St Louis, 2009, Mosby, p 1001; George-Gay B, Chernecky CC: In Clinical medical-surgical nursing: a decision-making reference, ed 1, Philadelphia, 2002, Saunders; Schroeder ML: Principles and practice of transfusion medicine, ed 10. In Lee GR, Foerster J, Lukens J et al, editors: Wintrobe's clinical hematology, vol 1, Baltimore, 1999, Lippincott Williams & Wilkins, pp 817-874.

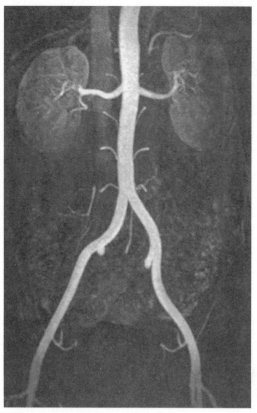

FIGURE 7-2
Magnetic resonance angiography (MRA) of the aorta and lower extremity arterial circulation. (From Adam A: Grainger & Allison's diagnostic radiology, ed 5, London, 2008, Churchill Livingstone.)

TABLE 7-8 Complications of Contrast Arteriography

Cause	Complication
Puncture site or catheter related	Hemorrhage/hematoma Pseudoaneurysm Arteriovenous fistula Atheroembolism Local thrombosis
Contrast agent related	Major (anaphylactoid) sensitivity reaction Minor sensitivity reactions Vasodilation/hypotension Nephrotoxicity Hypervolemia

From Belkin M, Owens CD, Whittemore AD et al: Peripheral arterial occlusive disease. In Townsend CM, Beauchamp RD, Evers BM et al, editors: Sabiston textbook of surgery: the biological basis of modern surgical practice, ed 18, Philadelphia, 2007, Saunders.

- Is the patient unable to complete daily activities secondary to fatigue?
- Is there a patient or family history of anemia or other blood disorders, cancer, hemorrhage, or systemic infection?
- Is there a history of blood transfusion?
- Is there a history of chemotherapy, radiation therapy, or other drug therapy?
- Has there been an environmental or occupational exposure to toxins?

- Have there been night sweats, chills, or fever?
- Is the patient easily bruised?
- Is wound healing delayed?
- Is there excessive bleeding or menses?

Other relevant data include the patient's diet (for the evaluation of vitamin- or mineral-deficiency anemia), history of weight loss (as a warning sign of cancer or altered metabolism), whether the patient abuses alcohol (a cause of anemia with chronic use), and race (some hematologic conditions have a higher incidence in certain races).

Inspection

During the hematologic evaluation, the patient is observed for the following[13,16,17]:

- General appearance (for lethargy, malaise, or apathy)
- Degree of pallor or flushing of the skin, mucous membranes, nail beds, and palmar creases. Pallor can be difficult to assess in dark-skinned individuals. In these individuals, lips, tongue, mucosa, and nail beds should be monitored.
- Presence of petechiae (purplish, round, pinpoint, nonraised spots caused by intradermal or subcutaneous hemorrhage) or ecchymosis (bruising)
- Respiratory rate

Palpation

The examination performed by the physician includes palpation of lymph nodes, liver, and spleen as part of a general physical examination. For specific complaints, the patient may receive more in-depth examination of a body system. Table 7-9 summarizes abnormal hematologic findings by body system on physical examination.

The physical therapist may specifically examine the following:

- The presence, location, and severity of bone or joint pain using an appropriate pain scale (see Chapter 21)
- Joint range of motion and integrity, including the presence of effusion or bony abnormality
- Presence, location, and intensity of paresthesia
- Blood pressure and heart rate for signs of hypovolemia (see Palpation in the Vascular Evaluation section for a description of vital sign changes with hypovolemia)

Laboratory Studies

In addition to the history and physical examination, the clinical diagnosis of hematologic disorders is based primarily on laboratory studies.

Complete Blood Cell Count. The standard complete blood cell (CBC) count consists of a red blood cell (RBC) count, white blood cell (WBC) count, WBC differential, hematocrit (Hct) measurement, hemoglobin (Hgb) measurement, and platelet (Plt) count (Table 7-10). Figure 7-3 illustrates a common method used by the medical-surgical team to document portions of the CBC in progress notes. If a value is abnormal, it is usually circled within this "sawhorse" figure.

Physical Therapy Considerations

- The most important thing to consider when looking at hemoglobin values is the patient's oxygen supply versus

TABLE 7-9 Signs and Symptoms of Hematologic Disorders by Body System

Body System	Sign/Symptom	Associated Condition
Cardiac	Tachycardia	Anemia, hypovolemia
	Palpitations	Anemia, hypovolemia
	Murmur	Anemia, hypovolemia
	Angina	Anemia, hypovolemia
Respiratory	Dyspnea	Anemia, hypovolemia
	Orthopnea	Anemia, hypovolemia
Musculoskeletal	Back pain	Hemolysis
	Bone pain	Leukemia
	Joint pain	Hemophilia
	Sternal tenderness	Leukemia, sickle cell disease
Nervous	Headache	Severe anemia, polycythemia, metastatic tumor
	Syncope	Severe anemia, polycythemia
	Vertigo, tinnitus	Severe anemia
	Paresthesia	Vitamin B_{12} anemia, malignancy
	Confusion	Severe anemia, malignancy, infection
Visual	Visual disturbances	Anemia, polycythemia
	Blindness	Thrombocytopenia, anemia
Gastrointestinal, urinary, and reproductive	Dysphagia	Iron-deficiency anemia
	Abdominal pain	Lymphoma, hemolysis, sickle cell disease
	Splenomegaly or hepatomegaly	Hemolytic anemia
	Hematemesis, melena	Thrombocytopenia and clotting disorders
	Hematuria	Hemolysis and clotting disorders
	Menorrhagia	Iron-deficiency anemia
Integumentary	Petechiae	Iron-deficiency anemia
	Ecchymosis	Hemolytic, pernicious anemia
	Flushing	Iron-deficiency anemia
	Jaundice	Hemolytic anemia
	Pallor	Conditions with low hemoglobin

Data from Black JM, Matassarin-Jacobs E, editors: Medical-surgical nursing: clinical management for continuity of care, ed 5, Philadelphia, 1997, Saunders.

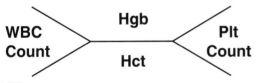

FIGURE 7-3
Illustration of portions of the complete blood cell count in shorthand format. *Hct,* Hematocrit; *Hgb,* hemoglobin; *Plt,* platelet; *WBC,* white blood cell.

demand. Decreased Hgb levels can reduce oxygen transport capacity and subsequently reduce the oxygen supply, which can reduce a patient's endurance level.

- It is important to consider the trends in the Hgb and Hct levels. If Hct/Hgb levels are low at baseline, these patients may be able to tolerate activity. However, patients with acutely low levels of Hct/Hgb may or may not tolerate increased activity.
- A physical therapist should be aware of signs and symptoms of hypoxia to major organs: brain, heart, and kidneys.
- Monitoring of tolerance and modifications in the therapeutic plan may be indicated with low levels of Hct/Hgb.[18] Hct is accurate in relation to fluid status; therefore Hct may be falsely high if the patient is dehydrated and falsely low if the patient is fluid overloaded.[11]

- Hct is approximately three times the Hgb value.
- A low Hct may cause the patient to experience weakness, dyspnea, chills, or decreased activity tolerance, or it may exacerbate angina.
- Patients with cancer such as leukemia or patients who are receiving cancer treatment will most likely present with lower Hct and Hgb values; therefore the therapist should proceed with caution in these patients.
- The term *pancytopenia* refers to a significant decrease in RBCs, all types of WBCs, and platelets.
- The term *neutropenia* refers to an abnormal decrease in WBCs, particularly neutrophils.
- The term *leukocytosis* refers to an abnormal increase in circulating WBCs.
- The term *thrombocytopenia* refers to a significant decrease in platelets.
- The term *thrombocytosis* refers to an abnormal increase in platelets.

Erythrocyte Indices. RBC, Hct, and Hgb values are used to calculate three erythrocyte indices: (1) mean corpuscular volume (MCV), (2) mean corpuscular Hgb, and (3) mean corpuscular Hgb concentration (Table 7-11). At most institutions, these indices are included in the CBC.

Erythrocyte Sedimentation Rate. The erythrocyte sedimentation rate (ESR), often referred to as the *sed rate,* is a

TABLE 7-10 Complete Blood Cell Count: Values and Interpretation*

Test	Description	Value	Indication/Interpretation
Red blood cell (RBC) count	Number of RBCs per µl of blood	Female: 4.2-5.4 million/µl Male: 4.7-6.1 million/µl	Blood loss, anemia, polycythemia. Elevated RBC count may increase risk of venous stasis or thrombi formation. Increased: polycythemia vera, dehydration, severe chronic obstructive pulmonary disease, acute poisoning. Decreased: anemia, leukemia, fluid overload, recent hemorrhage.
White blood cell (WBC) count	Number of WBCs per µl of blood	$5\text{-}10 \times 10^3$ (5000-10,000)	Presence of infection, inflammation, allergens, bone marrow integrity. Monitors response to radiation or chemotherapy. Increased: leukemia, infection, tissue necrosis. Decreased: bone marrow suppression.
WBC differential	Proportion (%) of the different types of WBCs (out of 100 cells)	Neutrophils 55%-70% Lymphocytes 20%-40% Monocytes 2%-8% Eosinophils 1%-4% Basophils 0.5%-1%	Presence of infectious states. Detect and classify leukemia.
Hematocrit (Hct)	Percentage of RBCs in whole blood	Female: 37%-47% Male: 42%-52%	Blood loss and fluid balance. Increased: polycythemia, dehydration. Decreased: anemia, acute blood loss, hemodilution.
Hemoglobin (Hgb)	Amount of hemoglobin in 100 ml of blood	Female: 12-16 g/100 ml Male: 14-18 g/100 ml	Blood loss, bone marrow suppression. Increased: polycythemia, dehydration. Decreased: anemia, recent hemorrhage, fluid overload.
Platelets (Plt)	Number of platelets in µl of blood	$150\text{-}450 \times 10^9$ 150,000-450,000 µl	Thrombocytopenia. Increased: polycythemia vera, splenectomy, malignancy. Decreased: anemia, hemolysis, DIC, ITP, viral infections, AIDS, splenomegaly, with radiation or chemotherapy.

Data from Elin RJ: Laboratory reference intervals and values. In Goldman L, Bennett JC, editors: Cecil textbook of medicine, vol 2, ed 21, Philadelphia, 2000, Saunders, p 2305; Matassarin-Jacobs E: Assessment of clients with hematologic disorders. In Black JM, Matassarin-Jacobs E, editors: Medical-surgical nursing: clinical management for continuity of care, ed 5, Philadelphia, 1997, Saunders, p 1465; Mosby's diagnostic and laboratory test reference, ed 8, St Louis, 2007, Mosby.

AIDS, Acquired immunodeficiency syndrome; *DIC,* disseminated intravascular coagulation; *ITP,* idiopathic thrombocytopenic purpura.

*Lab values vary among laboratories. RBC, hemoglobin, and platelet values vary with age and gender.

TABLE 7-11 Erythrocyte Indices: Values and Interpretation*

Test	Description	Value	Interpretation
Mean corpuscular volume (MCV) (Hct × 10/RBC)	Mean size of RBCs in a sample of blood	80-100 µm³	Increased by macrocytic, folic acid, or vitamin B_{12} deficiency anemias; liver disease; and recent alcohol use. Decreased by microcytic, iron-deficiency, and hypochromic anemias; thalassemia; and lead poisoning.
Mean corpuscular hemoglobin (MCH) (Hgb × 10/RBC)	Amount of Hgb in one RBC	26-34 pg/cell	Increased by macrocytic anemia. Decreased by microcytic anemia. Low mean corpuscular hemoglobin indicates Hgb deficiency.
Mean corpuscular hemoglobin concentration (MCHC) (Hgb/Hct × 100)	Proportion of each RBC occupied by Hgb	31-37 g/dl	Increased by spherocytosis (small round RBC). Decreased by microcytic, hypochromic, and iron-deficiency anemias and thalassemia.

Data from Elin RJ: Laboratory reference intervals and values. In Goldman L, Bennett JC, editors: Cecil textbook of medicine, vol 2, ed 21, Philadelphia, 2000, Saunders, p 2305; Matassarin-Jacobs E: Assessment of clients with hematologic disorders. In Black JM, Matassarin-Jacobs E, editors: Medical-surgical nursing: clinical management for continuity of care, ed 5, Philadelphia, 1997, Saunders, p 1466; and Pagana KD, Pagana TJ: Mosby's diagnostic and laboratory test reference, ed 10, St Louis, 2011, Mosby, pp 830-833.

Hct, Hematocrit; *Hgb,* hemoglobin; *RBC,* red blood cell.

*Lab values vary among laboratories.

measurement of how fast RBCs fall in a sample of anticoagulated blood. Normal values vary widely according to laboratory method. According to the Westergren method, the normal value for males is up to 15 mm per hour and the normal value for females is up to 20 mm per hour.[11]

The ESR is a reflection of acute-phase reaction in inflammation and infection. A limitation of the test is that it lacks sensitivity and specificity for disease processes. In addition, ESR cannot detect inflammation as quickly or as early as some other tests.[19]

ESR may be elevated in systemic infection, collagen vascular disease, and human immunodeficiency virus. It is a fairly reliable indicator of the course of disease. In general, as the disease worsens, the ESR increases; as the disease improves, the ESR decreases.[11] ESR may be decreased in the presence of sickle cell disease, polycythemia, or liver disease or carcinoma.

> ✎ **CLINICAL TIP**
> ESR is often normal in patients with connective tissue disease or neoplasms; heparin falsely increases the results.[19]

Peripheral Blood Smear. A blood sample may be examined microscopically for alterations in size and shape of the RBCs, WBCs, and platelets. RBCs are examined for size, shape, and Hgb distribution. WBCs are examined for proportion and the presence of immature cells. Finally, platelets are examined for number and shape.[20] Peripheral blood smear results are correlated with the other laboratory tests to diagnose hematologic disease.

Coagulation Profile. Coagulation tests assess the blood's ability to clot. The tests used to determine clotting are prothrombin time (PT) and partial thromboplastin time (PTT).

An adjunct to the measurement of PT is the international normalized ratio (INR). The INR was created to ensure reliable and consistent measurement of coagulation levels among all laboratories. The INR is the ratio of the patient's PT to the standard PT of the laboratory, raised by an exponent (the sensitivity index of the reagent) provided by the manufacturer.[21]

> ✎ **CLINICAL TIP**
> Because INR is more reliable and provides consistent measurement of coagulation levels, the INR value is used more often than PT.

The PT, PTT, and INR are used in clinical conditions in which an increased risk of thrombosis is present—for example, treatment of deep venous thrombosis (DVT), thrombosis associated with prosthetic valves, and atrial fibrillation (Table 7-12).[22]

> ✎ **CLINICAL TIP**
> When confirming an order for physical therapy in the physician's orders, the therapist must be sure to differentiate between the order for physical therapy and the blood test (i.e., the abbreviations for both physical therapy and prothrombin time are PT).

TABLE 7-12 Coagulation Profile

Test	Description	Value*	Indication/Interpretation
Prothrombin time (PT)	Examines the extrinsic and common clotting factors I, II, V, VII, and X	PT 11-12.5 seconds	Used to assess the adequacy of warfarin (Coumadin) therapy or to screen for bleeding disorders Increased: Coumarin therapy, liver diseases, bile duct obstruction, diarrhea, salicylate intoxication, DIC, hereditary factor deficiency, alcohol use, or drug interaction Decreased: Diet high in fat or leafy vegetables, or drug interaction
INR	Reflects standardized reporting of prothrombin time (PT) so that results are comparable among laboratories	0.8-0.11	Refer to Prothrombin time (PT)
Partial thromboplastin time (PTT) (activated PTT [aPTT] is a rapid version of PTT)	Examines the intrinsic and common clotting factors I, II, V, VIII, IX, X, XI	PTT 60-70 seconds aPTT 30-40 seconds	Used to assess the adequacy of heparin therapy and to screen for bleeding disorders Increased: Heparin or coumarin therapy, liver disease, vitamin K or congenital clotting factor deficiency, DIC Decreased: Extensive cancer, early DIC

Data from Pagana KD, Pagana TJ: Blood studies. In Mosby's manual of diagnostic and laboratory tests, St Louis, 1998, Mosby; Mosby's diagnostic and laboratory test reference, ed 8, St Louis, 2007, Mosby.
DIC, Disseminated intravascular coagulation.
*Values for PT and PTT vary between laboratories.

D-Dimer. The D-dimer assay provides (a highly specific) measurement of the amount of fibrin degradation. D-dimer tests have high sensitivity (95% to 99%) but are nonspecific (40% to 60%). Thrombotic problems such as DVT, pulmonary embolism (PE), and thrombosis of malignancy are associated with high levels of D-dimer. The test accurately identifies patients with DVT because its high sensitivity translates into a high negative predictive value. In other words, if the D-dimer test result is negative, the patient has a very low likelihood of having DVT. However, a positive D-dimer test result is less helpful because there are multiple conditions that may lead to elevated D-dimer titers, including advanced age, recent surgery, infection, inflammatory states and elevated liver enzyme levels. It is a simple and confirmatory test for disseminated intravascular coagulation (DIC). Levels of D-dimer can increase when a fibrin clot is lysed by thrombolytic therapy.[11,23]

> ✎ **CLINICAL TIP**
>
> A normal D-dimer value excludes pulmonary embolus in 30% of patients,[19] although a negative D-dimer result does not rule out the possibility of a pulmonary embolism. False-negative D-dimers are not uncommon for pulmonary emboli.[19]

Lymphatic Evaluation

Relevant history should include cancer and/or cancer treatment, trauma, and surgery, and onset of swelling at birth and/or puberty (primary lymphedema).[3] Clinical evaluation should include a detailed description of skin integrity, use of body diagrams, both anterior-posterior (AP) and lateral to draw unusual body contours. This description should also include presence of edema or fibrosis on the trunk quadrants, the head, and the neck, as well as on the limbs, and the location and condition of scars, fibrotic area, and open wounds. Circumferential measurements accurately assess the shape and contour of a limb. Circumferential measurements should be taken at consistent locations/sites relative to the anatomical landmarks for reliable comparison between limbs and overtime. Volumetric measurement is a useful to measure the actual volume of the limb and is more helpful in cases of bilateral extremity edema, when no "normal" limb can be used for comparison. Both volumetric measurements and girth measurements have been shown to be reliable, but the two methods cannot be reliably interchanged.[24]

> ✎ **CLINICAL TIP**
>
> Care should be taken to avoid indenting the edematous tissue with the tape measure during circumferential measurements.

Health Conditions

This section is divided into a discussion of vascular, hematologic, and lymphatic disorders.

Vascular Disorders

Vascular disorders are classified as arterial, venous, or combined arterial and venous disorders. Clinical findings differ between arterial and venous disorders, as described in Table 7-13.

Arterial Disorders

Atherosclerosis. Atherosclerosis is a diffuse and slowly progressive process characterized by areas of hemorrhage and the cellular proliferation of monocytes, smooth muscle, connective tissue, and lipids. The development of atherosclerosis begins early in life. In addition to the risk factors listed in Box 7-1, a high level of an inflammatory biomarker, C-reactive protein, has been identified as a good predictive marker for early identification of atherosclerosis.[25] Waist circumference and weight gain are the strongest predictors of early atherosclerosis in healthy adults.[26]

Atherosclerosis is the underlying cause of approximately 90% of all myocardial infarction and a large proportion of strokes and ischemic gangrenes.[27]

Clinical manifestations of atherosclerosis result from decreased blood flow through the stenotic areas. Signs and symptoms vary according to the area, size, and location of the lesion, along with the age and physiologic status of the patient. As blood flows through a stenotic area, turbulence will occur beyond the stenosis, resulting in decreased blood perfusion past the area of atherosclerosis. Generally, a 50% to 60% reduction in blood flow is necessary for patients to present with symptoms (e.g., pain). Turbulence is increased when there is an increase in blood flow to an area of the body, such as the lower extremities during exercise. When atherosclerosis develops slowly, collateral circulation develops to meet the needs.[24] A patient with no complaint of pain at rest may therefore experience leg pain (intermittent claudication [IC]) during walking or exercise as a result of decreased blood flow and the accumulation of metabolic waste (e.g., lactic acid).[4,28,29]

BOX 7-1   Risk Factors for Atherosclerosis

Reversible	Irreversible
Hypertension (controlled)	Male gender
Glucose intolerance and Diabetes (controlled)	Strong family history
Lipid abnormalities (controlled)	Genetic abnormalities
High LDL cholesterol	
Low HDL cholesterol	
Hypertriglyceridemia	
Cigarette smoking	
Obesity	
Sedentary lifestyle	
Cocaine	
Depression	

Data from Bryant RA, Nix DP: Acute and chronic wounds, ed 3, St Louis, 2007, Mosby; Kumar V: Robbins and Cotran pathologic basis of disease, ed 7, St Louis, 2005, Saunders; Crawford MH, DiMarco JP, Paulus WJ: Crawford: Cardiology, ed 3, St Louis, 2009, Mosby, Inc.

HDL, High-density lipoprotein; *LDL,* low-density lipoprotein.

TABLE 7-13 Comparison of Clinical Findings of Arterial and Venous Disorders

Clinical Finding	Arterial Disorders	Venous Disorders
Edema	May or may not be present	Present Worse at the end of the day Improves with elevation
Muscle mass	Reduced	Unaffected
Pain	Intermittent claudication Cramping Worse with elevation	Aching pain Exercise improves pain Better with elevation Cramping at night Paresthesias, pruritus (severe itching) Leg heaviness, especially at end of day
Pulses	Decreased to absent Possible systolic bruit	Usually unaffected, but may be difficult to palpate if edema is present
Skin	Absence of hair Small, painful ulcers on pressure points, especially lateral malleolus Normal toenails Tight, shiny skin Thickened toenails	Broad, shallow, painless ulcers of the ankle and lower leg
Color	Pale Dependent cyanosis	Brown discoloration Dependent cyanosis
Temperature	Cool	May be warm in presence of thrombophlebitis
Sensation	Decreased light touch Occasional itching, tingling, and numbness	Pruritus

Data from Black JM, Matassarin-Jacobs E, editors: Luckmann and Sorensen's medical-surgical nursing: a psychophysiologic approach, ed 4, Philadelphia, 1993, Saunders, p 1261.

The following are general signs and symptoms of atherosclerosis[30]:

- Peripheral pulses that are slightly reduced to absent.
- Presence of bruits on auscultation of major arteries (i.e., carotid, abdominal aorta, iliac, and femoral).
- Coolness and pallor of skin, especially with elevation.
- Presence of ulcerations, atrophic nails, and hair loss.
- Increased blood pressure.
- Subjective reports of continuous burning pain in the lower extremities at rest that is aggravated with elevation (ischemic pain) and relieved with placing the leg over the edge of the bed.[24] Pain at rest is usually indicative of severe (80% to 90%) arterial occlusion.
- Subjective reports of calf or lower-extremity pain, ache or cramp induced by walking (intermittent claudication) and relieved by rest.

✎ CLINICAL TIP

The distance a person can walk before the onset of pain indicates the degree of circulatory inadequacy (e.g., two blocks or more is mild, one block is moderate, one half block or less is severe).[24] Progression of ambulation distance in the patient with intermittent claudication can be optimized if ambulation is performed at short, frequent intervals (i.e., before the onset of claudicating pain).

Symptoms similar to intermittent claudication may have a neurologic origin from lumbar canal stenosis or disc disease. These symptoms are referred to as pseudoclaudication or neurologic claudication. Table 7-14 outlines the differences between true claudication and pseudoclaudication.[31]

All patients with claudication should be strongly advised to stop smoking. The beneficial effect of exercise training in patients with IC is well proven. The improvement in walking distance has been reported to be between 30% and 200%. A specific exercise program gives a more marked improvement than if the patient tries to exercise on his or her own. The greatest improvement in walking distance until pain develops seems to occur with an exercise duration of longer than 30 minutes per session and a frequency of at least three sessions per week. Walking should be used as a mode of exercise, and it should be performed at nearly maximum pain. The program should last at least 6 months.[27]

Medications that have been used in managing intermittent claudication include pentoxifylline and cilostazol.[32]

Treatment of atherosclerotic disease is based on clinical presentation and can range from risk-factor modifications (e.g., low-fat diet, increased exercise, and smoking cessation) to pharmacologic therapy (e.g., anticoagulation and thrombolytics) to surgical resection and grafting. Modification of risk factors has been shown to be the most effective method to lower the risk of morbidity (heart attack or stroke) from atherosclerosis.[33,34]

Aneurysm. An aneurysm is a localized dilatation or outpouching of the vessel wall that results from degeneration and weakening of the supportive network of protein fibers with a concomitant loss of medial smooth muscle cells. Aneurysms

TABLE 7-14 Differentiating True Intermittent Claudication from Pseudoclaudication

Characteristic of Discomfort	Intermittent Claudication	Pseudoclaudication
Activity-induced	Yes	Yes or no
Location	Unilateral buttock, hip, thigh, calf, and foot	Back pain and bilateral leg pain
Nature	Cramping Tightness Tiredness	Same as with intermittent claudication or presence of tingling, weakness, and clumsiness
Occurs with standing	No	Yes
Onset	Occurs at the same distance each time with walking on level surface Unchanged or decreased distance walking uphill Unchanged or increased distance walking downhill	Occurs at variable distance each time with walking on level surfaces Increased distance when walking uphill Decreased distance walking downhill
Relieved by	Stopping activity	Sitting

Data from Young JR, Graor RA, Olin JW et al, editors: Peripheral vascular diseases, St Louis, 1991, Mosby, p 183; Fritz JM: Spinal stenosis. In Placzek JD, Boyce DA, editors: Orthopaedic physical therapy secrets, Philadelphia, 2001, Hanley & Belfus, p 344.

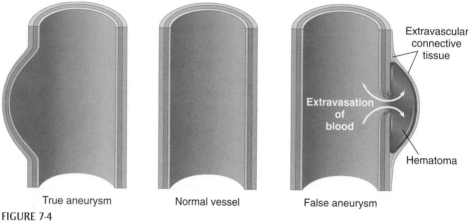

FIGURE 7-4

True and false aneurysms. *Center*, Normal vessel. *Left*, True aneurysm. The wall bulges outward and may be attenuated but is intact. *Right*, False aneurysm. The wall is ruptured, and there is a collection of blood (hematoma) that is bounded externally by adherent extravascular tissues. (From Kumar V: Robbins and Cotran pathologic basis of disease, ed 8, Philadelphia, 2010, Saunders.)

most commonly occur in the abdominal aorta or iliac arteries, followed by the popliteal, femoral, and carotid vessels.[28,33,35,36] The exact mechanism of aneurysm formation is not fully understood but includes a combination of the following:

- Genetic abnormality in collagen (e.g., with Marfan's syndrome)
- Aging and natural degeneration of elastin
- Increased proteolytic enzyme activity
- Atherosclerotic damage to elastin and collagen

A true aneurysm is defined as a 50% increase in the normal diameter of the vessel[36] and involves weakening of all three layers of the arterial wall. True aneurysms are also generally fusiform and circumferential in nature. False and saccular aneurysms are the result of trauma from dissection (weakness or separation of the vascular layers) or clot formation (Figure 7-4). They primarily affect the adventitial layer.[35]

Abdominal aortic aneurysm is dilatation of the abdominal aorta to more than 3 cm in diameter. These aneurysms can be infrarenal, juxtarenal or suprarenal, according to the relationship to the renal arteries.[27]

Approximately 80% of the aneurysms are identified incidentally on abdominal ultrasound, computed tomography (CT) scan, magnetic resonance imaging (MRI), or plain x-ray.[37] Aneurysms will rupture if the intraluminal pressure exceeds the tensile strength of the arterial wall. Rupture is mostly likely to occur in aneurysms that are 5 cm or larger.[24]

> ✎ **CLINICAL TIP**
>
> Abdominal aortic aneurysms are frequently referred to as *AAA*, *A³*, or *triple A* in the clinical setting.

Physical Therapy Considerations. The following are additional clinical manifestations of aneurysms:

- Popliteal aneurysm presents as a pulsating mass, 2 cm or more in diameter. Femoral aneurysms presents as a pulsating mass in the femoral area on one or both sides.[24] In thin individuals, an aortic aneurysm may be seen as a pulsating swelling in the upper abdomen.[27]

- Ischemic manifestations (described earlier in the Atherosclerosis section), if the aneurysm impedes blood flow. Most abdominal aneurysms are asymptomatic, but intermittent or constant pain in the form of mild to severe mid-abdominal or lower back discomfort is present in some form in 25% to 30% of cases. Groin or flank pain may be experienced because of increasing pressure on other strutures.[24] Most of the aneurysms are relatively asymptomatic until an embolus dislodges from the aneurysm or the aneurysm ruptures.[36]
- Cerebral aneurysms, commonly found in the circle of Willis, present with increased intracranial pressure and its sequelae (see Chapter 6 for more information on intracranial pressure).[35]
- Aneurysms that result in subarachnoid hemorrhage are also discussed in Chapter 6.
- Low back pain (aortic aneurysms can refer pain to the low back).
- Dysphagia (difficulty swallowing) and dyspnea (breathlessness) resulting from the enlarged vessel's compressing adjacent organs.

Surgical resection and graft replacement are generally the desired treatments for aneurysms.[38] However, endovascular repair of abdominal aneurysms is demonstrating favorable results. Endovascular repair involves threading an endoprosthesis through the femoral artery to the site of the aneurysm. The endoprosthesis is then attached to the aorta, proximal to the site of the aneurysm, and distal to the iliac arteries. This effectively excludes the aneurysm from the circulation, which minimizes the risk of rupture.[36] Non–surgical candidates must have blood pressure and anticoagulation management.[38]

Aortic Dissection. Aortic dissection is caused by an intimal tear, which allows creation of a false lumen between the media and adventitia. A history of Marfan's syndrome or hypertension is usually present.[39] Aortic dissection occurs at least twice as frequently in men than in women.[7] Signs and symptoms generally reflect the type of aortic dissection (whether type A or type B [Figure 7-5]) and the extent of cardiovascular involvement.[40] Signs and symptoms of aortic dissection include[40]:

- Pain: Sudden and excruciating pain in the chest (90% of the patients) or the upper back is the most common initial symptom. Another important characteristic of the pain is its tendency to migrate to the neck, abdomen, or groin, generally following the path of dissection.
- Shock: Cardiogenic or hypovolemic shock may be secondary to cardiac tamponade from aortic rupture into the pericardium, dissection or compression of the coronary arteries, acute aortic regurgitation, or acute blood loss.
- Syncope.
- Hypertension: More than 50% of patients with distal dissection are hypertensive, and severe hypertension with diastolic pressure as high as 160 mm Hg may be encountered with distal dissection. Severe hypertension may be due to renal ischemia.
- Reduced or absent pulses.
- Murmur of aortic regurgitation. This may be present in 50% of the patients with proximal dissection and may occur

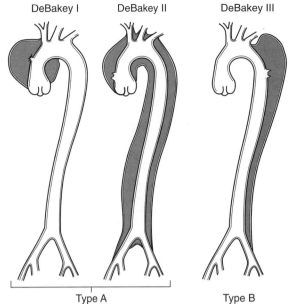

FIGURE 7-5
Classification of aortic dissections. **A,** Dissection of ascending aorta (type A). **B,** Dissection of descending aorta (type B). (From Kumar V: Robbins and Cotran pathologic basis of disease, ed 8, Philadelphia, 2010, Saunders.)

because of widening of the aortic annulus or actual disruption of the aortic valve leaflets.

- Pleural effusions: Pleural effusion, which occur most frequently in the left chest, can be caused by the rupture of the dissection into the pleural space or by weeping of fluid from the aorta as the result of an inflammatory reaction to the dissection.[41]
- Neurological manifestations (cerebrovascular accident and, rarely, altered consciousness, coma).

> ✎ **CLINICAL TIP**
>
> The pain of aortic dissection may mimic that of myocardial ischemia.[41]

The chest radiograph may be the first clue to the diagnosis of aortic dissection, but the findings on the chest radiograph are nonspecific, subject to interobserver variability and in many cases completely normal.[7]

Electrocardiogram (ECG) findings in these patients are nonspecific.[7,39] Transesophageal echocardiography (TEE) and CT scan are the primary diagnostic tests used by most institutions to diagnose aortic dissection.[42] TEE is highly accurate for the evaluation and diagnosis of acute aortic dissection, with sensitivity (98%) and specificity (94% to 97%). Contrast CT is also highly accurate for diagnosing aortic dissection, with sensitivity and specificity of 95% to 98%. MRI is a highly accurate noninvasive technique for evaluating aortic dissection but is rarely used as the initial test for diagnostic evaluation of acute dissection. MRI is known to have high sensitivity (95% to 100%) and specificity (94% to 98%) for the detection of aortic dissection.[7]

TABLE 7-15 Sources of Peripheral Emboli

Source	Percentage
Cardiac	80%
Atrial fibrillation	50%
Myocardial infarction	25%
Other	5%
Noncardiac	10%
Aneurysmal disease	6%
Proximal artery	3%
Paradoxical emboli	1%
Other or idiopathic	10%

From Belkin M, Owens CD, Whittemore AD et al: Peripheral arterial occlusive disease. In Townsend CM, Beauchamp RD, Evers BM et al, editors: Sabiston textbook of surgery: the biological basis of modern surgical practice, ed 18, Philadelphia, 2007, Saunders.

Management includes stabilizing the patient, aggressive control of blood pressure, and pain control. Patients may be managed medically or surgically, depending on the site of the dissection and the patient's comorbidities.

Arterial Thrombosis. Arterial thrombosis occurs in areas of low or stagnant blood flow, such as atherosclerotic or aneurysmal areas. The reduced or turbulent blood flow in these areas leads to platelet adhesion and aggregation, which then activates the coagulation cycle to form a mature thrombus (clot). Blood flow may then be impeded, potentially leading to tissue ischemia with subsequent clinical manifestations.[35,38]

Arterial Emboli. An arterial embolus is a fragment of thrombus, fat, atherosclerotic plaque, bacterial vegetation, or air that mobilizes within the arterial vessels and obstructs flow distal to the embolus.[43] Arterial emboli arise from areas of stagnant or disturbed blood flow in the heart or aorta. Acute arterial embolus is a surgical emergency. The likelihood of limb salvage decreases after 4 to 6 hours.[42] The most common sources of arterial emboli are listed in Table 7-15.

Areas in which arterial emboli tend to lodge and interrupt blood flow are arterial bifurcations and areas narrowed by atherosclerosis (especially in the cerebral, mesenteric, renal, and coronary arteries). Signs and symptoms of thrombi, emboli, or both depend on the size of the occlusion, the organ distal to the clot, and the collateral circulation available.[35]

When arterial thrombosis or embolism is suspected, the affected limb must be protected by proper positioning below the horizontal plane, and protective skin care must be provided. Heat or cold application and massage are to be avoided.[24] Treatment of thrombi, emboli, or both includes anticoagulation with or without surgical resection of the atherosclerotic area that is predisposing the formation of thrombi, emboli, or both. Medical management of arterial thrombosis can also include antithrombotic drugs (e.g., tissue factor or factor Xa inhibitors) or combined antithrombotic therapy with aspirin, a thienopyridine and warfarin, or both.[44]

Hypertension. Hypertension is an elevated arterial blood pressure, both systolic and diastolic, that is abnormally sustained at rest (Table 7-16).

TABLE 7-16 Hypertension as It Relates to Different Age Groups

Age	Normal Blood Pressure (Systolic/Diastolic)	Hypertensive Blood Pressure (Systolic/Diastolic)
Infants	80/40	90/60
Children	100/60	120/80
Teenagers (age 12-17 years)	115/70	130/80
Adults ≥18 years	<120/<80	(Prehypertension) 120-139/80-89 (Stage 1 hypertension) 140-159/90-99 (Stage 2 hypertension) ≥160/≥100

Data from Bullock B: Pathophysiology: adaptations and alterations in function, ed 4, Philadelphia, 1996, Lippincott-Raven, p 517; Chobanian A, et al: The seventh report of the Joint National Committee on Prevention, Detection, Evaluation and Treatment of High Blood Pressure. The JNC 7 report, Hypertension 2003, 42:1206-1252, 2003.

Hypertension is frequently asymptomatic; this creates a significant health risk for affected people.[24] Signs and symptoms that can result from hypertension and its effects on target organs are described in Table 7-17.

Two general forms of hypertension exist: essential and secondary. *Essential* or *idiopathic hypertension* is an elevation in blood pressure that results without a specific medical cause but is related to the following risk factors[35,45]:
- Genetic predisposition
- Smoking
- Sedentary lifestyle
- Type A personality
- Obesity
- Diabetes mellitus
- Diet high in fat, cholesterol, and sodium
- Atherosclerosis
- Imbalance of vasomediator production, nitric oxide (vasodilator), and endothelin (potent vasoconstrictor)

Secondary hypertension results from a known medical cause, such as renal disease and others listed in Table 7-18. If the causative factors are treated sufficiently, systolic blood pressure may return to normal limits.[35]

A rise in diastolic blood pressure from a sitting to standing position suggests essential hypertension, whereas a fall in blood pressure from the sitting to standing position indicates secondary hypertension.[9]

Management of hypertension consists of behavioral (e.g., diet, smoking cessation, activity modification) and pharmacologic intervention to maintain blood pressure within acceptable parameters. Pharmacologic treatment can likely be deferred in hypertensive patients who regularly participate in aerobic exercise. Exercise high in intensity and duration has a beneficial effect in the management of hypertension, and the antihypertensive effect of regular training can be maintained as long as 3 years.[46] The primary medications used are diuretics and

TABLE 7-17 Hypertensive Effects on Target Organs

Organ	Hypertensive Effect	Clinical Manifestations
Brain	Cerebrovascular accident	Area of brain involved dictates presentation. May include severe occipital headache, paralysis, speech and swallowing disturbances, or coma
	Encephalopathy	Rapid development of confusion, agitation, convulsions, and death
Eyes	Blurred or impaired vision	Nicking (compression) of retinal arteries and veins, at the point of their junction
	Encephalopathy	Hemorrhages and exudates on visual examination
		Papilledema
Heart	Myocardial infarction	Electrocardiographic changes
		Enzyme elevations
	Congestive heart failure	Decreased cardiac output
		Auscultation of S3 or gallop
		Cardiomegaly on radiograph
	Myocardial hypertrophy	Increased angina frequency
		ST- and T-wave changes on electrocardiogram
	Dysrhythmias	Ventricular or conduction defects
Kidneys	Renal insufficiency	Nocturia
		Proteinuria
		Elevated blood urea nitrogen and creatinine levels
	Renal failure	Fluid overload
		Accumulation of metabolites
		Metabolic acidosis

Data from Bullock B: Pathophysiology: adaptations and alterations in function, ed 4, Philadelphia, 1996, Lippincott-Raven, p 522.

TABLE 7-18 Causes of Secondary Hypertension

Origin	Description
Coarctation of the aorta	Congenital constriction of the aorta at the level of the ductus arteriosus, which results in increased pressure (proximal to the area) of constriction and decreased pressure (distal to the area) of constriction
Cushing's disease or syndrome	See Pituitary Gland in Chapter 10
Oral contraceptives	May be related to an increased secretion of glucocorticoids from adrenal or pituitary dysfunction
Pheochromocytoma	Tumor of the adrenal medulla causing increased catecholamine secretion
Primary aldosteronism	Increased aldosterone secretion primarily as result of an adrenal tumor
Renin-secreting tumors	See Adrenal Gland in Chapter 10
Renovascular disease	Parenchymal disease, such as acute and chronic glomerulonephritis Narrowing stenosis of renal artery as a result of atherosclerosis or congenital fibroplasia

Data from Bullock B: Pathophysiology: adaptations and alterations in function, ed 4, Philadelphia, 1996, Lippincott-Raven, p 517.

angiotensin-converting enzyme inhibitors along with beta blockers, calcium channel blockers, and vasodilators.[35,47-49] A summary of these medications, their actions, and their side effects can be found in Chapter 19, Tables 19-3 and 19-3a.

Hypertensive crisis is a medical emergency. It occurs when the blood pressure is high enough to threaten target organs acutely. Hypertensive emergency requires admission to an intensive care unit and parenteral therapy.[50]

Physical Therapy Considerations
- Hypertension is a risk factor for heart attack, stroke, and kidney failure.
- Systolic blood pressure gradually increases through life. Diastolic blood pressure increases until 50 to 60 years of age.
- Women typically have lower blood pressure than men until after menopause.[51]
- Physical exertion increases blood pressure acutely and decreases resting blood pressure over time.[51]
- Blood pressure is usually lowest in the morning when metabolic rate is the lowest, rises throughout the day, and peaks in late afternoon when the person is mentally awake and physically active.[51]
- Knowledge of medication schedule may facilitate activity tolerance by having optimal blood pressures at rest and with activity.
- Review and clarify any strict blood pressure parameters that the physician has designated for patient because some patients need to have higher or lower systolic pressures than expected normal ranges.
- When the blood pressure measurement reveals an elevated blood pressure, make sure the cuff size is right for the patient's arm, take the blood pressure in the opposite extremity, and then notify the team.

- In certain patient populations (e.g., patients who have had mastectomies, patients with a peripherally inserted central catheter [PICC] line) there are restrictions on taking blood pressure in the upper extremities. In these cases, blood pressure can be taken in the lower extremities.
- In patients receiving antihypertensive therapy, keep in mind the signs and symptoms of low blood pressure, such as dizziness, confusion, syncope, restlessness, or drowsiness, especially in elderly patients.
- Patients can present with an elevated blood pressure when they are apprehensive, in pain, and under stress. Keep this in mind, and try to calm the patient (by applying a wet washcloth on the forehead and/or neck and by distracting the patient through talking). Repeat the measurement in a few minutes for an accurate representation of blood pressure.

Systemic Vasculitis. Systemic vasculitis is a general term referring to the inflammation of arteries and veins that progresses to necrosis, leading to a narrowing of the vessels. Although the specific cause of many of these disorders is not known, infectious organisms, drugs, tumors, and allergic reactions are some of the defined triggers. Pathogenetic factors include immune complex disease, antineutrophil cytoplasmic antibodies, anti–endothelial cell antibodies, and cell-mediated immunity. The major ischemic manifestations of vasculitis are defined by the type and size of blood vessels involved and the tissue and organ damage caused by the ischemia related to the vascular occlusion.[52] The secondary manifestations of vasculitis are numerous and may include thrombosis, aneurysm formation, hemorrhage, arterial occlusion, weight loss, fatigue, depression, fever, and generalized achiness that is worse in the morning. The recognized forms of vasculitis are discussed in the following sections.[29,53-55]

Polyarteritis Nodosa. Polyarteritis nodosa (PAN) is an acute necrotizing vasculitis of medium-sized and small arteries.[52] Most cases present with an unknown etiology; however, the hepatitis B virus has been emerging as one of the more common causative factors.[54] PAN usually begins with nonspecific symptoms, which may include malaise, fatigue, fever, myalgias, and arthralgias. Skin lesions are common, and a majority of patients have vasculitic neuropathy.[56] The most frequently involved organs are the kidney, heart, liver, and gastrointestinal tract, with symptoms representative of the dysfunction of the involved organ. Aneurysm formation with destruction of the medial layer of the vessel is the hallmark characteristic of PAN. Pulmonary involvement can occur; however, most cases of vasculitis in the respiratory tract are associated with Wegener's granulomatosis.

Current management of PAN includes corticosteroid therapy with or without concurrent cytotoxic therapy with cyclophosphamide (Cytoxan). Antiviral agents may also be used if there is an associated viral infection. Elective surgical correction of PAN is not feasible, given its diffuse nature. Patients diagnosed with PAN have a 5-year survival rate of 12% without medical treatment and 80% with treatment.[53,54]

Wegener's Granulomatosis. Wegener's granulomatosis is a granulomatous necrotizing disease that affects small- and medium-sized blood vessels throughout the body, with primary manifestations in the upper respiratory tract, lungs, and kidneys. The etiology is unknown; diagnosis and treatment are still in development. It occurs most commonly in the fourth and fifth decades of life and affects men and women with equal frequency.[39] Pulmonary signs and symptoms mimic those of pneumonia (i.e., fever, productive cough at times with negative sputum cultures, and chest pain).[47,54] The 1-year mortality rate is 90% without therapy, 50% with corticosteroid therapy, and 10% with combined corticosteroid and cytotoxic therapy.[54]

Treatment of Wegener's granulomatosis may consist of a combination of immunosuppressive agents and corticosteroids (methotrexate and prednisone, respectively). Antiinfective agents may also be prescribed if there is associated respiratory tract infection.[31,34]

Thromboangiitis Obliterans. Thromboangiitis obliterans (Buerger's disease) is a vasculitis (inflammatory and thrombotic process) affecting the peripheral blood vessels (both arteries and veins), primarily in the extremities.[24] It is found mainly in young men ages 20 to 45 years and is directly correlated with a heavy smoking history.[4,35,53] If abstinence from tobacco is adhered to, the disease takes a favorable course. If smoking is continued, the disease progresses, leading to gangrene and small-digit amputations.[57] The disease is characterized by segmental thrombotic occlusions of the small- and medium-sized arteries in the distal lower and upper extremities. The thrombotic occlusions consist of microabscesses that are inflammatory in nature, suggesting a collagen or autoimmune origin, although the exact etiology is still unknown.[35,53] Rest pain is common, along with intermittent claudication that occurs more in the feet than in the calf region.[3] The diagnosis is made by invasive and noninvasive methods. The noninvasive methods include physical exam, Doppler ultrasound, plethysmography, and ankle-brachial index (ABI). The invasive methods include magnetic resonance angiography (MRA), other forms of angiography, and spiral CT.[58]

Treatment of Buerger's disease can include smoking cessation, corticosteroids, prostaglandin E_1 infusion, vasodilators, hemorheologic agents, antiplatelet agents, and anticoagulants.[35,53]

Giant Cell Arteritis. Giant cell arteritis (GCA) is another granulomatous inflammatory disorder of an unknown etiology. It predominantly affects the large arteries and is characterized by destruction of the internal elastic lamina. Two clinical presentations of GCA have been recognized: temporal arteritis and Takayasu's arteritis.[35] Temporal artery biopsy (TAB) is the "gold standard" for the diagnosis of GCA and ESR, C-reactive protein, and platelet count are the primary serologic markers. Color ultrasonography of the temporal arteries detects characteristic signs of vasculitis with a high sensitivity and specificity. Vision loss is the most dreaded complication of GCA, and when it occurs it tends to be profound and permanent.[59]

Temporal arteritis is a more common and mild presentation of GCA that occurs after 50 years of age. The onset of arteritis is usually sudden, with severe, continuous, unilateral, throbbing headache and temporal pain as the first symptoms. The pain may radiate to the occipital area, face, or side of the neck. Visual disturbances range from blurring to diplopia to visual loss. Irreversible blindness may occur in the course of the disease from involvement of the ophthalmic artery.

Other symptoms include enlarged, tender temporal artery, scalp sensitivity, and jaw claudication (pain in response to chewing, talking or swallowing) when involvement of the external carotid artery causes ischemia of the masseter muscles; pain is relieved by rest.[59] Polymyalgia rheumatica, a clinical syndrome characterized by pain on active motion and acute onset of proximal muscular stiffness, is frequently associated with temporal arteritis. The primary treatment for temporal arteritis is prednisone.[31,54]

Takayasu's arteritis generally affects young Asian women but has been known to occur in both genders in African Americans and Hispanics as well. It is a form of generalized GCA that primarily involves the upper extremities and the aorta and its major branches. The pulmonary circulation is involved in approximately 50% of cases of Takayasu's artertitis.[56] Lower-extremity involvement is less common. Management of Takayasu's arteritis may consist of prednisone and cyclophosphamide, along with surgical intervention if the disease progresses to aneurysm, gangrene, or both.[31]

Raynaud's Disease. Raynaud's disease is an episodic vasospastic disorder characterized by digital color change (white to blue to red—reflecting the vasoconstriction, cyanosis, and vasodilation process, respectively) with exposure to cold environment or emotional stress. Numbness, tingling, and burning pain may also accompany the color changes. However, despite these vasoconstrictive episodes, peripheral pulses remain palpable. If idiopathic, it is called *Raynaud's disease*. If associated with a possible precipitation systemic or regional disorder (autoimmune diseases, myeloproliferative disorders, multiple myeloma, cryoglobulinemia, myxedema, macroglobulinemia, or arterial occlusive disease), it is called *Raynaud's phenomenon*.[4,31,47]

In Raynaud's disease, the disease is symmetric by rule; in Raynaud's phenomenon, the changes may be most noticeable in one hand or even in one or two fingers only. Infrequently, the feet and toes are involved. Between attacks, the affected extremities may be entirely normal. The incidence of disease is estimated to be as high as 10% in the general population. An abnormality of the sympathetic nervous system has long been implicated in the etiology of Raynaud's disease; recently, research has focused on the theory of up-regulation of vascular smooth muscle α_2-adrenergic receptors. The distinction between Raynaud's disease and Raynaud's phenomenon is meant to reflect a difference in prognosis. Whereas Raynaud's disease is benign and often controllable, Raynaud's phenomenon may

progress to atrophy of the terminal fat pads and development of fingertip gangrene. Women 16 to 40 years of age are most commonly affected, especially in cold climates or during the winter season. Raynaud's disease is usually benign, causing mild discomfort on exposure to cold and progressing very slightly over the years. The prognosis of Raynaud's phenomenon is that of the associated disease.[39] Areas generally affected are the fingertips, toes, and the tip of the nose.[4,31,47]

Management of Raynaud's disease and Raynaud's phenomenon may consist of any of the following: conservative measures to ensure warmth and protection of the body and extremities; regular exercise; diet rich in fish oils and antioxidants (vitamins C and E); pharmacologic intervention, including calcium channel blockers and sympatholytics; conditioning and biofeedback; acupuncture; and sympathectomy.[31,39,60]

Complex Regional Pain Syndrome. Complex regional pain syndrome (CRPS) is a rare disorder of the extremities characterized by autonomic and vasomotor instability. Use of the former name of this entity, reflex sympathetic dystrophy (RSD), is now discouraged because the precise role of the sympathetic nervous system is unclear and dystrophy is not an inevitable sequela of the syndrome.

The presenting symptom is constant, extreme pain that occurs after the healing phase of minor or major trauma, fractures, surgery, or any combination of these. Injured sensory nerve fibers may transmit constant signals to the spinal cord that result in increased sympathetic activity to the limbs. Affected areas initially present as dry, swollen, and warm but then progress to being cold, swollen, and pale or cyanotic. It occurs in all age groups and equally in both sexes and can involve either the arms or the legs.[39]

Three stages have been defined (Steinbrocker classification), although all patients may not have evolved through the stages or proceed in a temporal fashion.[52,57]

- Stage 1 (acute—occurring within hours to days after the injury): Pain, tenderness, edema, and temperature changes predominate.
- Stage 2 (dystrophic—3 to 6 months after the injury): Pain extends beyond the area affected; loss of hair and dystrophic nails become apparent. Muscle wasting, osteoporosis, and decreased range of motion may occur.
- Stage 3 (atrophic or chronic—6 months after injury): Atrophy, demineralization, functional impairment, and irreversible damage are present.

Management of CRPS may consist of any of the following[31,61-64]:

- Physical or occupational therapy, or both (cornerstone therapy)
- Pharmacologic sympathetic blocks
- Surgical sympathectomy
- Spinal cord electrical stimulation
- Baclofen drug administration
- Prophylactic vitamin C administration after sustaining fractures
- Bisphosphonate administration

The prognosis partly depends on the stage in which the lesions are encountered and the extent and severity of associated

> ✎ **CLINICAL TIP**
>
> At the time of an exacerbation, gently rewarm fingers or toes as soon as possible by placing hands in the axilla, wiggle fingers or toes, and move or walk around to improve circulation. If possible, run warm water over the affected body part until normal color returns.[24]

organic disease. Early treatment offers the best prognosis for recovery.[39]

Compartment Syndrome. Compartment syndrome is a condition in which the circulation within a closed compartment is compromised by an increase in pressure within the compartment, causing necrosis of muscles and nerves and eventually of the skin because of excessive swelling. Volkmann ischemic contracture is a sequela of untreated or inadequately treated compartment syndrome in which necrotic muscle and nerve tissue has been replaced with fibrous tissue.[65]

Compartment syndrome can occur after traumatic injuries, which include fractures, crush injuries, hematomas, penetrating injuries, circumferential burn injury, electrical injuries, and revascularization procedures. External factors, such as casts and circular dressings that are too constrictive, may also lead to compartment syndrome.[28,31,66] Compartment syndrome can also occur as a chronic condition that develops from overuse associated with strenuous exercise. Diagnosis of compartment syndrome is established by measuring compartment pressures. Normal tissue pressure is between 0 and 8 mm Hg. Compartment pressures of 32 to 37 mm Hg can cause compression of capillaries.[66]

Permanent muscle damage can begin after 4 to 12 hours of ischemia. Nerves appear to be more sensitive than muscle to the effects of increased pressure, and damage can occur after approximately 8 hours of pressure elevation.[67]

A common symptom of compartment syndrome is pain associated with tense, tender muscle groups that worsens with palpation or passive movement of the affected area. Numbness or paralysis may also be accompanied by a gradual diminution of peripheral pulses. Pallor, which indicates tissue ischemia, can progress to tissue necrosis if appropriate management is not performed.[28,31,66]

Management of compartment syndrome consists of preventing prolonged external compression of the involved limb, limb elevation, and, ultimately, fasciotomy (incisional release of the fascia) if compartment pressures exceed 37 to 52 mm Hg. Mannitol can also be used to help reduce swelling.[28,31,66]

Physical Therapy Considerations

- Patient, staff, and family education on proper positioning techniques can reduce the risk of swelling and subsequent compartment syndrome.
- In cases when compartment syndrome is present:
  - Elevation of the affected limb must be discontinued, and the limb should be placed no higher than the heart level.
  - Circumferential bandages must be removed.[68]
- The physical therapist should delineate any range-of-motion precautions that may be present after fasciotomies that cross a joint line.

Venous Disorders

Varicose Veins. Varicose veins are chronic dilations of the veins that first result from a weakening in the venous walls, which then lead to improper closure of the valve cusps. Incompetence of the valves further exacerbates the venous dilatation. The prevalence of varicose veins in Western populations was estimated in one study to be about 25% to 30% in women and

10% to 20% in men.[57] Varicose veins can be either primary or secondary. Primary varicose veins originate in the superficial veins—the saphenous veins and their branches—whereas secondary varicose veins occur in the deep and perforating veins. Primary varicose veins tend to run in families, affect both legs, and are twice as common in females as in males. Usually, secondary varicose veins occur in only one leg. Both types are more common in middle adulthood.

Primary varicose veins can result from congenital weakness of the valves or venous wall; from conditions that produce prolonged venous stasis, such as pregnancy or wearing tight clothing; or from occupations that necessitate standing for an extended period. Secondary varicose veins result from disorders of the venous system, such as deep vein thrombophlebitis, trauma, and occlusion.[9]

Risk factors include female gender, pregnancy, family history, prolonged standing, and history of phlebitis.[39]

Patients generally complain of itchy, tired, heavy-feeling legs after prolonged standing.[28,69] Large varicose veins are unsightly and may produce anxiety and cause major lifestyle changes. Trauma to a varicose vein may result in severe bleeding, particularly in older adults, as their skin may be atrophic.[70]

Management of varicose veins may consist of any of the following: behavioral modifications (e.g., avoiding prolonged sitting or standing and constrictive clothing), weight loss (if there is associated obesity), elevating the feet for 10 to 15 minutes 3 or 4 times a day, gradual exercise, applying well-fitting support stockings in the morning, showering or bathing in the evening, sclerotherapy (to close dilated veins), ambulatory phlebectomy, endovenous ablation, and surgical ligation and stripping of incompetent veins.[28,57,69]

Venous Thrombosis. Venous thrombosis can occur in the superficial or deep veins (DVT) and can result from a combination of venous stasis, injury to the endothelial layer of the vein, and hypercoagulability (Box 7-2).Venous stasis of the lower extremities occurs as a consequence of immobility, whereas

---

BOX 7-2 Risk Factors for Deep Venous Thrombosis

- Surgery and immobilization
- Obesity
- Hospital stay in a critical care area
- Pregnancy and postpartum period
- Heart failure or respiratory failure
- Tobacco use
- Central venous catheters, pacemakers, and defibrillators
- Use of oral contraceptives or hormone replacement therapy
- Cancer and chemotherapy
- Prolonged airline travel
- Diabetes
- Trauma
- Hypertension
- Varicose veins
- Stroke and spinal cord injury
- Increasing age

Data from Hill KM: Careful assessment and diagnosis can prevent complications of DVT, *Clin Updates*, May 2007.

hypercoagulability may occur as a result of inflammation, malignancy, or tissue damage of intimal walls. Thrombus formation usually occurs in legs, but its incidence in upper extremities is growing, particularly because of increasing use of subclavian venous catheters.[71]

DVT places the patient at risk for PE, recurrent thrombosis, and postphlebitic syndrome. There are two types of thrombus: (1) mural thrombus, where the thrombus is attached to the wall of the vein but does not occlude the vessel lumen, and (2) occlusive thrombus, which begins by attachment to the vessel wall and progresses to completely occlude the vessel lumen.[24,28]

There are two types of venous thrombosis: superficial (saphenous vein in the lower extremity) and deep (usually of the femoral or iliac veins of the lower extremities and pelvis).[24] Superficial venous thrombosis of the upper extremity can occur, although it is less common and is seen in people with systemic illness in the presence of an indwelling central venous catheter, malignancy or less often hemodialysis.[24]

A DVT proximal to the calf is associated with higher risk of PE. Clinical studies indicate a strong association between DVT and PE. As many as 50% of patients who have a proximal DVT develop a PE, and among those who have a clinically significant PE, 70% have evidence of DVT.[72]

Signs and symptoms of venous thrombosis can include the following[31,73]:

- Pain and swelling distal to the site of thrombus
- Redness and warmth in the area around the thrombus
- Dilated veins
- Low-grade fever
- A dull ache or tightness in the region of DVT

> ✎ **CLINICAL TIP**
>
> Patients with DVT in a lower extremity may complain of pain around the general area of the thrombus with weight bearing, though clinical presentation of DVT varies and physical exams are only 30% accurate.[71] Physical therapy intervention for patients with suspected DVT should be withheld until cleared by the medical-surgical team.

The primary imaging study to identify patients with DVT now is ultrasonography. It is relatively inexpensive, noninvasive, and widely available. Ultrasound is considered to be 97% sensitive and 96% specific for symptomatic patients with suspected DVT of the proximal leg. The sensitivity of ultrasound for calf DVT is well below 90%.[56] Other diagnostic methods include venography and impedance plethysmography. MRI is developing a growing role in the diagnosis of DVT, with a sensitivity of 97% and specificity of 95%.[40] The Wells clinical decision rule (CDR) for DVT, as described in the Vascular Tests section, has been shown to be a reliable and valid tool for clinical assessment and predicting the risk of DVT in the lower extremity.[24,56]

Patients admitted to the hospital and/or undergoing surgery are often on DVT prophylaxis, which includes mechanical and pharmacological approaches[72]; lower-extremity elevation or application of compression stockings (elastic or sequential pneumatic), or both, if bed rest is required; and anticoagulation medications (intravenous heparin or oral warfarin [Coumadin]). There are several recommendations to prevent DVT. Prolonged sitting increases blood viscosity, hematocrit, and serum lactate. Primary prevention of DVT is through the use of early mobilization for low-risk individuals and prophylactic use of anticoagulants in people at moderate to high risk for DVT.[24] It is important for postoperative patients to initiate early ambulation, stay hydrated, wear nonrestrictive clothing, and exercise their calf muscles frequently to reduce venous stasis and improve venous return.[56] Routine use of elastic stockings in all postoperative patients along with the use of sequential compression also help in prevention of DVTs.[24]

The initial treatment for DVT is anticoagulation with unfractionated heparin (heparin) and low-molecular-weight heparin (LMWH) such as enoxaparin or fondaparinux (Arixtra) for at least 5 days and until the INR is at or above 2.0 for two consecutive days.[74]

> ✎ **CLINICAL TIP**
>
> Physical therapists should be cautious for the signs and symptoms of unusual bleeding in patients who are on anticoagulation after the diagnosis of DVT.

Heparin blocks the extension of thrombus and reduces the risk of further emboli. It does not actively lyse a clot, but allows the body's own fibrinolytic mechanism to operate over a period several days to weeks. After initial anticoagulation with heparin, warfarin (Coumadin) and fondaparinux (Arixtra) are used. Fondaparinux is more effective at decreasing the risk of DVT after orthopedic surgery than LMWH. It is recommended for patients to have at least 3 to 6 months of treatment for an initial event of DVT. Patients with first occurrence of DVT should receive 3 months of therapy in the setting of an identifiable risk factor or surgery; patients with idiopathic DVT should receive 6 months of therapy.[74]

If a patient cannot be anticoagulated, a device called an *inferior vena cava (IVC) filter* can prevent lower extremity thrombi from embolizing to the lungs. The primary indications for IVC filter placement include contraindications to anticoagulation, recurrent embolism while on adequate therapy, and significant bleeding complications during anticoagulation. IVC filters are sometimes placed in the setting of massive PE when it is believed that any further emboli might be lethal. More recently, temporary filters have been used in patients in whom the risk of bleeding appears to be short-term; such devices can be removed up to 2 weeks later.[56] IVC filters prevent

> ✎ **CLINICAL TIP**
>
> Homans' sign (pain in the upper calf with forced ankle dorsiflexion) has been used as a screening tool for venous thrombosis, but it is an insensitive and nonspecific test (sensitivity and specificity are only about 50%) that has a very high false-positive rate.[40]

approximately 97% of symptomatic PEs that originate from the lower extremities.[75] Management of venous thrombosis may also consist of thrombolytic therapy (streptokinase and urokinase), or both, and surgical thrombectomy (limited uses).[28] However, the use of thrombolytic therapy is not recommended for an isolated DVT.[40]

Traditionally, all patients with the diagnosis of DVT were required to be on bed rest for the first few days because of the fear of dislodging clots that may result in pulmonary embolism. However, with the introduction of LMWH, known by the generic name of lovenox, selected stable patients are able to be treated on an outpatient basis and are discharged home on LMWH. Recent literature review shows that bed rest has no influence on the risk of developing PEs. The incidence of new PE and risk of thrombus propagation is not increased in patients with uncomplicated DVT who are mobilized early; however, there may be an increased risk of acute PE among patients with DVT and known PE when ambulation begins early, so these patients require careful consideration. Early ambulation of patients with DVT, anticoagulation, and use of compression stockings lead to a more rapid resolution of pain and swelling associated with DVT, reduce the risk of extension of proximal DVT, and decrease the incidence, severity, and recurrence of postthrombotic syndrome, in addition to preventing venous stasis. Early ambulation is recommended in patients who have not been diagnosed with PE in the setting of DVT and who do not have cardiopulmonary impairment. Current evidence suggests that patients with DVT who are receiving appropriate anticoagulation could be considered for early ambulation, within the first 24 hours, provided they have adequate cardiopulmonary reserve and no evidence of PE.[76-78] Use of a compression stocking while ambulating has an added advantage, and compression stockings are reported to help with pain relief and leg circumference.[40,79-81]

Pulmonary Embolism. PE is the primary complication of venous thrombosis, with emboli commonly originating in the lower extremities. About 75% to 90% of PEs originate from the lower extremities; the rest originate from the right atrium and upper extremities,[75] as well as the pelvic venous plexus. Mechanical blockage of a pulmonary artery or capillary, depending on clot size, results in an acute ventilation-perfusion mismatch that leads to a decrease in partial pressure of oxygen and oxyhemoglobin saturation, which ultimately manifests as tissue hypoxia. Chronic physiologic sequelae from PE include pulmonary hypertension, chronic hypoxemia, and right congestive heart failure. Refer to the Laboratory Studies section for details on the D-dimer test. Refer to Chapter 4 for more details on ventilation-perfusion mismatches, as well as the respiratory sequelae (dyspnea, chest pain, hemoptysis, and tachypnea) of PE.[28,82]

Management of PE consists of prevention of venous thrombosis formation (see the Venous Thrombosis section), early detection, and thorough anticoagulation therapy with standard heparin or LMWH. Thrombolytic therapy has also been used in patients with PE. The placement of an inferior vena cava filter is indicated when patients cannot be anticoagulated or when there is recurrence of PE despite anticoagulation.[28,82]

> ✎ **CLINICAL TIP**
>
> Physical therapy intervention should be discontinued immediately if the signs and symptoms of an acute PE arise during an examination or treatment session.

Chronic Venous Insufficiency and Postphlebitic Syndrome. Chronic venous insufficiency and postphlebitic syndrome are similar disorders that result from venous outflow obstruction, valvular dysfunction from thrombotic destruction of veins, or both. Valvular dysfunction is generally the most significant cause of either disorder. Figure 7-6 illustrates the venous valves and the normal function of the valves.

Within 5 years of sustaining a DVT, approximately 50% of patients develop signs of these disorders. The hallmark characteristics of both chronic venous insufficiency and postphlebitic syndrome are the following[1,8,28,58,83]:

- Chronic swollen limbs, which becomes worse while the limbs are in a dependent position.
- Skin changes such as the following are common: (1) hemosiderin staining or hemosiderosis, a classic indicator of venous disease, is a discoloration of soft tissue that results when extravasated RBCs break down and release the pigment hemosiderin, resulting in a gray-brown pigmentation of the skin (also called hyperpigmentation or tissue staining) and (2) lipodermatosis (fibrosis or hardening of the soft tissue in the lower leg), which is indicative of long-standing venous disease.
- Venous stasis ulceration
- Management of these disorders may consist of any of the following: leg elevation above the level of the heart 2 to 4 times daily for 10 to 15 minutes; application of proper elastic supports (knee length preferable); skin hygiene; avoidance of crossing legs, poorly fitting chairs, garters, and sources of pressure above the legs (e.g., tight girdles); elastic compression stockings; pneumatic compression stockings (if the patient needs to remain in bed); exercise to aid muscular

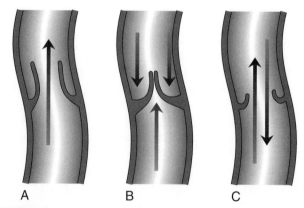

FIGURE 7-6

Venous valves. **A,** Open valves allow forward blood flow. **B,** Closed valves prevent backflow. **C,** Incompetent valves are unable to fully close, causing blood to flow backward and producing venous insufficiency. (Redrawn from Bryant R, Nix D: Acute and chronic wounds: current management concepts, ed 3, St Louis, 2007, Mosby.)

pumping of venous blood; surgical ligation of veins; and wound care to venous ulcers. Refer to Chapter 12 for more information on wound care.[1,28,83]

> ### ✎ CLINICAL TIP
>
> Caution should be taken in providing compressive dressings and elevating the lower extremities of patients who have arterial insufficiency, diabetes mellitus, or congestive heart failure.

Combined Arterial and Venous Disorders

Arteriovenous Malformations. Arteriovenous malformations (AVMs) involve shunting of blood directly from the artery to the vein, bypassing the capillary bed. The presence of an arteriovenous fistula in the AVM is usually the cause of the shunt. The majority of AVMs occur in the trunk and extremities, with a certain number of cases also presenting in the cerebrovascular region.[53]

Signs of AVMs may include the following[53]:

- Skin color changes (erythema or cyanosis)
- Venous varices
- Edema
- Limb deformity
- Skin ulceration
- Pulse deficit
- Bleeding
- Ischemic manifestations in involved organ systems

Hematologic Disorders

Erythrocytic Disorders

Disorders of RBCs are generally categorized as a decrease or an increase in the number of RBCs in the circulating blood.

Anemia. Anemia is defined as a significant reduction in the mass of circulating red blood cells. As a result, the oxygen binding capacity of blood is diminished. Because the blood volume is normally maintained at a nearly constant level, anemic patients have a decrease in the concentration of red cells or hemoglobin in peripheral blood.[56] Anemia can be described according to etiology as (1) a decrease in RBC production, (2) abnormal RBC maturation, or (3) an increase in RBC destruction.[13] Anemia can also be described according to morphology based on RBC size or color.[84] RBCs that are of normal size are normocytic; RBCs that are smaller than normal are microcytic; and RBCs that are larger than normal are macrocytic. RBCs of normal color are normochromic; RBCs of decreased color are microchromic. Some of the most common anemias are described in this section.

Posthemorrhagic Anemia. Posthemorrhagic anemia can occur with rapid blood loss from traumatic artery severance, aneurysm rupture, or arterial erosion from malignant or ulcerative lesions, or as a result of surgery. Blood loss results in a normocytic, normochromic anemia.

The signs and symptoms of posthemorrhagic anemia depend on the amount of blood loss and may include the following[85]:

- With 20% to 30% blood volume loss: Dizziness and hypotension when not at rest in a recumbent position; tachycardia with exertion.
- With 30% to 40% blood volume loss: Thirst, dyspnea, diaphoresis, cold and clammy skin, hypotension and tachycardia, decreased urine output, clouding or loss of consciousness when at rest in a recumbent position.
- With 40% to 50% blood volume loss: A severe state of shock with the potential for death ensues.

Management of posthemorrhagic anemia may consist of any of the following: control of bleeding at the source, intravenous and oral fluid administration, blood and blood product transfusion, and supplemental oxygen.[14,84,86]

Iron-Deficiency Anemia. Iron-deficiency anemia is the most common cause of anemia (Box 7-3), affecting at least one third of the world's population.[58,87] When iron loss exceeds iron intake for a time long enough to deplete the body's iron stores, insufficient iron is available for normal Hgb production. Iron deficiency is characterized by hypochromic microcytic anemia.[87]

The average American diet contains 10 to 15 mg of iron per day, of which 10% is absorbed via the stomach, duodenum, and upper jejunum. Menstrual blood loss in women plays a major role in iron metabolism. Women with heavy menstrual losses should absorb 3 to 4 mg of iron from the diet each day.[39] Serum ferritin is the preferred initial diagnostic test and is a good indicator of the available iron stores in the body. A ferritin level less than 10 mcg/L is diagnostic of iron-deficiency anemia. Often, the iron-deficiency anemia is asymptomatic if the onset is insidious.[11,88,89]

Signs and symptoms of iron-deficiency anemia include the following[70,87]:

- Easy fatigability, tachycardia, palpitations, and dyspnea on exertion
- Dizziness, headache and irritability
- Dysphagia (Plummer-Vinson syndrome, formation of esophageal webs)
- Softening and spooning of nails; pale earlobes, palms, and conjunctivae (severe anemia)
- Concave or spoon shaped nails (koilonychia)[87]
- Many iron-deficient patients develop pica, which is the craving to eat unusual substances such as dirt or ice

---

> ### BOX 7-3 Causes of Iron Deficiency
>
> - Deficient diet
> - Decreased absorption
> - Increased requirements
> - Pregnancy
> - Lactation
> - Blood loss
> - Gastrointestinal
> - Menstrual
> - Blood donation
> - Hemoglobinuria
> - Iron sequestration

Data from McPhee SJ, Papadakis MA, Tierney LM: Current medical diagnosis and treatment, ed 46, New York, 2007, McGraw-Hill Medical.

Management of iron-deficiency anemia consists of a medical workup to identify possible blood loss site, iron supplementation, or nutritional counseling.[14,84,86,90] Iron supplementation during pregnancy is almost always required.[39]

Vitamin B₁₂ Anemia. Decreased levels of vitamin B_{12} cause the production of macrocytic, normochromic RBCs. Vitamin B_{12} deficiency is commonly caused by poor absorption of vitamin B_{12} from enteritis or iliac disease. It is less commonly associated with Crohn's disease and pancreatic insufficiency. Because vitamin B_{12} is present in all foods of animal origin, dietary vitamin B_{12} insufficiency is extremely rare and is seen only in vegans. The most common cause of vitamin B_{12} deficiency is associated with pernicious anemia. *Pernicious anemia* is caused by the absence of intrinsic factor available to bind to vitamin B_{12}.[39] In addition to the general presentation of anemia, the signs and symptoms of vitamin B_{12} deficiency may include the following:

- Pale skin and mild icterus (a yellow discoloration of the skin, mucous membranes, and sclerae of the eyes, caused by greater than normal amounts of bilirubin in the blood)[91]
- Anorexia and diarrhea
- Oral ulceration

Early neurologic symptoms include decreased vibratory sensation, loss of proprioception, and ataxia.[92] Later involvement results in spasticity, hyperactive reflexes, and a positive Romberg's sign. These neurologic symptoms result from the formation of a demyelinating lesion of the neurons of the spinal cord and cerebral cortex.[70]

Vitamin B_{12} deficiency is diagnosed by clinical presentation, low serum vitamin B_{12} levels, elevated lactate dehydrogenase and MCV values, and positive urine sampling (Schilling test). Neurologic symptoms are reversible if the onset is less than 6 months.[55] Management of vitamin B_{12} anemia consists of lifelong vitamin B_{12} supplementation and nutritional counseling.[14,84,86]

✎ CLINICAL TIP

Patients who receive monthly vitamin B_{12} injections may have improvements in their alertness and activity tolerance for a few days after the injection. Therefore physical therapy intervention and goal setting should accommodate these changes.

Folic Acid Anemia. Decreased folic acid (folate) causes the production of macrocytic, normochromic RBCs. The most common cause of folic acid deficiency is inadequate dietary intake. Patients who are alcoholic or anorexic, pregnant women, and patients who do not eat fresh produce and those who overcook their food are candidates for folate deficiency.[90] The common occurrence of folic acid deficiency during the growth spurts of childhood and adolescence and during the third trimester of pregnancy is explained by the increased demands for folate required for DNA synthesis in these circumstances.[24] The presentation of folic acid anemia is similar to vitamin B_{12} deficiency anemia, except there are no neurologic sequelae. Folic acid anemia is diagnosed by clinical presentation, a low serum folate level, and elevated lactate and MCV values.[93] Management of folic acid anemia consists of folic acid supplementation.[90]

Aplastic Anemia. Aplastic anemia is characterized by a decreased RBC production secondary to bone marrow damage. The bone marrow damage either causes irreversible changes to the stem cell population, rendering these cells unable to produce RBCs, or alters the stem cell environment, which inhibits RBC production. The exact mechanism of stem cell damage is unknown; however, present theories include exposure to radiation and chemotherapy or pharmacologic agents, the presence of infection or malignancy, or as an autoimmune response.[94] RBCs are normochromic and normocytic or macrocytic. WBC and platelet counts are also decreased. The hallmark of aplastic anemia is pancytopenia.[39] Definitive diagnosis is by bone marrow biopsy.

Signs and symptoms of aplastic anemia may include the following:

- Bleeding is the most common symptom (easy bruisability, gum bleeds, nose bleeds, petechiae, hematuria, heavy menstrual flow, fecal blood).
- Fatigue and dyspnea.
- Pallor is common and is observed on the mucosal membranes and palmar surfaces.
- Fever or infection.
- Sore throat.

Management of aplastic anemia may include any of the following: investigation and removal of causative agent; red blood cell and platelet transfusion; immunosuppression; bone marrow transplantation and peripheral stem cell transplantation; corticosteroids; and antibiotics. Aplastic anemia can be fatal if untreated.*

Hemolytic Anemia. Hemolysis is the destruction or removal of red blood cells from the circulation before their normal life span of 120 days. Hemolysis can be a lifelong process. It most often presents as anemia when the formation of the RBCs cannot match the pace of RBC destruction. The two types of hemolytic anemia are *extravascular* and *intravascular* hemolytic anemia. Extravascular hemolytic anemia involves the destruction of RBCs outside of the circulation, usually in the spleen and liver.[96] This condition is usually the result of an inherited defect of the RBC membrane or structure, but it can be an autoimmune process in which antibodies in the blood cause RBC destruction through mononuclear phagocytosis.

Intravascular hemolytic anemia is the destruction of RBC membrane within the circulation. It results in the deposition of Hgb in plasma. This may occur because of a genetic enzyme deficit, the attack of oxidants on RBCs, or infection. It may also occur traumatically when RBCs are torn apart at sites of blood flow turbulence, near a tumor, through prosthetic valves, or with aortic stenosis.

Signs and symptoms of hemolytic anemia may include:
- Fatigue and weakness
- Nausea and vomiting

---

*References 9,14,39,84,86,87,95.

- Fever and chills
- Decreased urine output
- Jaundice
- Abdominal or back pain and splenomegaly (intravascular only)

Management of hemolytic anemia may include any of the following: investigation and removal of the causative factor, fluid replacement, blood transfusion, corticosteroids, or splenectomy.[14,84,86]

Sickle Cell Anemia. Sickle cell anemia is an autosomal homozygous (hemoglobin SS or HgSS) recessive trait characterized by RBCs that become sickle (crescent)-shaped when deoxygenated. Over time, cells become rigid and occlude blood vessels, thus causing tissue ischemia and infarction. The risk of cerebrovascular accident and infarction of other organs or muscles is high. Symptoms and physical findings of sickle cell anemia may include:

- Jaundice, nocturia, hematuria, pyelonephritis, renal failure, splenohepatomegaly.
- Retinopathy or blindness.
- Chronic nonhealing ulcers of the lower extremity.
- Systolic murmur and an enlarged heart.
- Paresthesias.
- Acute painful episodes that affect long bones and joints, with the low back being the most frequent site of pain. Other parts of the body affected are the scalp, face, jaw, abdomen, and pelvis. The pain is usually nociceptive (secondary to tissue damage) and is sharp and throbbing in nature.[97]

A complication of sickle cell anemia that may require hospitalization is pain crisis, intense pain in any major organ or body area. Pain crisis is usually treated with parenteral opioids.[97] Lasting from 4 to 6 days to weeks, pain crisis can be precipitated by infection, dehydration, hypoxia, sleep apnea, exposure to cold, or menstruation, or it may be of unknown etiology.[98]

> ### ✎ CLINICAL TIP
> Tachycardia may be the first change observed when monitoring vital signs during sickle cell crisis, usually accompanied by a sense of fatigue, generalized weakness, loss of stamina, and exertional dyspnea.[24]

Acute chest syndrome (ACS) is a situation that requires hospital admission. The patient presents with chest pain, dyspnea, hypoxemia, and infiltrates on chest x-ray, perhaps with pleural effusion.[99] ACS may be caused by intrapulmonary sickling, sickle cell emboli, or bone marrow or fat embolism, or by infection.[99] The ACS is currently defined as a new infiltrate on chest radiograph associated with one or more symptoms, such as fever, cough, sputum production, tachypnea, dyspnea, or new-onset hypoxia.[100] ACS is the leading cause of death in adolescents and adults with sickle cell disease.[16]

Management of sickle cell anemia may include the prevention or supportive treatment of symptoms with rest; hydration; analgesia; supplemental oxygen; incentive spirometry; use of corticosteroids or cytotoxic agents, such as hydroxyurea[62];

partial RBC exchange; and psychosocial support.[14,84,86,94,100] The average life expectancy of a patient with sickle cell anemia is 40 to 50 years.[90] Note that sickle cell anemia is differentiated from sickle cell trait. A patient with sickle cell trait has a heterozygous trait of Hgb that is asymptomatic for the signs and symptoms of anemia, although RBCs may sickle under the conditions of high altitude, strenuous exercise, or anesthesia.[94] No treatment is usually necessary; however, genetic counseling is a reasonable strategy.[39]

> ### ✎ CLINICAL TIP
> The use of oximetry can help the physical therapist and patient monitor RBC oxygenation and gauge exercise intensity.

Anemia of Chronic Diseases. The term *anemia of chronic disease* (ACD) designates an anemia syndrome typically found in patients with chronic infections, inflammatory disorders, or neoplastic disorders. ACD occurs in approximately 50% of hospitalized patients, as identified by laboratory studies. ACD has also been observed in acute trauma and critical care patients.

The clinical features are those of the causative condition. The diagnosis should be suspected in patients with chronic diseases and is confirmed by low serum level, low total iron-binding capacity, and normal or increased serum ferritin.

In most cases, no treatment is necessary. Purified recombinant erythropoietin is effective for treatment of anemia of renal failure or anemia related to cancer and inflammatory conditions.[87]

Polycythemia. Polycythemia is a chronic disorder characterized by excessive production of RBCs, platelets, and myelocytes. As these increase, blood volume, blood viscosity, and Hgb concentration increase, causing excessive workload for the heart and congestion of some organs.[16] The three types of polycythemia are *primary polycythemia (polycythemia vera), secondary polycythemia,* and *relative polycythemia.*

1. Primary polycythemia, or polycythemia vera, is an acquired myeloproliferative disorder[39] that causes an increase in the number of RBCs, WBCs, and platelets.[101] The origin of this disease is unknown; however, there is an autonomous overproduction of erythroid stem cells from bone marrow leading to increased blood viscosity and expanded blood volume. Thus there is a risk for thrombus formation and bleeding.[90] Primary polycythemia may convert to chronic myelogenous leukemia or myelofibrosis. The hallmark of polycythemia vera is a hematocrit above normal, at times greater than 60%.[39]
2. Secondary polycythemia is the overproduction of RBCs owing to a high level of erythropoietin. The increased erythropoietin level is a result of either altered stem cells (which automatically produce erythropoietin or erythropoietin-secreting tumors, such as hepatoma or cerebellar hemangioblastoma)[89] or chronic low oxygenation of tissues, in which the body attempts to compensate for hypoxia. The latter is common in individuals with chronic obstructive pulmonary disease, cardiopulmonary disease, or exposure to high altitudes.

3. Relative polycythemia is the temporary increase in RBCs secondary to decreased fluid volume (dehydration), as with excessive vomiting, diarrhea, or excessive diuretic use, or after a burn injury.

Signs and symptoms of polycythemia may include[42]:

- Headache, dizziness, blurred vision, and vertigo, all a result of hypervolemia
- Venous thrombosis, a result of hyperviscosity
- Bleeding from the nose, gastrointestinal bleeding, and spontaneous bruising, all a result of platelet dysfunction
- Fatigue
- Paresthesia in the hands and feet
- Splenomegaly (polycythemia vera only)

Management of polycythemia includes phlebotomy as the main therapy. Blood is withdrawn from the vein to decrease blood volume and decrease hematocrit to 45%. Every 2 to 4 days, 250 to 500 ml of blood is removed, depending on the age of the patient, with a goal for the hematocrit to be below 42% for females and 45% for males.[16,56] Other treatments used in polycythemia are myelosuppressive therapy (hydroxyurea); interferon[30]; antiplatelet therapy (aspirin); radiophosphorus (for primary polycythemia); smoking cessation; and fluid resuscitation (for relative polycythemia).

Neutropenia. Neutropenia is defined as an absolute neutrophil count (ANC) of less than $1500/\mu l$ and is calculated from the WBC differential: ANC = WBC (cells/μl) × percent (polymorphonuclear neutrophils + bands) divided by 100.[102] A variety of bone marrow disorders (e.g., leukemia) and nonmarrow conditions (e.g., immunologic peripheral destruction, sepsis, or hypersplenism) or chemotherapy may cause neutropenia. Neutropenia is considered mild (ANC between 1000 and $1500/\mu l$), moderate (ANC between 500 and $1000/\mu l$), or severe (ANC less than $500/\mu l$).[103] The risk of infection, typically bacterial, is related to the severity of the neutropenia, with the risk of infection increasing at $1000/\mu l$.[103] Usual signs of inflammatory responses to infection may be absent in a neutropenic patient; however, fever in a neutropenic patient should always be assumed to be of infectious origin. Refer to Chapter 14 for more information on neutropenia.

Medical therapy consists of symptomatic management of fever, discontinuation of causative drugs, broad-spectrum antibiotics or antifungal agents to treat infection, good dental hygiene, the administration of myeloid growth factor, and hematopoietic cell transplantation.[39,103]

Thrombocytic Disorders

Disseminated Intravascular Coagulation. DIC involves the introduction of thromboplastic substances into the circulation that initiate a massive clotting cascade accompanied by fibrin, plasmin, and platelet activation. It is a complex and paradoxic disorder characterized by both hemorrhage and thrombus formation (Table 7-19). First, fibrin is deposited in the microcirculation, leading to organ ischemia and the destruction of RBCs as they pass through these deposits. Second, platelets and clotting factors are consumed and hemorrhage occurs. Plasmin is activated to further decrease clotting factor, and

TABLE 7-19 Common Signs and Symptoms of Disseminated Intravascular Coagulation

System	Related to Hemorrhage	Related to Thrombi
Integumentary	Bleeding from gums, venipunctures, and old surgical sites; epistaxis; ecchymoses	Peripheral cyanosis, gangrene
Cardiopulmonary	Hemoptysis	Dysrhythmias, chest pain, acute myocardial infarction, pulmonary embolus, respiratory failure
Renal	Hematuria	Oliguria, acute tubular necrosis, renal failure
Gastrointestinal	Abdominal distention, hemorrhage	Diarrhea, constipation, bowel infarct
Neurologic	Subarachnoid hemorrhage	Altered level of consciousness, cerebral vascular accident

From Urden LD, Stacy KM, Lough ME: Thelan's critical care nursing: diagnosis and management, ed 5, St Louis, 2006, Mosby.

fibrin further inhibits platelet function, which further increases bleeding.

DIC, either acute or chronic, is always a secondary process mediated by inflammatory cytokines.[104] DIC may be mild and self-limiting or may be severe, and it is often associated with critical illness.[105] The onset of acute DIC usually occurs in the presence of illness within hours or days of the initial injury or event. This condition is associated with severe infection and gram-negative sepsis. Other causes of DIC include trauma, burn injury, shock, tissue acidosis, antigen-antibody complexes, or the entrance of amniotic fluid or placenta into the maternal circulation.[89] Organ failure is common.[6] Chronic DIC is associated with hemangioma and other cancers (particularly pancreatic or prostate cancer), systemic lupus erythematosus, or missed abortion. DIC is a life-threatening condition with high mortality and requires immediate medical attention.[6]

The diagnostic workup for DIC includes platelet count (thrombocytopenia), PT and activated partial thromboplastin time (aPTT) (prolonged), INR (elevated), fibrinogen level (decreased), and presence of D-dimer.[106] The D-dimer has high sensitivity and specificity for diagnosing DIC.[6]

✎ **CLINICAL TIP**

Inflate the blood pressure cuff only as high as needed to obtain a reading. Frequent blood pressure readings may cause bleeding under the cuff, particularly for patients with thrombocytic disorders, so rotate arm use to reduce repeated trauma.

Management of DIC may include treatment of the causative condition; hemodynamic and cardiovascular support, which includes fluid management, oxygen supplementation, and invasive monitoring; blood and blood product transfusion for active bleeding; heparin therapy (this is controversial); and recombinant protein factor therapy (experimental).[16,104]

Hemophilia. Hemophilia is a disease characterized by excessive spontaneous hemorrhaging at mucous membranes, into joint spaces (hemarthrosis) and muscles, or intracranially. It is the result of a genetic deficiency of a clotting factor. There are four basic types[107]:

1. Hemophilia A is characterized by the lack of factor VIII and is inherited as an X-linked recessive trait.
2. Hemophilia B (Christmas disease) is characterized by the lack of factor IX and is inherited as an X-linked recessive trait.
3. Hemophilia C is characterized by the lack of factor XI and is inherited as an autosomal recessive trait.
4. von Willebrand's disease is characterized by the lack of factor VIII and is inherited as an autosomal dominant trait.

Patients with mild hemophilia experience bleeding only with trauma or after surgical procedures, whereas patients with severe hemophilia may bleed with minor trauma or spontaneously.[90]

Hemophilia A, when severe, is characterized by excessive bleeding into various organs of the body. Soft-tissue hematomas and hemarthroses leading to severe, crippling hemarthropathy are highly characteristic of the disease. Muscle hemorrhages can be more insidious and massive than joint bleeding and most often involve the flexor muscle groups.[24] Bleeding into joints accounts for approximately 75% of bleeding episodes in severely affected patients with hemophilia A.[108] The knee is the most frequently affected joint, followed by the ankle, elbow, hip, shoulder, and wrist. Joints with at least four bleeds in 6 months are called target joints. When the blood is introduced into the joint, the joint becomes distended, causing swelling, pain, warmth and stiffness.[24] In seriously affected patients, major hemorrhages may dissect through tissue planes, ultimately leading to compromise of vital organs. However, bleeding episodes are intermittent, and some patients do not hemorrhage for weeks or months.[109]

Symptoms and physical findings of bleeding episode from hemophilia may include

- Petechiae, purpura, and ecchymosis.
- Hematoma. (Intramuscular hematomas are common in hemophilia A, bleeding into the psoas muscle is common,

> ✎ **CLINICAL TIP**
>
> Patients with psoas hematoma will present with severe pain, usually around the buttocks, and their primary complaint is usually the inability to get comfortable in any position. A large iliopsoas hemorrhage can cause displacement of the kidney and ureter and can compress the neurovascular bundle. Iliopsoas bleeds are considered a medical emergency requiring immediate physician referral.[24]

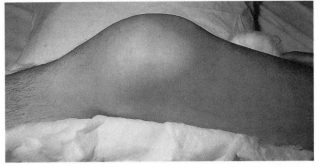

FIGURE 7-7
Acute hemarthrosis of the knee is a common complication of hemophilia. (From Forbes CD, Jackson WF: Color atlas and text of clinical medicine, ed 3, London, 2003, Mosby.)

and femoral nerve involvement may be partial or complete.[110])

- Disorientation.
- Convulsions.
- Tachycardia, tachypnea, and hypotension.
- Intracranial bleeding is the major cause of death for all age groups of hemophiliacs.[6]
- Pain.

Patients with acute hemarthrosis have pain, with objective findings of warmth, a tense effusion, tenderness, and limitation of motion, and the joint is usually held in flexion. Acute hemarthrosis of the knee is a common complication of hemophilia (Figure 7-7). It may be confused with acute infection unless the patient's coagulation disorder is known. Patients with subacute or chronic arthritis (related to hemophilia) have chronically swollen joints, which are usually painless and slightly warm to touch.[111] Repeated hemarthrosis causes joint deformity and radiologic changes.

Management of hemophilia may include any of the following: methods to stop active bleeding (e.g., direct pressure), supportive therapy depending on the location of the bleed (e.g., joint debridement), factor replacement therapy, and pain management.[94]

> ✎ **CLINICAL TIP**
>
> Watch for signs of joint effusion (warmth and edema) in patients with hemophilia who are prone to hemarthrosis, especially during weight-bearing activities.

Thalassemia. Thalassemia is an autosomal-recessive disease characterized by abnormal formation of Hgb chains in RBCs, resulting in RBC membrane damage and abnormal erythropoiesis and hemolysis.

Hgb is composed of two alpha and two beta chains. α-Thalassemia is a defect in alpha-chain synthesis in which one (alpha trait), two (α-thalassemia minor), or three (Hgb H disease) genes are altered. Each type of α-thalassemia varies in presentation from a lack of symptoms (alpha trait and minor) to chronic severe hemolytic anemia (Hgb H).[89] β-Thalassemia minor is a defect in beta-chain synthesis in one of two beta chains and is usually asymptomatic. β-Thalassemia major is a severe reduction or absence in beta-chain production that results in severe anemia, growth failure, bony deformities, hepatosplenomegaly, and jaundice with a life expectancy of 20 to 30 years from complications of heart failure, cirrhosis, and endocrinopathy.[90]

Patients with thalassemia are classified as having thalassemia minor, thalassemia intermedia, or thalassemia major, depending on the severity of their anemia. Patients with thalassemia minor generally have little or no hematologic disease. Patients with thalassemia intermedia may require occasional transfusions. Patients with thalassemia major require lifelong chronic RBC transfusion to maintain adequate hemoglobin levels.[58]

Management of the thalassemia may include folate supplementation, blood transfusion, iron-chelating agents, and splenectomy.[90]

Thrombocytopenia. Thrombocytopenia is an acute or chronic decrease in the number of platelets (less than 150,000/μl) in the circulation. It can result from decreased platelet production (caused by infection, drug or immune responses, or blood vessel damage), increased platelet destruction (caused by malignancy, antiplatelet antibodies, or the use of myelosuppressive drugs), or altered platelet distribution (caused by cardiac surgery–induced hypothermia, portal hypertension, or splenomegaly).[107]

Signs and symptoms of thrombocytopenia may include[112]:
- Bleeding of nose, gums, or puncture sites or blood in emesis, urine, or stool
- Ecchymosis and petechiae
- Tachycardia and tachypnea
- Signs of increased intracranial pressure if a cranial bleed is present
- Renal failure
- Splenomegaly

Management of thrombocytopenia may include treatment of the causative factor; immunosuppressive therapy; anticoagulants in plasma transfusion or plasmapheresis; corticosteroids; or splenectomy.[107]

Physical Therapy Considerations. A physical therapist should implement fall precautions for the patient who is thrombocytopenic during all physical therapy interventions; patients with thrombocytopenia should be educated about the fall risk precautions and the potential for bleeding.

Blood pressure cuffs and similar devices must be used with caution. Elastic support stockings must be thigh high, never knee high. Mechanical compression with a pneumatic pump and soft-tissue mobilization are avoided unless approved by a physician.[24]

Heparin-Induced Thrombocytopenia. Heparin-induced thrombocytopenia (HIT) is the most common type of drug-induced thrombocytopenia and one of the most common causes of thrombocytopenia in hospitalized patients.[39] Heparin can have a dramatic thrombocytopenic effect, usually 5 to 10 days after the initiation of heparin therapy. The clinical presentation of HIT is distinct and may include[113]:
- Large, bilateral lower-extremity DVT
- Upper-extremity DVT at a venous catheter site

- Skin lesions at the injection site
- Aortic or ileofemoral thrombus with limb ischemia
- Pulmonary embolism
- An acute systemic reaction to heparin

HIT may be type I (the asymptomatic aggregation of platelets) or type II (an immune response resulting in platelet activation and venous or arterial thrombi).[114] Type I is more common than type II, and type II is associated with greater risk of life-threatening thrombosis.[115] HIT is diagnosed by clinical presentation, a platelet count less than 100×10^9/L, and a positive platelet aggregation test. Heparin-PF 4 antibody testing is recommended for patients suspected to have HIT.[116] Management of HIT starts with the immediate discontinuation of heparin and initiation of fast-acting, nonheparin alternative anticoagulation. The direct thrombin inhibitors argatroban, lepirudin, and bivalirudin are nonheparin anticoagulants that inhibit thrombin without interaction with heparin-PF4 antibodies.[116] Management of HIT also includes plasmapheresis and immunoglobulin therapy, in addition to supportive therapies for alteration in skin integrity and pain.[114]

Thrombotic Thrombocytopenic Purpura. Thrombotic thrombocytopenic purpura (TTP) is the rapid accumulation of thrombi in small blood vessels. TTP is primarily seen in young adults 20 to 50 years of age.[90] The etiology of TTP is unknown; however, it is associated with bacterial or viral infections, estrogen use, certain drug use, pregnancy, and autoimmune disorders such as acquired immunodeficiency syndrome.[90] The diagnosis of TTP is made by thrombocytopenia, anemia, and elevated serum lactate dehydrogenase. The coagulation tests are normal.[39]

Signs and symptoms of TTP may include:
- Hemolytic anemia, thrombocytopenia
- Fatigue and weakness
- Fever
- Pallor, rash, petechiae
- Waxing and waning headache, confusion, altered consciousness from lethargy to coma
- Hemiparesis and seizures
- Abdominal pain and tenderness due to pancreatitis
- Acute renal failure

Management of TTP may include emergent large-volume plasmapheresis; plasma exchange; antiplatelet agents; corticosteroids; immunosuppressive agents; or splenectomy if not refractory to initial therapy or if the condition recurs.[90]

Idiopathic Thrombocytopenic Purpura. Idiopathic thrombocytopenic purpura (ITP) is an autoimmune disorder in which an IgG autoantibody is formed that binds to the platelets. Platelets are not destroyed by direct lysis; rather, destruction takes place in the spleen without subsequent enlargement (splenomegaly). An enlarged spleen should lead one to doubt the diagnosis of ITP.

Patients are systemically well and usually not febrile. The hallmark of the disease is thrombocytopenia. The bone marrow will appear normal, and coagulation studies will be entirely normal.

The common symptoms are of bleeding and include epistaxis, oral bleeding, menorrhagia, purpura, and petechiae. Most patients will require treatment, but some patients will have spontaneous remissions. Treatment is usually with corticosteroids, most commonly with prednisone and in some cases with immunoglobulins. Splenectomy is the most definitive treatment for ITP, and most patients will ultimately undergo splenectomy. Platelet transfusions are rarely used in the treatment of ITP because exogenous platelets will survive no better than the patient's own and will usually last less than a few hours.[39]

Lymphatic Disorders

Lymphedema

Lymphedema is a chronic disorder characterized by an abnormal collection of lymph fluid in the tissues of one or more body regions. The most common cause for the accumulation of the fluid is a mechanical insufficiency of the lymphatic system. Lymphedema can be classified as primary or secondary. *Primary (idiopathic) lymphedema* is caused by a condition that is congenital or hereditary. In this case, the lymph node or the lymph vessel formation is abnormal. *Secondary (acquired) lymphedema* is caused by injury to one or more components of the lymphatic system in some other manner, when some of the lymphatic system is blocked, dissected, fibrosed, or damaged.

Lymphedema can develop in any part of the body or limb(s). The severity of lymphedema is graded using the scale from the International Society of Lymphology, as described in Table 7-20.

Signs and symptoms of lymphedema include:
- Swelling distal to or adjacent to the area where lymph system function has been impaired
- Symptoms usually not relieved by elevation

- Pitting edema in early stages and nonpitting edema in later stages, when fibrotic changes occur
- Fatigue and heaviness, pressure, tightness, tingling, and numbness in the affected region—causing tremendous discomfort
- Fibrotic changes in the skin
- Increased circumferential limb girth
- Loss of range of motion

Diagnosis of lymphedema can be made without the use of special diagnostic tests. It is beyond the scope of this text to discuss the diagnosis of lymphedema in detail. However, when evaluating a patient with suspected lymphedema, cardiac, renal, thyroid, and arteriovenous disease must be ruled out medically. Management includes manual lymphatic drainage and lymphedema bandaging. Early intervention is of significance.

The physical therapist should have special training to treat this patient population. Manual lymphatic drainage is a specialized manual therapy technique that affects primarily superficial lymphatic circulation. Manual lymphatic drainage improves lymph transport capacity, redirects lymph flow toward collateral vessels, and mobilizes excess lymph fluid.

> ### ✎ CLINICAL TIP
> Patients, particularly those with primary lymphedema of the lower extremities, should be evaluated for abdominal and genital edema before undergoing any treatment to reduce the extremity lymphedema to avoid the complication of moving more fluid to an already overloaded abdominal area.[24]

Lymphedema bandaging is a highly specialized form of bandaging that uses multiple layers of unique padding materials and short stretch bandages to create a supportive structure for edematous and lymphedematous body segments. It is commonly used in between the manual lymphatic drainage treatments.[3]

Management

The management of vascular disorders includes pharmacologic therapy and vascular surgical procedures. Hematologic disorders may be managed with pharmacologic therapy, as well as with nutritional therapy and blood product transfusion.

Pharmacologic Therapy

Common drug classifications for the management of vascular and hematologic disorders include:
- Anticoagulants (see Chapter 19, Table 19-2)
- Antiplatelet agents (see Chapter 19, Table 19-4)
- Thrombolytic agents (see Chapter 19, Table 19-7)
- Colony-stimulating factors (Chapter 19, Table 19-24)

Anticoagulation Therapy

The standard INR goal for anticoagulation therapy with warfarin (Coumadin) is 1.5 to 2.5 times a control value and is

TABLE 7-20 Stages of Lymphedema

Stage 0 (latent lymphedema)	Lymph transport capacity is reduced; no clinical edema is present
Stage 1	Accumulation of protein-rich pitting edema. Reversible with elevation; area affected may be normal size on waking in the morning. Increases with activity, heat, and humidity
Stage 2	Accumulation of protein-rich nonpitting edema with connective scar tissue. Irreversible; does not resolve overnight; increasingly more difficult to pit. Clinical fibrosis is present. Skin changes present in severe stage 2
Stage 3 (lymphostatic elephantiasis)	Accumulation of protein-rich edema with significant increase in connective tissue and scar tissue. Severe nonpitting fibrotic edema. Atrophic changes (hardening of dermal tissue, skin folds, skin papillomas, and hyperkeratosis)

Data from Goodman CC: The hematologic system. In Goodman CC, Boissonnault WG, editors: Pathology: implications for the physical therapist, ed 3, Philadelphia, 2009, Saunders.

TABLE 7-21 Therapeutic Values for International Normalized Ratio (INR)

INR 2.0-3.0	Prophylaxis of venous thrombosis (high-risk surgery)
	Treatment of venous thrombosis and pulmonary embolism
	Prevention of systemic embolism
	Tissue heart valves
	Valvular heart disease
	Atrial fibrillation
	Recurrent systemic embolism
	Cardiomyopathy
INR 2.5-3.5	Acute myocardial infarction
	Mechanical prosthetic heart valve replacement

Data from Goldman L, Ausiello D: Cecil textbook of medicine, ed 24, St Louis, 2012, Saunders; Gibbar-Clements T, Shirrell D, Dooley R et al: The challenge of warfarin therapy, Am J Nurs 100:38-40, 2000.

categorized by condition or clinical state[117] according to the values in Table 7-21.

Physical Therapy Considerations

The physical therapist should understand some basic concepts of anticoagulation therapy to intervene safely and estimate length of stay.

- The physician will determine the PT/INR and PTT goal for each patient. This goal is documented in the medical record. The patient remains in a hospital setting until the goal is reached.
- The therapeutic effect of heparin or LMWH is reached within minutes or hours, whereas the effect of warfarin is reached in 3 to 5 days; thus heparin or LMWH is usually prescribed before warfarin. The dose of heparin or LMWH is increased or decreased depending on the PTT goal, then the patient is transitioned to warfarin as indicated.
- The terms *subtherapeutic* and *supertherapeutic* imply a coagulation level below or above the anticoagulation goal, respectively.
- A subtherapeutic PT/INR or PTT indicates a risk for thrombus formation, whereas a supertherapeutic level indicates a risk for hemorrhage.
- Supertherapeutic anticoagulation is rapidly reversed by vitamin K or fresh-frozen plasma.
- Anticoagulant agents are temporarily discontinued before surgery to minimize bleeding intraoperatively or postoperatively.
- The physical therapist should always monitor the patient who is taking anticoagulants for signs and symptoms of bleeding, as bleeding can occur even if the PT/INR is therapeutic.[117]

Blood Product Transfusion

Blood and blood products are transfused to replenish blood volume, maintain oxygen delivery to tissues, or maintain proper coagulation.[118] The need for blood transfusion should be dependent on the patient's symptoms. It has been reported that refrigerated, banked blood loses its ability to deliver oxygen in a short period of time.[119] Table 7-22 lists the most common transfusion products and the rationale for their use. Blood may be autologous (patient donates own blood) or homologous (from a volunteer donor).

Before transfusing blood or blood products, the substance to be given must be typed and crossed. This process ensures that the correct type of blood is given to a patient to avoid adverse reactions. A variety of transfusion reactions can occur during or after the administration of blood products (Table 7-23). These blood transfusion reactions are usually not fatal, but they can extend a patient's length of stay. Blood transfusions are a form of liquid tissue transplant and it can cause significant immunosuppression. This effect is known as TRIM (transfusion-related immunomodulation), and it happens every time a patient receives blood. Transfusion reactions can be nonimmunologic and are caused by the physical and chemical properties of the transfused blood.[120] There is a threat of transmitting infectious diseases via a blood transfusion.[119]

In addition to these reactions, complications of blood transfusion include air embolism (if the blood is pumped into the patient) or circulatory overload (from a rapid increase in volume). Circulatory overload occurs when the rate of blood (fluid) transfusion is greater than the circulation can accommodate. Signs and symptoms include tachycardia, cough, dyspnea, crackles, headache, hypertension, and distended neck veins. To prevent circulatory overload during a transfusion, intravenous fluids may be stopped, or a diuretic (e.g., furosemide [Lasix]) may be given. Delayed adverse transfusion reactions include iron overload, graft-versus-host disease, hepatitis, human immunodeficiency virus 1 infection, or delayed hemolytic reaction (approximately 7 to 14 days posttransfusion).[121]

Physical Therapy Considerations

- If the patient is receiving blood products, the physical therapist should observe the patient for signs or symptoms, or both, of transfusion reaction before initiating physical therapy intervention.
- Depending on the medical status of the patient, the therapist may defer out-of-bed or vigorous activities until the transfusion is complete. On average, the transfusion of a unit of blood takes 3 to 4 hours.
- Defer physical therapy intervention during the first 15 minutes of a blood transfusion as most blood transfusion reactions occur within this time frame.
- During a blood transfusion, vital signs are usually taken every 15 to 30 minutes by the nurse and posted at the bedside.
- After a blood transfusion, it takes 12 to 24 hours for the Hgb and Hct to increase.[50]

Vascular Surgical Procedures

Surgical management of coronary vascular disorders, such as angioplasty, arthrectomy, and stent placement, is described in Chapter 3 under Percutaneous Revascularization Procedures. These same techniques are also used in peripheral arteries rather than coronary arteries. This section therefore concentrates on embolization therapy, transcatheter thrombolysis/thrombectomy,

TABLE 7-22 Common Blood Products and Their Clinical Indications and Outcomes

Product	Content	Clinical Indications	Outcome
Whole blood	Blood cells and plasma	Acute major blood loss in setting of hypotension, tachycardia, tachypnea, pallor, and decreased Hct and Hgb. To treat oxygen-carrying deficit (RBC) and volume expansion (plasma). When more than 10 units of blood are required in a 24-hour period. Whole blood is rarely used.	Resolution of signs and symptoms of hypovolemic shock or anemia. Hct should increase 3% in a nonbleeding adult (per unit transfused).
Red blood cells (RBCs)	RBCs only	Acute or chronic blood loss. To treat oxygen-carrying deficit in setting of tachycardia, tachypnea, pallor, fatigue, and decreased Hct and Hgb. Anemia without need for volume expansion.	Resolution of signs and symptoms of anemia. Hct should increase 3% in a nonbleeding adult (per unit transfused).
Platelets (Plts)	Concentrated platelets in plasma	To restore clotting function associated with or after blood loss. To increase platelet count in a bleeding patient with platelet <100,000, in advance of a procedure with platelet <50,000, or prophylactically with platelet <10,000.	Resolution of thrombocytopenia. Prevention or resolution of bleeding. Platelets should increase by 5000 in a 70-kg adult (per unit).
Fresh-frozen plasma (FFP)	All plasma components, namely blood factors and protein	To replace or increase coagulation factor levels. Acute disseminated intravascular coagulation. Thrombotic thrombocytopenic purpura. Factor XI deficiency. Liver disease Rapid reversal of warfarin therapy.	Improved or adequate coagulation levels or factor assays. One unit of FFP should increase the level of any clotting factor by 2% to 3%.
Albumin	Albumin cells with few globulins and other proteins	Volume expansion in situations when crystalloid (saline or Ringer's lactate) is inadequate such as shock, major hemorrhage, or plasma exchange. Acute liver failure. Burn injury.	Acquire and maintain adequate blood pressure and volume support.
Plasma protein fraction (PPF)	Albumin, globulins, and plasma proteins	See Albumin, above.	See Albumin, above.
Cryoprecipitate	Factors VIII and XIII, von Willebrand's factor, and fibrinogen in plasma	Replacement of these factor deficiencies. Replacement of fibrinogen when an increase in volume would not be tolerated with FFP. Bleeding associated with uremia.	Correction of these factor or fibrinogen deficiencies. Cessation of bleeding in uremic patients.

Data from U.S. Department of Health and Human Services, National Institutes of Health: National Blood Resource Education Programs transfusion therapy guidelines for nurses, September 1990; Churchill WH: Transfusion therapy, Sci Am Med 4, 2001; Current medical diagnosis and treatment, 2007; Avoiding bad blood. Key steps to safe transfusions, Nursing made incredibly easy! 2(5):20-28, 2004.

Hct, Hematocrit; *Hgb,* hemoglobin.

endarterectomy, bypass grafting, and aneurysm repair and replacement with synthetic grafts. Endovascular procedures are becoming more and more common in patients with peripheral arterial disease. The basic concept of most endovascular procedures is to obtain percutaneous access to a blood vessel and then to gain access across the lesion (either stenosis or aneurysm) with a guidewire.[122]

Embolization Therapy

Embolization* therapy is the process of purposely occluding a vessel with Gelfoam, coils, balloons, polyvinyl alcohol, and various glue-like agents, which are injected as liquids and then solidify in the vessel. Embolization therapy is performed with a specialized intravascular catheter after angiographic evaluation has outlined the area to be treated.

Indications for embolization therapy include disorders characterized by inappropriate blood flow, such as AVMs or, less commonly, persistent hemoptysis. Complications of embolization therapy include tissue necrosis, inadvertent embolization of normal tissues, and passage of embolic materials through arteriovenous communications.[38]

Transcatheter Thrombolysis and/or Thrombectomy

Transcatheter thrombolysis is the process of directly infusing thrombolytic agents such as urokinase and tissue plasminogen activator (tPA) into occluded vessels. The indications for this procedure include lysis of clot in thrombosed bypass grafts,

---

*The term *embolization* is general and can refer to a pathologic occlusion of a vessel by fat, air, or a dislodged portion of a thrombus, or to the therapeutic procedure described in this section. The context in which embolization is discussed must be considered to avoid confusion.

TABLE 7-23 Acute Adverse Blood Reactions

Reaction	Cause	Signs and Symptoms	Onset
Febrile reaction	Patient's blood (anti-leukocyte antibodies) is sensitive to transfused plasma protein, platelets, or white blood cells.	Chills followed by low-grade fever, headache, nausea and vomiting, flushed skin, muscle pain, anxiety (mild). Hypotension, tachycardia, tachypnea, cough (severe).	During transfusion or up to 24 hours posttransfusion
Allergic reaction	Patient's blood (IgE, IgG, or both) is sensitive to transfused plasma protein.	Hives, flushed or itchy skin, and bronchial wheezing (mild). Tachypnea, chest pain, cardiac arrest (severe).	Within minutes of starting transfusion
Septic reaction	Transfused blood components are contaminated with bacteria.	Rapid onset of high fever, hypotension, chills, emesis, diarrhea, abdominal cramps, renal failure, shock.	Within minutes to 30 minutes after transfusion
Acute hemolytic reaction	Patient's blood and transfused blood are not compatible, resulting in red blood cell destruction.	Fever with or without chills is the most common manifestation. Tachycardia, hypotension, tachypnea, cyanosis, chest pain, headache or backache, acute renal failure, cardiac arrest.	Within minutes to hours after transfusion
Anaphylactic reaction	Patient is deficient in IgA and develops IgA antibody to transfused components.	Hives (mild). Wheezing or bronchospasm, anxiety, cyanosis, nausea, emesis, bloody diarrhea, abdominal cramps, shock, cardiac arrest (severe).	Within a few seconds of starting transfusion
Transfusion-related acute lung injury	Transfusion of antibodies in donor plasma is reactive with recipient granulocytes.	Chills, fever, chest pain, hypotension, cyanosis; chest radiograph shows florid pulmonary edema.	Within several hours after transfusion

Data from Linker CA: Blood. In Tierney LM, McPhee SJ, Papadakis MA, editors: Current medical diagnosis and treatment 2001, Stamford, CT, 2001, Appleton & Lange pp 505-558; Kozier B, Erb G, Blais K et al., editors: Fundamentals of nursing: concepts, process and practice, ed 8, Redwood City, CA, 2007, Benjamin-Cummings, p 110; Larison PJ, Cook LO: Adverse effects of blood transfusion. In Harmening DM, editor: Modern blood banking and transfusion practices, Philadelphia, 1999, FA Davis; U.S. Department of Health and Human Services, National Institutes of Health: National Blood Resource Education Programs transfusion therapy guidelines for nurses, September 1990.

Ig, Immunoglobulin.

acute carotid occlusions, and acute or chronic peripheral arterial ischemia. Patients with an acute thrombotic arterial occlusion are considered ideal candidates for lytic therapy.[123] There is considerable debate about the indication of thrombolysis in the setting of acute DVT. The tip of the catheter is introduced into the center of the thrombus, and a low dose of thrombolytic agent is administered. The catheter is left in place for extended periods of time to allow for the clot to lyse properly.[124] This procedure may also include angioplasty, if warranted, to open a stenotic area. By injecting the thrombolytic agent into the area of occlusion, transcatheter thrombolysis has fewer systemic complications of hemorrhage compared to intravenous infusion of thrombolytic agents.[12] The major risk for thrombolytic therapy is bleeding.[56]

Thrombectomy is a method to lyse or remove an extensive thrombus in the lower extremity. This is an immediate but invasive method of restoring perfusion. Two main categories of the devices/catheters are used: "contact" and "noncontact" devices. The contact catheters come in direct contact with the vessel wall. The noncontact catheters use a pressurized fluid to break up the clot, which is then extracted by the catheter.[123]

Peripheral Vascular Bypass Grafting

To reperfuse an area that has been ischemic from peripheral vascular disease, two general bypass grafting procedures (with many specific variations of each type) can be performed. The area of vascular occlusion can be bypassed with an inverted portion of the saphenous vein or with a synthetic material, such as Gore-Tex, Dacron, or Lycra. (The synthetic graft is referred to as a *prosthetic graft*.) Vascular surgeons generally describe and illustrate in the medical record what type of procedure was performed on the particular vascular anatomy. The terminology used to describe each bypass graft procedure indicates which vessels were involved. (For example, a fem-pop bypass graft involves bypassing an occlusion of the femoral artery with another conduit to the popliteal artery distal to the area of occlusion.) After a bypass procedure, patients require approximately 24 to 48 hours (depending on premorbid physiologic status and extent of surgery) to become hemodynamically stable and are usually monitored in an intensive care unit setting. Figures 7-8 and 7-9 illustrate two vascular bypass procedures.

Complications that can occur after bypass grafting include the following[28]:

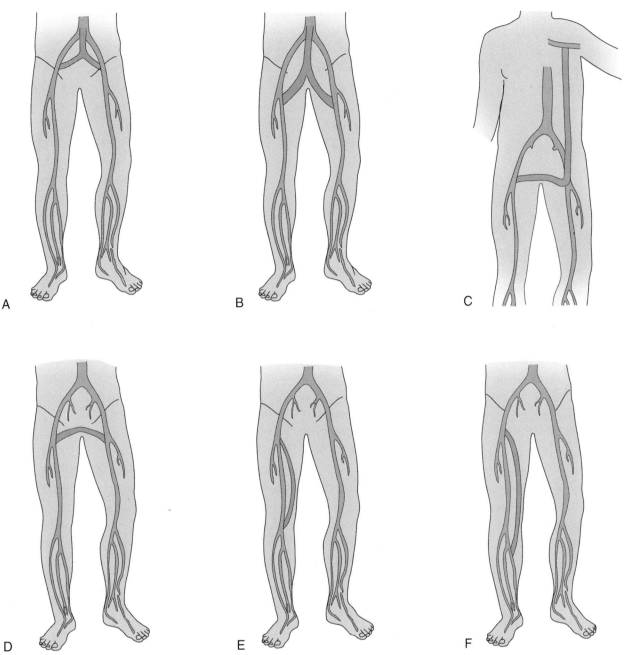

FIGURE 7-8
Peripheral arterial bypass procedures. **A,** Aortoiliac bypass. **B,** Aortobifemoral bypass. **C,** Axillobifemoral bypass. **D,** Femorofemoral bypass. **E,** Femoropopliteal bypass. **F,** Femorotibial bypass. (From Urden LD, Stacy KM, Lough ME: Thelan's critical care nursing: diagnosis and management, ed 6, St Louis, 2010, Mosby.)

- Hemorrhage (at graft site or in gastrointestinal tract)
- Thrombosis
- Pseudoaneurysm formation at the anastomosis
- Infection
- Renal failure
- Sexual dysfunction
- Spinal cord ischemia
- Colon ischemia

Endarterectomy

Endarterectomy is a process in which the stenotic area of an artery wall is excised and the noninvolved ends of the artery are reanastomosed. It can be used to correct localized occlusive vascular disease, commonly in the carotid arteries, eliminating the need for bypassing the area.[38]

> ✎ **CLINICAL TIP**
> The abbreviation CEA is often used to refer to a carotid endarterectomy procedure.

Aneurysm Repair and Reconstruction

Aneurysm repair and reconstruction involve isolating the aneurysm by clamping off the vessel proximal and distal to the

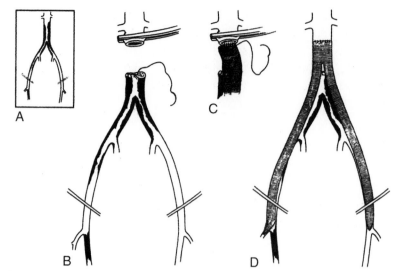

FIGURE 7-9
Aortofemoral graft. **A,** Schematic illustration of a preoperative aortogram. **B,** A segment of diseased aorta is resected, and the distal aortic stump is oversewn. **C,** End-to-end proximal anastomosis. **D,** Completed reconstruction. (From Rutherford RB, editor: Vascular surgery, ed 5, Philadelphia, 2000, Saunders.)

aneurysm, excising the aneurysm, and replacing the aneurysmal area with a synthetic graft (Figure 7-10). Performing the procedure before the aneurysm ruptures (elective surgery) is preferable to repairing a ruptured aneurysm (emergency surgery) because a ruptured aneurysm presents an extremely challenging and difficult operative course owing to the hemodynamic instability from hemorrhage. The cross-clamp time of the vessels is also crucial because organs distal to the site of repair can become ischemic if the clamp time is prolonged.

The surgical repair of AAAs can be accomplished by a transperitoneal or retroperitoneal approach. Transperitoneal repair via a midline laparotomy incision is the most widely used approach.[37]

The endovascular procedure is less invasive and is associated with good technical success and fair overall patency.[37] Complications that may occur after aneurysm repair are similar to those discussed in the Peripheral Vascular Bypass Grafting section.[28]

Physical Therapy Considerations

- Incisions should be inspected before and after physical therapy interventions to assess the patency of the incision, as drainage or weeping may occur during activity. If drainage or weeping occurs, stop the current activity and inspect the amount of drainage. Provide compression, if appropriate, and notify the nurse promptly. Once the drainage is stable or under the management of the nurse, document the incidence of drainage accordingly in the medical record.

- Abdominal incisions or other incisional pain can limit a patient's cough effectiveness and lead to pulmonary infection. Diligent attention to position changes, deep breathing, assisted coughing, and manual techniques (e.g., percussion and vibration techniques as needed) can help prevent pulmonary infections.

- Grafts that cross the hip joint, such as aortobifemoral grafts, require clarification by the surgeon regarding the amount of flexion allowed at the hip.

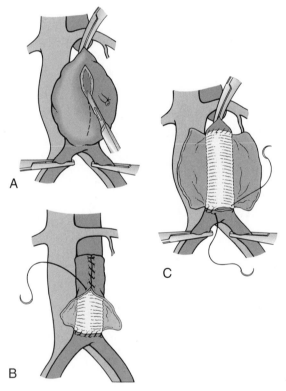

FIGURE 7-10
Surgical repair of an abdominal aortic aneurysm. **A,** Incising the aneurysmal sac. **B,** Insertion of synthetic graft. **C,** Suturing native aortic wall over synthetic graft. (From Lewis SM, Heitkemper MM, Dirksen SR, editors: Medical-surgical nursing, assessment and management of clinical problems, ed 6, St Louis, 2004, Mosby.)

- The patient with an incision on the medial aspect of the lower extremity (typically from a vascular graft procedure) will have a tendency to externally rotate the hip when resting in bed. This is particularly true if the incision is lengthy and crosses the knee joint. The physical therapist should promote neutral leg position, with or without elevation as directed by the surgeon, and educate the patient and caregivers on the importance of avoiding the "frog-leg" position.

- After a patient is cleared for out-of-bed activity, specific orders from the physician should be obtained regarding weight bearing on the involved extremities, particularly those with recent bypass grafts.

- Patients may also have systolic blood pressure limitations postoperatively to maintain adequate perfusion of the limb or to ensure the patency of the graft area. Blood pressures that are below the specified limit may decrease perfusion, whereas pressures above the limit may lead to graft damage. Thorough vital sign monitoring before, during, and after activity is essential.[13]

- Patients who have undergone bypass grafting procedures should have improved peripheral pulses; therefore any reduction in the strength of distal peripheral pulses that occurs after surgery should be brought to the attention of the nurse and physician.

Physical Therapy Management for Patients with Vascular and Hematologic Disorders

The primary goals of physical therapy for patients with vascular and hematologic disorders are to optimize functional mobility and activity tolerance. In addition to these goals, patients with vascular disorders require patient education to prevent skin breakdown and DVT formation, manage edema, and prevent joint contractures and muscle shortening. Patients with hematologic disorders may require patient education for activity modification, pain management, or fall prevention (especially if the patient is at risk of bleeding or on anticoagulant therapy). Progression of activity tolerance in patients with hematologic disorders does not occur at the same rate as in patients with normal blood composition; therefore the time frame for goal achievement may need to be lengthened.

Patients who have either vascular and/or hematologic dysfunction will potentially have overlapping needs. For simplicity, however, the following intervention guidelines are divided.

Physical Therapy Interventions for Patients with Vascular Disorders

For patients with peripheral vascular disease, comorbidities such as coronary artery disease, cerebrovascular disease, diabetes mellitus, and chronic obstructive pulmonary disease are likely to be present; therefore being watchful for signs and symptoms of angina or stroke in conjunction with monitoring vital signs, pulmonary limitations, and blood glucose levels is essential. This patient population also has the potential for sensory impairments; consequently, sensory testing is an important component of the physical therapy evaluation as well as patient education on frequent skin checks.

For patients who are being evaluated for a possible diagnosis of aortic dissection, the physical therapist may need to modify or defer physical therapy intervention until the definitive diagnosis is established. The patient's presentation and hemodynamic status should be taken into consideration in the decision-making process. Once the diagnosis is made, the option of medical or surgical treatment should be a guide to the physical therapist's plan of care. In either case, if the patient is seen for physical therapy, vital signs should be monitored continuously, the presenting symptoms should be kept in mind, and any changes in the vital signs or in the symptoms should be reported to the medical team.

Peripheral edema can result from a variety of disorders, including venous insufficiency, liver disease, renal insufficiency or renal failure, and heart failure; therefore the physical therapist should perform a thorough review of the patient's medical history before performing any edema management techniques. For example, limb elevation may be helpful in chronic venous insufficiency but may be detrimental in acute congestive heart failure. For patients with a diagnosis of DVT, use of compression stockings should be emphasized.

Physical Therapy Interventions for Patients with Hematologic Disorders

For patients who have hematologic dysfunction, the physical therapist should monitor the patient's CBC and coagulation profile on a daily basis and follow the trend[24] to determine the potential risk for bruising or bleeding, for thrombus formation, and for altered oxygen-carrying capacity at rest and with exertion. To gain insight into the hemostatic condition of the patient, determine (1) whether the abnormal blood laboratory values are expected or consistent with the patient's medical-surgical status, (2) the relative severity (mild, moderate, or severe) of the abnormal laboratory values, (3) the patient's presentation and clinical symptoms, and (4) whether the patient has a medical history or predisposing condition that could be exacerbated by the abnormal laboratory values.

The physical therapist must determine the need to modify or defer physical therapy intervention in the setting of abnormal blood laboratory values, most commonly alterations in Hct, platelet, and PT/INR. The patient's diagnosis, presentation, and medical intervention must be taken into consideration for patients with low H&H (hemoglobin and hematocrit), especially postoperative patients and those who are critically ill. Monitoring of vital signs and oxygen saturation at rest and with activity is crucial in patients with low H&H because the hemodynamic sequelae of alterations in blood volume or viscosity may be subtle or insidious in onset and first noticed by the physical therapist in response to exercise.

Exercise guidelines for patients with thrombocytopenia vary among hospitals. Decreased platelets are associated with risk of life-threatening hemorrhage. Physical therapy interventions must be tailored to the individual's platelet levels. General rules regarding exercises that should be performed are as follows:

- Spontaneous central nervous system, gastrointestinal, and/or respiratory tract bleeding may occur when platelet count is below 10,000 mm³.

- Activities of daily living, active range of motion, and ambulation with physician approval for platelet count of less than 20,000 mm³.

- Active range of motion and walking as tolerated, low-intensity exercise with no weights or resistance up to 2 pounds, stationary bicycling (no resistance) for platelet count of 20,000 to 50,000 mm^3.

- Progressive resistive exercise, ambulation, or stationary bicycling (with resistance) for a platelet count of 50,000 to 150,000 mm.[3,4,24]

For an INR greater than 3.5 (the standard highest level for anticoagulation), consult with the nurse or physician before physical therapy intervention and modify treatment accordingly. Observe the patient for the signs and symptoms of thrombus formation or bleeding during physical therapy intervention. Immediately report any abnormalities to the nurse. The risk of bleeding increases as INR value reaches 4 and even more sharply when the INR is higher than 5. When considering physical therapy for patients with elevated INR in this range, two scenarios should be considered: (1) is the patient already actively bleeding internally or externally, and (2) will the patient experience trauma during physical therapy that will lead to bleeding?

If INR is less than 4, the patient should participate in physical therapy and regular exercise program if allowed in a particular facility and/or approved by the primary care physician. Advancing the exercise program or increasing the exercise intensity should wait for the INR to be within therapeutic range. If the INR is between 4 and 5, resistive exercises should be held and light exercise should be continued. Unsteady gait in an ambulatory patient should be addressed with appropriate assistive device. All necessary precautions should be taken to avoid a fall.[126]

Mobilization of a patient who has an INR value more than 5 should be dependent on the patient's presentation (age, prior level of function [PLOF], current functional status, cognitive status, and current medical condition), the medical intervention for the high INR, and institutional guidelines along with the risk/benefit of physical therapy intervention. If the INR is more than 6, the medical team may consider bed rest until the INR is corrected. The INR is usually corrected in 2 days.[126]

Although the preceding guidelines offer direction, there are often no specific numeric protocols delineated in respective facilities; thus the decision to modify or defer physical therapy is often based on the clinical picture as well as the quantitative data. For example, a patient may have a low platelet count but is hemodynamically stable without signs of active bleeding. The physical therapist may therefore decide to continue to mobilize the patient out of bed. Conversely, if a patient with a low platelet count has new hemoptysis, the physical therapist may then defer manual chest physical therapy techniques, such as percussion.

The physical therapist should also consider the fall risk when mobilizing a patient with abnormal laboratory values (Hct, INR, Plt), versus the benefit of mobilizing the patient. For example, an elderly patient who has a high INR with an unsteady gait pattern and cognitive impairments is at a higher risk for falling than is a young adult with a high INR and a steady gait. At the same time, the negative effects of bed rest on the patient are significant. Complications related to bed rest, such as pulmonary compromise, muscle weakness, and functional decline,[125] are taken into consideration when making the decision to mobilize a patient. In this case, the physical therapist needs to modify the physical therapy intervention based on the goals for that particular patient (i.e., walking versus sitting out of bed in a chair).

Ultimately consultation and collaboration with other members of the medical team will help facilitate the clinical decision making and optimize the plan of care and safety for the patient.

References

1. Black JM, Matassarin-Jacobs E, editors: Luckmann and Sorensen's medical-surgical nursing: a psychophysiologic approach, ed 4, Philadelphia, 1993, Saunders, p 1286.
2. Marieb EN: Blood. In Marieb EN, editor: Human anatomy and physiology, ed 9, Redwood City, CA, 2012, Benjamin-Cummings, pp 584-611.
3. O'Sullivan SB, Schmitz TJ: Physical rehabilitation, ed 5, Philadelphia, 2007, FA Davis.
4. Knight CA: Peripheral vascular disease and wound care. In SB O'Sullivan, TJ Schmitz, editors: Physical rehabilitation: assessment and treatment, ed 4, Philadelphia, 2001, FA Davis, pp 583-608.
5. Bickley LS, Szilagyi PG: Bates' guide to physical examination and history taking, ed 10, Philadelphia, 2008, Lippincott Williams & Wilkins.
6. Hodgson JM, Mueller DK, Van Norman GA: Deep vein thrombosis. First consult, 2008. http://www.mdconsult.com.
7. Zipes DP: Braunwald's heart disease: a textbook of cardiovascular medicine, ed 9, Philadelphia, 2011, Saunders.
8. Bryant RA, Nix DP: Acute and chronic wounds: current management concepts, ed 4, St Louis, 2012, Mosby.
9. Mills EJ: Handbook of medical-surgical nursing, ed 4, Philadelphia, 2006, Lippincott Williams & Wilkins.
10. Seidel HM, Ball JW, Dains JE et al: Mosby's guide to physical examination, ed 7, St Louis, 2010, Mosby.
11. Pagana KD, Pagana TJ: Mosby's diagnostic and laboratory test reference, ed 10, St Louis, 2010, Mosby.
12. Fahey VA, editor: Vascular nursing, ed 4, Philadelphia, 2003, Saunders.
13. Hillman RS, Ault KA, editors: Hematology in clinical practice: a guide to diagnosis and management, ed 5, New York, 2010, McGraw-Hill, p 17.
14. Goodman CC, Snyder TK: Overview of hematology: signs and symptoms. In Goodman CC, Snyder TK, editors: Differential diagnosis in physical therapy: musculoskeletal and systemic conditions, ed 5, Philadelphia, 2012, Saunders, p 114.
15. Matassarin-Jacobs E: Assessment of clients with hematologic disorders. In Matassarin-Jacobs E, Black JM, editors: Medical-surgical nursing: clinical management for continuity of care, ed 5, Philadelphia, 1997, Saunders, pp 1461-1468.
16. Swearingen PL: Manual of medical-surgical nursing care. nursing interventions and collaborative management, ed 7, St Louis, 2010, Mosby.
17. Dorland WA: Dorland's illustrated medical dictionary, ed 29, Philadelphia, 2000, Saunders.
18. Boissonnault W: Primary care for the physical therapist: examination and triage, ed 2, St Louis, 2011, Saunders.
19. Chernecky CC, Berger BJ: Laboratory tests and diagnostic procedures, ed 5, Philadelphia, 2008, Saunders.

20. Perkins SL: Examination of the blood and bone marrow, ed 10. In Lee GR, Foerster J, Lukens J, editors: Wintrobe's clinical hematology, vol 1, Baltimore, 1999, Williams & Wilkins, pp 9-35.
21. Zieve PD, Waterbury L: Thromboembolic disease. In Barker LR, Burton JR, Zieve PD, editors: Principles of ambulatory medicine, ed 7, Baltimore, 2006, Williams & Wilkins, pp 642-651.
22. Pilszeck F, Rifkin WD, Walerstein S: Overuse of prothrombin and partial thromboplastin coagulation tests in medical inpatients, Heart Lung 34(6):402-405, 2005.
23. Glasheen JJ: Hospital medicine secrets, Philadelphia, 2006, Mosby.
24. Goodman, CC: The hematologic system. In Goodman CC, Boisonnault WG, editors: Pathology: implications for the physical therapist, ed 3, Philadelphia, 2009, Saunders.
25. Ridker PM, Stampfer MJ, Rifai N: Novel risk factors for systemic atherosclerosis: a comparison of C-reactive protein, fibrinogen, homocysteine, lipoprotein(A), and standard cholesterol screening as predictors of peripheral arterial disease, JAMA 285(19):2481, 2001.
26. Stamatelopoulos KS, Lekakis JP, Vamvakou G et al: The relative impact of different measures of adiposity on markers of early atherosclerosis, Int J Cardiol 119(2):139-146, 2007.
27. Crawford MH, DiMarco JP, Paulus WJ: Cardiology, ed 3, Philadelphia, 2009, Mosby.
28. Hallet JW, Brewster DC, Darling RC, editors: Handbook of patient care in vascular surgery, ed 3, Boston, 1995, Little, Brown.
29. McCance KL, Huether SE, editors: Pathophysiology: the biologic basis for disease in adults and children, ed 6, 2009, St Louis, Mosby, p 1001.
30. Thompson JM, McFarland GK, Hirsch JE et al: Clinical nursing, ed 5, St Louis, 2002, Mosby.
31. Young JR, Graor RA, Olin JW et al, editors: Peripheral vascular diseases, St Louis, 1991, Mosby.
32. Tjon JA, Reimann LE: Treatment of intermittent claudication with pentoxifylline and cilostazol, Am J Health Syst Pharm 58(6):485-493, 2001.
33. Weiner SD, Reis ED, Kerstein MD: Peripheral arterial disease: medical management in primary care practice, Geriatrics 56(4):20, 2001.
34. Tierney S, Fennessy F, Hayes DB: ABC of arterial and vascular disease. Secondary prevention of peripheral vascular disease, BMJ 320(7244):1262-1265, 2000.
35. Bullock BL, editor: Pathophysiology: adaptations and alterations in function, ed 4, Philadelphia, 1996, Lippincott-Raven, p 524.
36. Thompson MM, Bell PRF: Arterial aneurysms (ABC of arterial and venous disease), BMJ 320(7243):1193, 2000.
37. Townsend CM, Beauchamp RD, Evers MB et al: Townsend: Sabiston textbook of surgery, the biological basis of modern surgical practice, ed 19, St Louis, 2012, Saunders.
38. Strandness DE, Breda AV, editors: Vascular diseases: surgical and interventional therapy, vols 1 and 2, New York, 1994, Churchill Livingstone.
39. McPhee SJ, Papadakis MA, Tierney LM: Current medical diagnosis and treatment, ed 52, New York, 2012, McGraw-Hill Professional.
40. Wolfson AB, Hendey GW, Hendry PL et al: Harwood-Nuss' clinical practice of emergency medicine, ed 5, Philadelphia, 2009, Lippincott Williams & Wilkins.
41. Parsons: Critical care secrets, ed 4, St Louis, 2007, Mosby.
42. Marx JA, Adams J, Rosen P et al: Rosen's emergency medicine: concepts and clinical practice, ed 7, St Louis, 2009, Mosby.
43. Monahan FD, Green C, Neighbors M: Manual of medical-surgical nursing, ed 7, St Louis, 2010, Mosby.
44. Rauch U, Osende JI, Fuster V et al: Thrombus formation on atherosclerotic plaques: pathogenesis and clinical consequences, Ann Intern Med 134(3):224, 2001.
45. Brown MJ: Science, medicine, and the future. Hypertension, BMJ 314(7089):1258-1261, 1997.
46. Ketelhut RG et al: Regular exercise as an effective approach in antihypertensive therapy. Med Sci Sports Exerc 36(1):4-8, 2004.
47. Smeltzer SC, Bare BG, editors: Brunner and Suddarth's textbook of medical-surgical nursing, ed 12, Philadelphia, 2009, Lippincott Williams & Wilkins, p 722.
48. Mulrow CD, Pignone M: What are the elements of good treatment for hypertension? (Evidence-based management of hypertension), BMJ 322(7294):1107, 2001.
49. Hyman DJ, Pavlik VN: Self-reported hypertension treatment practices among primary care physicians, Arch Intern Med 160(15):2281, 2000.
50. George-Gay B, Chernecky CC: Clinical medical-surgical nursing: a decision-making reference, ed 1, Philadelphia, 2002, Saunders.
51. Cameron MH, Monroe LG: Physical rehabilitation for the physical therapist assistant, St Louis, 2010, Saunders.
52. Paget SA, Gibofsky A, Beary JF et al: Hospital for special surgery manual of rheumatology and outpatient orthopedic disorders: diagnosis and therapy, ed 5, Philadelphia, 2005, Lippincott Williams & Wilkins.
53. Moore WS, editor: Vascular surgery: a comprehensive review, ed 6, Philadelphia, 2001, Saunders, p 90.
54. Easton DM: Systematic vasculitis: a difficult diagnosis in the elderly. Physician Assist 25(1):37, 2001.
55. Kallenberg CGM, Cohen Tervaert CGM: What is new in systemic vasculitis? Ann Rheum Dis 59(11):924, 2000.
56. Goldman L, Ausiello D: Cecil textbook of medicine, ed 24, St Louis, 2012, Saunders.
57. Ferri, FF: Ferri's clinical advisor 2012: instant diagnosis and treatment, Philadelphia, 2012, Mosby, p 56A.
58. Nettina SM: Lippincott manual of nursing practice. Part 2—cardiovascular health, ed 8, Philadelphia, 2006, Lippincott Williams & Wilkins.
59. Falardeau J: Giant cell arteritis, Neurol Clin 28(3):581-591, 2010.
60. Mawdsley A: The big freeze. (Treating Raynaud's phenomenon.), Chem Druggist, S4, 1998.
61. Wittink H: Adjuvant physical therapy versus occupational therapy in patients with reflex sympathetic dystrophy/complex regional pain syndrome type I, Phys Ther 81(1):753, 2001.
62. Schwartzman RJ: New treatments for reflex sympathetic dystrophy, N Engl J Med 343(9):654-656, 2000.
63. Zollinger PE, Tuinebreijer WE, Kreis RW et al: Effect of vitamin C on frequency of reflex sympathetic dystrophy in wrist fractures: a randomised trial, Lancet 354(9195):2025, 1999.
64. Adami S, Fossaluzza V, Gatti D et al: Bisphosphonate therapy of reflex sympathetic dystrophy syndrome, Ann Rheum Dis 56(3):201-204, 1997.
65. Canale ST, Daugherty K, Bones L: Campbell's operative orthopedics, ed 11, Philadelphia, 2003, Mosby.
66. Tumbarello C: Acute extremity compartment syndrome, J Trauma Nurs 7(2):30, 2000.
67. Monahan FD, Neighbors M, Green C: Manual of medical-surgical nursing, ed 7, St Louis, 2010, Mosby.
68. Love C: A discussion and analysis of nurse-led pain assessment for the early detection of compartment syndrome, J Orthop Nurs 2(3):160-167, 2010.
69. London NJ, Nash R: ABC of arterial and venous disease. Varicose veins, BMJ 320(7246):1391, 2000.
70. Buttaro TM, Trybulski J, Bailey PP et al: Primary care: a collaborative practice, ed 4, St Louis, 2012, Mosby.

71. Meguid C: Best practice for deep vein thrombosis prophylaxis, J Nurse Pract 7(7):582-587, 2011.

72. Anaya DA, Nathens AB: Thrombosis and coagulation: deep vein thrombosis and pulmonary embolism prophylaxis, Surg Clin North Am 85(6):1163-1177, 2005.

73. Tepper SH, McKeough DM: Deep venous thrombosis: risks, diagnosis, treatment interventions and prevention, Acute Care Perspect 9, 2000.

74. First Consult: Deep vein thrombosis. Latest updates November 10, 2011.

75. Pretorius ES, Solomon JA: Radiology secrets plus, ed 3, Philadelphia, 2010, Mosby.

76. Aldrich D, Hunt DP: When can the patient with deep venous thrombosis begin to ambulate? Phys Ther 84(3):268-273, 2004.

77. Gay V, Hamilton R, Heiskell S et al: Influence of bedrest or ambulation in the clinical treatment of acute deep vein thrombosis on patient outcomes: a review and synthesis of the literature, Medsurg Nurs 18(5):293-299, 2009.

78. Kahn SR, Shirer I, Kearon C: Physical activity in patients with deep venous thrombosis: a systematic review, Thromb Res 122:763-773, 2008.

79. Trujillo-Santos J et al: Bed rest or ambulation in the initial treatment of patients with acute deep vein thrombosis or pulmonary embolism, Chest 127(50):1631-1636, 2005.

80. Partsch H et al: Immediate ambulation and leg compression in the treatment of deep vein thrombosis, Disease Month 51(2-3):135-140, 2005.

81. Partsch H et al: Compression and walking versus bedrest in the treatment of proximal deep venous thrombosis with low molecular weight heparin, J Vasc Surg 32:861-869, 2000.

82. Saunders CS: Improving survival in pulmonary embolism, Patient Care 34(16):50, 2000.

83. Coats U: Management of venous ulcers, Crit Care Nurse Q 21(2):14-23, 1998.

84. Purtillo DT, Purtillo RP, editors: A survey of human diseases, ed 2, Boston, 1989, Little, Brown, p 287.

85. Lee GR: Acute posthemorrhagic anemia, ed 10. In Lee GR, Foerster J, Lukens J, editors: Wintrobe's clinical hematology, vol 2, Baltimore, 1999, Williams & Wilkins, pp 1485-1488.

86. Erythrocyte disease. In AE Belcher, editor: Blood disorders, St Louis, 1993, Mosby, p 51.

87. McPherson RA, Pincus MR: Henry's clinical diagnosis and management by laboratory methods, ed 22, Philadelphia, 2011, Saunders.

88. Killip S, Bennett JM, Chambers MD: Iron deficiency anemia, Am Fam Physician 75(5):671-678, 2007.

89. The hematopoietic and lymphoid systems. In Kumar V, Cotran R, Robbins SL, editors: Basic pathology, ed 9, Philadelphia, 2012, Saunders, pp 340-392.

90. Linker CA: Blood. In Tierney LM, McPhee SJ, Papadakis MA, editors: Current medical diagnosis and treatment 2001, Stamford, CT, 2001, Appleton & Lange, pp 505-558.

91. Mosby's dictionary of medicine, nursing & health professions, ed 7, St Louis, 2006, Mosby.

92. Lehne RA: Drugs for deficiency anemias. In Lehne RA, editor: Pharmacology for nursing care, ed 7, Philadelphia, 2009, Saunders, pp 589-602.

93. Roper D, Stein S, Payne M et al: Anemias caused by impaired production of erythrocytes. In Rodak BF, editor: Diagnostic hematology, Philadelphia, 1995, Saunders, p 181.

94. Sheppard KC: Nursing management of adults with hematologic disorders. In Beare PG, Myers JL, editors: Adult health nursing, ed 3, St Louis, 1998, Mosby, pp 670-711.

95. Hoffman R, Benz EJ Jr, Shattil SJ et al: Hematology: basic principles and practice, ed 5, Philadelphia, 2008, Churchill Livingstone.

96. Dhaliwal G, Cornett P, Tierney LM Jr: Hemolytic anemia, Am Fam Physician 69(11):2599-2606, 2004.

97. Ballas SK: Pain management of sickle cell disease, Hematol Oncol Clin North Am 19(5):785-802, 2005.

98. Painful events. In Reid CD, Charach S, Lubin B, editors: Management and therapy of sickle cell disease, ed 3, 1995, National Institutes of Health Pub 25-2117, p 35.

99. Acute chest syndrome. In Reid CD, Charach S, Lubin B, editors: Management and therapy of sickle cell disease, ed 3, 1995, National Institutes of Health Pub 25-2117, p 47.

100. Johnson CS: Sickle cell disease, Hematol Oncol Clin North Am 19(5):xi-xiii, 2005.

101. Babior BM, Stossel TP: In Hematology: a pathophysiological approach, ed 3, New York, 1994, Churchill Livingstone, p 359.

102. Coates TD, Baehner RL: Laboratory evaluation of neutropenia and neutrophil dysfunction. UpToDate. http://www.uptodate.com. Last accessed June 26, 2008.

103. Baehner RL: Overview of neutropenia. UpToDate. http://www.uptodate.com. Last accessed June 26, 2008.

104. Levi M, De Jonge E: Current management of disseminated intravascular coagulation. Hosp Pract (Off Ed) 35:59-66, 2000.

105. Matassarin-Jacobs E: Nursing care of clients with hematologic disorders. In Matassarin-Jacobs E, Black JM, editors: Medical-surgical nursing: clinical management for continuity of care, ed 5, Philadelphia, 1997, Saunders, pp 1469-1532.

106. Urden LA, Stacy KM, Lough ME: Thelan's critical care nursing: diagnosis and management, ed 6, 2009, St Louis, Mosby.

107. Thrombolytic disorders. In Belcher AE, editor: Blood disorders, St Louis, 1993, Mosby, p 112.

108. Gilbert MS: Musculoskeletal complications of haemophilia: the joint, Haemophilia 6(Suppl 1):34-37, 2000.

109. Lichtman M, Beutler E, Williams W et al: In Williams hematology, ed 7, New York, 2006, McGraw-Hill Professional.

110. Greer J, Forester J, Lukens J: Winthrobe's clinical hematology, ed 11, vols 1 and 2, Philadelphia, 2003, Lippincott Williams & Wilkins.

111. Harris ED Jr, Budd RC, Genovese M et al: Kelly's textbook of rheumatology, ed 8, Philadelphia, 2008, Saunders.

112. Horrell CJ, Rothman J: Establishing the etiology of thrombocytopenia, Nurse Pract 25:68-77, 2000.

113. Warkentin TE: Clinical picture of heparin-induced thrombocytopenia. In Warkentin TE, Greinacher A, editors: Heparin-induced thrombocytopenia, New York, 1999, Marcel Dekker, pp 43-73.

114. Jerdee AI: Heparin-associated thrombocytopenia: nursing implications, Crit Care Nurs 18:38-43, 1998.

115. Meyer JP: Heparin-induced thrombocytopenia, BJU Int 99:728-730, 2007.

116. Levy JH, Hursting M: Heparin-induced thrombocytopenia, a prothrombotic disease, Hematol Oncol Clin North Am 21(1):65-88, 2007.

117. Gibbar-Clements T, Shirrell D, Dooley R et al: The challenge of warfarin therapy, Am J Nurs 100:38-40, 2000.

118. Harkness GA, Dincher JR, editors: Medical-surgical nursing: total patient care, ed 9, St Louis, 1996, Mosby, p 656.

119. Joint Commission perspectives on patient safety: a Joint Commission Resources publication: A new look at blood transfusion, 2007.

120. Schroeder ML: Principles and practice of transfusion medicine, ed 10. In Lee GR, Foerster J, Lukens J, editors: Wintrobe's clinical hematology, vol 1, Baltimore, 1999, Williams & Wilkins, pp 817-874.

121. U.S. Department of Health and Human Services, National Institutes of Health: National blood resource education

programs. Transfusion therapy guidelines for nurses, September 1990.

122. Mulholland MW, Lillemore KD, Doherty GM et al: In Greenfield's surgery: scientific principles and practice, ed 4, Philadelphia, 2005, Lippincott Williams & Wilkins.

123. Schmittling ZC, Hodgson KJ: Thrombolysis and mechanical thrombectomy for arterial disease, Surg Clin North Am 5(84):1237-1266, 2004.

124. Hallett J, Mills J, Earnshaw J Reekers JA, Rooke T et al: Comprehensive vascular and endovascular surgery, ed 2, St Louis, 2009, Mosby.

125. Einhorn CS: Deciding activity level for an acute post-surgical patient with and elevated risk of bleeding, J Acute Care Phys Ther 3(1):164-170, 2012.

126. Tuzson A: How high is too high? INR and acute care physical therapy, Acute Care Perspect, Spring 2009.

Gastrointestinal System

Jaime C. Paz

CHAPTER OBJECTIVES

The objectives of this chapter are to provide the following:

1. An understanding of the structure and function of the gastrointestinal (GI) system
2. Information on the clinical evaluation of the GI system, including physical examination and diagnostic studies
3. An overview of the various diseases and disorders of the GI system
4. Information on the management of GI disorders, including pharmacologic therapy and surgical procedures
5. Guidelines for physical therapy intervention in patients with GI diseases and disorders

PREFERRED PRACTICE PATTERNS

The most relevant practice patterns for the diagnoses discussed in this chapter, based on the American Physical Therapy Association's *Guide to Physical Therapist Practice*, second edition, are as follows:

- Primary Prevention/Risk Reduction for Skeletal Demineralization: 4A
- Impaired Aerobic Capacity/Endurance Associated with Deconditioning: 6B
- Primary Prevention/Risk Reduction for Integumentary Disorders: 7A

Please refer to Appendix A for a complete list of the preferred practice patterns, as individual patient conditions are highly variable and other practice patterns may be applicable.

Disorders of the gastrointestinal (GI) system can have numerous effects on the body, such as decreased nutrition, anemia, and fluid imbalances. These consequences may, in turn, affect the activity tolerance of a patient, which will ultimately influence many physical therapy interventions. In addition, physical therapists must be aware of pain referral patterns from the GI system that may mimic musculoskeletal symptoms (Table 8-1).

Body Structure and Function

The basic structure of the GI system is shown in Figure 8-1, with the primary and accessory organs of digestion and their respective functions described in Tables 8-2 and 8-3.

Clinical Evaluation

Evaluation of the GI system involves combining information gathered through history, physical examination, and diagnostic studies.

History

Before performing the physical examination, the presence or absence of items related to GI pathology (Box 8-1) is ascertained through patient interview, questionnaire completion, or chart review. Please see Chapter 2 for a description of the general medical record review.

TABLE 8-1 Gastrointestinal System Pain Referral Patterns

Structure	Segmental Innervation	Areas of Pain Referral
Esophagus	T4-T6	Substernal region Upper abdomen
Stomach	T6-T10	Upper abdomen Middle and lower thoracic spine
Small intestine	T7-T10	Middle thoracic spine
Pancreas	T6-T10	Upper abdomen Upper and lower thoracic spine
Gallbladder	T7-T9	Right upper abdomen Right, middle, and lower thoracic spine
Liver	T7-T9	Right, middle, and lower thoracic spine Right cervical spine
Common bile duct	T6-T10	Upper abdomen Middle lumbar spine
Large intestine	T11–L1	Lower abdomen Middle lumbar spine
Sigmoid colon	T11-T12	Upper sacral region Suprapubic region Left lower quadrant of abdomen

From Boissonault WG, Bass C: Pathological origins of trunk and neck pain: part I. Pelvic and abdominal visceral disorders, J Orthop Sports Phys Ther 12:194, 1990.

TABLE 8-2 Structure and Function of the Primary Organs of Digestion

Structure	Function
Oral cavity	Entrance to the gastrointestinal system; mechanical and chemical digestion begins here
Pharynx	Involved in swallowing and mechanical movement of food to esophagus
Esophagus	Connects mouth to the stomach, transports and disperses food
Stomach (cardia, fundus, body, pylorus)	*Mechanical functions:* storage, mixing, and grinding of food and regulation of outflow to small intestine *Exocrine functions:* secretion of hydrochloric acid, intrinsic factor, pepsinogen, and mucus necessary for digestion *Endocrine functions:* secretion of hormones that trigger the release of digestive enzymes from the pancreas, liver, and gallbladder into the duodenum
Small intestine (duodenum, jejunum, ileum)	*Duodenum:* neutralizes acid in food transported from the stomach and mixes pancreatic and biliary secretions with food *Jejunum:* absorbs nutrients, water, and electrolytes *Ileum:* absorbs bile acids and intrinsic factors to be recycled in the body—necessary to prevent vitamin B_{12} deficiency
Large intestine (cecum; appendix; ascending, transverse, descending, and sigmoid colon; rectum; anus)	Absorbs water and electrolytes Stores and eliminates indigestible material as feces

Data from Scanlon JC, Sanders T, editors: Essentials of anatomy and physiology, ed 2, Philadelphia, 1993, FA Davis, p 362; Patton KT: Anatomy & physiology (with media), ed 7, St Louis, 2009, Mosby, pp 837-863.

TABLE 8-3 Structure and Function of the Accessory Organs of Digestion

Structure	Function
Teeth	Break down food to combine with saliva.
Tongue	Provides taste sensations by cranial nerve VII (taste). Keeps the food between the teeth to maintain efficient chewing action for food to mix with saliva.
Salivary glands	Produce saliva, which is necessary to dissolve food for tasting and moisten food for swallowing.
Liver	Regulates serum levels of fats, proteins, and carbohydrates. Bile is produced in the liver and is necessary for the absorption of lipids and lipid-soluble substances. The liver also assists with drug metabolism and red blood cell and vitamin K production.
Gallbladder	Stores and releases bile into the duodenum via the hepatic duct when food enters the stomach.
Pancreas	Exocrine portion secretes bicarbonate and digestive enzymes into duodenum. Endocrine portion secretes insulin, glucagon, and numerous other hormones into the bloodstream, all of which are essential in regulating blood glucose levels.
Spleen*	Filters out foreign substances and degenerates blood cells from the bloodstream. Also stores lymphocytes.

Data from Scanlon JC, Sanders T, editors: Essentials of anatomy and physiology, ed 2, Philadelphia, 1993, FA Davis; Patton KT: Anatomy & physiology (with media), ed 7, St Louis, 2009, Mosby, pp 837-863.

*The spleen is not part of the gastrointestinal system but is located near other gastrointestinal components in the abdominal cavity.

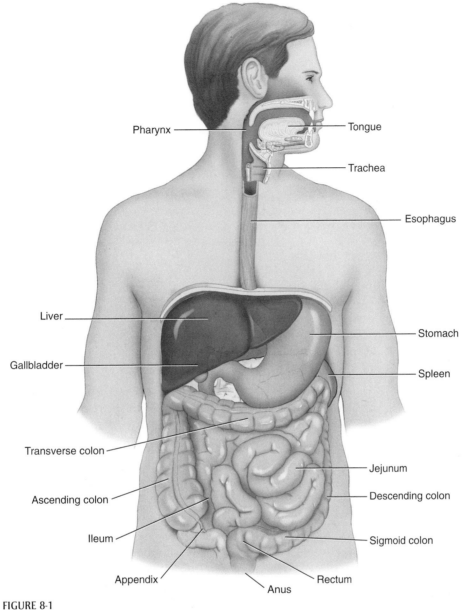

Pharynx — — Tongue

— Trachea

— Esophagus

Liver — — Stomach

Gallbladder — — Spleen

Transverse colon —

— Jejunum

Ascending colon — — Descending colon

Ileum — — Sigmoid colon

Appendix — — Rectum
Anus

FIGURE 8-1
Schematic representation of the gastrointestinal system.

Physical Examination

Physical examination of the abdomen consists of inspection, auscultation, percussion, and palpation. Physicians and nurses usually perform this examination on a daily basis in the acute care setting; however, physical therapists can also perform this examination to help delineate between systemic and musculoskeletal pain.

Inspection

Figure 8-2 demonstrates the abdominal regions associated with organ location. During inspection, the physical therapist should note asymmetries in size and shape in each quadrant, umbilicus appearance, and presence of abdominal scars indicative of previous abdominal procedures or trauma.[1]

✎ CLINICAL TIP

The physical therapist should document any changes in abdominal girth, especially enlargement. In addition, the nurses and physicians should be notified. Abdominal enlargement may hinder the patient's respiratory and mobility status. Observe for abdominal distention in postoperative patients (especially orthopedic) taking narcotics (this can be an early sign of reduced gastrointestinal motility).[2]

The physical therapist should also note the presence of incisions, tubes, and drains during inspection, because these may require particular handling or placement during mobility exercises.

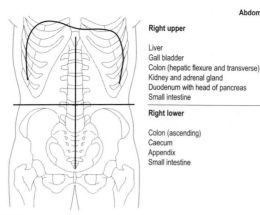

Abdominal Quadrants

Right upper	Left upper
Liver	Stomach
Gall bladder	Spleen
Colon (hepatic flexure and transverse)	Pancreas
Kidney and adrenal gland	Kidney and adrenal gland
Duodenum with head of pancreas	Colon (splenic flexure and transverse)
Small intestine	Small intestine (jejunum)

Right lower	Left lower
Colon (ascending)	Colon (descending)
Caecum	Sigmoid colon
Appendix	Small intestine
Small intestine	

FIGURE 8-2

The four abdominal quadrants, showing the viscera found in each. (From Palastanga N, Soames RW: Anatomy and human movement: structure and function, ed 6, Edinburgh, 2012, Churchill Livingstone.)

BOX 8-1   Items Associated with Gastrointestinal Pathology

Signs and Symptoms	Stool and Urine Characteristics	Associated Disorders
Nausea and vomiting	Change in stool color	History of hernia
Hemoptysis		History of hepatitis or other liver diseases
Constipation	Change in urine color	
Diarrhea	Hematochezia (bright red blood in stool)	
Jaundice		
Heartburn		Drug and alcohol abuse
Abdominal pain	Melena (black, tarry stools)	
Dysphagia		Fatty food intolerance
Odynophagia (painful swallowing)		Thyroid dysfunction
		Diabetes mellitus

Data from Koopmeiners MB: Screening for gastrointestinal system disease. In WG Boisonnault, editor: Examination in physical therapy practice, New York, 1991, Churchill Livingstone, p 113; Goodman CC: The gastrointestinal system. In Goodman CC, Boisonnault WG, editors: Pathology: implications for the physical therapist, Philadelphia, 1998, Saunders, pp 456-460; McQuaid K: Approach to the patient with gastrointestinal disease. In Goldman L, Schafer AI, editors: Goldman's Cecil medicine, ed 24, Philadelphia, 2011, Saunders, pp 828-844.

Auscultation

The abdomen is auscultated for the presence or absence of bowel sounds and bruits (murmurs) to help evaluate gastric motility and vascular flow, respectively. Bowel sounds can be altered postoperatively, as well as in cases of diarrhea, intestinal obstruction, paralytic ileus, and peritonitis. The presence of bruits over the aorta or the renal, iliac, or femoral arteries may be indicative of vascular disease.[3]

Percussion

Mediate percussion is used to evaluate liver and spleen size and borders, as well as to identify ascitic fluid, solid- or fluid-filled masses, and air in the stomach and bowel.[3] The technique for mediate percussion is described in the Physical Examination section of Chapter 4.

Palpation

Light palpation and deep palpation are used to identify abdominal tenderness, muscular resistance, and superficial organs and masses. The presence of rebound tenderness (i.e., abdominal pain worsened by a quick release of palpatory pressure) is an indication of possible peritoneal irritation and requires immediate medical attention. Muscle guarding during palpation may also indicate a protective mechanism for underlying visceral pathology.[3,4]

Diagnostic Studies

Discussion of the diagnostic evaluation for the GI system is divided into (1) the examination of the GI tract and (2) the examination of the hepatic, biliary, pancreatic, and splenic systems. Examination of the GI tract includes the esophagus, stomach, and intestines (small and large). Table 8-4 summarizes the laboratory tests used to measure functional aspects of secretion, digestion, absorption, and elimination within the GI tract.[5-12] Table 8-5 summarizes diagnostic procedures used to visualize the GI tract.

Examination of the hepatic (liver), biliary (gallbladder and cystic ducts), pancreatic, and splenic systems involves numerous laboratory tests and diagnostic procedures, which are often performed concurrently to fully delineate the etiology of a patient's clinical presentation. Because of the common location of these organs and shared access to the biliary tree, disease or dysfunction in one organ can often extend into the other organs.[13,14]

> ✎ **CLINICAL TIP**
>
> Laboratory tests used to examine the liver are frequently referred to as *liver function tests* or LFTs.

Hepatocellular disease results in cellular damage in the liver, which causes increased levels of the following enzymes: aspartate aminotransferase (AST; previously called serum glutamic-oxaloacetic transaminase), alanine aminotransferase (ALT;

TABLE 8-4 Laboratory Tests for the Gastrointestinal System*

Test	Description

Carcinoembryonic antigen (CEA)
    Reference value:
    Adult nonsmoker <2.5 ng/ml
    Adult smoker: up to 5 ng/ml
	Purpose: protein used to monitor recurrence of colorectal cancer and response to antineoplastic therapy for both colorectal and breast cancer. Presence of CEA in other body fluids maybe indicative of metastasis.

Gastrin Reference value: 0-180 pg/ml	Hormone that stimulates the release of gastric acid in stomach. Purpose: to confirm the diagnosis of Zollinger-Ellison syndrome and monitor for recurrence of gastrinoma (gastrin-producing tumor).

Helicobacter pylori tests
 	
    Stool sample
    Reference value: negative for *H. pylori* antigen
    Serologic test
    Reference value: immunoglobulin G negative
    Urea breath test
    Reference value: negative
    Tissue biopsy
    Reference value: negative for *H. pylori*
	Purpose: to confirm the diagnosis of *H. pylori* infection, which is the cause of most peptic ulcers and chronic gastritis and is a carcinogen for gastric carcinoma.
	Purpose: to identify presence of *H. pylori* antigen.
	
	Purpose: to identify the presence of immunoglobulin G antibody to *H. pylori* in the blood.
	Purpose: to identify the presence of *H. pylori* in the stomach.
	
	Purpose: to visualize *H. pylori* bacteria.
	A tissue biopsy is obtained during an endoscopy procedure and microscopically examined.

5-Hydroxyindoleacetic acid (5-HIAA) Reference value: 1-9 mg/24 hr (urine sample)	Purpose: to diagnose a carcinoid tumor and provide ongoing evaluation of tumor stability. 5-HIAA is a urinary metabolite of serotonin and is produced by most carcinoid tumors found in the appendix, intestine, or lung.

Lactose tolerance test (oral lactose tolerance test)
    Reference value:
    Blood glucose >20 mg/dl
	Purpose: to identify lactose intolerance or lactase deficiency as a cause of abdominal cramps and diarrhea, as well as to help identify the cause of malabsorption or maldigestion syndrome.
	An oral dose of lactose is provided to a fasting patient, and serial blood samples are measured.
	Minimal rise in blood glucose or urine lactose levels indicates lactose intolerance and/or lactase deficiency.

Occult blood (fecal occult blood test, FOBT, FOB, Guaiac smear test) Reference value: negative	Purpose: a screening tool for early diagnosis of colon cancer. Three stool specimens over several days are collected and examined for the presence of occult (nonvisible) blood in the feces, which can be indicative of adenocarcinoma and premalignant polyps in the colon.
Serotonin (5-hydroxytryptamine) Reference value: 50-200 ng/ml (blood)	Purpose: to detect a carcinoid tumor. Venous blood levels of serotonin are measured, as carcinoid tumors secrete excess amounts of serotonin.

Data from Pagana KD, Pagana TJ: Mosby's diagnostic and laboratory test reference, ed 9, St Louis, 2009, Mosby; Lab Tests Online: http://labtestsonline.org. Accessed July 12, 2012.

*Words or abbreviations in parentheses are synonyms for the test names.

previously called serum glutamate pyruvate transaminase), and lactate dehydrogenase (LD).[14,15]

Hepatocellular dysfunction can be identified when bilirubin levels are elevated or when clotting times are increased (denoted by an increased prothrombin time and the international normalized ratio [INR]). The liver produces clotting factors, and therefore an increased prothrombin time or INR implicates impaired production of coagulation factors. Refer to Chapter 7 for more details on coagulation tests.

Cholestasis is the impairment of bile flow from the liver to the duodenum and results in elevations of the following serum enzymes: alkaline phosphatase (ALP), aspartate transaminase (previously known as γ-glutamine-oxaloacetic transaminase or γ-glutamyl transpeptidase), and 5′-nucleotidase.[14,15]

Table 8-6 summarizes the laboratory tests performed to measure hepatic, biliary, and pancreatic function. Table 8-7 summarizes the diagnostic procedures performed to visualize these organs.

Additional diagnostic procedures used to evaluate the GI system are laparoscopy, magnetic resonance imaging (MRI), and positron emission tomography (PET) scans. These methods are described in the following sections.

Laparoscopy

Laparoscopy is the insertion of a laparoscope (a fiberoptic tube) into the abdominal cavity through a small incision in the periumbilical area. To perform this procedure, a local anesthetic is given, and gas (i.e., nitric oxide or carbon dioxide) is infused into the abdominal cavity to allow better visualization and manipulation of the scope.[16] Box 8-2 describes the diagnostic and therapeutic interventions that may be performed with a laparoscope.

Magnetic Resonance Imaging

The use of MRI of the GI system is primarily indicated for imaging of the liver for hepatic tumors, iron overload, and

TABLE 8-5 Diagnostic Procedures for the Gastrointestinal (GI) System*

Test	Description
Barium enema (BE) Reference value: No lesions, deficits, or abnormalities of the colon are noted.	Purpose: to investigate and identify pathologic conditions that change the structure or function of the colon (large bowel). The colon is emptied of feces, and contrast medium (barium) is instilled rectally. Fluoroscopic and x-ray images are then taken to identify the presence of any structural anomalies as well as polyps, tumors, and diverticula.
Barium swallow (esophagography) Reference value: No structural or functional abnormalities are visualized.	Purpose: to identify pathologic conditions that change the structure or function of the esophagus. The patient takes repeated swallows of barium liquid while x-ray and fluoroscopic images are taken in vertical, semivertical, and horizontal positions to examine the passage of contrast medium during swallowing and peristaltic movement of the esophagus.
Colonoscopy (lower panendoscopy) Reference value: No abnormalities of structure or mucosal surface are visualized in the colon or terminal ileum.	Purpose: to perform routine screening of the colon for the presence of polyps or tumors and to investigate the cause of chronic diarrhea, bleeding, or other undiagnosed GI complaints. Patients are sedated, and an endoscope is inserted into the rectum and passed through the various parts of the colon. Tissue biopsy may be performed during this procedure.
Computed tomography of the GI tract (CT scan, computed axial tomography [CAT])	Purpose: to detect intra-abdominal abscesses, tumors, infarctions, perforation, obstruction, inflammation, and diverticulitis. Metastases to the abdominal cavity can also be detected. Intravenous or oral contrast may be used during the procedure.
Esophageal function studies: Manometry Reference value: Lower esophageal sphincter (LES) pressure: 12-25 mm Hg. Esophageal pH (acid reflux) Reference value: pH between 4 and 4.5. Acid perfusion test (Bernstein test) Reference value: Negative.	Purpose: to evaluate esophageal motor disorders that could be causing dysphagia, for placement of intraluminal devices, and for preoperative evaluation of patients who are being considered for antireflux surgery to rule out other possible diagnoses. Purpose: to evaluate changes in esophageal pH levels via capsule that is implanted into esophageal mucosa 5-6 cm above the gastroesophageal junction. Monitoring takes place over 24- 48 hours. Purpose: to determine that heartburn is of esophageal rather than cardiac origin. Hydrochloric acid is instilled into the esophagus through the endoscope or nasogastric tube. Complaints of heartburn with acid instillation confirm the esophageal origin.
Esophagogastroduodenoscopy (EGD, upper gastrointestinal endoscopy) Reference value: No abnormal structures or functions are observed in the esophagus, stomach, or duodenum.	Purpose: to identify and biopsy tissue abnormality; to evaluate the esophagus, stomach, and duodenum to investigate the cause of upper GI bleeding, dysphagia, dyspepsia, gastric outlet obstruction, gastric ulcers, or epigastric pain. An endoscope is passed through the mouth into the esophagus to the stomach, pylorus, and upper duodenum. Tissue biopsy can be performed during the procedure.
Gallium scan (gallium-67 imaging, total body scan) Reference value: No structural or functional abnormalities are visualized.	Purpose: to locate malignancy, metastases, sites of inflammation, infection, and abscess. A radionuclide is injected intravenously with images taken in the following time frames: 4-6 hours later to identify infectious or inflammatory disease as well as benign or malignant tumors. 24, 48, and 72 hours later to identify and/or monitor presence of pathology.
Gastrografin study	Purpose: Similar to barium swallow, except Gastrografin (diatrizoate) is used as an imaging agent.
GI bleeding scan (GI scintigraphy, abdominal scintigraphy) Reference value: No evidence of focal bleeding.	Purpose: to evaluate the presence, source, or both, of GI bleeding. Radionuclide-labeled red blood cells are injected intravenously, followed by intermittent imaging studies of the abdomen and pelvis for up to 24 hours.
KUB (kidneys, ureters, bladder) x-ray	Purpose: to provide x-ray image of abdomen. Kidneys, ureters, bladder, and small and large intestines are visualized, and resulting images can be used in assisting with diagnosis of conditions to these organs.
Paracentesis and peritoneal fluid analysis (abdominal paracentesis, peritoneal tap) Reference value: Clear, odorless, pale yellow.	Purpose: To help delineate the cause of peritoneal effusion. The peritoneal cavity is accessed with either a long thin needle or a trocar and stylet with the patient under local anesthesia. Peritoneal fluid is collected and examined. Peritoneal tissue biopsy can also be performed during this procedure for cytologic studies required for the differential diagnosis of tuberculosis, fungal infection, and metastatic carcinoma.
Sigmoidoscopy (proctoscopy, anoscopy) Reference value: No tissue abnormalities are visualized in the sigmoid colon, rectum, or anus.	Purpose: Sigmoidoscopy is used as a screening tool for the anus, rectum, and sigmoid colon for cancer and to investigate the cause of rectal bleeding or monitor inflammatory bowel disease. Proctoscopy is used to view the anus and rectum. Anoscopy is used to investigate the anus.
Upper GI (UGI) series and small bowel series (small bowel follow-through) Reference value: No structural or functional abnormalities are found.	Purpose: to detect disorders of structure or function of the esophagus, stomach and duodenum, and jejunum and ileum (the latter two are for the small bowel series). Imaging studies of all these areas are performed while the patient drinks a barium solution. Passage of the barium through these structures can take from 30 minutes to 6 hours.

Data from Malarkey LM, McMorrow ME, editors: Nurse's manual of laboratory tests and diagnostic procedures, Philadelphia, 2000, Saunders, pp 432-468; Pagana KD, Pagana TJ: Mosby's diagnostic and laboratory test reference, ed 9, St Louis, 2009, Mosby; Andreoli TE, Benjamin IJ, Griggs RC et al: Andreoli and Carpenter's Cecil essentials of medicine, ed 8, Philadelphia, 2010, Saunders.

*Words or abbreviations in parentheses are synonyms for the test names.

TABLE 8-6 Laboratory Tests for the Hepatic, Biliary, and Pancreatic Systems*

Test	Involved Systems	Purpose
Alanine aminotransferase (ALT, serum glutamic-pyruvic transaminase [GPT], SGPT) Reference value: 4-36 IU/L	Hepatic	To detect hepatocellular disease. Very specific in detecting acute hepatitis from viral, toxic, or drug-induced causes.
Alkaline phosphatase (ALP, total alkaline phosphatase [T-ALP]) Reference value: 0.5-2.0 King-Armstrong units/dl	Hepatic, biliary	Nonspecific indicator of liver disease, bone disease, or hyperparathyroidism. Sensitive test for metastatic lesions to liver.
Alkaline phosphatase isoenzymes (ALP$_1$)	Hepatic, biliary	Used to distinguish between liver and bone pathology when total serum ALP is elevated. There are ALP isoenzymes for both liver (ALP$_1$) and bone (ALP$_2$).
Alpha fetoprotein (AFP, α-fetoprotein) Reference value: <40 ng/ml	Hepatic, biliary	A tumor marker for hepatocellular cancer in nonpregnant adults. AFP normally exists during pregnancy; otherwise, levels are very low.
Ammonia (NH$_3$) Reference value: 10-80 mcg/dl	Hepatic	To evaluate or monitor liver disease, hepatoencephalopathy, and the effects of impaired portal vein circulation. Ammonia is a by-product of protein metabolism and is converted to urea in the liver.
Amylase, serum Reference value: 30-220 U/L	Pancreatic	To assist in diagnosis of acute pancreatitis and traumatic injury to the pancreas or as surgical complication of the pancreas.
Amylase, urine Reference values: 6.5-48.1 U/hr (1-hr test) 5000 U/24 hr (24-hr test)	Pancreatic	To confirm diagnosis of acute pancreatitis when serum amylase levels are normal or borderline elevated.
Aspartate aminotransferase (AST, serum glutamate oxaloacetate transaminase [GOT], SGOT, transaminase) Reference value: 0-35 U/L	Hepatic	To assist in diagnosis of suspected hepatocellular disease. AST is highly concentrated in the liver, but it is also present in skeletal muscle, kidney, and pancreas.
Bilirubin Reference values: Total, 0.3-1.2 mg/dl Direct (conjugated), 0.1-0.2 mg/dl Indirect (unconjugated), 0.2-0.8 mg/dl	Hepatic, biliary	Used to evaluate liver function, diagnose jaundice, and monitor progression of jaundice. Total bilirubin is the sum of direct and indirect bilirubin. Elevation in direct (conjugated) bilirubin or indirect (unconjugated) bilirubin helps to determine cause of jaundice.
Carbohydrate antigen 19-9 (CA 19-9) Reference value: <37 U/ml	Hepatic, pancreatic	An associated tumor marker used in the diagnosis and treatment surveillance of pancreatic and hepatobiliary cancer.
Ceruloplasmin (enzyme involved in metabolism of iron) Reference value: 18-45 mg/dl	Hepatic	Used to help establish a diagnosis of Wilson disease.
Fecal fat (fecal lipids, quantitative fat, 72-hr stool collection, quantitative stool fat) Reference value: 2-6 g/24 hr	Pancreatic, biliary	To identify steatorrhea (high levels of fat in the feces). This can be caused by gallstones, pancreatic duct obstruction, cystic fibrosis, and small intestine disease.
Gamma-glutamyltransferase (γ-glutamyl-transferase [GT], γ-glutamyl-transpeptidase [GGT, GGTP, GTP]) Reference values: Male, 8-38 U/liter Female, 5-38 U/liter	Hepatic, biliary, pancreatic	Detects liver cell dysfunction and is sensitive to cholangitis, biliary obstruction, or cholecystitis.
Hepatitis panel Reference value: negative (no presence of antibodies)	Hepatic	Distinguishes among the three common types of viral hepatitis (HAV, HBV, HCV). Presence of distinct antibodies or antigens for a specific virus will help confirm the diagnosis and assist with treatment planning.

Continued

TABLE 8-6 Laboratory Tests for the Hepatic, Biliary, and Pancreatic Systems*—cont'd

Test	Involved Systems	Purpose
Lipase Reference value: <160 U/L	Pancreatic	Used to diagnose pancreatitis and pancreatic disease. Lipase is a digestive enzyme used to digest fatty acids. Elevated levels indicate onset of acute pancreatitis.
5′-Nucleotidase (5′N, 5′-NT) Reference value: 2-17 IU/L	Hepatic	An enzyme specific to the liver. Elevated levels help to identify extrahepatic or intrahepatic diseases.
Protein electrophoresis Reference value: albumin, 3.5-5.0 g/dl	Hepatic	To identify: presence of abnormal proteins (multiple myeloma) or absence of normal proteins (liver disease) and to detect high/low amounts of different protein groups.
Serum proteins (albumin) Reference value: 3.5-5.0 g/dl	Hepatic	Provides general information about nutritional status, the oncotic pressure of the blood, and the losses of protein associated with liver, renal, skin, or intestinal diseases.
Sweat test (sweat chloride, cystic fibrosis sweat test, iontophoresis sweat test) Reference value: Sodium: <70 mEq/L Chloride: <50 mEq/L	Pancreatic	Gold standard test used to diagnose cystic fibrosis in children, as these children have higher contents of sodium and chloride in their sweat.

Data from Knight JA: Liver function tests: their role in the diagnosis of hepatobiliary diseases, J Infus Nurs 28(2):108-117, 2005; Parad RB, Comeau AM, Dorkin HL et al: Sweat testing infants detected by cystic fibrosis newborn screening, J Pediatr 147(3 Supp 1):S69-S72, 2005; Davies JC: New tests for cystic fibrosis, Paediatr Respir Rev 7(S1:S141-S143, 2006; Pagana KD, Pagana TJ: Mosby's diagnostic and laboratory test reference, ed 9, St Louis, 2009, Mosby; Lab Tests Online: http://labtestsonline.org. Accessed July 12, 2012.
*Words or abbreviations in parentheses are synonyms for the test names.

TABLE 8-7 Diagnostic Procedures for the Hepatic, Biliary, Pancreatic, and Splenic Systems*

Test	Purpose
Computed tomography (CT) of the liver, biliary tract, pancreas, and spleen	Used to identify the presence of tumor, abscess, cyst, sites of bleeding, or hematoma in these organs. Contrast medium may be used with CT scan of the liver and pancreas.
Endoscopic retrograde cholangiopancreatography and pancreatic cytology (ECRP)	Used to investigate the cause of obstructive jaundice, persistent abdominal pain, or both. Generally identifies stones in the common bile duct as well as chronic pancreatitis and duodenal cancer.
Gallbladder nuclear scanning (hepatobiliary scintigraphy, cholescintigraphy, DISIDA scanning, HIDA [heptoiminodiacetic acid] scan)	Purpose: to examine the gallbladder and the biliary ducts leading out of it. Radionuclide material is injected into the patient, absorbed by the liver, and excreted through biliary ducts; can diagnose obstructions in the ducts.
Liver biliary biopsy, percutaneous	To diagnose pathologic changes in the liver and monitor disease progression.
Liver-spleen scan	A radionuclide is injected intravenously, and imaging of the liver and spleen is performed. Used to confirm and evaluate suspected hepatocellular disease and enlargement of the liver or spleen.
Magnetic resonance cholangiopancreatography (MRCP)	Imaging test used to visualize gallbladder, biliary ducts, and pancreatic ducts. Can identify obstructions (stones) and other pathology in the gallbladder and ducts. It is the imaging modality of choice for suspected cases of primary sclerosing cholangitis.
Ultrasound of the liver, biliary tract, pancreas and spleen	Imaging tool for examining the liver, spleen, gallbladder, and pancreas. Cyst, abscess, hematoma, primary neoplasm, and metastatic disease can be detected in the liver as well as gallstones and pancreatic abscesses and tumors.

Data from Knight JA: Liver function tests: their role in the diagnosis of hepatobiliary diseases, J Infus Nurs 28(2):108-117, 2005; Parad RB, Comeau AM, Dorkin HL et al: Sweat testing infants detected by cystic fibrosis newborn screening, J Pediatr 147(3 Supp 1):S69-S72, 2005; Davies JC: New tests for cystic fibrosis, Paediatr Respir Rev 7(S1:S141-S143, 2006; Fulcher AS: MRCP and ERCP in the diagnosis of common bile duct stones, Gastrointest Endosc 56(6 Supp 1):S178-S182, 2002; Taylor ACF, Little AF, Hennessy OF et al: Prospective assessment of magnetic resonance cholangiopancreatography for noninvasive imaging of the biliary tree, Gastrointest Endosc 55(1):17-22, 2002; Miller AH, Pepe PE, Brockman CR et al: ED ultrasound in hepatobiliary disease, J Emerg Med 30(1):69-74, 2006; Kalimi R, Gecelter GR, Caplin D et al: Diagnosis of acute cholecystitis: sensitivity of sonography, cholescintigraphy, and combined sonography-cholescintigraphy, J Am Coll Surg 193(6):609-613, 2001; Pagana KD, Pagana TJ: Mosby's diagnostic and laboratory test reference, ed 9, St Louis, 2009, Mosby; Ferri's clinical advisor 2013, St Louis, 2012, Mosby.
*Words or abbreviations in parentheses are synonyms for the test names.

BOX 8-2 Laparoscopic Utilization

Diagnostic	Therapeutic
Acute abdominal/pelvic pain	Cholecystectomy (gallbladder removal)
Chronic abdominal/pelvic pain	Appendectomy
Suspected advanced cancer	Hernia repair
Abdominal mass of uncertain etiology	Tubal ligation
Unexplained infertility	Oophorectomy
	Gastrectomy
	Colectomy
	Vagotomy
	Gastric bypass

Data from Sheipe M: Breaking through obesity with gastric bypass surgery, Nurse Pract 31(10):12-21, 2006; Pagana KD, Pagana TJ: Mosby's diagnostic and laboratory test reference, ed 9, St Louis, 2009, Mosby, pp 589-592.

hepatic and portal venous occlusion.[17] Otherwise, computed tomography scans are preferred for the visualization of other abdominal organs.[18] Good success, however, has been reported recently in using MRI for defining tissue borders for managing and resecting colorectal tumors.[19,20] MRI has also been successful in helping to delineate the etiology of cirrhosis between alcohol abuse and viral hepatitis.[21]

Positron Emission Tomography

PET is the use of positively charged ions and computer technology to create color images of organs and their functions. Combination technology using both PET and CT scanning is also available. Clinical uses of PET for the GI system include evaluation of pancreatic function and GI cancer.[22,23]

Health Conditions

GI disorders can be classified regionally by the structure involved and may consist of the following:
- Motility disorders
- Inflammation or hemorrhage
- Enzymatic dysfunction
- Neoplasms
- Morbid obesity

Esophageal Disorders

Physical therapists should be aware of any positioning precautions for patients with esophageal disorders that may exacerbate their dysphagia or gastroesophageal reflux disease (GERD).

Dysphagia

Dysphagia, or difficulty swallowing, can occur from various etiologies (Table 8-8) and is generally classified by its location as either *oropharyngeal dysphagia* occurring in the pharynx or upper esophagus, or *esophageal dysphagia* occurring in the esophageal body or lower esophageal sphincter.[24]

The following characteristics of dysphagia should also be noted to aid in the diagnosis:

TABLE 8-8 Classification and Possible Etiologies of Dysphagia

Classification	Possible Etiology
Oropharyngeal	Neuromuscular: stroke, Parkinson's disease, multiple sclerosis, myasthenia gravis, head trauma, dementia, Bell's palsy, tumors of the central nervous system Structural: oropharyngeal tumor, infection of pharynx or neck, thyromegaly, esophageal webs, cleft palate
Esophageal	Neuromuscular: achalasia, diffuse esophageal spasm, hypertensive lower esophageal sphincter, scleroderma Structural: peptic stricture, esophageal rings or webs, diverticuli, tumors, foreign bodies, vascular compression, mediastinal masses, spinal osteophytes, mucosal injury from infection or gastric reflux

Data from Satpathy HK: Dysphagia. In Ferri F, editor: Ferri's clinical advisor 2013, St Louis, 2012, Mosby.

- Does it occur with ingestion of solids, liquids, or both?
- Is it accompanied by pain?
- Is it intermittent, constant, or progressive?
- Does the patient complain of regurgitation/reflux or coughing while eating?
- The location at which the food becomes stuck should also be noted.[24]

Diagnosis can be established with imaging studies such as video fluoroscopy, modified barium swallow study, endoscopy, CT, and MRI. The primary goal of treatment includes airway protection and maintenance of nutrition with specific strategies employed once a definitive etiology is established.[25]

Esophageal Motility Disorders and Angina-like Chest Pain

Poor esophageal motility from neuromuscular dysfunction can result in dysphagia, chest pain, or heartburn. Achalasia, GERD, and distal esophageal spasm (DES) are the most common causes of primary esophageal motility disorders.[26]

Achalasia is a neuromuscular disorder of esophageal motility characterized by impaired lower esophageal sphincter (LES) relaxation and aperistalsis (absence of peristalsis) in the smooth muscle of the esophagus. Innervation to both the LES and the smooth muscle is thought to be disrupted, resulting in loss of motility. In addition to the aforementioned symptoms, clinical manifestations may include chest pain, regurgitation, hiccups, halitosis, weight loss, and aspiration pneumonia. All patients with achalasia will have solid food dysphagia with variable degrees of liquid aphasia. Treatment is aimed at compensating for poor esophageal emptying by reducing LES pressure with pharmacologic therapy, forceful dilation, or surgical myotomy.[26,27]

Distal esophageal spasm is characterized by the occurrence of normal peristalsis with intermittent nonperistaltic, simultaneous contractions of the body of the esophagus. Clinical manifestations include intermittent chest pain with or without eating that may be similar in character to angina, described as squeezing or crushing in nature, radiating to the jaw, neck, arms, or midline of the back.[26] The etiology is unknown, and management is directed at smooth muscle relaxation with pharmacologic agents along with behavior modification and biofeedback.[26,28]

Gastroesophageal Reflux Disease

GERD is characterized by gastric acid backflow into the esophagus as a result of an incompetent lower esophageal sphincter. Clinical manifestations include complaints of heartburn (especially with sour or bitter regurgitation), nausea, gagging, cough, or hoarseness. Two episodes of heartburn and/or complications from regurgitation per week defines the presence of GERD.[29] Although the exact etiology of GERD is unknown, tobacco abuse, along with the consumption of alcohol, coffee, peppermint, or chocolate, has been associated with this inappropriate relaxation. Esophageal and gastric motility disorders may also contribute to GERD, as may hiatal hernia and/or obesity. Gastroesophageal reflux is a strong predisposing factor for developing esophageal adenocarcinoma. Depending on the severity of GERD, treatment can range from dietary modifications (avoid risk factors and eat small frequent meals in an upright position) to weight reduction, antacids, proton pump inhibitors, H_2 blockers, or surgery.[30,31] Advancements in Nissen fundoplication have shown good long-term outcomes in improving GERD symptoms.[29,32]

Barrett's Esophagus

Barrett's esophagus is a condition in which columnar epithelium replaces the normal stratified squamous mucosa of the distal esophagus. According to the American Gastrointestinal Association, "intestinal metaplasia is required for the diagnosis of Barrett's esophagus as intestinal metaplasia is the only type of esophageal columnar epithelium that is clearly associated with malignancy."[33] Barrett's esophagus is generally associated with chronic GERD. The mechanism of cellular metaplasia is thought to occur from chronic inflammatory injury from acid and pepsin that refluxes from the stomach into the distal esophagus.[34,35] Barrett's esophagus is also a strong predisposing factor for developing esophageal adenocarcinoma, the incidence of which rose in the 1990s.[35-37]

Associated signs and symptoms include dysphagia, esophagitis, ulceration, perforations, strictures, bleeding, or adenocarcinoma.[35] Treatment for Barrett's esophagus includes controlling symptoms of GERD and healing reflux esophagitis. For patients with confirmed high-grade dysplasia within Barrett's esophagus, endoscopic eradication therapy with radiofrequency ablation, photodynamic therapy, or endoscopic mucosal resection is recommended.[33]

Esophageal Varices

Varices are dilated blood vessels in the esophagus caused by portal hypertension and may result in hemorrhage that necessitates immediate medical and, usually, invasive management.[38] Alcohol abuse is an associated risk factor.[39] Refer to the Cirrhosis section later in this chapter for more information on portal hypertension and alcoholic cirrhosis.

Esophageal Cancer

A description of esophageal cancers with respect to evaluation and management can be found in the Cancers in the Body Systems section in Chapter 11.

✎ **CLINICAL TIP**

Patients who have undergone esophagectomy may likely have chest tubes. Please refer to Chapter 18, Table 18-7 for chest tube management.

Stomach Disorders

Gastrointestinal Hemorrhage

Bleeding in the GI system can occur in either the upper GI system (upper gastrointestinal bleed [UGIB]) or in the lower GI system (lower gastrointestinal bleed [LGIB]). A UGIB occurs in the esophagus, stomach, or duodenum; an LGIB occurs in the colon and anorectum. A UGIB can result from one or more of the following: gastric or duodenal ulcers, gastric erosion, and gastric or esophageal varices. An LGIB can result from one or more of the following: (1) inflammatory bowel disease (e.g., diverticulitis), (2) ischemic colitis, (3) anal and rectal lesions (e.g., hemorrhoids), and (4) ulcerated polyps or colorectal cancer.[40-42]

GI bleeds can be small and require minimal to no intervention or very severe and constitute medical emergencies because of hemodynamic instability that can lead to shock. Hematemesis or dark brown ("coffee-ground") emesis (vomitus), hematochezia (passage of blood from the rectum), and melena (black, tarry stools) from acid degradation of hemoglobin are the primary clinical manifestations of GI bleeds.[42]

Patients requiring management are generally stabilized hemodynamically with intravenous (IV) fluids, blood transfusions, or both before the cause of bleeding can be fully delineated. Nasogastric tubes (see Chapter 18) are typically used in the stabilization and management of UGIB. Management is targeted at the causative factors that resulted in either UGIB or LGIB. Endoscopy, colonoscopy, or sigmoidoscopy can be performed to help evaluate or treat the source of upper or lower GI hemorrhage.[41-43]

✎ **CLINICAL TIP**

Patients with GI bleeding will need their complete blood count and coagulation profiles reviewed frequently in order to determine parameters for physical therapy management.

Gastritis

Gastritis is the general term used to describe diffuse inflammatory lesions in the mucosal layer of the stomach. Gastritis can be subdivided as erosive, nonerosive, or specific types based on histological features and those found endoscopically.[44]

Common causes of gastritis include *Helicobacter pylori (H. pylori)* infection, use of aspirin or nonsteroidal antiinflammatory drugs (NSAIDs), alcohol use, radiation, Crohn's disease, and sarcoidosis. Clinical manifestations include abdominal pain, nausea, and vomiting typically occurring when gastritis has led to ulceration; otherwise patients may be asymptomatic. Symptoms of upper GI bleed may also be present if ulceration occurs. Management of gastritis consists of addressing the underlying cause with antimicrobial agents in the case of *H. pylori* infection and acid suppression therapy.[24,45-48]

Peptic Ulcer Disease

Peptic ulcer disease (PUD) is an ulceration in the stomach (gastric ulcer) or duodenum (duodenal ulcer) resulting from an imbalance between various mucosa-damaging substances and mucosal protective factors. The two primary causes of PUD are *H. pylori* infection and NSAID use. Other factors that can contribute to PUD include incompetent LES, bile acids, impaired bicarbonate secretion, decreased blood flow to gastric mucosa, cigarette smoking, and alcohol use.[24,49-52]

Clinical manifestations of PUD include abdominal pain located in the epigastric region that is burning, gnawing, or "hunger-like" in quality. Pain can occur 2 to 5 hours after a meal or at night (between midnight and 3 AM), which can awaken patients. Relief of pain can occur immediately after a meal, and pain is rarely constant. Ulcer pain can also radiate to the low back region. Hemorrhage occurs in approximately 15% of patients with PUD.[24]

Management of PUD includes lifestyle changes (smoking cessation and discontinuation of aspirin or alcohol use), discontinuing NSAID use, and beginning proton pump inhibitor or H2 blocker therapy and/or antimicrobial therapy for *H. pylori*.[24,52]

Zollinger-Ellison Syndrome

Zollinger-Ellison syndrome (ZES) is a rare syndrome that includes gastric acid hypersecretion, caused by a gastrin-producing tumor (gastrinoma) in the pancreas and duodenum. Symptoms include abdominal pain, heartburn, diarrhea, nausea, and weight loss. Diagnosis of ZES is often delayed given the similarity to PUD or GERD. Management is primarily directed at surgical resection of the gastrinoma, along with decreasing gastric acid hypersecretion.[53-55]

Gastric Emptying Disorders

Abnormal gastric emptying is described as either decreased or increased emptying. Decreased gastric emptying is also referred to as *gastric retention* or *gastroparesis* and may result from or be associated with (1) pyloric stenosis as a consequence of peptic ulcers, (2) diabetes mellitus, (3) diabetic ketoacidosis, (4) electrolyte imbalance, (5) autonomic neuropathy, (6) gastric surgery, and (7) malignancy.[56,57] Addressing the primary cause as well as pharmacologic intervention to promote gastric motility is indicated for patients with decreased gastric emptying disorders.[57]

Enhanced gastric emptying (also known as *dumping syndrome*) is associated with an interruption of normal digestive sequencing that result from vagotomy, gastrectomy, gastric bypass, or surgery for PUD. Gastric peristalsis, mixing, and grinding are

disturbed, resulting in rapid emptying of liquids, slow or increased emptying of solids, and prolonged retention of indigestible solids.[56] With enhanced gastric emptying, blood glucose levels are subsequently low and can result in signs and symptoms of anxiety, sweating, intense hunger, dizziness, weakness, and palpitations. Nutritional and pharmacologic management are the usual treatment choices.[57]

Gastric Cancer

The most common malignant neoplasms found in the stomach are adenocarcinomas, which arise from normal or mucosal cells. Benign tumors are rarely found but include leiomyomas and polyps. For a more detailed discussion of gastric oncology, see the Cancers in the Body Systems section in Chapter 11.

Intestinal Disorders

Appendicitis

Inflammation of the appendix of the large intestine can be classified as acute, gangrenous, or perforated. Acute appendicitis involves an inflamed but intact appendix. Gangrenous appendicitis is the presence of focal or extensive necrosis accompanied by microscopic perforations. Perforated appendicitis is a gross disruption of the appendix wall and can lead to serious complications if it is not managed promptly.[58] The etiology of appendicitis includes a combination of obstruction in the appendix lumen coupled with infection, with bacterial or viral invasion the more common occurrence.[58,59]

Signs and symptoms of appendicitis may include[59]:
- Right lower quadrant, epigastric, or periumbilical abdominal pain that fluctuates in intensity
- Abdominal tenderness in the right lower quadrant at McBurney's point, located approximately one third of the distance from the right anterior superior iliac crest to the umbilicus[60]
- Vomiting with presence of anorexia
- Constipation and failure to pass flatus
- Low-grade fever (no greater than 102°F or 39°C)

Management of appendicitis involves timely and accurate diagnosis of acute appendicitis to prevent perforation. Treatment choices include antimicrobial agents with definitive management consisting of surgical appendectomy.[58]

Diverticular Disease

Diverticulosis is the presence of diverticula, which is an outpocketing, or herniation, of the mucosa of the large colon through the muscle layers of the intestinal wall. Diverticular disease occurs when the outpocketing becomes symptomatic. Diverticulitis is the result of inflammation and localized peritonitis that occurs after the perforation of a single diverticulum.[59,61,62]

Signs and symptoms of diverticular disease include the following[59,63]:
- Achy, left lower quadrant pain and tenderness (pain intensifies with acute diverticulitis)
- Urinary frequency

- Fever and elevated white blood cell count (acute diverticulitis)
- Constipation, bloody stools, or both
- Nausea, vomiting, anorexia

Management of diverticular disease includes any of the following[59,61,63,64]:

- Dietary modifications (e.g., increased fiber)
- IV fluids
- Pain medications
- Antimicrobial agents
- Invasive management with percutaneous abscess drainage, laparoscopic colectomy or sigmoid resection, or use of the DaVinci robot with minimally invasive procedures

Hernia

Abdominal Hernia. An abdominal hernia is an abnormal protrusion of bowel that is generally classified by the area where the protrusion occurs. These include the following areas: (1) linea alba, (2) inguinal, (3) femoral, (4) ventral or incisional, and (5) umbilical.[65,66] A hernia is referred to as *reducible* when its contents can be replaced within the surrounding musculature and is *irreducible* or *incarcerated* when it cannot. A *strangulated* hernia has compromised circulation with potential to be fatal. Signs and symptoms of abdominal herniation include[66]:

- Abdominal distention, nausea, and vomiting
- Observable bulge with position changes, coughing, or laughing
- Paresthesia if nerve compression occurs with hernia
- Pain of increasing severity with fever, tachycardia, and abdominal rigidity (if the herniated bowel is strangulated)

Management of herniation includes any of the following[66-68]:

- "Watchful waiting" in asymptomatic cases
- Surgical repair with a laparoscope
- Open surgical reinforcement of weakened area with mesh, wire, or fascia
- Temporary colostomy in cases of intestinal obstruction

Hiatal Hernia. A hiatal hernia is an abnormal protrusion of the stomach upward through the esophageal hiatus of the diaphragm.[69] Causative risk factors for a hiatal hernia are similar to those for abdominal hernia. Clinical manifestations mimic those of GERD, including heartburn-like epigastric pain that usually occurs after eating and with recumbent positioning, dysphagia, chest pain, dyspnea, or hoarseness.[69]

Management of hiatal hernia can include behavior modifications, such as avoiding reclining after meals, drinking caffeine or alcohol, and smoking tobacco. Eating small, frequent, bland meals with a high fiber content may also be beneficial. Pharmacologic intervention typically includes acid-reducing

---

✎ CLINICAL TIP

Positions associated with bronchopulmonary hygiene or functional mobility may exacerbate pain in patients who have a hernia, particularly a hiatal hernia. Therefore careful modification of these interventions will be necessary for successful completion of these activities.

---

medications. In certain cases, when these measures have proven ineffective, surgical management of the hiatal hernia can be performed laparoscopically or with open procedures.[69]

Intestinal Obstructions

Failure of intestinal contents to be propelled forward, in either the small or large intestine, can be caused by mechanical or functional obstructions.

Mechanical Obstruction. Blockage of the bowel by adhesion, herniation, volvulus (twisting of bowel on itself), tumor, inflammation, impacted feces, or invagination (intussusception) of a bowel segment into an adjacent segment (much like a telescope) constitutes mechanical obstruction.[70,71]

Functional Obstructions (Paralytic Ileus). Paralytic ileus is defined as "functional inhibition of propulsive bowel activity."[72] Obstructions may result from abdominal surgery, intestinal distention, hypokalemia, peritonitis, severe trauma, spinal fractures, ureteral distention, or use of narcotics.

Signs and symptoms of intestinal obstructions include the following[73]:

- Sudden onset of crampy abdominal pain that may be intermittent as peristalsis occurs
- Abdominal pain and/or distention
- Nausea, vomiting
- Obstipation (inability to pass gas or stool)
- Localized tenderness
- High-pitched or absent bowel sounds (depending on extent of obstruction)
- Tachycardia and hypotension in presence of dehydration or peritonitis
- Bloody stools

Management of intestinal obstructions includes any of the following[72-75]:

- Insertion of a nasogastric tube in cases of severe abdominal distention or intractable vomiting
- Restoration of intravascular volume
- Surgical resection (laparoscopic technique or open laparotomy) of mechanical obstructions from adhesions, necrosis, tumor, or unresolved inflammatory lesions, particularly if the obstruction is in the large intestine
- Colostomy placement and eventual colostomy closure (colostomy closure is also referred to as *colostomy takedown*)

Constipation can occur after major orthopedic surgery (e.g., total joint arthroplasty) as a result of frequent narcotic use for adequate pain control.[2] Early mobilization with this population (and all postoperative surgical populations) can help to lessen the likelihood of this complication. Abdominal distention will also have an impact on other patient functions that may affect how well patients are able to progress with their physical therapy treatment. The ability to take deep breaths, reach for objects, and perform bed mobility will be that much more difficult with the extra girth associated with abdominal distention.

Intestinal Ischemia

Ischemia within the intestinal tract can be acute or chronic, with most cases occurring either in the colon or in areas supplied by the superior mesenteric artery.[76] Another form of intestinal ischemia is called ischemic colitis. It can result from many factors, such as thrombosis or emboli to the superior mesenteric artery; intestinal strangulation; chronic vascular insufficiency; hypotension; oral contraceptives (combined with history of thrombophilic defects)[77]; NSAIDs; and vasoconstrictors, such as vasopressin and dihydroergotamine. Methamphetamine and cocaine have vasoconstrictive properties that can also lead to intestinal ischemia. Significant ischemia that is not managed in a timely manner can lead to intestinal necrosis or gangrene and prove to be a life-threatening situation.[78]

Signs and symptoms of intestinal ischemia include[76]:
- Abdominal pain ranging from colicky pain to a steady severe ache, depending on the severity of ischemia
- Nausea and vomiting
- Diarrhea or rectal bleeding
- Rebound tenderness, abdominal distention, and muscle guarding
- Tachycardia, hypotension, and fever (with necrosis)

Management of intestinal ischemia includes any of the following[76,79]:
- Revascularization procedures, including balloon angioplasty and bypass grafting
- Resection of necrotic segments with temporary colostomy or ileostomy placement and subsequent reanastomosis of functional segments as indicated
- Antiinfective agents
- Vasodilators or vasopressors (blood perfusion enhancement)
- Anticoagulation therapy
- IV fluid replacement
- Insertion of nasogastric tube
- Analgesic agents

Irritable Bowel Syndrome

Irritable bowel syndrome (IBS), also referred to as *irritable* or *spastic colon*, is characterized by inconsistent motility of the large bowel (i.e., constipation or diarrhea). Diagnostic criteria includes abdominal pain or discomfort that persists for at least 3 days per month in the past 3 months associated along with two or more of the following[80]:
- Defecation relieves or improves pain
- Onset is associated with a change in the frequency of bowel movement
- Onset is associated with a change in the form or appearance of the stool

Motility of the large bowel can be affected by emotions; history of physical or sexual abuse; certain foods, such as milk products; neurohumoral agents; GI hormones; toxins; prostaglandins; and colon distention.[81,82] Some evidence suggests that patients with IBS may have bacterial overgrowth in their small intestines.[83]

Additional signs and symptoms of IBS include[81]:
- Diffuse abdominal pain, reports of feeling bloated, or both
- Constipation or diarrhea
- Correlation of GI symptoms with eating, high emotional states, or stress
- No weight loss
- Tender sigmoid colon on palpation

Management of IBS includes any of the following[80,81,84]:
- Laxatives or antidiarrheal (loperamide) agents
- Antispasmodic agents
- Dietary modifications, including a high-fiber diet
- Counseling or psychotherapy with or without antidepressants
- Antibiotic therapy

Malabsorption Syndromes

Malabsorption syndrome is a general term for disorders that are characterized by the small intestine's failure to absorb or digest carbohydrates, proteins, fats, water, vitamins, and electrolytes.[85] This syndrome is associated with patients who have manifestations of acquired immunodeficiency disease. The nutritional deficits that result from malabsorption can lead to other chronic disorders, such as anemia or osteoporosis. Malabsorption syndromes can result from any of the following[86,87]:
- Pancreatic insufficiency (chronic pancreatitis, carcinoma)
- Crohn's disease (see the Crohn's Disease section)
- Celiac disease (small intestine mucosal damage from glutens [e.g., wheat, barley, rye, and oats])
- Parasitic infection
- Liver disease
- Whipple's disease (infection of the small intestine by *Tropheryma whipplei* bacteria)

Signs and symptoms of malabsorption syndromes include[85,88]:
- Diarrhea, steatorrhea (excessive fat excretion), or both
- Anorexia and weight loss
- Abdominal bloating
- Bone pain

Management of malabsorption syndromes includes any of the following[88,89]:
- Antidiarrheal agents
- Antibiotic therapy
- Dietary modifications and nutritional support
- Fluid hydration, electrolyte, vitamin, and mineral support

Peritonitis

Peritonitis is general or localized inflammation in the peritoneal cavity and may be acute, chronic, septic or aseptic, and primary or secondary. Etiologies for primary peritonitis include bacterial infection with secondary peritonitis typically occurring as a result of ascites, perforation of the GI tract, gangrene of the bowel, trauma, and surgical irritants.[4,90,92]

Signs and symptoms of peritonitis include[4,91]:
- Constant abdominal pain
- Fever, nausea, and/or vomiting
- Abdominal guarding with diffuse tenderness and rigidity
- Abdominal distention
- Diminished or absent bowel sounds
- Rebound tenderness
- Tachycardia, hypotension

Management of peritonitis includes any of the following[4,90,91]:
- Laparoscopic evaluation, with or without subsequent surgical correction of primary etiology

- Antibiotic therapy
- Fluid management with electrolytes and colloids
- Pain management
- Nasogastric suctioning
- Invasive monitoring of central hemodynamic pressures

Crohn's Disease

Crohn's disease is one form of idiopathic inflammatory bowel disease (IBD) that can occur in any part of the GI system. The small intestine, particularly the ileum and the proximal portion of the colon, is most commonly involved, whereas the esophagus and stomach are rarely affected. Suspected causes of Crohn's disease include genetic predetermination, exaggerated immunologic mechanisms, infectious agents, psychological issues, dietary factors, smoking, and environmental factors.[92,93]

Signs and symptoms of Crohn's disease may include the following[93]:

- Constant crampy abdominal pain, often in right lower quadrant, not relieved by bowel movement
- Right lower quadrant abdominal mass
- Diarrhea, weight loss
- Low-grade fever
- Fistula formation

Management of Crohn's disease includes any of the following[92-94]:

- Antiinflammatory medications (corticosteroids)
- Antibiotics
- Immune modulators
- IV fluids and dietary modification and support (possible total parenteral nutrition use)
- Nasogastric suctioning
- Activity limitations (in acute phases)
- Surgical resection of involved area, either by open laparotomy or video laparoscopy, with or without need for ileostomy or stoma

Complications of Crohn's disease can include[93]:

- Intestinal obstruction, possibly leading to fistula, abscess, or perforations in the intestine
- Inflammation of the eyes, skin, and mucous membranes
- Arthritis, ankylosing spondylitis
- Gallstones
- Vitamin B_{12} deficiency
- Thromboembolism

Ulcerative Colitis

Ulcerative colitis is a chronic idiopathic inflammatory disease of the intestine (IBD) limited to the mucosal layer of the colon and rectum. The definitive etiology of ulcerative colitis is unknown, but suspected causes are similar to those of Crohn's disease. Inflammation can be mild, moderate, or severe.[92,95,96]

Signs and symptoms of ulcerative colitis include[95,96]:

- Crampy lower abdominal pain that is relieved by a bowel movement
- Small, frequent stools to profuse diarrhea (mild to severe)
- Rectal bleeding
- Fever
- Fatigue with anorexia and weight loss

- Dehydration
- Tachycardia

Management of ulcerative colitis includes any of the following[95,96]:

- Antiinflammatory medications, including steroids and mesalamine suppositories
- Immunomodulatory agents.
- Antibiotics.
- Surgical resection of the entire diseased colon and rectum can provide a cure for ulcerative colitis as well as prevent colorectal cancer.
- Other surgical options include subtotal colectomy with ileostomy, colectomy with ileorectal anastomosis, protocolectomy with various types of ileostomy.
- Dietary modification and support (possible total parenteral nutrition use).
- Activity limitations.
- Iron supplements, blood replacement, or both.
- Antidiarrheal agents.

Related manifestations of ulcerative colitis may include[96]:

- Arthritis, ankylosing spondylitis, osteomalacia, osteoporosis
- Inflammation of the eyes, skin, and mucous membranes
- Hepatitis, bile duct carcinoma
- Anemia, leukopenia, or thrombocytopenia

Polyps

Polyps of the colon are mucosal lesions that project within the bowel and consist of four types: adenomatous, hyperplastic, harmartomatous, and inflammatory. Adenomatous polyps have the most potential to become a precursor to colorectal cancer.[97,98]

Signs and symptoms of polyps include[97,98]:

- Rectal bleeding (occult or overt)
- Constipation or diarrhea
- Crampy pain in the lower abdomen

Management of polyps includes[97-99]:

- Screening and modification of risk factors for colorectal cancer, such as obesity, smoking, and excessive alcohol consumption for patients over the age of 50
- Colonoscopy, flexible sigmoidoscopy, proctosigmoidoscopy, endoscopy, or barium enema for detection of the polyp
- Tissue biopsy to determine its malignancy potential
- Polypectomy with electrocautery
- Surgical resection, if indicated, with or without ileostomy

Intestinal Tumors

Benign or metastatic neoplasms of the intestine include colonic adenomas (polyps), villous or papillary adenomas, lipomas, leiomyomas, and lymphoid hyperplasia. Tumors affect motility and absorption functions in the intestine (see the Cancers in the Body Systems section in Chapter 11 for further details).

Anorectal Disorders

Disorders of the anus and rectum generally involve inflammation, obstruction, discontinuity from the colon, perforations, or tumors. The most common disorders are (1) hemorrhoids, (2) anorectal fistula, (3) anal fissure, (4) imperforate anus, and (5) rectal prolapse. Signs and symptoms include pain with defecation and bloody stools. Management is supportive according to the disorder, and surgical correction is performed as necessary.[71,87]

Morbid Obesity

Obesity is a complex disorder with many contributing metabolic, psychological, and genetic factors.[100] It is defined as a chronic disease characterized by an excess of body fat.[101] The medical standard for measuring obesity is body mass index (BMI).[101] BMI is determined by dividing the person's weight in kilograms by their height in meters squared.[101] A normal BMI is 18.5 to 24.9, overweight is 25 to 29.9, and obese is 30 or more.[102]

Comorbidities such as type 2 diabetes, cardiovascular disease, dyslipidemia, obstructive sleep apnea, degenerative joint disease, renal disease, cholelithiasis, depression, and cancer have been linked to morbid obesity.[103-105] Conservative treatment involves weight loss measures such as diet modifications and behavioral and lifestyle changes; however, these measures have shown up to a 90% relapse in weight gain.[106] Therefore bariatric (weight loss) surgery is recommended in these scenarios (assuming that the patient is medically and psychologically appropriate for the surgery). Bariatric surgery is indicated for patients with a BMI greater than 40 kg/m^2 or a BMI greater than 35 kg/m^2 with related comorbid conditions.[105]

Bariatric surgical options include[100,105,107]:
- Gastric bypass: Roux-en-Y and resectional gastric bypass
- Adjustable gastric banding
- Vertical banded gastroplasty
- Biliopancreatic diversion
- Sleeve gastrectomy

All of these bariatric procedures can be performed either through open laparotomy or laparoscopically, except for the biliopancreatic diversion, which is typically performed as an open procedure.[105] One year after bariatric surgery, weight loss is positively associated with patients who participated in an exercise program.[108] Improved functional capacity and quality of life, measured by 6-minute walk distance and SF-36, respectively, have also been reported in patients 3 and 6 months after gastric bypass surgery.[109]

Physical Therapy Considerations

- To improve patient safety and mobility, use of specialized bariatric equipment (e.g., gait/transfer belts, walkers, and beds) and assistance from several qualified personnel is recommended.[110-113]
- Early and frequent ambulation is recommended beginning 2 to 6 hours postoperatively and occurring every 2 to 4 hours while awake.
- Exercise should be terminated if the following occur[114-116]:
  - Increase in systolic pressure of 20 mm Hg or more
  - Decrease in diastolic pressure of 20 mm Hg or more
  - Heart rate increase or decrease by more than 20 beats per minute
  - Severe dyspnea or paradoxical breathing
  - Dizziness
  - Excessive sweating
  - Patient report of feeling faint

- To prevent pulmonary complications, active breathing exercises and airway clearance techniques should be performed.[110,117]
- To optimize skin integrity, consistent and diligent skin inspection is essential for bariatric patients, especially in areas such as surgical incision sites and skin fold because decreased mobility and poor vascular supply to adipose tissue can facilitate the development of integumentary impairments.[110,118]

For more information, refer to the review by Hinkle.[118a]

Liver and Biliary Disorders

The liver is the only organ in the body with regenerative properties[119]; therefore patients with acute liver inflammation will heal well if given the proper rest and medical treatment. Physical therapists should aim not to overfatigue these patients with functional activities to help promote proper healing of the liver.

Hepatitis

Hepatic inflammation and hepatic cell necrosis may be acute or chronic and may result from viruses, autoimmune diseases, alcohol, and Wilson's disease (a rare copper metabolism disorder).[120] Viral hepatitis is the most common type of hepatitis and can be classified as hepatitis A, B, C, D, E, F, or G (i.e., HAV, HBV, HCV, HDV, HEV, HFV, and HGV or HGBV, respectively).[121]

Hepatitis A, B, and C are the most common types of viral hepatitis. Hepatitis A is transmitted via the fecal-oral route, mostly from contaminated water sources, is typically self-limiting, and has vaccination available. Hepatitis B is more common than hepatitis C, but both are transmitted through blood and body fluids. Acute viral hepatitis generally resolves with appropriate medical management, but in some cases, hepatitis B and C can become chronic and result in end-stage cirrhosis or hepatocellular carcinoma.[122]

Signs and symptoms of hepatitis include[121]:
- Abrupt onset of malaise
- Muscle weakness
- Fever
- Poor appetite, weight loss, or anorexia
- Nausea, abdominal discomfort, and pain
- Headache
- Jaundice
- Dark-colored urine

Management of hepatitis includes any of the following[121,122]:
- Adequate periods of rest
- Vaccinations (only for HAV, HBV, HDV)
- Fluid and nutritional support
- Removal of precipitating irritants (e.g., alcohol and toxins)

✎ **CLINICAL TIP**

Health care workers who are exposed to blood and body fluids during patient contact must ensure that they are properly vaccinated against hepatitis B.[123] This includes receiving periodic measurements of antibody titers to the viruses and supplementation with booster shots as needed to maintain appropriate immunity against these infections.

- Antiinflammatory agents
- Antiviral agents

Cirrhosis

Cirrhosis is a chronic disease state that is characterized by hepatic parenchymal cell destruction and necrosis, and regeneration with fibrosis or scar tissue formation. The fibrosis that occurs in the liver reduces its ability to synthesize plasma proteins (albumin), clotting factors, and bilirubin. The primary complications that can occur from cirrhosis include portal hypertension (Figure 8-3), ascites, jaundice, impaired clotting ability, hepatic encephalopathy, and variceal bleeding.[90,124,125]

Cirrhosis may result from a variety of etiologies, including[125]:

- Alcohol or drug abuse
- Viral hepatitis
- Hemochromatosis
- Wilson's disease
- Alpha$_1$-antitrypsin deficiency
- Biliary obstruction
- Venous outflow obstruction
- Cardiac failure
- Malnutrition
- Pancreatitis

Signs and symptoms of cirrhosis include[90,125]:

- Recent weight loss or gain
- Fatigability
- Jaundice
- Lower-extremity edema
- Anorexia, nausea, or vomiting

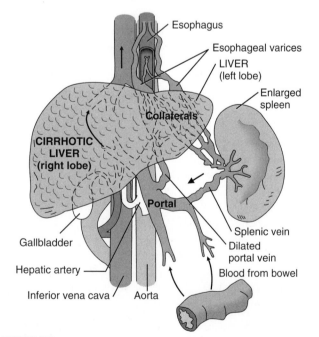

HEART

FIGURE 8-3
Portal hypertension. (From Goodman CC, Fuller KS, Boissonnault WG, editors: Pathology: implications for the physical therapist, ed 3, St Louis, 2009, Saunders.)

- Fever
- Decreased urine output (urine dark yellow or amber)
- Associated GI manifestations of esophageal varices, bowel habit changes, and GI bleeding
- Altered mental status
- Flapping tremor (asterixis)
  Management of cirrhosis includes[125]:
- Supportive care, including IV fluids, whole blood and blood products, colloid (albumin), vitamin and electrolyte replacement, and dietary and behavioral modifications (eliminate alcohol consumption)
- Medical (beta-blockade and corticosteroids) or surgical correction (or both) of primary etiology or secondary complications as indicated
- Paracentesis to drain peritoneal edema (ascites)
- Supplemental oxygen
- Liver transplantation (see Chapter 14)

Hepatic Encephalopathy and Coma

Acute and chronic liver diseases, particularly cirrhosis, may lead to neuropsychiatric manifestations that may progress from hepatic encephalopathy to pre-coma to coma. The majority of neuropsychiatric manifestations are linked to multiple factors such as ammonia intoxication, inflammatory cytokines, benzodiazepine-like compounds as well as infections, GI bleeding, use of sedatives, dehydration, and electrolyte imbalance.[90,126,127]

Signs and symptoms of hepatic encephalopathy include a combination of impaired mental status and neuromuscular dysfunction occurring over a period of hours to days. Altered consciousness may be present and includes a number of symptoms ranging from changes in personality to disorientation, sleep disturbance, stupor, and coma.[126,127] Table 8-9 provides an overview of the evaluation for severity levels associated with hepatic encephalopathy.

Management of hepatic encephalopathy and coma may consist of any of the following[126,127]:

- Administering nonabsorbable disaccharides, such as lactulose and lactitol, which is the mainstay of treatment to help reduce ammonia levels
- Correction of fluid and electrolyte or acid-base imbalances, or both
- Supplemental oxygen
- Removal of any precipitating substances
- Ammonia detoxicants such as L-ornithine-L-aspartate
- Nutritional support
- Antiinfective agents
- Artificial liver support devices such as bioartificial liver support (BAL)

Cholecystitis with Cholelithiasis

Cholecystitis is acute or chronic inflammation of the gallbladder. It is associated with obstruction by gallstones in 90% of cases.[128] Gallstone formation (cholelithiasis) is associated with three factors: gallbladder hypomobility, supersaturation of bile with cholesterol, and crystal formation from an increased concentration of insoluble bilirubin in the bile. Cholelithiasis can

TABLE 8-9 West Haven Criteria of Altered Mental Status in Hepatic Encephalopathy

Grade	Consciousness	Intellect and Behavior	Neurologic Findings
0	Normal	Normal	Normal; impaired psychomotor testing
1	Mild lack of awareness	Shortened attention span; impaired addition or subtraction	Mild asterixis or tremor
2	Lethargic	Disoriented; inappropriate behavior	Obvious asterixis; slurred speech
3	Somnolent but arousable	Gross disorientation; bizarre behavior	Muscular rigidity and clonus; hyperreflexia
4	Coma	Coma	Decerebrate posturing

Data from Ferenci P, Lockwood A, Mullen K et al: Hepatic encephalopathy—definition, nomenclature, diagnosis, and quantification: final report of the working party at the 11th World Congresses of Gastroenterology, Vienna, 1998. Hepatology 35:716-721, 2002 in Sundaram V, Shaikh OS: Hepatic encephalopathy: pathophysiology and emerging therapies, Med Clin North Am 93:819-836, 2009.

lead to secondary bacterial infection that further exacerbates the cholecystitis.[129-131]

Signs and symptoms of cholecystitis include[129,130]:

- Severe abdominal pain in the right upper quadrant (RUQ) with possible pain referral to the interscapular region
- Rebound tenderness and abdominal rigidity
- Jaundice
- Anorexia
- Nausea, vomiting, or both
- Fever
- Murphy's sign (inhibited inspiration on palpation) in RUQ

Management of cholecystitis includes any of the following[129-131]:

- Laparoscopic cholecystectomy or cholecystostomy (temporary drain placement in the gallbladder until obstruction is relieved)
- Gallstone dilution therapy with chenodeoxycholic and ursodeoxycholic acid
- Antiinfective agents
- Pain management
- IV fluids
- Insertion of nasogastric tube

Pancreatic Disorders

Pancreatitis

Inflammation of the pancreas can be acute or chronic. The incidence of acute pancreatitis is rising, and the clinical sequelae are potentially severe, including progression to chronic pancreatitis, development of adult respiratory distress syndrome (ARDS), and/or shock. This section therefore focuses on acute pancreatitis. Acute pancreatitis can be categorized as necrotizing or interstitial. Pancreatitis involves an exaggerated release and activity of pancreatic enzymes into the peritoneal cavity, along with autodigestion of pancreatic parenchyma. The exact trigger to this process is unknown, but the most common contributing factors are gallstones and alcohol and drug abuse.[132,133] Other contributing factors also include[132,133]:

- Trauma
- Endoscopic retrograde cholangiography (see Table 8-7)
- Metabolic disorders (hyperlipidemia, hypercalcemia)
- Vasculitis

- Pancreatic obstruction
- Autoimmune pancreatitis
- Medications
- Postoperative sequelae from abdominal or cardiothoracic surgery

Signs and symptoms of acute pancreatitis include[132,133]:

- Steady, dull abdominal pain in the epigastrium, left upper quadrant, or periumbilical area often radiating to back, chest, and lower abdomen. Pain can be exacerbated by food, alcohol, vomiting, and resting in the supine position.
- Nausea, vomiting, and abdominal distention
- Fever, tachycardia, and hypotension (in acute cases)
- Jaundice
- Abdominal tenderness or rigidity
- Diminished or absent bowel sounds

Management of acute pancreatitis includes any of the following[132,133]:

- Pain management, generally with narcotics, possibly through patient-controlled analgesia (see Chapter 21)
- IV fluid and electrolyte replacement
- Eliminating oral food intake and providing alternative nutritional support, such as total parenteral nutrition
- Surgical correction or resection of obstructions such as cholecystectomy
- Nasogastric suctioning
- Supplemental oxygen and mechanical ventilation (as indicated)
- Invasive monitoring (in more severe cases)

Management

General management of GI disorders may consist of any of the following: pharmacologic therapy, nutritional support, dietary modifications, and surgical procedures. Nutritional support and dietary modifications are beyond the scope of this book. This section focuses on pharmacologic therapy and surgical procedures. A discussion of physical therapy intervention is also included.

Pharmacologic Therapy

Medications used to treat GI disorders can be broadly categorized as (1) those that control gastric acid secretion and (2) those that normalize gastric motility. Refer to Chapter 19 for an overview of these medications (Table 19-25, Antacids; Table 19-26, Antidiarrheal Medications; Table 19-27, Antispasmodic Medications; Table 19-28, Cytoprotective Medications; Table IV-29, Histamine-2 Receptor Antagonists [H2RAs]; Table 19-30 Laxatives; and Table 19-31, Proton Pump Inhibitors). Other medications that do not fall into these categories are mentioned in specific sections under Health Conditions, earlier in the chapter.

Surgical Procedures

Surgical intervention is indicated in GI disorders when medical intervention is insufficient (Table 8-10). The location and extent of incisions depend on the exact procedure. The decision to perform either an open laparotomy or a laparoscopic repair will depend on physician preference based on surgical difficulty and documented outcomes of specific techniques. Many open laparotomy procedures requiring large abdominal incisions are being replaced with laparoscopic procedures. Laparoscopic procedures have been shown to reduce hospital length of stay, many postoperative complications, or both.[61,129,134,135] Postoperative complications may include pulmonary infection, wound infection, and bed rest deconditioning. Refer to Chapter 20 for further descriptions of the effects of anesthesia.

With all colostomies, an external, plastic pouch is placed over the stoma in which the patient's stool collects. Patients are instructed on proper care and emptying of their colostomy pouch. This procedure can be performed in the ascending, transverse, or sigmoid portions of the colon, with sigmoid colostomies being the most commonly performed.

Physical Therapy Considerations

- Before any mobility treatment, the physical therapist should ensure that the colostomy pouch is securely closed and adhered to the patient. When possible, coordinate with the nurse or the patient to empty the colostomy bag before therapy to fully minimize accidental spills.
- Patients who are experiencing abdominal pain from recent surgical incisions may be more comfortable in the side-lying position (if allowed) to help relieve skin tension on the recent incision.
- Instructing the patient to bend his or her knees up while the head of the bed is being lowered may also decrease incisional discomfort.
- Patients with new colostomies may have difficulty accepting the new device, and therapists will need to be respectful of the patient's time frame for adjustment.

Physical Therapy Management

The following are general goals and guidelines for the physical therapist when working with the patient who has GI dysfunction. These guidelines should be adapted to a patient's specific needs.

Goals

The primary physical therapy goals for this patient population are similar to those of other patients in the acute care setting:

(1) to optimize functional mobility, (2) to maximize activity tolerance and endurance, and (3) to prevent postoperative pulmonary and integumentary complications.

Guidelines for Physical Therapy Management

In addition to considerations described in earlier sections of this chapter, further guidelines include, but are not limited to, the following:

1. Patients with GI dysfunction can have increased fatigue levels as a result of poor nutritional status. Therefore consider the patient's fatigue level with treatment planning and setting of goals.
   a. Consultation with the nutritionist is helpful in gauging the appropriate activity prescription, which is based on the patient's caloric intake, particularly in patients with chronic liver disease.[136] It is difficult to improve the patient's strength or endurance if his or her caloric intake is insufficient for the energy requirements of exercise.
   b. Review the patient's laboratory values to determine treatment parameters for that session.[137] Refer to Chapters 7 and 14 for pertinent sections on complete blood count, coagulation profile, and lab value guidelines for activity.
2. Patients with GI dysfunction may have certain positioning precautions.
   a. Dysphagia can be exacerbated in supine positions and may also lead to aspiration pneumonia.[138]
   b. Portal hypertension can be exacerbated in the supine position because of gravitational effects on venous flow.
   c. If the patient has associated esophageal varices from portal hypertension, then the risk of variceal rupture may be increased in this position as well.
   d. Patients with portal hypertension and esophageal varices should also avoid maneuvers that create a Valsalva effect, such as coughing. The increase in intraabdominal pressure from Valsalva maneuvers can further exacerbate the esophageal varices.[139] (Huffing, instead of coughing, may be more beneficial in these situations.)
3. Nonpharmacologic pain management techniques from the physical therapist may benefit patients who have concurrent diagnoses of rheumatologic disorders and GI dysfunction.
   a. Because NSAIDs are a causative risk factor for many inflammatory and hemorrhagic conditions of the GI system, these medications typically are weaned or discontinued from the patient with any exacerbation of these conditions.
   b. Therefore patients who were reliant on NSAIDs for pain management before admission for their rheumatologic conditions may have limitations in functional mobility as a result of altered pain management.
4. Patients with ascites or large abdominal incisions are at risk for pulmonary complications. Ascites and surgical incisions create ventilatory restrictions for the patient.[136,140,141]
   a. In addition, these conditions can hinder cough effectiveness and functional mobility, both of which can further contribute to pulmonary infection.

TABLE 8-10 Common GI Surgical Procedures

Appendectomy	Removal of the appendix. Performed either through open laparotomy or laparoscopically.
Cholecystectomy	Removal of the gallbladder. Generally performed laparoscopically.
Colectomy	Resection of a portion of the colon. The name of the surgical procedure generally includes the section removed (e.g., transverse colectomy is resection of the transverse colon). A colectomy may also have an associated colostomy or ileostomy. Performed either through open laparotomy or laparoscopically.
Colostomy	A procedure used to divert stool from a portion of the diseased colon to the exterior. There are three general types of colostomies: end, double-barrel, and loop colostomy.
End (Brooke) colostomy	Involves bringing the functioning end of the intestine (the section of bowel that remains connected to the upper GI tract) out onto the surface of the abdomen and forming the stoma by cuffing the intestine back on itself and suturing the end to the skin.
Double-barrel colostomy	Two separate stomas are formed on the abdominal wall. The proximal stoma is the functional end that is connected to the upper GI tract and will drain stool. The distal stoma, also called a *mucous fistula*, is connected to the rectum to drain small amounts of mucus material. This is most often a temporary colostomy.
Loop colostomy	Created by bringing a loop of bowel through an incision in the abdominal wall. An incision is made in the bowel to allow the passage of stool through the loop colostomy. Also used as a temporary colostomy.
Fundoplication	Upper curve of stomach (fundus) is wrapped around the esophagus at its juncture with the stomach. Helps to reinforce the esophageal sphincter in situations of hernia and/or manage GERD to prevent acid reflux.[32]
Gastric bypass	Creation of a small gastric pouch to limit oral intake in restrictive and malabsorptive disorders.[105,107]
Roux-en-Y	Creation of a gastric pouch with 20-30 ml capacity via stapling, with stoma that is attached to jejunum (distal stomach and proximal small bowel bypassed). Performed open and laparoscopically (Figure 8-4).[105,107]
Vertical banded gastroplasty	Creates a small gastric pouch via permanent stapling, with an outlet from the pouch that is restricted by a band or ring that slows emptying of food to the small intestine (see Figure 8-4).[105,106]
Adjustable gastric banding	Creates a small pouch in the upper stomach using an adjustable silicone band, with a resulting narrow outlet to the small intestine (see Figure 8-4).[105,107]
Gastrectomy	Removal of a portion (partial) or all (total) of the stomach. Indicated for gastric cancer and peptic ulcer disease. Partial gastrectomy may either be a Billroth I or Billroth II procedure.
Billroth I (gastroduodenostomy)	Resection of the pyloric portion of the stomach and anastomosis with the duodenum.
Billroth II (gastrojejunostomy)	Resection of the distal portion of the stomach and the duodenum and anastomosis with the jejunum.
Ileostomy	A procedure similar to a colostomy and performed in areas of the ileum (distal portion of the small intestine). A continent ileostomy is another method of diverting stool that, instead of draining into an external pouch, drains either into more distal and functioning portions of the intestine or into an internal pouch that is surgically created from the small intestine.
Resection and reanastomosis	The removal (resection) of a nonfunctioning portion of the GI tract and the reconnection (reanastomosis) of proximal and distal GI portions that are functional. The name of the procedure will then include the sections that are resected or reanastomosed—for example, a pancreaticojejunostomy is the joining of the pancreatic duct to the jejunum after a dysfunctional portion of the pancreas is resected.
Whipple procedure (pancreaticoduodenectomy)	Consists of en bloc removal of the duodenum, a variable portion of the distal stomach and the jejunum, gallbladder, common bile duct, and regional lymph nodes. This removal is followed by pancreaticojejunostomy, choledochojejunostomy, and gastrojejunostomy. This procedure is reserved for the patient with severe or unremitting chronic pancreatitis or pancreatic cancer.
GI Transplantation	Approved transplant procedures for patients with irreversible intestinal failure include isolated intestinal, combined liver-small intestine and multivisceral transplantation. Refer to Chapter 14 for a description of transplant considerations.

Data from Cox, JA, Rogers, MA, Cox, SD: Treating benign colon disorders using laparoscopic colectomy, AORN J 73(2), 2001, 375; Beckingham IJ: ABC of diseases of liver, pancreas, and biliary system, gallstone disease, BMJ 322(7278):91, 2001; Pedersen AG, Petersen OB, Wara P et al: Randomized clinical trial of laparoscopic versus open appendicectomy, Br J Surg 88(2), 200-205, 2001; McMahon AJ, Fischbacher CM, Frame SH, et al: Impact of laparoscopic cholecystectomy: a population-based study, Lancet 356(9242):1632, 2000; Ben-David K, Sarosi GA: Appendicitis. In Feldman M, Friedman LS, Brandt LJ, editors: Sleisenger and Fordtran's gastrointestinal and liver disease, ed 9, Philadelphia, 2010, Saunders, pp 2059-2071; Julka K, Ko CW: Infectious diseases and the gallbladder, Infect Dis Clin N Am 24:885-898, 2010; Cima RR, Pemberton JH: Ileostomy, colostomy and pouches. In Feldman M, Friedman LS, Brandt LJ, editors: Sleisenger and Fordtran's gastrointestinal and liver disease, ed 9, Philadelphia, 2010, Saunders, pp 2015-2025; Mann BD: Surgery: a competency-based companion, Philadelphia, 2011, Saunders; Colquitt JL, Picot J, Loveman E, Clegg AJ: Surgery for obesity, Cochrane Database Syst Rev 2009(2):CD003641, 2009. doi:10.1002/14651858.DC006341.pub3.; Abrams P, Abu-Elmagd K, Felmet K et al: Intestinal and multivisceral transplantation. In Vincent JL, Abraham E, Moore FA et al, editors: Textbook of critical care, ed 6, St Louis, 2011, Elsevier, pp 1443-1453.

COMMON BARIATRIC PROCEDURES

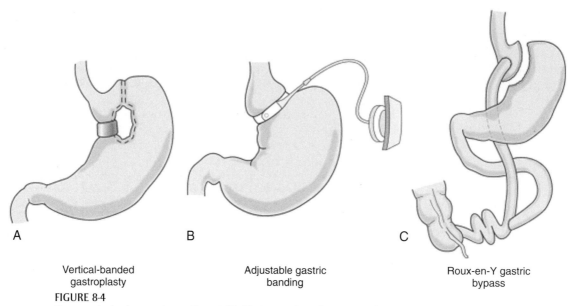

A	B	C
Vertical-banded gastroplasty	Adjustable gastric banding	Roux-en-Y gastric bypass

FIGURE 8-4

Common bariatric procedures. (From Still CD, Jensen GL: Obesity. In Rakel RE, Bope ET, editors: Conn's current therapy, ed 60, Philadelphia, 2008, Saunders.)

b. Effective pain management before physical therapy intervention, along with diligent position changes, instruction on incisional splinting during deep breathing and coughing, and early mobilization with or without assistive devices, will help prevent the development of pulmonary complications and deconditioning.[142]

References

1. McQuaid K: Approach to the patient with gastrointestinal disease. In Goldman L, Schafer AI, editors: Goldman's Cecil medicine, ed 24, Philadelphia, 2011, Saunders.
2. Panus PC, Katzung B, Jobst EE et al: Opioid analgesics and antagonists. In Pharmacology for the physical therapist, New York, 2009, McGraw-Hill.
3. Seidel HM, Ball JW, Dains JE et al: Mosby's guide to physical examination, ed 5, St Louis, 2003, Mosby, pp 525-583.
4. Skipworth RJE, Fearon KCH: Acute abdomen: peritonitis, Surgery (Oxford) 23(6):204-207, 2005.
5. Malarkey LM, McMorrow ME, editors: Nurse's manual of laboratory tests and diagnostic procedures, Philadelphia, 2000, Saunders, pp 412-431, 469-549.
6. Naghibalhossaini F, Ebadi P: Evidence for CEA release from human colon cancer cells by an endogenous GPI-PLD enzyme, Cancer Lett 234(2), 2006, 158-167, 2006.
7. Oh DS, Wang HS, Ohning GV et al: Validation of a new endoscopic technique to assess acid output in Zollinger-Ellison syndrome, Clin Gastroenterol Hepatol 4(12):1467-1473, 2006.
8. Ricci C, Holton J, Vaira D: Diagnosis of *Helicobacter pylori*: invasive and non-invasive tests, Best Pract Res Clin Gastroenterol 21(2):299-313, 2007.
9. Van der Horst-Schrivers ANA, Post WJ, Kema IP et al: Persistent low urinary excretion of 5-HIAA is a marker for favourable survival during follow-up in patients with disseminated midgut carcinoid tumours, Eur J Cancer 43(18):2651-2657, 2007.
10. Tornblom H, Lindberg G, Nyberg B et al: Full-thickness biopsy of the jejunum reveals inflammation and enteric neuropathy in irritable bowel syndrome, Gastroenterology 123(6):1972-1979, 2002.
11. Lee KJ, Inoue M, Otani T et al: Colorectal cancer screening using fecal occult blood test and subsequent risk of colorectal cancer: a prospective cohort study in Japan, Cancer Detect Prev 31(3):3-11, 2007.
12. Anjaneyulu V, Shankar-Swarnalatha G, Chandra-Sekhar Rao S: Carcinoid tumor of the gall bladder, Ann Diagn Pathol 11(2):113-116, 2007.
13. Malarkey LM, McMorrow ME, editors: Nurse's manual of laboratory tests and diagnostic procedures, Philadelphia, 2000, Saunders, p 469.
14. Knight JA: Liver function tests: their role in the diagnosis of hepatobiliary diseases, J Infus Nurs 28(2):108-117, 2005.
15. Kapelman B: Approach to the patient with liver disease. In Sachar DB, Waye JD, Lewis BS, editors: Pocket guide to gastroenterology, Baltimore, 1991, Williams & Wilkins, p 90.
16. Laparoscopy. In Pagana KD, Pagana TJ: Mosby's diagnostic and laboratory test reference, ed 9, St Louis, 2009, Mosby, pp 589-592.
17. MRI and MRC reveals distinct features in rare type of liver cancer, Hepatitis Wkly, April 23, 2001.
18. Modahl L, Digumarthy SR, Rhea JT et al: Emergency department abdominal computed tomography for nontraumatic abdominal pain: optimizing utilization, J Am Coll Radiol 3(11):860-866, 2006.
19. Beets-Tan RGH, Beets GL, Vliegen RFA et al: Accuracy of magnetic resonance imaging in prediction of tumour-free resection margin in rectal cancer surgery, Lancet 357(9255):497, 2001.
20. Goh V, Padhani AR, Rasheed S: Functional imaging of colorectal cancer angiogenesis, Lancet Oncol 8(3):245-255, 2007.

21. Brancatelli G, Federle MP, Ambrosini R et al: Cirrhosis: CT and MRI imaging evaluation, Eur J Radiol 91:57-69, 2007.

22. Kwon RS, Sahani DV, Brugge WR: Gastrointestinal cancer imaging, Gastroenterology 128(6):1538-1553, 2005.

23. Mittra E, Quon A: Positron emission tomography/computer tomography: the current technology and applications, Radiol Clin North Am 47:147-160, 2009.

24. Lowell MJ: Esophagus, stomach and duodenum. In Marx JA, Hockberger RS, Walls RM, editors: Rosen's emergency medicine, ed 7, St Louis, 2009, Mosby, pp 1137-1152.

25. Satpathy HK: Dysphagia. In Ferri's clinical advisor 2013, St Louis, 2013, Mosby.

26. Kahrilas PJ, Pandolfino JE: Esophageal neuromuscular function and motility disorders. In Feldman M, Friedman LS, Brandt LJ, editors: Sleisenger and Fordtran's gastrointestinal and liver disease, ed 9, St Louis, 2012, Saunders, pp 677-705.

27. Boeckxstaens GEE: Achalasia, Best Pract Res Clin Gastroenterol 21(4):595-608, 2007.

28. Sifrim D, Fornari F: Non-achalasic motor disorders of the oesophagus, Best Pract Res Clin Gastroenterol 21(4):575-593, 2007.

29. Ferri F: Gastroesophageal reflux disease. In Ferri F, editor: Ferri's clinical advisor 2013, St Louis, 2013, Mosby.

30. Pace B, Lynm C, Glass RM: Gastroesophageal reflux disease, JAMA 285(18):2408, 2001.

31. Richter JE: Gastroesophageal reflux disease, Best Pract Res Clin Gastroenterol 21(4):609-631, 2007.

32. Kelly JJ, Watson DI, Chin KF et al: Laparoscopic Nissen fundoplication: clinical outcomes at 10 years, J Am Coll Surg 205(4):570-575, 2007.

33. The AGA Institute Medical Position Panel: American Gastrointestinal Association medical position statement on the management of Barrett's esophagus, Gastroenterology 140:1084-1091, 2011.

34. Morales TG, Sampliner RE: Barrett's esophagus, Arch Intern Med 159(13):1411, 1999.

35. Atherfold PA, Jankowski JA: Molecular biology of Barrett's cancer, Best Pract Res Clin Gastroenterol 20(5):813-827, 2006.

36. Spechler SJ, Lee E, Ahnen D et al: Long-term outcome of medical and surgical therapies for gastroesophageal reflux disease: follow-up of a randomized controlled trial, JAMA 285(18):2331, 2001.

37. Jankowski JA, Harrison RF, Perry I et al: Barrett's metaplasia, Lancet 356(9247):2079, 2000.

38. Lo GH: The role of endoscopy in secondary prophylaxis of esophageal varices, Clin Liver Dis 14(2):307-323, 2010.

39. Miller WO, van Ness MM: Esophageal varices. In van Ness MM, Chobanian SJ, editors: Manual of clinical problems in gastroenterology, Boston, 1994, Little, Brown, p 195.

40. Lucas BD: A practical approach to acute lower GI bleeding, Patient Care 34(4):23, 2000.

41. Meaden C, Makin AJ: Diagnosis and treatment of patients with gastrointestinal bleeding, Curr Anaesth Critical Care 15(2):123-132, 2004.

42. Jensen DM: Gastrointestinal hemorrhage and occult gastrointestinal bleeding. In Goldman L, Schafer AI, editors: Goldman's Cecil medicine, ed 24, Philadelphia, 2011, Saunders, pp 857-862.

43. Hines SE: Current management of upper GI tract bleeding, Patient Care 34(2):20, 2000.

44. Ferri F: Gastritis. In Ferri F, editor: Ferri's clinical advisor 2013, St Louis, 2013, Mosby.

45. McManus TJ: Helicobacter pylori: an emerging infectious disease, Nurse Pract 25(8):40, 2000.

46. de Boer WA, Tytgat GNJ: Treatment of Helicobacter pylori infection, BMJ 320(7226):31, 2000.

47. Wolle K, Malfertheiner P: Treatment of Helicobacter pylori, Best Pract Res Clin Gastroenterol 21(2):315-324, 2007.

48. Jain KS, Shah AK, Bariwal J et al: Recent advances in proton pump inhibitors and management of acid-peptic disorders, Bioorg Med Chem 15(3):1181-1205, 2007.

49. Lai LH, Sung JJY: Helicobacter pylori and benign upper digestive disease, Best Pract Res Clin Gastroenterol 21(2):261-279, 2007.

50. Jones MP: The role of psychosocial factors in peptic ulcer disease: beyond Helicobacter pylori and NSAIDs, J Psychosom Res 60(4):407-412, 2006.

51. Majumdar D, Atherton J: Peptic ulcers and their complications, Surgery (Oxford) 24(3):110-114, 2006.

52. Ferri F: Peptic ulcer disease. In Ferri F, editor: Ferri's clinical advisor 2013, St Louis, 2013, Mosby.

53. Mark DH, Norton JA: Surgery to cure the Zollinger-Ellison syndrome, JAMA 282(14):1316, 1999.

54. Hoffman KM, Furukawa M, Jensen RT: Duodenal neuroendocrine tumors: classification, functional syndromes, diagnosis and medical treatment, Best Pract Res Clin Gastroenterol 19(5):675-697, 2005.

55. Morrow EH, Norton JA: Surgical management of Zollinger-Ellison syndrome: state of the art, Surg Clin North Am 89:1091-1103, 2009.

56. Tack J: Gastric motor disorders, Best Pract Res Clin Gastroenterol 21(4):633-644, 2007.

57. Blanton WP, Oviedo JA, Wolfe MM: Diseases of the stomach and duodenum. In Andreoli TE, Benjamin IJ, Griggs RC et al, editors: Andreoli and Carpenter's Cecil essentials of medicine, ed 8, Philadelphia, 2010, Saunders.

58. Ben-David K, Sarosi GA: Appendicitis. In Feldman M, Friedman LS, Brandt LJ, editors: Sleisenger and Fordtran's gastrointestinal and liver disease, ed 9, Philadelphia, 2010, Saunders, pp 2059-2071.

59. Dominguez EP, Sweene, JF, Choi YU: Diagnosis and management of diverticulitis and appendicitis, Gastroenterol Clin North Am 35(2):367-391, 2006.

60. Manfredi RA, Ranniger C: Appendicitis. In Adams JG, Barton ED, Collings J et al, editors: Emergency medicine, Philadelphia, 2008, Saunders, pp 371-377.

61. Cox JA, Rogers MA, Cox SD: Treating benign colon disorders using laparoscopic colectomy, AORN J 73(2):375, 2001.

62. Ferri F: Diverticular disease (diverticulosis, diverticulitis). In Ferri F, editor: Ferri's clinical advisor 2013, St Louis, 2013, Mosby.

63. Touzios JG, Dozios EJ: Diverticulosis and acute diverticulitis, Gastroenterol Clin North Am 38:513-525, 2009.

64. Ferzoco LB, Raptopoulous V, Silen W: Acute diverticulitis, N Engl J Med 338(21):1521-1526, 1998.

65. Sinha R, Rajiah P, Tiwary P: Abdominal hernias: imaging review and historical perspectives, Curr Probl Diagn Radiol 36(1):30-42, 2007.

66. Malangoni MA, Rosen MJ: Hernias. In Townsend CM, Beauchamp RD, Evers BM et al, editors: Sabiston textbook of surgery, ed 19, Philadelphia, 2012, Saunders, pp 1114-1140.

67. Kingsnorth A, LeBlanc K: Hernias: inguinal and incisional, Lancet 362(9395):1561-1571, 2003.

68. Gray SH, Hawn MT, Itani KMF: Surgical progress in inguinal and ventral incisional hernia repair, Surg Clin North Am 88:17-26, 2008.

69. Brady MF: Hiatal hernia. In Ferri F, editor: Ferri's clinical advisor 2013, St Louis, 2013, Mosby.

70. Macutkiewicz C, Carlson G: Acute abdomen: intestinal instruction, Surgery (Oxford) 23(6):208-212, 2005.

71. Turner JR: The gastrointestinal tract. In Kumar V, Abbas AK, Fausto N et al, editors: Robbins and Cotran pathologic basis of disease, professional edition, ed 8, Philadelphia, 2009, Saunders.

72. Luckey A, Livingston E, Tache Y: Mechanisms and treatment of postoperative ileus, Arch Surg 138:206-214, 2003, 2003.

73. Turnage RH, Heldman M: Intestinal obstruction. In Feldman M, Friedman LS, Brandt LJ, editors: Sleisenger and Fordtran's gastrointestinal and liver disease, ed 9, Philadelphia, 2010, Saunders, pp 2105-2120.

74. Franklin ME, Gonzalez JJ, Miter DB et al: Laparoscopic diagnosis and treatment of intestinal obstruction, Surg Endosc 18:26-30, 2004.

75. Schuster TG, Montie JE: Postoperative ileus after abdominal surgery, Urology 59(4):465-471, 2002.

76. Brandt LJ, Feuerstadt P: Intestinal ischemia. In Feldman M, Friedman LS, Brandt LJ, editors: Sleisenger and Fordtran's gastrointestinal and liver disease, ed 9, Philadelphia, 2010, Saunders, pp 2027-2048.

77. van Vlitjmen EF, Brouwer JL, Veeger NJ et al: Oral contraceptives and the absolute risk of venous thromboembolism in women with single or multiple thrombophilic defects. Results from a retrospective family cohort study, Arch Intern Med 167(3):282-289, 2007.

78. Scharff JR, Longo WE, Vartanian SM et al: Ischemic colitis: spectrum of disease and outcome, Surgery 134(4):624-629, 2003.

79. Cangemi JR, Picco MF: Intestinal ischemia in the elderly, Gastroenterol Clin North Am 38:527-540, 2009.

80. Ferri F: Irritable bowel syndrome. In Ferri F, editor: Ferri's clinical advisor 2013, St Louis, 2013, Mosby.

81. Spiller R: Clinical update: irritable bowel syndrome, Lancet 369(9573):1586-1588, 2007.

82. Hasler WL: Traditional thoughts on the pathophysiology of irritable bowel syndrome, Gastroenterol Clin North Am 40:21-43, 2011.

83. Voelker R: Bacteria and irritable bowel, JAMA 285(4):401, 2001.

84. Jailwala J, Imperiale TF, Kroenke K: Pharmacologic treatment of the irritable bowel syndrome: a systematic review of randomized, controlled trials, Ann Intern Med 133(2):136, 2000.

85. Kierszenbaum AL, Tres LL: Histology and cell biology, an introduction to pathology, ed 3, Philadelphia, 2011, Saunders.

86. Bartusek D, Valek V, Husty J et al: Small bowel ultrasound in patients with celiac disease: retrospective study, Eur J Radiol 63(2):302-306, 2007.

87. Disease of the Alimentary Tract. In Stevens A, Lowe J, Scott I, editors: Core pathology, ed 3, 2008, Elsevier.

88. Tsai PM, Duggan C: Malabsorption syndromes. In Strain J, editor: Encyclopedia of human nutrition, St Louis, 2005, Elsevier, pp 196-203.

89. Schiller LR: Diarrhea and malabsorption in the elderly, Gastroenterol Clin North Am 38:481-502, 2009.

90. Krige JE, Beckingham IJ: ABC of diseases of liver, pancreas, and biliary system: portal hypertension—2. Ascites, encephalopathy, and other conditions, BMJ 322(7283):416-418, 2001.

91. Prather C: Inflammatory and anatomic diseases of the intestine, peritoneum, mesentery, and omentum. In Goldman L, Schafer AI, editors: Goldman's Cecil medicine, ed 24, Philadelphia, 2011, Saunders, pp 921-928.

92. Blumberg RS, Strober W: Prospects for research in inflammatory bowel disease, JAMA 285(5):643, 2001.

93. Sands BE, Siegel CA: Crohn's disease. In Feldman M, Friedman LS, Brandt LJ, editors: Sleisenger and Fordtran's gastrointestinal and liver disease, ed 9, Philadelphia, 2010, Saunders, pp 1941-1973.

94. Schreiber S: Safety and efficacy of recombinant human interleukin 10 in chronic active Crohn's disease, JAMA 285(11):1421, 2001.

95. Ho GT, Lees C, Satsangi J: Ulcerative colitis, Medicine 35(5) 277-282, 2007.

96. Osterman MT, Lichtenstein GR: Ulcerative colitis. In Feldman M, Friedman LS, Brandt LJ, editors: Sleisenger and Fordtran's gastrointestinal and liver disease, ed 9, Philadelphia, 2010, Saunders, pp 1975-2012.

97. Colorectal polyps: latest guidelines for detection and follow-up, Consultant 41(3):364, 2001.

98. Management of colonic polyps and adenomas. The Society for Surgery of the Alimentary Tract (SSAT) patient guidelines. http://www.ssat.com/cgi-bin/polyps.cgi. Accessed July 13, 2012.

99. Levin B, Lieberman DA, McFarland B et al: Screening and surveillance for the early detection of colorectal cancer and adenomatous polyps, 2008: A joint guideline from the American Cancer Society, the U.S. Multi-Society Task Force on Colorectal Cancer, and the American College of Radiology, CA 58:130-160, 2008.

100. Gallagher S: Taking the weight off with bariatric surgery, Nursing 34(3):58-63, 2004.

101. Blackwood HS: Obesity: a rapidly expanding challenge, Nurs Manage 35(5):27-36, 2004.

102. Huang IC, Frangakis C, Wu AW: The relationship of excess body weight and health-related quality of life: evidence from a population study in Taiwan, Int J Obes 30(8):1250-1259, 2006.

103. Madan AK, Orth W, Ternovits CA et al: Metabolic syndrome: yet another co-morbidity gastric bypass helps cure, Surg Obes Related Dis 2(1):48-51, 2006.

104. Jamal MK, DeMaria EJ, Johnson JM et al: Impact of major co-morbidities on mortality and complications after gastric bypass, Surg Obes Related Dis 1(6):511-516, 2005.

105. Colquitt JL, Picot J, Loveman E et al: Surgery for obesity, Cochrane Database Syst Rev (2):CD003641, 2009.

106. Miller K: Obesity: surgical options, Best Pract Res Clin Gastroenterol 18(6):1147-1165, 2004.

107. Sheipe M: Breaking through obesity with gastric bypass surgery, Nurse Pract 31(10):12-21, 2006.

108. Livhitis M, Mercado C, Yermilov I et al: Exercise following bariatric surgery: systematic review, Obes Surg 20:657-665, 2010.

109. Tompkins J, Bosch PR, Chenowith R et al: Changes in functional walking distance and health-related quality of life after gastric bypass surgery, Phys Ther 88:928-935, 2008.

110. Davidson JE, Kruse MW, Cox DH et al: Critical care of the morbidly obese, Crit Care Nurs Q 26(2):105-116, 2003.

111. Baptiste A: Technology solutions for high-risk tasks in critical care, Crit Care Nurs Clin North Am 19(2):177-186, 2007.

112. Baptiste A, Evitt C, Kelleher V et al: Safe bariatric patient handling toolkit, Bariatric Nurs Surg Patient Care 2(1):17-46, 2007.

113. Muir M, Archer-Heese G: Essentials of a bariatric patient handling program, Online J Issues Nurs 14(1):1-8, 2009.

114. Genc A, Ozyurek S, Koca U et al: Respiratory and hemodynamic responses to mobilization of critically ill obese patients, Cardiopulm Phys Ther J 23(1):14-18, 2012.

115. Petering R, Webb CW: Exercise, fluid, and nutrition recommendations for the postgastric bypass exerciser, Curr Sports Med Rep 8(2):92-97, 2009.

116. Harrington JM, Wells CL: Cardiovascular and pulmonary considerations of the obese patient for the rehabilitation clinician, Bariatric Nurs Surg Patient Care 2(4):267-280, 2007.

117. Forti E, Ike D, Barbalho-Moulim B et al: Effects of chest physiotherapy on the respiratory function of postoperative gastroplasty patients, Clinics 67(7):683-689, 2009.

118. Wilson JA, Clark JJ: Obesity: impediment to wound healing, Crit Care Nurs Q 26(2):119-132, 2003.

118a. Hinkle C, Buchanan A, Paz J: Physical therapy management of patient status post bariatric surgery in acute care: a systematic review, *JACPT,* 2013 (in press).

119. The liver as an organ. In Hall JE, editor: Guyton and Hall textbook of medical physiology, ed 12, Philadelphia, 2011, Saunders, pp 837-839.

120. Pawlotsky JM, McHutchinson J: Chronic viral and autoimmune hepatitis. In Goldman L, Schafer AI, editors: Goldman's Cecil medicine, ed 24, Philadelphia, 2011, Saunders, pp 973-979.

121. Curry MP, Chopra S: Acute viral hepatitis. In Mandell GL, Bennett JE, Dolin R, editors: Mandell, Douglas and Bennett's principles and practice of infectious disease, ed 7, Philadelphia, 2009, Churchill Livingstone, pp 577-1592.

122. Gludd LL, Gludd C: Meta-analyses on viral hepatitis, Infect Dis Clin North Am 23:315-330, 2009.

123. Vaccine information statement: hepatitis B vaccine. U.S. Department of Health and Human Services, Centers for Disease Control. http://www.cdc.gov/vaccines/pubs/vis/downloads/vis-hep-b.pdf. Accessed July 16, 2012.

124. Cardenas A, Gines P: Management of complications of cirrhosis in patients awaiting liver transplantation, J Hepatol 42(1 Supp 1):S124-S133, 2005.

125. Ferri F: Cirrhosis. In Ferri F, editor: Ferri's clinical advisor 2013, St Louis, 2013, Mosby.

126. McAvoy NC, Hayes PC: Hepatic encephalopathy, Medicine 35(2):108-111, 2007.

127. Sundaram V, Shaikh OS: Hepatic encephalopathy: pathophysiology and emerging therapies, Med Clin North Am 93:819-836, 2009.

128. Zeimet A, McBride DR, Basilan R et al: Infectious diseases. In Rakel RR, Rakel DP, editors: Textbook of family medicine, ed 8, Philadelphia, 2011, Saunders, pp 207-247.

129. Beckingham IJ: ABC of diseases of liver, pancreas, and biliary system. Gallstone disease, BMJ 322(7278):91, 2001.

130. Yusoff IF, Barkun JS, Barkun AN: Diagnosis and management of cholecystitis and cholangitis, Gastroenterol Clin North Am 32(4):1145-1168, 2003.

131. Julka K, Ko CW: Infectious diseases and the gallbladder, Infect Dis Clin North Am 24:885-898, 2010.

132. Siva S, Pereira SP: Acute pancreatitis, Medicine 35(3):171-177, 2007.

133. Forsmark CE: Pancreatitis. In Goldman L, Schafer AI, editors: Goldman's Cecil medicine, ed 24, Philadelphia, 2011, Saunders, pp 938-944.

134. Pedersen AG, Petersen OB, Wara P et al: Randomized clinical trial of laparoscopic versus open appendicectomy, Br J Surg 88(2):200-205, 2001.

135. McMahon AJ, Fischbacher CM, Frame SH et al: Impact of laparoscopic cholecystectomy: a population-based study, Lancet 356(9242):1632, 2000.

136. Stockton KA: Exercise training in patients with chronic liver disease. Physiother Theory Pract 17:29-38, 2001.

137. Acute Care Section, American Physical Therapy Association: Lab values interpretation resources. Update 2012. http://www.acutept.org/associations/11622/files/labvalues.pdf. Accessed March 20, 2012.

138. Dean E: Oxygen transport deficits in systemic disease and implications for physical therapy, Phys Ther 77(2):187-202, 1997.

139. Dib N, Oberti F, Cales P: Current management of the complications of portal hypertension: variceal bleeding and ascites, CMAJ 174(10):1433-1443, 2006.

140. Brooks-Brunn JA: Postoperative atelectasis and pneumonia, Heart Lung 24:94-115, 1995.

141. Christensen EF, Schultz P, Jensen OV et al: Postoperative pulmonary complications and lung function in high-risk patients: a comparison of three physiotherapy regimens after upper abdominal surgery in general anesthesia, Acta Anaesth Scand 35:97-104, 1991.

142. Basse L, Raskov HH, Jakobsen DH et al: Accelerated postoperative recovery programme after colonic resection improves physical performance, pulmonary function and body composition, Brit J Surg 89:446-453, 2002.

Genitourinary System

Jaime C. Paz

CHAPTER OBJECTIVES

The objectives of this chapter are the following:

1. Provide a basic understanding of the structure and function of the genitourinary system
2. Provide information about the clinical evaluation of the genitourinary system, including physical examination and diagnostic studies
3. Describe the various health conditions of the genitourinary system
4. Provide information about the management of genitourinary disorders, including renal replacement therapy and surgical procedures
5. Give guidelines for physical therapy management in patients with genitourinary diseases and disorders

PREFERRED PRACTICE PATTERNS

The most relevant practice patterns for the diagnoses discussed in this chapter, based on the American Physical Therapy Association's *Guide to Physical Therapist Practice*, second edition, are as follows:

- Primary Prevention/Risk Reduction for Skeletal Demineralization: 4A
- Impaired Aerobic Capacity/Endurance Associated with Deconditioning: 6B
- Primary Prevention/Risk Reduction for Integumentary Disorders: 7A

Please refer to Appendix A for a complete list of the preferred practice patterns, as individual patient conditions are highly variable and other practice patterns may be applicable.

The regulation of fluid and electrolyte levels by the genitourinary system is an essential component of cellular and cardiovascular function. Imbalance of fluids, electrolytes, or both can lead to blood pressure changes or impaired metabolism that can ultimately influence the patient's activity tolerance (see Chapter 15). Genitourinary structures can also cause pain that is referred to the abdomen and back. To help differentiate neuromuscular and skeletal dysfunction from systemic dysfunction, physical therapists need to be aware of pain referral patterns from these structures (Table 9-1).

Body Structure and Function

The genitourinary system consists of two kidneys, two ureters, one urinary bladder, and one urethra. The genitourinary system also includes the reproductive organs: the prostate gland, testicles, and epididymis in men, and the uterus, fallopian tubes, ovaries, vagina, external genitalia, and perineum in women. Of these reproductive organs, only the prostate gland and uterus are discussed in this chapter.

The anatomy of the genitourinary system is shown in Figure 9-1. An expanded, frontal view of the kidney is shown in Figure 9-2. The functional unit of the kidney is the *nephron*, with approximately 1 million nephrons in each kidney. Urine is formed in the nephron through a process consisting of glomerular filtration, tubular reabsorption, and tubular secretion.[1]

The following are the primary functions of the genitourinary system[2]:

- Excretion of cellular waste products (e.g., urea and creatinine [Cr],) through urine formation and micturition (voiding).
- Regulation of blood volume by conserving or excreting fluids.

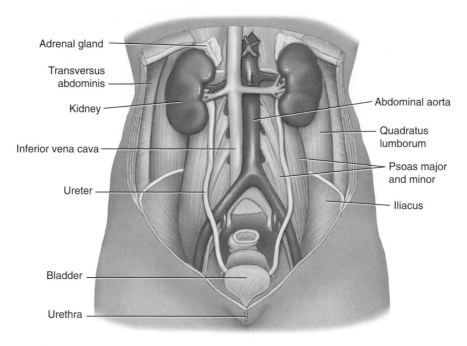

FIGURE 9-1
Schematic illustration of the genitourinary system, including trunk musculature.

TABLE 9-1 Segmental Innervation and Pain Referral Areas of the Urinary System

Structure	Segmental Innervation	Possible Pain Referral Area
Kidney	T10-L1	Lumbar spine (ipsilateral flank) Upper abdomen
Ureter	T11-L2, S2-S4	Groin Upper and lower abdomen Suprapubic region Scrotum Medial and proximal thigh Thoracolumbar region
Urinary bladder	T11-L2, S2-S4	Sacral apex Suprapubic region Thoracolumbar region

From Boissonault WG, Bass C: Pathological origins of trunk and neck pain: part 1. Pelvic and abdominal visceral disorders, J Orthop Phys Ther 12:194, 1990.

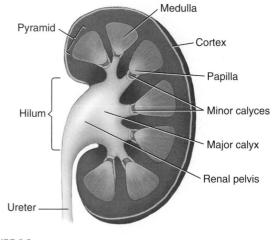

FIGURE 9-2
Renal cross-section.

- Electrolyte regulation by conserving or excreting minerals.
- Acid-base balance regulation (H^+ [acid] and HCO_3^- [base] ions are reabsorbed or excreted to maintain homeostasis).
- Arterial blood pressure regulation. Sodium excretion and renin secretion maintain homeostasis. Renin is secreted from the kidneys during states of hypotension, which results in formation of angiotensin I and II. Angiotensin causes vasoconstriction to help increase blood pressure. Angiotensin also triggers the release of aldosterone, resulting in conservation of water by the kidney.
- Erythropoietin secretion (necessary for stimulating red blood cell production).

The brain stem controls micturition through the autonomic nervous system. Parasympathetic fibers stimulate voiding, whereas sympathetic fibers inhibit it. The internal urethral sphincter of the bladder and the external urethral sphincter of the urethra control flow of urine.[3]

Clinical Evaluation

Evaluation of the genitourinary system involves the integration of patient history, physical findings, and laboratory data.

Physical Examination

History

Patients with suspected genitourinary pathology often present with characteristic complaints or subjective reports. Therefore a detailed history, thorough patient interview, review of the patient's medical record, or a combination of these provides a good beginning to the diagnostic process for possible genitourinary system pathology. The description of pain can offer clues as to its source: renal pain can be described as aching and dull in nature, whereas urinary pain is generally described as colicky (occurring in wavelike spasms) and/or intermittent.[4]

Changes in voiding habits or a description of micturition patterns are also noted during patient history and are listed here[4-6]:

- Dysuria (painful burning or discomfort during urination)
- Nocturia (urinary frequency, more than once, at night)
- Incomplete bladder emptying
- Difficulty initiating urinary stream
- Hematuria (blood in urine)
- Frequency (greater than every 2 hours)
- Hesitancy (weak or interrupted stream)
- Proteinuria (urine appears foamy)
- Oliguria (very low urine output, such as less than 400 ml in a 24-hour period)

✎ CLINICAL TIP

As a side effect of the medication phenazopyridine (Pyridium), a patient's urine may turn rust-colored and be misinterpreted as hematuria.[7] Pyridium is prescribed in the treatment of urinary pain and urgency. However, any new onset of possible hematuria should always be alerted to the medical team for proper delineation of the cause.

Observation

The presence of abdominal or pelvic distention, peripheral edema, incisions, scars, tubes, drains, and catheters should be noted when performing patient inspection, because these may reflect current pathology and recent interventions. Refer to Chapter 18 for more information on medical equipment. The physical therapist must handle external tubes and drains carefully during positioning or functional mobility treatments.

✎ CLINICAL TIP

Patients with genitourinary disorders may also present with skin changes, such as pallor or rough, dry skin.[6] Take caution in handling patients with skin changes from dehydration to prevent any skin tears that can lead to infection formation.

Palpation

The kidneys and a distended bladder are the only palpable structures of the genitourinary system. Distention or inflammation of the kidneys results in sharp or dull pain (depending on severity) with palpation.[6,8]

Percussion

Pain and tenderness that are present with fist percussion of the kidneys can be indicative of kidney infection or polycystic

kidney disease. Fist percussion is performed by placing one hand along the costovertebral angle of the patient and striking the dorsal surface of that hand with a closed fist of the examiner's other hand.[6] Direct percussion with a closed fist may also be performed over the costovertebral angles. The patient should feel a "thud" but not pain or tenderness.[8]

Auscultation

Auscultation is performed to examine the blood flow to the kidneys from the abdominal aorta and the renal arteries. The presence of bruits (murmurs) can indicate impaired perfusion to the kidneys, which can lead to renal dysfunction. Placement of the stethoscope is generally in the area of the costovertebral angles and the four abdominal quadrants. Refer to Chapter 8, Figure 8-2, for a diagram of the abdominal quadrants.[6,8]

Diagnostic Tests*

Urinalysis

Urinalysis is a very common diagnostic tool used not only to examine the genitourinary system, but also to help evaluate for the presence of other systemic diseases. Urine specimens can be collected by bladder catheterization or suprapubic aspiration of bladder urine, or by having the patient void into a sterile specimen container. Urinalysis is performed to examine[6,9,10]:

- Urine color, appearance, and odor
- Specific gravity, osmolarity, or both (concentration of urine ranges from 1.005 to 1.030)
- pH (4.6 to 8.0)
- Presence of glucose, ketones, proteins, bilirubin, urobilinogen, occult blood, red blood cells, white blood cells, crystals, casts, bacteria or other microorganisms
Urine abnormalities are summarized in Table 9-2.

✎ CLINICAL TIP

If the patient is having his or her urine collected (to measure hormone and metabolite levels), the physical therapist should have the patient use the predesignated receptacle in situations when the patient needs to urinate during a physical therapy session: this will ensure that the collection is not interrupted. The predesignated receptacle can be a urinal for men or a collection "hat" placed on the toilet or commode for women. If micturition occurs during a PT session, do not discard the urine, as it may be necessary to record or process the sample. Urine output (UO) may also be collected throughout the day to measure the patient's urine output relative to the patient's fluid intake (input). This provides a general estimate of the patient's renal function. Measurements of the patient's input and output are often abbreviated I/Os.

*The reference range of various laboratory values can vary among different facilities. Be sure to verify the reference values located in the laboratory test section of the medical record.

TABLE 9-2 Urine Abnormalities

Abnormality	Etiology
Glycosuria (presence of glucose)	Hyperglycemia and probable diabetes mellitus.
Proteinuria (presence of proteins)	Proteins are usually too large to be filtered; therefore permeability has abnormally increased. Can occur with diabetes, acute or chronic kidney disease, nephrotic syndrome, congestive heart failure, systemic lupus erythematosus.
Hematuria (presence of blood and red blood cells)	Possible urinary tract bleeding or kidney diseases (calculi, cystitis, neoplasm, glomerulonephritis, or miliary tuberculosis).
Bacteriuria (presence of bacteria)	Generally indicates urinary tract infection. Urine is generally cloudy in appearance, with the possible presence of white blood cells.
Ketonuria (presence of ketones)*	Can result from diabetes, fasting or starvation, a high-protein diet, and alcoholism.
Bilirubinuria (presence of bilirubin)	Usually an early indicator of liver disease and hepatocellular jaundice.
Crystals (end products of food metabolism)	Can occur with renal stones, gout, parathyroid or malabsorption abnormalities.

Data from Bates P: Nursing assessment: urinary system. In Lewis SM, Heitkemper MM, Dirksen SR, editors: Medical-surgical nursing: assessment and management of clinical problems, ed 5, St Louis, 2000, Mosby, pp 1241-1255; Abdomen. In Seidel HM, Ball JW, Dains JE, et al, editors: Mosby's guide to physical examination, ed 5, St Louis, 2003, Mosby, p 551; Weigel KA, Potter CK: Assessment of the renal system. In Monahan FD, Neighbors M, Sands JK, editors: Phipps' medical-surgical nursing: health and illness perspectives, ed 8, St Louis, 2008, Mosby, pp 943-960; Pagana KD, Pagana TJ: Mosby's diagnostic and laboratory test reference, ed 9, St Louis, 2009, Mosby.

*Ketones are formed from protein and fat metabolism, and trace amounts in the urine are normal.

Creatinine Tests

Two measurements of Cr (end product of muscle metabolism) are performed: measurements of plasma Cr and Cr clearance. Plasma Cr is measured by drawing a sample of venous blood. Increased levels are indicative of decreased renal function. The reference range of plasma Cr is 0.5 to 1.2 mg/dl.[10]

Cr clearance, also called a 24-hour urine test, specifically measures glomerular filtration rate. Decreased clearance (indicated by elevated levels of plasma creatinine relative to creatinine levels in the urine) indicates decreased renal function. The reference range of Cr clearance is 87 to 139 ml per minute.[10]

Estimated Glomerular Filtration Rate

The 24-hour urine collection necessary to measure creatinine clearance has become time consuming and expensive to perform, resulting in a prediction equation for glomerular filtration rate (eGFR). This estimate includes the patient's age, gender,

ethnicity, and serum (blood) creatinine with a reference value of greater than 60 ml/min/1.73 m^2.[10]

Blood Urea Nitrogen

As an end product of protein and amino acid metabolism, increased blood urea nitrogen (BUN) levels can be indicative of any of the following: decreased renal function or fluid intake, increased muscle (protein) catabolism, increased protein intake, congestive heart failure, or acute infection. Levels of BUN need to be correlated with plasma Cr levels to implicate renal dysfunction, because BUN level can be affected by decreased fluid intake, increased muscle catabolism, increased protein intake, and acute infection. Alterations in BUN and Cr level can also lead to an alteration in the patient's mental status. The reference range of BUN is 10 to 20 mg/dl in adults.[6,9,10]

> ✎ **CLINICAL TIP**
> Noting BUN and Cr levels on a daily basis for any changes may help explain changes in the patient's mental status, participation in physical therapy sessions, or both.

Radiographic Examination

Kidneys, Ureters, and Bladder X-Ray. An x-ray of the kidneys, ureters, and bladder (a procedure often abbreviated as "KUB") is generally performed as an initial screening tool for genitourinary disorders. The size, shape, and position of the renal, ureteral, and bladder structures are delineated to help identify renal calculi (kidney stones), tumor growth or shrinkage (chronic pyelonephritis), and calcifications in the bladder wall. A KUB can also be performed when internal hemorrhage is suspected after major traumatic incidents. Identification of any of these disorders requires further evaluation.[6,9,11]

Pyelography. Radiopaque dyes are used to radiographically examine the urinary system. Two types of tests are performed: intravenous pyelography (IVP) and retrograde urography.

Intravenous pyelography consists of (1) taking a baseline radiograph of the genitourinary system, (2) intravenous injection of contrast dye, and (3) sequential radiographs to evaluate the size, shape, and location of urinary tract structures and to evaluate renal excretory function. The location of urinary obstruction or cause of nontraumatic hematuria may be also be identified with this procedure.[6,9,11]

Retrograde urography consists of passing a catheter or cystoscope into the bladder and then proximally into the ureters before injecting the contrast dye. This procedure is usually performed in conjunction with a cystoscopic examination and is indicated when urinary obstruction or trauma to the genitourinary system is suspected. Evaluation of urethral stent or catheter placement can also be performed with this procedure.[5,6,9,11]

Renal Arteriography. Renal arteriography consists of injecting radiopaque dye into the renal artery (arteriography) through a catheter that is inserted into the femoral or brachial artery. Arterial blood supply to the kidneys can then be examined radiographically. Indications for arteriography include suspected aneurysm, renal artery stenosis, renovascular hypertension and trauma, palpable renal masses, chronic pyelonephritis, renal abscesses, and determination of the suitability of a (donor) kidney for renal transplantation.[9-12]

> ✎ **CLINICAL TIP**
>
> Patients who are scheduled for procedures involving contrast dye are generally restricted from eating or drinking 8 hours before the procedure. A patient who is scheduled for an afternoon procedure may therefore be fatigued earlier in the day and may want to defer a scheduled therapy session. Modifying the intended therapy session and respecting the person's wishes at this time are both suitable alternatives.

Bladder Examination: Cystoscopy

Cystoscopy consists of passing a flexible, fiberoptic scope through the urethra into the bladder to examine the bladder neck, urothelial lining, and ureteral orifices. The patient is generally placed under general or local anesthesia during this procedure. Cystoscopy is performed to directly examine the prostate in men, bladder, urethra, and ureters, as well as to examine the causes of urinary dysfunction and for removal of small tumors.[9,10]

> ✎ **CLINICAL TIP**
>
> Patients may experience urinary frequency or dysuria after cystoscopic procedures; therefore the therapist should be prepared for sudden interruptions during a therapy session that is conducted the same day after this diagnostic procedure.

Cystometry (Cystometrogram)

Cystometry is used to evaluate motor and sensory function of the bladder in patients with incontinence or evidence of neurologic bladder dysfunction. The procedure consists of inserting a catheter into the bladder, followed by saline instillation and pressure measurements of the bladder wall.[6,10,11]

Renal Scanning

The structure, function, and perfusion of the kidneys can be examined with a nuclear scan using different radioisotopes for different testing procedures and structures.[10]

Ultrasonography Studies

Ultrasound is used to (1) evaluate kidney size, shape, and position; (2) determine the presence of kidney stones, cysts, and prerenal collections of blood, pus, lymph, urine, and solid masses; (3) identify the presence of a dilated collecting system; and (4) help guide needle placement for biopsy or drainage of a renal abscess or for placement of a nephrostomy tube.[9] It is the test of choice to help rule out urinary tract obstruction.[11]

Computed Tomography Scan

Indications for computed tomography (CT) of the genitourinary system include defining renal parenchyma abnormalities and

differentiating solid mass densities as cystic or hemorrhagic. Kidney size and shape, as well as the presence of cysts, abscesses, tumors, calculi, congenital abnormalities, infections, hematomas, and collecting system dilation, can also be assessed with CT.[5,9-11]

Magnetic Resonance Imaging and Angiography

Multiple uses for magnetic resonance imaging (MRI) and angiography (MRA) include imaging the renal vascular system, staging of renal cell carcinoma, identifying bladder tumors and their local metastases, and distinguishing between benign and malignant prostate tumors.[9,10]

Biopsies

Renal Biopsy. A renal biopsy consists of examining a small portion of renal tissue that is obtained percutaneously with a needle to determine the pathologic state and diagnosis of a renal disorder, monitor kidney disease progression, evaluate response to medical treatment, and assess for rejection of a renal transplant. A local anesthetic is provided during the procedure, and accuracy of biopsy location is improved when guided by ultrasound, fluoroscope, or CT scanning.[6,9-11]

Bladder, Prostate, and Urethral Biopsies. Bladder, prostate, and urethral biopsies involve taking tissue specimens from the bladder, prostate, and urethra with a cystoscope, or needle aspiration via the transrectal or transperineal approach. Biopsy of the prostate can also be performed through an open biopsy procedure, which involves incising the perineal area and removing a wedge of prostate tissue. Examination for pain, hematuria, and suspected neoplasm are indications for these biopsies.[9]

Health Conditions

Renal System Dysfunction

Acute Kidney Injury

Acute kidney injury (AKI) (formerly known as acute renal failure [ARF]) can result from a variety of causes and is defined as an abrupt or rapid deterioration in renal function that results in a rise in serum creatinine levels or blood urea nitrogen with or without decreased urine output occurring over hours or days.[13] There are three types of AKI, categorized by their etiology: prerenal, intrinsic, and postrenal.[13-15]

Prerenal AKI is caused by a decrease in renal blood flow from reduced cardiac output, dehydration, hemorrhage, shock, burns, or trauma.[13,14]

Intrinsic AKI involves primary damage to kidneys and is caused by acute tubular necrosis (ATN), glomerulonephritis, acute pyelonephritis, atheroembolic renal disease, malignant hypertension, nephrotoxic substances (e.g., aminoglycoside antibiotics or contrast dye), or blood transfusion reactions.[13]

Postrenal AKI involves obstruction distal to the kidney and can be caused by urinary tract obstruction by renal stones, obstructive tumors, or benign prostatic hypertrophy.[13,14,16-19]

Two primary classification criteria have been developed to monitor the progression and severity of AKI: Risk, Injury,

TABLE 9-3   **Risk, Injury, Failure, Loss, End-Stage Kidney Disease (RIFLE) Classification**

Class	Glomerular Filtration Rate (GFR) Criteria	Urine Output Criteria
Risk	GFR decrease > 25% or serum creatinine × 1.5	<0.5 ml/kg/hr × 6 hr
Injury	GFR decrease > 50% or serum creatinine × 2	<0.5 ml/kg/hr × 12 hr
Failure	GRF decrease 75% or serum creatinine × 3 or serum creatinine ≥4 mg/dl with an acute rise > 0.5 mg/dl	<0.3 ml/kg × 24 hr or anuria × 12 hr
Loss	Complete loss of kidney function >4 weeks (persistent acute renal failure)	
End-stage kidney disease	End-stage kidney disease >3 months	

Data from Bellomo R, Ronco C, Kellum JA et al: Acute renal failure—definition, outcome measures, animal models, fluid therapy and information technology needs: the Second International Consensus Conference of the Acute Dialysis Quality Initiative (ADQI) Group, Crit Care 8:R204-R212, 2004.

✎ **CLINICAL TIP**

Patients who have AKI may have the phrase "due to void" used when the medical team is awaiting urine output after Foley catheterization. Voluntary voiding in sufficient amounts may contribute to discharge planning.

Failure, Loss, End-Stage Kidney Disease (RIFLE) (Table 9-3) and Acute Kidney Injury Network (AKIN) classification (Table 9-4).

Clinical manifestations of AKI are based upon the specific type and can include the following[13-19]:

- Hypovolemic symptoms of thirst, hypotension, and decreased urine output
- Acid-base imbalance
- Electrolyte imbalance
- Infection
- Anemia
- Peripheral edema
- Pulmonary vascular congestion, pleural effusion
- Cardiomegaly, gallop rhythms, elevated jugular venous pressure
- Hepatic congestion
  Management of AKI includes any of the following:
- Treatment of the primary etiology, including antimicrobial agents if applicable
- Treatment of life-threatening conditions associated with AKI
- Optimize hemodynamics and fluid status
- Balance acid-base and electrolytes, particularly potassium levels

TABLE 9-4   **Acute Kidney Injury Network (AKIN) Classification**

Classes	Serum Creatinine (sCr) Criteria	Urinary Output Criteria
1	sCr increase × 1.5 or sCr increase > 0.3 mg/dl from baseline	<0.5 ml/kg/hr >6 hr
2	sCr increase × 2 from baseline	<0.5 ml/kg/hr > 12 hr
3	sCr increase × 3 or sCr increase > 4 mg/dl with an acute increase > 0.5 mg/dl	<0.5 ml/kg > 24 hr or anuria × 12 hr

Data from Mehta RL, Kellum JA, Shah SV et al: Acute Kidney Injury Network: report of an initiative to improve outcomes in acute kidney injury, Crit Care 11:R31, 2007.

- Peritoneal dialysis, hemodialysis, continuous renal replacement therapy as necessary (refer to the Renal Replacement Therapy section)
- Transfusions and blood products
- Nutritional support

Chronic Kidney Disease

Chronic kidney disease (CKD) is an irreversible reduction in renal function that occurs as a slow, insidious process from a large number of systemic diseases that injure the kidney or from intrinsic disorders of the kidney. The renal system has considerable functional reserve, and as many as 50% of the nephrons can be destroyed before symptoms occur. Progression of CKD to complete renal failure is termed *end-stage kidney disease* (ESKD). At this point, renal replacement therapy (RRT) is required for patient survival.[14,20]

CKD can result from primary renal disease or other systemic diseases. Primary renal diseases that cause CKD are polycystic kidney disease, chronic glomerulonephritis, chronic pyelonephritis, arthroembolic renal disease, and chronic urinary obstruction. The two primary systemic diseases that are associated with CKD are type 2 diabetes and hypertension.[21] Other systemic diseases that can result in CKD include gout, systemic lupus erythematosus, amyloidosis, nephrocalcinosis, sickle cell anemia, scleroderma, and human immunodeficiency virus.[14] Complications of CKD are similar to those of AKI, including anemia and hypertension, but can also include bone pain and extraosseous calcification.[20] Patients with CKD are staged based on the severity of their disease (as measured by GFR), from the United States Kidney Disease Outcomes Quality Initiative (KDOQI). Stage 1 is normal kidney function, whereas renal replacement therapy (RRT) is recommended in stage 5.[21]

Management of CRF includes conservative management or RRT.[21,22]

Conservative management includes the following[16,17,22,23]:
- Nutritional support, dietary modifications (salt and protein restrictions)
- Smoking cessation
- Calcium carbonate and vitamin supplements
- Erythropoietin for anemia

- Allopurinol therapy
- Hyperkalemia correction
- Avoiding use of nonsteroidal antiinflammatory drugs, acetaminophen, bisphosphonates, oral estrogens or herbal therapies
  Renal replacement therapy includes the following:
- Peritoneal dialysis or hemodialysis to maintain fluid and electrolyte balance
- Renal transplantation (see Chapter 14)

> ✎ **CLINICAL TIP**
>
> Patients who are on bed rest or have yet to begin consistently ambulating are likely to be put on anticoagulants. For patients with chronic renal disease, unfractionated heparin is the preferred medication to use for venous thromboembolism prophylaxis. Because most medicines, including anticoagulants, are eliminated through the kidneys, patients with renal disease may have a higher likelihood of bleeding if anticoagulant dosing is not titrated closely.[24] Therefore monitor the patients' clotting times before moving them.

Pyelonephritis

Pyelonephritis is an acute or chronic inflammatory response in the kidney, particularly the renal pelvis, from bacterial, fungal, or viral infection. It can be classified as acute or chronic.

Acute Pyelonephritis. Acute pyelonephritis is frequently associated with concurrent cystitis (bladder infection). The common causative agents are bacterial, including *Escherichia coli*, *Proteus*, *Klebsiella*, *Enterobacter*, *Pseudomonas*, *Serratia,* and *Citrobacter*. Predisposing factors for acute pyelonephritis include urine reflux from the ureter to the kidney (vesicoureteral reflux), kidney stones, pregnancy, neurogenic bladder, catheter or endoscope insertion, and female sexual trauma. Women are more prone to acute pyelonephritis than men.[17,22,25] Spontaneous resolution of acute pyelonephritis may occur in some cases without intervention.

Signs and symptoms of acute pyelonephritis include any of the following[26]:

- Sudden onset of fever and chills
- Pain and/or tenderness with deep palpatory pressure of one or both costovertebral (flank) areas
- Urinary frequency, dysuria and urgency
- Possible hematuria, pyuria (presence of white blood cells [leukocytes])
- Nausea, vomiting, and diarrhea
  Management of acute pyelonephritis includes any of the following[26]:
- Antibiotic therapy commonly includes ciprofloxacin (Cipro), ampicillin (Omnipen), levofloxacin, norfloxacin, ceftriaxone, trimethoprim/sulfamethoxazole (TMP-SMX), or ofloxacin.
- In complicated cases requiring hospitalization, bed rest, intravenous fluids, and antipyretic agents are also indicated.[26]

> ✎ **CLINICAL TIP**
>
> Kidney infection (pyelonephritis) may be referred to as an "upper UTI" or urinary tract infection.

Chronic Pyelonephritis. Chronic pyelonephritis is characterized by chronic interstitial inflammation and scarring resulting in destruction of nephrons. Chronic pyelonephritis is a cause of CKD and is categorized into two forms, reflux-associated and obstructive. Reflux-associated is the most common form and occurs when there is a reflux of urine from the bladder resulting in kidney scarring. Obstructive chronic pyelonephritis occurs from recurrent episodes of kidney infection that result from distal obstruction.[27]

Signs and symptoms of chronic pyelonephritis will not be present without renal insufficiency. Once renal insufficiency occurs, the patient will be symptomatic and similar to those described earlier in the AKD and CKD sections. If recurrent bouts of acute pyelonephritis are present, then a history of intermittent symptoms of fever, flank pain, and dysuria may be reported.[26]

Management of chronic pyelonephritis includes any of the following[26]:

- Treatment of primary etiology and preserving renal function
- Prolonged antimicrobial therapy to maximize effectiveness

Glomerular Diseases

Injury to the glomeruli with subsequent inflammation can result from a variety of situations, either from primary kidney disorders or as a secondary consequence of systemic diseases such as systemic lupus erythematosus, amyloidosis, Wegener's granulomatosis, diabetes mellitus, or hypertension. Primary glomerulonephritis may be idiopathic, be drug induced, or result from streptococcal infection. Approximately 25% of glomerulonephritis will result in CKD. Primary glomerulonephritis can include acute nephritic syndrome, postinfectious glomerulonephritis, and chronic glomerulonephritis. Immunoglobulin A (IgA) nephropathy or Berger's disease is a form of idiopathic glomerulonephritis and is the most common type worldwide.[28,29]

Glomerular diseases can result in any of these five major syndromes[29]:

- Nephritic syndrome, manifested by hematuria, azotemia, proteinuria, oliguria, edema, and hypertension
- Rapidly progressive glomerulonephritis, manifested by acute nephritis, proteinuria, and acute kidney failure
- Nephrotic syndrome, manifested by proteinuria (>3.5 g/day), hypoalbuminemia, hyperlipidemia, lipiduria
- Chronic kidney failure, manifested by azotemia (high nitrogen levels) and uremia progressing for months to years
- Isolated urinary abnormalities, manifested by subnephrotic proteinuria and/or glomerular hematuria
  Regardless of the type of glomerulonephritis, common signs and symptoms may include[28,29]:
- Edema
- Joint pain

- Oral ulcers or malar rash
- Dark urine
- Hypertension
- Heart murmurs
- Skin pallor
- Abdominal and/or back tenderness

Management for acute glomerulonephritis can include non-pharmacological strategies, such as diet or fluid restrictions, or medical management including diuretics, electrolyte correction, antimicrobials, and/or immunosuppression.[28]

Acute Interstitial Nephritis

A hypersensitivity reaction, commonly induced by medications (methicillin or nonsteroidal antiinflammatory drugs) or infections, can result in inflammation of the renal interstitium and tubules, which is referred to as acute *interstitial nephritis (AIN) or acute tubulointerstitial nephritis*. Physical findings of AIN include the following[30]:

- Leukocyturia
- Mild hematuria
- Mild proteinuria

Management of interstitial nephritis includes any of the following[16,30,31]:

- Fluid and nutritional support
- Removal of causative medications while treating primary infection (as indicated)
- Renal replacement therapy (as indicated)

Nephrolithiasis

Nephrolithiasis is characterized by renal calculi (kidney stones) that form in the renal pelvis. There are four primary types of kidney stones, which are categorized according to the stone-forming substances: (1) calcium, (2) struvite (composed of magnesium, ammonium, and phosphate), (3) uric acid, and (4) cystine.[32] Many factors contribute to stone formation and include the following[33]:

- Dietary factors (high protein, organ meats, salt, spinach, rhubarb, beet, black tea intake)
- Hyperparathyroidism, sarcoidosis, metabolic syndrome, diabetes mellitus
- Medications (carbonic anhydrase inhibitors, triamterene, indinavir, and vitamin C or D)

Signs and symptoms of kidney stones include the following[33]:

- Colicky pain in the flank and/or lower abdominal region, with possible radiation into the groin, depending on the stone location. (Pain increases greatly as the stone passes through the ureters.)
- Hematuria, urinary frequency.
- Nausea and vomiting.
- Fever.
- Variable urine pH.
- Variable levels of serum calcium, chloride, phosphate, carbon dioxide, uric acid, and Cr.

After identification of the stones by noncontrast CT scan, management of kidney stones includes any of the following[32,33]:

- Analgesics (NSAIDs) and fluids.
- Reduction in dietary consumption of predisposing factors described earlier.
- Alpha1 antagonists and calcium channel blockers may enhance passage of stones.
- Ureteroscopic stone manipulation or in situ extracorporeal shock wave lithotripsy (ECSWL) in cases where stones do not pass spontaneously.

Diabetic Nephropathy

Approximately 40% of people with type 1 or type 2 diabetes will develop diabetic nephropathy, which is the primary cause of patients starting renal replacement therapy.[34] The presence of proteinuria (>0.5 g/24 hr) defines diabetic neuropathy, and, ideally, screening for kidney dysfunction should occur at the time of diagnosis for type 2 diabetes. Microalbuminuria levels help to establish the diagnosis of nephropathy with random urine samples, a technique recommended by the American Diabetes Association. Risk factors include sustained hyperglycemia, hypertension, smoking, dyslipidemia, and diets high in protein and fat. Patients with diabetic nephropathy are also at high risk for cardiovascular disease, and therefore routine screening for coronary heart disease, carotid disease, peripheral artery disease, and atherosclerotic renal-artery stenosis should occur.[34]

Signs and symptoms of diabetic nephropathy include the following[34]:

- Microalbuminuria
- Decreased glomerular filtration rate
- Retinopathy
- Manifestations of AKI or CKD as noted in earlier sections.

Management of diabetic nephropathy includes any of the following[16,35,36]:

- Strict glycemic control (refer to the Diabetes Mellitus section in Chapter 10)
- Management of risk factors including hypertension, smoking, and dyslipidemia including behavioral and medical strategies (see Chapter 3)
- Nutritional support
- Renal replacement therapy

Renal Artery Stenosis

Renal artery stenosis (RAS) commonly results from atherosclerotic disease and concomitant risk factors for vascular disease such as advancing age, elevated cholesterol, smoking, and systemic hypertension.[37] Population-based studies in the United States report that more than 70% of older patients with 60% occlusion of the renal artery have clinical manifestations of cardiovascular disease.[38] Additional but less common causes of RAS include fibromuscular dysplasia or systemic disease. Decreased renal perfusion results in renovascular hypertension, which can worsen preexisting systemic hypertension.[37]

Signs and symptoms of renal artery stenosis include the following[37,39]:

- Unexplained hypertension
- Flank or upper abdominal pain
- Abdominal bruits

- Peripheral or pulmonary edema
- Acute kidney injury after initiating angiotensin-converting enzyme (ACE) inhibitor or angiotensin receptor blocker therapy[40,41]

Diagnosis can be established by renal duplex ultrasonography, MRA, CT angiography, and invasive digital subtraction renal angiography (which is the gold standard for diagnosis).[40,41]

Management of renal artery stenosis includes any of the following[39]:

- Antihypertensive agents (ACE inhibitors or angiotensin receptor blockers, in appropriate cases).
- Antiplatelet therapy with aspirin.
- Glycemic and lipid control.
- Renal replacement therapy as indicated.
- Surgery: Angioplasty with stent placement has not been shown to have better results than medical therapy in controlling blood pressure or recovery of renal function.[41]

Renal Vein Thrombosis

Renal vein thrombosis (RVT) is an uncommon disorder, primarily seen in children, that is caused by severe dehydration. In adults who are postoperative or have sustained trauma are also at risk for RVT, along with adults who may have a hypercoagulable state, renal tumors extending into the renal vein, or nephrotic syndrome. Renal vein occlusion can increase renal vein pressure, creating a decrease in renal artery blood flow.[42] Diagnosis is confirmed with renal Doppler ultrasound, CT scan, or MRI.

Signs and symptoms of renal vein thrombosis include the following[42]:

- Flank or loin pain
- Fever
- Manifestations of acute kidney injury, including oliguria
- Gross hematuria

RVT can be managed with systemic anticoagulants or catheter-directed thrombolytic therapy with urokinase or tissue plasminogen activator.[42]

Lower Urinary Tract Dysfunction

Cystitis

Inflammation of the urinary bladder may occur acutely or extend to a chronic situation. Acute cystitis commonly occurs from urinary tract infections (UTIs) resulting from pathogens such as *Escherichia coli*, *Staphylococcus saprophyticus*, *Proteus*, *Klebsiella*, and *Enterobacter*. Urinary tract infections are also common causes of kidney infections (pyelonephritis). Prostatic enlargement, cystocele of the bladder, calculi (stones), or tumors can also result in cystitis.[43,44]

A variant of cystitis is chronic pelvic pain syndrome, which occurs predominantly in women and results in severe suprapubic pain, urinary frequency, hematuria, and dysuria without evidence of infection.[43]

Signs and symptoms of acute cystitis include the following[43,44]:

- Urinary frequency and urgency (as often as every 15 to 20 minutes)
- Dysuria
- Lower abdominal or suprapubic pain
- Urinalysis may reveal pyuria, hematuria, and bacteriuria

Management of cystitis includes antimicrobial treatment for approximately 3 days or less depending on the exact agent prescribed.[44]

Urinary Calculi

Urinary calculi are stones (urolithiasis) that can form anywhere in the urinary tract outside of the kidneys and are mostly composed of calcium oxalate and phosphate.[27] Formation of stones, symptoms, and management are similar to that of kidney stones (see the Nephrolithiasis section for further details on the formation and clinical presentation of kidney stones).

Neurogenic Bladder

A neurogenic bladder is characterized by dysfunctional voiding as a result of neurologic injury that interferes with urine storage or voluntary coordinated voiding.[45] Control of the bladder occurs at multiple levels throughout the central nervous system, and consequently injury at one or more of these levels can result in voiding dysfunction. The range of symptoms of neurogenic bladder can include suprapubic or pelvic pain, urinary incontinence to urinary retention, incomplete voiding, paroxysmal hypertension with diaphoresis (autonomic dysreflexia), urinary tract infection, and occult decline in kidney function.[45]

Management consists of addressing the primary neurologic disturbance (as able) and providing antimicrobial agents for any associated infection in order to preserve kidney function.[45] A progressive approach also includes[46]:

- Bladder retraining, fluid regulation, and pelvic floor exercises
- Antimuscarinic agents (desmopressin)
- Antimuscarinic agents plus clean intermittent self-catheterization (CISC)
- Antimuscarinic agents plus CISC and botulinum toxin (BoNT/A)
- Indwelling catheterization with or without antimuscarinic agents, BoNT/A, and/or possible surgery

Urinary Incontinence

Incontinence of urine can be transient or acute and can result from situations such as fluid imbalance, stool impaction, impaired mobility, delirium, and side effects of medications. Inadequate resolution of these factors and/or repeated episodes

---

> ✎ **CLINICAL TIP**
>
> If patients are incontinent of urine, observe whether bed linens and/or the hospital gown is soiled before a physical therapy session, as these need to be changed in order to minimize skin breakdown. A condom catheter (for men) or adult incontinence undergarments (for men and women) can be applied before mobility treatment to aid in completion of the session.

TABLE 9-5 Types of Chronic Urinary Incontinence

Type	Description	Common Causes
Stress	Loss of urine that occurs involuntarily in situations associated with increased intraabdominal pressure, such as with laughing, coughing, or exercise	Urethral sphincter dysfunction, or weakness in pelvic floor muscles
Urge	Leakage of urine because of inability to delay voiding after a sensation of bladder fullness is perceived	Neurologic disorders, spinal cord injury, or detrusor overactivity
Mixed	Combination of stress and urge symptoms	Combination of stress and urge causes above
Overflow	Leakage of urine from mechanical forces or urinary retention from an overdistended bladder	Anatomic obstruction by prostate, stricture, or cystocele Diabetes mellitus or spinal cord injury Neurologic disorders, detrusor failure
Functional	The inability to void because of cognitive or physical impairments, psychological unwillingness, or environmental barriers	Mobility and/or cognitive impairment(s)

Adapted from Stiles M, Walsh: Care of the elderly patient. In Rakel RE, Rakel DP, editors: Textbook of family medicine, ed 8, Philadelphia, 2011, Saunders, p 49.

can contribute to chronic urinary incontinence.[47] Table 9-5 provides a summary of the different types of chronic urinary incontinence. Management of the various types of chronic incontinence may include scheduled voiding, pelvic floor exercises, antimuscarinic drugs, surgical intervention, and catheterization.[47]

Prostate Disorders

Benign Prostatic Hyperplasia

Benign prostatic hyperplasia (BPH) is characterized by an increased number of epithelial and stromal cells in the prostate gland and may contribute to lower urinary tract symptoms (LUTS) in men over the age of 40.[48] Digital rectal examination can detect benign enlargement or abnormalities that may be associated with prostate cancer. In the presence of microscopic hematuria, CT urogram and cystoscopy is recommended, along with laboratory tests such as measurement of serum prostate antigen (PSA).[49] Enlargement of the prostate from BPH can result in urinary tract obstruction; however, factors such as those described in Table 9-5 are also contributing issues to LUTS in both men and women.[48] Thus there are overlapping signs and symptoms of BPH and LUTS, including[48,50]:

- Frequency of micturition, urgency
- Urge incontinence
- Decreased force and caliber of urinary stream
- Straining to void, hesitancy
- Postvoid dribble
- Nocturia, dysuria and hematuria

Management of BPH includes any of the following[48,51]:

- Alpha$_1$-adrenergic blocking agents act to relax the smooth muscle in the neck of the bladder to facilitate voiding. Currently prescribed agents include tamsulosin (Flomax) and prazosin (Minipress). Other medications include doxazosin (Cardura), terazosin (Hytrin), and alfuzosin (Uroxatral).
- 5α-Reductase enzyme inhibitor used to inhibit male hormones to the prostate, causing the gland to shrink over time. Agents include finasteride (Proscar) and dutasteride (Avodart).

- Antiinfective agents (if there is associated infection).
- Intermittent catheterization (as necessary).

Surgical options include transurethral incision of the prostate (TUIP), transurethral resection of the prostate (TURP), transurethral needle ablation of the prostate (TUNA), or open prostatectomy.

Prostatitis

Prostatitis is an inflammation of the prostate gland. It can be divided into four categories: (1) acute bacterial, (2) chronic bacterial, (3) chronic pelvic pain syndrome, and (4) asymptomatic prostatitis. Causative pathogens for acute and chronic bacterial prostatitis can include *E. coli*, *Pseudomonas aeruginosa*, *Klebsiella*, *Proteus*, and *Enteroccocus*.[52]

Signs and symptoms of prostatitis include the following[52]:

- Suprapubic, perineal, or low back pain
- Fever, chills, malaise, nausea and vomiting
- Increased urinary frequency or urgency to void
- Painful urination (dysuria)
- Difficulty initiating a stream, interrupted voiding, or incomplete emptying
- Sexual dysfunction

Management of prostatitis includes any of the following[52]:

- Antimicrobial agents (for bacterial prostatitis)
- Alpha$_1$-adrenergic blocking agents or antiinflammatory agents
- Antipyretics
- Invasive management as a last resort

Endometriosis

Endometriosis is the second most common cause of dysmenorrhea and can be a confounding source of musculoskeletal pain. Aberrant growth of endometrial tissue occurs outside of the uterus, particularly in the dependent parts of the pelvis and ovaries. The incidence is greatest between the ages of 25 and 29. The exact nature of the pathogenesis and etiology are currently unknown. Several theories are available: (1) direct endometrial implantation due to retrograde menstrual flow into the pelvic cavity from the uterus, (2) transformation of multipotential cells into endometrium-like cells, (3) transport of endometrial cells by uterine vascular and lymphatic systems to distant sites, and (4) disorder of immune surveillance allowing growth of endometrial implants. Differential diagnosis of endometriosis may include pelvic inflammatory disease, ectopic pregnancy, appendicitis, hernia, irritable bowel syndrome, nerve entrapment, interstitial cystitis, or muscle strain. Laparoscopic examination will confirm the diagnosis of endometriosis.[53-55]

Signs and symptoms of endometriosis include the following[53-55]:

- Classic triad of dysmenorrhea, dyspareunia (pain with intercourse), and infertility
- Pelvic pain (hypogastric and perineal regions) related to the menstrual cycle
- Pain in the low back and lower extremities
- Intermittent constipation/diarrhea, dysuria, hematuria, and urinary frequency
- Abnormal bleeding (premenstrual spotting, menorrhagia)

Management of endometriosis includes any of the following[53-55]:

- Nonsteroidal antiinflammatory drugs for relief of symptoms associated with dysmenorrhea.
- Conservative therapies aimed at enhancing fertility (for those wishing to bear children).
- Hormonal therapy aimed at reducing hormone levels and cyclic stimulation of ectopic endometrial tissue. Agents used include estrogen-progesterone, progestins, and gonadotropin-releasing hormone (GnRH) agonists.
- Laparoscopic ablation of endometrial implants (ectopic tissue) with concurrent uterine nerve ablation to significantly reduce pain.
- Total abdominal hysterectomy and bilateral salpingo-oophorectomy (TAH-BSO) in women who no longer wish to bear children, followed by estrogen replacement therapy.

Management

The specific management of various genitourinary disorders is discussed earlier in the respective health conditions sections. This section expands on renal replacement therapy and surgical procedures. Guidelines for physical therapy management for patients who have genitourinary dysfunction are also discussed.

Renal Replacement Therapy

The primary methods of managing fluid and electrolyte balance in patients with AKI or CKD are peritoneal dialysis, intermittent hemodialysis, or continuous renal replacement therapy. For either type of dialysis (peritoneal or intermittent), the principles of diffusion, osmosis, and ultrafiltration to balance fluid and electrolyte levels are used. Diffusion is the movement of solutes, such as Cr, urea, or electrolytes, from an area of higher concentration to an area of lower concentration. Osmosis is the movement of fluid from an area of lesser solute concentration to an area of greater solute concentration. Ultrafiltration, the removal of water and fluid, is accomplished by creating pressure gradients between the arterial blood and the dialyzer membrane

or compartment.[56,57] Continuous renal replacement therapy (CRRT) is generally implemented in the critical care setting in patients with AKI.[58] Kidney transplantation is described in Chapter 14.

Peritoneal Dialysis

Peritoneal dialysis (PD) involves using the peritoneal cavity as a semipermeable membrane to exchange soluble substances and water between the dialysate fluid and the blood vessels in the abdominal cavity.[18,56,57] Dialysate fluid is instilled into the peritoneal cavity through an indwelling catheter. After the dialysate is instilled into the peritoneum, there is an equilibration period when water and solutes pass through the semipermeable membrane. Once equilibration is finished, then the peritoneal cavity is drained of the excess fluid and solutes that the failing kidneys cannot remove. Instillation, equilibration, and drainage constitute one exchange.[56,57] The process of peritoneal dialysis can range from 45 minutes to 9 hours, depending on the method of PD, and patients can have anywhere from 4 to 24 exchanges per day.[56]

There are two types of PD: automated PD (APD) and continuous ambulatory PD (CAPD). APD uses an automatic cycling device to control the instillation, equilibration, and drainage phases. CAPD is schematically represented in Figure 9-3.[56]

PD is indicated for patients with CKD, who may or may not be hospitalized. The choice to use PD versus intermittent hemodialysis is dependent on whether there is a functioning peritoneal cavity as well as the ability for the patient or care providers to manage the exchanges. In cases of AKI, intermittent hemodialysis or CRRT are preferable modalities.[58,59]

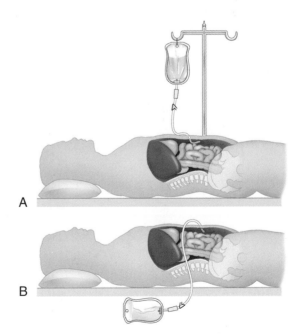

FIGURE 9-3
Schematic illustration of continuous ambulatory peritoneal dialysis. **A,** Instillation of dialysate fluid. **B,** Drainage of excess fluid and solutes.

Intermittent Hemodialysis

Kidney functions that are controlled by intermittent hemodialysis include (1) fluid volume, (2) electrolyte balance, (3) acid-base balance, and (4) filtration of nitrogenous wastes. The patient's arterial blood is mechanically circulated through semipermeable tubing that is surrounded by a dialysate solution in the dialyzer (artificial kidney). The dialysate fluid contains vital solutes to permit diffusion of electrolytes into or out of the patient's blood. As the patient's arterial blood is being filtered through the dialyzer, "clean" blood is returned to the patient's venous circulation.[57,58] Figure 9-4 illustrates this process.

Vascular access is attained either through cannula insertion (usually for temporary dialysis) or through an internal arteriovenous fistula (for chronic dialysis use), which is surgically created in the forearm. The arteriovenous fistula is created by performing a side-to-side, side-to-end, or end-to-end anastomosis between the radial or ulnar artery and the cephalic vein.

If a native fistula cannot be created, then a synthetic graft is surgically anastomosed between the arterial and venous circulation.[56] Figure 9-5 illustrates these various types of vascular access.

Patients who require intermittent hemodialysis for AKI are generally required to replace 2 to 3 liters of fluid per dialysis session in order to fully achieve clear waste products and achieve osmotic balance. This large amount of fluid exchange can promote hypotension and possible ischemia of nephrons in patients who are critically ill. Therefore, in the more unstable patient, continuous renal replacement therapy may be more suitable.[60]

Patients who require chronic intermittent hemodialysis usually have it administered three to four times per week, with each exchange lasting approximately 3 to 4 hours. The overall intent of this process is to extract up to 2 days' worth of excess fluid and solutes from the patient's blood.[18,61]

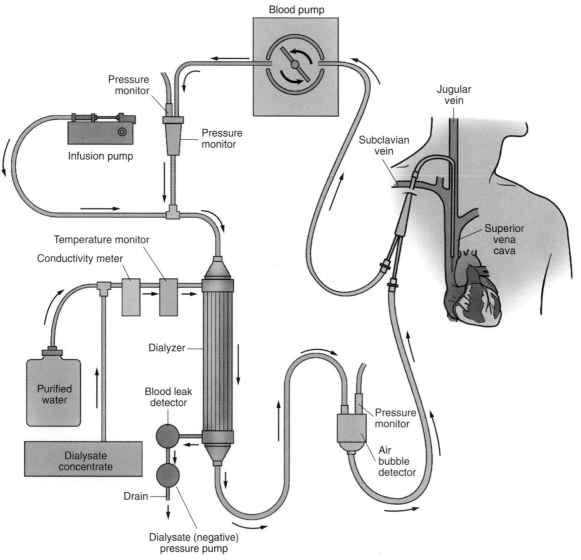

FIGURE 9-4
Schematic representation of hemodialysis. (From Thompson JM, McFarland GK, Hirsch JE, et al: Mosby's clinical nursing, ed 3, St Louis, 1993, Mosby, p 938.)

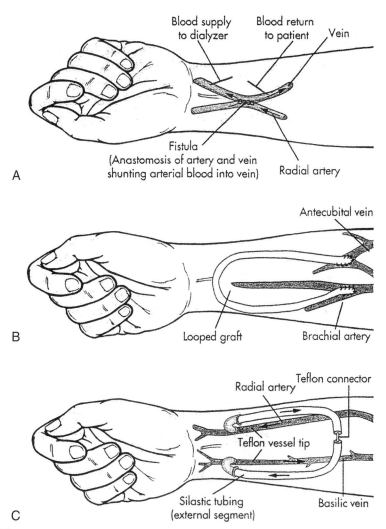

FIGURE 9-5
Methods of vascular access for hemodialysis. **A,** Internal arteriovenous fistula. **B,** Looped graft in forearm.
C, External cannula or shunt. (From Lewis SM, Heitkemper MM, Dirksen SR, editors: Medical-surgical
nursing: assessment and management of clinical problems, ed 6, St Louis, 2004, Mosby, p 1233.)

> ✎ **CLINICAL TIP**
>
> Pulmonary hygiene treatments can be performed during dialysis; however, this depends on the hemodynamic stability of the patient and is at the discretion of the nurse or physician. Extreme caution should be taken with the access site to prevent accidental disruption.

Continuous Renal Replacement Therapy

The purpose of CRRT is to provide a continuous mechanism that balances fluid and electrolytes as well as small and medium solutes from the body in a manner that mimics the natural function of the patient's native kidney. Because of the process involved with CRRT, it is frequently used in the critical care setting to stabilize and manage patients without the adverse effects of hypotension that can occur with intermittent hemodialysis. Predictable outcomes of CRRT include[58]:
- Hemodynamic stability
- Continuous control of fluid status

- Control of acid-base status and electrolyte, calcium, and phosphate balance
- Provision of protein-rich nutrition with excellent uremic control
- Prevention of intracerebral water fluctuations
- Minimal risk of infection

There are several techniques to achieve CRRT, which are outlined in Table 9-6. Vascular access is dependent on the specific type of CRRT indicated for the patient. Figure 9-6 provides an illustration of continuous venovenous hemofiltration.

> ✎ **CLINICAL TIP**
>
> The dialysis staff is generally nearby to monitor the procedure and is a valuable source of information regarding the patient's hemodynamic stability. Also, inquiring about the length of time for the hemodialysis may be helpful in scheduling therapy sessions.

TABLE 9-6 Continuous Renal Replacement Therapy (CRRT) Techniques

Types of CRRT	Description
Slow continuous ultrafiltration (SCUF)	Used for fluid control only Can have arteriovenous or venovenous modes
Continuous venovenous hemofiltration (CVVH)	Convective blood purification through a high-permeability membrane Arteriovenous mode also available
Continuous venovenous hemodialysis	Diffusive purification of blood through a low-permeability dialyzer For small molecule clearance only
Continuous venovenous hemodiafiltration (CVVHDF)	Diffusive and convective blood purification with a highly permeable membrane
Continuous high-flux dialysis (CVVHFD)	Diffusive and convective blood purification with a highly permeable membrane and an accessory pump to control ultrafiltration
Continuous plasma-filtration adsorption (CPFA)	A highly permeable plasma filter filters plasma, allowing it to pass through a bed of adsorbent material (carbon or resins) Fluid balance maintained throughout process

Data from Ronco C, Ricci Z, Bellomo R et al: Renal replacement therapy. In Vincent JL, Abraham E, Moore FA et al, editors: Textbook of critical care, ed 6, Philadelphia, 2011, Saunders, pp 894-901.

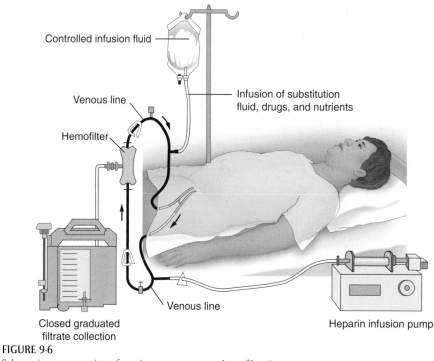

FIGURE 9-6
Schematic representation of continuous venovenous hemofiltration.

Surgical Interventions

Surgical interventions for genitourinary system disorders can be categorized broadly as procedures that remove diseased portions of the genitourinary tract or procedures that restore urinary flow. These interventions are briefly discussed in the following sections. Refer to Chapter 20 for general anesthesia and postoperative considerations.

Nephrectomy

There are three types of nephrectomy. The primary indications for removing a part or all of the kidney include renal cell carcinoma, polycystic kidney disease, severe traumatic injury to the kidney, and organ donation, as well as removing a failing

transplanted organ.[62,63] Nephrectomy can be performed as an open or laparoscopic procedure.[62-66] The types of nephrectomy and their definitions follow:

- *Radical nephrectomy*—removal of the entire kidney, a section of the ureter, the adrenal gland, and the fatty tissue surrounding the kidney.
- *Simple nephrectomy*—removal of the entire kidney with a section of the ureter. Generally performed when harvesting donor organs for kidney transplantation.
- *Partial nephrectomy*—only the infected or diseased portion of the kidney is removed.

Nephron-sparing surgery (NSS) is a term also used with partial nephrectomy and is indicated for patients with small, localized tumors. Minimally invasive techniques include laparoscopic and robotic partial nephrectomies as well as cryoablation and radiofrequency ablation to target localized masses.[66,67]

Prostatectomy

Prostatectomy is the surgical removal of a prostate gland with or without its capsule and is indicated for patients with acute urinary retention, recurrent or persistent urinary tract infections, significant bladder outlet obstruction that is not responsive to medical therapy, recurrent hematuria of prostatic origin, bladder calculi, and renal insufficiency secondary to obstruction. The procedure can be performed via open approach or through transurethral resection of the prostate (TURP).[68]

Urinary Incontinence Procedures

When conservative treatment of urinary stress incontinence is unsuccessful or not desired, surgical management is considered. Stress incontinence has been reported in as many as 78% of women with 30% opting for surgery. Procedures such as the Burch and Marshall-Marchetti-Kranz (MMK) retropubic urethropexies are aimed at reestablishing the anatomic support of the urethrovesical junction and proximal urethra in order to provide stability during increases in intraabdominal pressure. Sling procedures involve placement of synthetic mesh acting as a dynamic support in the midurethral region and can be performed via retropubic or transobturator approaches. Injection of urethral bulking agents, such as collagen and carbon beads, can also be performed to help support the urethra.[69]

Urinary Diversion

Procedures aimed at diverting urine flow are indicated for patients who have undergone cystectomy or have a diseased bladder. Obstructed ureters as well as total urinary incontinence are also indications. Urinary diversion involves creating a conduit from either the small or large intestine.[70] Figure 9-7 illustrates some methods of urinary diversion.

Physical Therapy Management

The following are general goals and guidelines for the physical therapist when working with patients who have genitourinary dysfunction. These guidelines should be adapted to a patient's specific needs.

The primary physical therapy goals in this patient population are similar to those of other patients in the acute care setting. These goals are to (1) optimize safe functional mobility, (2) maximize activity tolerance and endurance, and (3) prevent postoperative pulmonary complications.

General physical therapy management guidelines and considerations revolve around the normal functions of the genitourinary system that are disrupted by the various health conditions discussed earlier in this chapter. These include, but are not limited to, the following:

1. Evaluating laboratory values before examination or intervention can help the physical therapist decide which particular signs and symptoms to monitor as well as determine the parameters of the session.[71] Refer to Chapter 15 for more information on fluid and electrolyte imbalance.

2. The inability to regulate cellular waste products, blood volume, and electrolyte levels can result in:
   - Mental status changes from a buildup of ammonia, BUN, Cr, or a combination of these. If this situation occurs, then the therapist may choose to modify or defer physical therapy intervention, particularly educational activities that require concentration.
   - Disruption of excitable tissues such as peripheral nerves and skeletal, cardiac, and smooth muscle from altered levels of electrolytes.[72] If this situation occurs, then the therapist may need to reduce exercise intensity during muscle-strengthening activities. In addition, if peripheral neuropathy results in sensory deficits, then the therapist needs to take the appropriate precautions with the use of modalities and educate the patient on protective mechanisms to avoid skin breakdown.
   - Peripheral or pulmonary edema from inability to excrete excess body fluids.[72] Pulmonary edema can result in shortness of breath with activities and recumbent positioning. Peripheral edema can result in range-of-motion limitations and skin breakdown. Refer to Table 3-5 for a description of pitting edema, and see Chapter 4 for a description of pulmonary edema.
   - Fluid and electrolyte imbalance can also alter the hemodynamic responses to activity; therefore careful vital sign and symptom monitoring should always be performed.

3. Blood pressure regulation can be altered by the inability to excrete body fluids and activate the renin-angiotensin system.[72]

4. Activity tolerance can be reduced by the factors mentioned in this section, as well as anemia that can result from decreased erythropoietin secretion from kidneys, which is necessary for stimulating red blood cell production.[72]

5. Patients will likely demonstrate variable levels of fatigue when receiving RRT; some patients are more fatigued before a dialysis session, whereas others are more fatigued after a dialysis session. Hemodialysis sessions typically occur three times per week but may have different schedules depending on the patient situation.

6. Patients with CKD may present with concurrent clinical manifestations of diabetes mellitus, as diabetes mellitus is a strong contributing factor to this disorder. Refer to Chapter 10 for more information on diabetes mellitus.

7. As stated in the introduction to this chapter, patients with genitourinary dysfunction may have referred pain (see Table 9-1). Physical therapists can play a role in differentiating the source of a patient's back pain as well as possibly providing symptomatic management of this referred pain.

8. Patients who have undergone surgical procedures with abdominal incisions are less likely to perform deep breathing and coughing because of incisional pain. Diligent position changes, instruction on incisional splinting during deep breathing, and coughing, along with early mobilization, help prevent the development of pulmonary complications.[73-77]

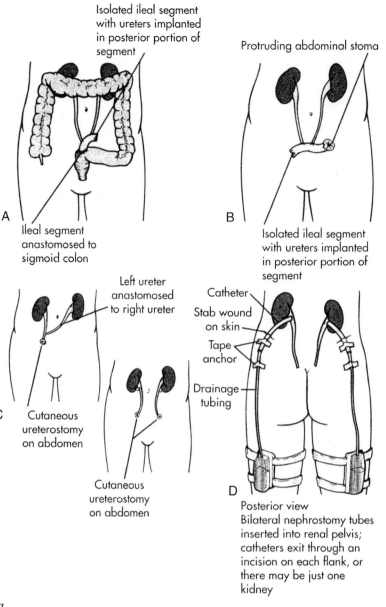

FIGURE 9-7
Methods of urinary diversion. **A,** Ureteroileosigmoidostomy. **B,** Ileal loop (or ileal conduit). **C,** Ureterostomy (transcutaneous ureterostomy and bilateral cutaneous ureterostomies). **D,** Nephrostomy. (From Lewis SM, Heitkemper MM, Dirksen SR, editors: Medical-surgical nursing: assessment and management of clinical problems, ed 6, St Louis, 2004, Mosby, p 1203.)

9. For patients who are ambulatory and present with urinary urgency, possibly from diuretic therapy, the use of a bedside commode may be a beneficial recommendation to minimize the incidences of incontinence.

10. Patients who are incontinent may benefit from a home exercise program, referral to a physical therapist who specializes in pelvic floor strengthening, or both on discharge from the hospital.

References

1. The urinary system. In Patton KT, Thibodeau GA, editors: Anatomy & physiology, ed 7, St Louis, 2010, Mosby.
2. Patton KT, Thibodeau GA, editors: Anatomy & physiology, ed 7, St Louis, 2010, Mosby.
3. Bullock BL: Normal renal and urinary excretory function. In Bullock BL, editor: Pathophysiology: adaptations and alterations in function, ed 4, Philadelphia, 1996, Lippincott, p 616.
4. Screening for urogenital disease. In Goodman CC, Kelly Snyder TE, editors: Differential diagnosis for physical therapists, ed 5, St Louis, 2013, Elsevier, pp 384-386.
5. McLinn DM, Boissonnault WG: Screening for male urogenital system disease. In Boissonnault WG, editor: Examination in physical therapy practice: screening for medical disease, New York, 1991, Churchill Livingstone, p 121.

6. Bates P: Nursing assessment: urinary system. In Lewis SM, Heitkemper MM, Dirksen SR, editors: Medical-surgical nursing: assessment and management of clinical problems, ed 5, St Louis, 2000, Mosby, pp 1241-1255.

7. Pyridium. http://www.rxlist.com/pyridium-drug/patient-images-side-effects.htm#sideeffects. Accessed June 7, 2012.

8. Abdomen. In Seidel HM, Ball JW, Dains JE et al, editors: Mosby's guide to physical examination, ed 5, St Louis, 2003, Mosby, pp 541-552.

9. Malarkey LM, McMorrow ME: Nurse's manual of laboratory tests and diagnostic procedures, ed 2, Philadelphia, 2000, Saunders, pp 38-48, 629-670.

10. Pagana KD, Pagana TJ: Mosby's diagnostic and laboratory test reference, ed 9, St Louis, 2009, Mosby.

11. Weigel KA, Potter CK: Assessment of the renal system. In Monahan FD, Neighbors M, Sands JK, editors: Phipps' medical-surgical nursing: health and illness perspectives, ed 8, St Louis, 2008, Mosby, pp 943-960.

12. Thompson FD, Woodhouse CRJ: Disorders of the kidney and urinary tract, London, 1987, Edward Arnold.

13. Cheng CM, Ponnusamy A, Anderton JG: Management of acute renal failure in the elderly patient, a clinician's guide, Drugs Aging 25(6):455-476, 2008.

14. Weigel KA, Potter CK, Green CJ: Kidney failure. In Monahan FD, Neighbors M, Sands JK, editors: Phipps' medical-surgical nursing: health and illness perspectives, ed 8, St Louis, 2008, Mosby, pp 1003-1039.

15. Sharfuddin AA, Weisbord SD, Palevsky PM et al: Acute kidney injury. In Taal MW, Chertow GM, Marsden PA et al, editors: Brenner and Rector's the kidney, ed 9, Philadelphia, 2011, Saunders, pp 1044-1085.

16. Renal system. In Thompson JM, McFarland GK, Hirsch JE et al, editors: Mosby's manual of clinical nursing practice, ed 2, St Louis, 1989, Mosby, p 1021.

17. Huether SE: Alterations of renal and urinary tract function. In McCance KL, Huether SE, editors: Pathophysiology: the biologic basis for disease in adults and children, ed 2, St Louis, 1994, Mosby, p 1212.

18. Dirkes SM: Continuous renal replacement therapy: dialytic therapy for acute renal failure in intensive care, Nephrol Nurs J 27(6):581, 2000.

19. Ford-Martin PA: Acute kidney failure. In Boyden K, Olendorf D, editors: Gale encyclopedia of medicine, Farmington Hills, Mich, 1999, Gale Group, p 33.

20. Mitch WE: Chronic kidney disease. In Goldman L, Schafer AI, editors: Goldman's Cecil medicine, ed 24, Philadelphia, 2012, Saunders, pp 810-818.

21. Schena FP: Management of patients with chronic kidney disease, Int Emerg Med 6(S1):S77-S83, 2011.

22. Boissonnault WG: Urinary tract disorders. In Goodman CC, Boissonnault WG, editors: Pathology: implications for the physical therapist, Philadelphia, 1998, Saunders, pp 532-546.

23. Ford-Martin PA: Chronic kidney failure. In Boyden K, Olendorf D, editors: Gale encyclopedia of medicine, Farmington Hills, Mich, 1999, Gale Group, p 716.

24. Lobo BL: Use of newer anticoagulants in patients with chronic kidney disease, Am J Health Syst Pharm 64:2017-2026, 2007.

25. Wright KD: Pyelonephritis. In Boyden K, Olendorf D, editors: Gale encyclopedia of medicine, Farmington Hills, Mich, 1999, Gale Group, p 2422.

26. Schaeffer AJ, Schaeffer EM: Infections of the urinary tract. In Wein AJ, editor: Campbell-Walsh urology, ed 10, Philadelphia, 2012, Saunders, pp 257-326.

27. Disease of the urinary system. In Stevens A, Lowe J. Scott I, editors: Core pathology, ed 3, 2008, Elsevier.

28. Ferri FF: Ferri's clinical advisor, Philadelphia, 2013, Mosby.

29. Alpers CE: The kidney. In Kumar V, Abbas AK, Fausto N et al, editors: Robbins and Cotran Pathologic basis of disease, professional edition, ed 8, Philadelphia, 2010, Saunders.

30. Falk RJ, Kahl CR: Glomerulonephritis and interstitial nephritis. In Vincent JL, Abraham E, Moore FA, et al, editors: Textbook of critical care, ed 6, St Louis, 2011, Saunders Elsevier, pp 916-917

31. Interstitial nephritis. In Glanze WD, Anderson LE, editors: Mosby's medical, nursing, and allied health dictionary, ed 5, St Louis, 1998, Mosby, p 48.

32. Ban KM, Easter JS: Selected urologic problems. In Marx JA, Hockberger RS, Walls RM et al, editors: Rosen's emergency medicine, ed 7, St Louis, 2010, Mosby, pp 1308-1313.

33. Emmett M, Fenves AZ, Schwartz JC: Approach to the patient with kidney disease. In Taal MW, Chertow GM, Marsden PA et al, editors: Brenner and Rector's the kidney, ed 9, Philadelphia, 2011, Saunders, pp 856-859.

34. Gross JL, de Azevedo MJ, Silveiro SP et al: Diabetic nephropathy: diagnosis, prevention and treatment, Diabetes Care 28:176-188, 2005.

35. Diabetic nephropathy, Diabetes Care 24(1):S69, 2001.

36. Evans TC, Capell P: Diabetic nephropathy, Clin Diabetes 18(1):7, 2000.

37. Textor SC: Renovascular hypertension and ischemic nephropathy. In Taal MW, Chertow GM, Marsden PA et al, editors: Brenner and Rector's the kidney, ed 9, Philadelphia, 2011, Saunders, pp 1752-1791.

38. Edwards MS, Hansen KJ, Craven TE et al: Associations between renovascular disease and prevalent cardiovascular disease in the elderly: a population-based study, Vasc Endovasc Surg 38:25-35, 2004.

39. Dubose TD, Santos RM: Vascular disorders of the kidney. In Goldman L, Schafer AI, editors: Goldman's Cecil medicine, ed 24, Philadelphia, 2012, Saunders pp 784-789.

40. Watnick S, Morrison G: Kidney disease. In Tierney LM, McPhee SJ, Papadakis MA, editors: Current medical diagnosis & treatment, ed 47, New York, 2008, McGraw-Hill, pp 785-815.

41. Wheatley K, Ives N, Gray R et al: Revascularization versus medical therapy for renal artery stenosis, N Engl J Med 2009; 361:1953-1962, 2009.

42. Greco BA, Dwyer JP, Lewis JB: Thromboembolic renovascular disease. In Floege J, Johnson RJ, Freehally J, editors: Comprehensive clinical nephrology, Philadelphia, 2010, Saunders, pp 770-771.

43. Kumar V, Abbas AK, Fausto N et al, editors: Robbins and Cotran pathologic basis of disease, professional edition, ed 8, Philadelphia, 2010, Saunders.

44. Carter C, Stallworth J, Holleman R: Urinary tract disorders. In Rakel RE, Rakel DP, editors: Textbook of family medicine, ed 8, Philadelphia, 2011, Saunders, pp 921-923.

45. Kaynan AM, Perkash I: Neurogenic bladder. In Frontera WR, Silver JK, Rizzo TD, editors: Essentials of physical medicine and rehabilitation, ed 2, Philadelphia, 2008, Saunders, pp 733-744.

46. Panicker JN, Fowler CJ, DasGupta R: Neurology. In Daroff RB, Fenichel GM, Jankovic J, editors: Bradley's neurology in clinical practice, ed 6, Philadelphia, 2012, Saunders, pp 668-687.

47. Stiles M, Walsh K: Care of the elderly patient. In Rakel RE, Rakel DP, editors: Textbook of family medicine, ed 8, Philadelphia, 2011, Saunders, pp 47-50.

48. Roehrborn CG: Benign prostatic hyperplasia: etiology, pathophysiology, epidemiology and natural history. In Wein AJ, Kavoussi LR, Novick AC et al, editors: Campbell-Walsh urology, ed 10, Philadelphia, 2011, Saunders, pp 2570-2621.

49. Paolone DR: Benign prostatic hyperplasia, Clin Geriatr Med 26(2):223-239, 2010.

50. Thorner DA, Weiss JP: Benign prostatic hyperplasia: symptoms, symptom scores, and outcome measures, Urol Clin North Am 36(4):417-429, 2009.

51. Moul JD: Men's health. In Bope ET, Kellerman RD, editors: Conn's current therapy, Philadelphia, 2012, Saunders, pp 967-980.

52. Sharp VJ, Takacs EB, Powell CR: Prostatitis: diagnosis and treatment, Am Fam Physician 82(4):397-406, 2010.

53. MacKay HT: Gynecology. In Tierney LM, McPhee SJ, Papadakis MA, editors: Current medical diagnosis & treatment, ed 47, New York, 2008, McGraw-Hill, pp 645-646.

54. Troyer MR: Differential diagnosis of endometriosis in a young woman with nonspecific low back pain, Phys Ther 87:801-810, 2007.

55. Kim WJ, Alvero R: Endometriosis. In Ferri F, editor: Ferri's clinical advisor 2013, St Louis, 2013, Mosby

56. Brunier B, Bartucci M: Acute and chronic renal failure. In Lewis SM, Heitkemper MM, Dirksen SR, editors: Medical-surgical nursing: assessment and management of clinical problems, ed 5, St Louis, 2000, Mosby, pp 1310-1330.

57. Urinary system disorders. In Gould BE, Dyer RM, editors: Pathophysiology for the health professions, ed 4, Philadelphia, 2011, Saunders, p 448.

58. Ronco C, Ricci Z, Bellomo R et al: Renal replacement therapy. In Vincent JL, Abraham E, Moore FA et al, editors: Textbook of critical care, 6, Philadelphia, 2011, Saunders, pp 894-901.

59. Chiu YW, Mehrotra R: The utilization and outcome of peritoneal dialysis. In Himmelfarb J, Sayegh MH, editors: Chronic kidney disease, dialysis and transplantation, ed 3, Philadelphia, 2010, Saunders, pp 405-417.

60. Dirkes S, Hodge K: Continuous renal replacement therapy in the adult intensive care unit: history and current trends, Crit Care Nurse 27(2):61-80, 2000.

61. Noble H: An aging renal population—is dialysis always the answer? Br J Nurs 20(9):545-549, 2011.

62. Bates P: Renal and urologic problems. In Lewis SM, Heitkemper MM, Dirksen SR, editors: Medical-surgical nursing: assessment and management of clinical problems, ed 5, St Louis, 2000, Mosby, pp 1290-1293.

63. Ford-Martin PA: Nephrectomy. In Boyden K, Olendorf D, editors: Gale encyclopedia of medicine, Farmington Hills, Mich, 1999, Gale Group, p 2040.

64. Fornara P, Doehn C, Frese R et al: Laparoscopic nephrectomy in young-old, old-old, and oldest-old adults, J Gerontol A Biol Sci Soc Sci 56(5):M287, 2001.

65. Sasaki TM: Is laparoscopic donor nephrectomy the new criterion standard? JAMA 284(20):2579, 2000.

66. Delacroix SE, Wood CG, Jonasch E: Renal neoplasia. In Taal MW, Chertow GM, Marsden PA et al, editors: Brenner and Rector's the kidney, ed 9, Philadelphia, 2011, Saunders, pp 1508-1536.

67. Kimura M, Baba S, Polasick TJ: Minimally invasive surgery using ablative modalities for localized renal mass, Int J Urol 17:215-227, 2010.

68. Han M, Partin AW: Retropubic and suprapubic open prostatectomy. In Wein AJ, Kavoussi LR, Novick AC et al, editors: Campbell-Walsh urology, ed 10, Philadelphia, 2011, Saunders, pp 2695-2705.

69. Wai CY: Surgical treatment for stress and urge urinary incontinence, Obstet Gynecol Clin North Am 36:509-519, 2009.

70. Dahl DM, McDougal WS: Use of intestinal segments in urinary diversion. In Wein AJ, Kavoussi LR, Novick AC et al, editors: Campbell-Walsh urology, ed 10, Philadelphia, 2011, Saunders, pp 2435-2442.

71. Lab values interpretation resource: update 2012. Acute Care Section, American Physical Therapy Association. http://www.acutept.org/associations/11622/files/labvalues.pdf. Accessed March 21, 2013.

72. Dean E: Oxygen transport deficits in systemic disease and implications for physical therapy, Phys Ther 77(2):187, 1997.

73. Brooks-Brunn JA: Postoperative atelectasis and pneumonia, Heart Lung 24:94-115, 1995.

74. Brooks-Brunn JA: Predictors of postoperative pulmonary complications following abdominal surgery, Chest 111:564-571, 1997.

75. Basse L, Raskov HH, Jakobsen DH et al: Accelerated postoperative recovery programme after colonic resection improves physical performance, pulmonary function and body composition, Br J Surg 89:446-453, 2002.

76. Olsén MF, Nordgren IH, Lönroth H et al: Randomized controlled trial of prophylactic chest physiotherapy in major abdominal surgery, Br J Surg 84:1535-1538, 1997.

77. Olsén MF, Lönroth H, Bake B: Effects of breathing exercises on breathing patterns in obese and non-obese subjects, Clin Physiol 19(3):251-257, 1999.

Jaime C. Paz
Jessika Vizmeg

CHAPTER OBJECTIVES

The objectives of this chapter are the following:

1. Provide an understanding of normal functions of the endocrine system, including the thyroid, pituitary, adrenal, and parathyroid glands, as well as the pancreas
2. Describe the clinical evaluation of these endocrine organs
3. Describe the health conditions associated with endocrine system dysfunction and subsequent medical management
4. Provide physical therapy guidelines for working with patients who have endocrine system dysfunction

PREFERRED PRACTICE PATTERNS

The most relevant practice patterns for the diagnoses discussed in this chapter, based on the American Physical Therapy Association's *Guide to Physical Therapist Practice*, second edition, are as follows:

- Primary Prevention/Risk Reduction for Skeletal Demineralization: 4A
- Impaired Aerobic Capacity/Endurance Associated with Deconditioning: 6B
- Primary Prevention/Risk Reduction for Integumentary Disorders: 7A

Please refer to Appendix A for a complete list of the preferred practice patterns, as individual patient conditions are highly variable and other practice patterns may be applicable.

The endocrine system consists of endocrine glands, which secrete hormones into the bloodstream, and target cells for those hormones. Target cells are the principal sites of action for the endocrine glands. Figure 10-1 displays the location of the primary endocrine glands.

The endocrine system has direct effects on cellular function and metabolism throughout the entire body, with symptoms of endocrine dysfunction, metabolic dysfunction, or both often mimicking those of muscle weakness.[1] Therefore it is important for the physical therapist to carefully distinguish the source (endocrine versus musculoskeletal) of these symptoms to optimally care for the patient. For example, complaints of weakness and muscle cramps can both result from hypothyroidism or inappropriate exercise intensity. If the therapist is aware of the patient's current endocrine system status, then inquiring about a recent medication adjustment may be more appropriate than adjusting the patient's exercise parameters.

As a group, the prevalence of endocrine and metabolic disorders is approximately 5% of the U.S. population.[2] An estimated deficit in endocrinologists to meet the demands of the population is projected through the year 2020.[2] According to the Centers for Disease Control and Prevention (CDC), approximately 1.7% of the diagnoses of patients admitted to the emergency room were classified as endocrine disorders,[3] 4.9% of ambulatory care visits are a result of endocrine or metabolic disorders,[4] and 5.3% of hospital discharges had endocrine or metabolic disorders listed as a primary diagnosis.[5]

General Evaluation of Endocrine Function

Measurement of endocrine function can be performed by examining (1) the endocrine gland itself, using imaging techniques, or (2) levels of hormones or hormone-related substances in the bloodstream or urine. When reviewing the medical record, it is important for the physical therapist to know that high or low levels of endocrine substances can indicate endocrine

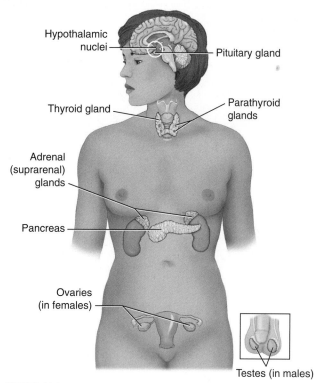

Hypothalamic nuclei

Pituitary gland

Thyroid gland

Parathyroid glands

Adrenal (suprarenal) glands

Pancreas

Ovaries (in females)

Testes (in males)

FIGURE 10-1
Schematic representation of the primary endocrine glands in women and men. (Courtesy Marybeth Cuaycong.)

dysfunction. A common method for assessing levels of hormone is radioimmunoassay (RIA).[6] RIA is an immunologic technique for comparing levels of radiolabeled hormone with unlabeled hormone, which compete for binding sites on a given antibody.

Another method of evaluation, referred to as *provocative testing*, can be classified into suppression or stimulation tests. Stimulation tests are used for testing endocrine hypofunction; suppression tests are useful for evaluating endocrine hyperfunction.[7] The most commonly used endocrine tests are discussed in this chapter. Clinicians should refer to their particular institution's laboratory values (generally located in the lab result section of the clinical record) for normal ranges of hormone or hormone-related substances referenced in their setting.

> ✎ **CLINICAL TIP**
>
> An imbalance of hormone levels may affect the patient's tolerance to activity. Familiarity with the endocrine tests and values can help the clinician gauge the intended treatment parameters (i.e., type, duration, frequency, and intensity) for the next session(s).

Thyroid Gland

Body Structure and Function

The thyroid gland secretes three hormones: thyroxine (T_4), triiodothyronine (T_3), and calcitonin, with T_4 and T_3 commonly

TABLE 10-1 Target Sites and Actions of Thyroid Gland Hormones

Hormone(s)	Target Site(s)	Actions
Thyroxine (T_4) and triiodothyronine (T_3)	Systemic	Increases metabolic rate; stimulates growth, and development of all cells, particularly of the nervous system; and enhances the effects of catecholamines
Thyrocalcitonin	Bone	Inhibits bone resorption Lowers blood levels of calcium

Data from Brashers VL, Jones RE: Mechanisms of hormonal regulation. In McCance KL, Huether SE, Brashers VL et al, editors: Pathophysiology: the biologic basis for disease in adults and children, ed 6, St Louis, 2010, Mosby, pp 697-726; Hall S: Prescribing in thyroid disease, Nurse Prescribing 8(8):382-387, 2010.

referred to as the thyroid hormones (Table 10-1). Thyroxine and triiodothyronine require the presence of adequate amounts of iodine to be properly synthesized. Therefore dietary deficiencies of iodine can hinder thyroid hormone production. The production and secretion of thyroid hormones are regulated by thyrotropin (also called thyroid-stimulating hormone [TSH]), which is secreted from the anterior pituitary gland. TSH levels are directly influenced by T_4 levels through a negative feedback loop. Thyrotropin is further regulated by thyrotropin-releasing hormone, which is secreted from the hypothalamus.[8-10]

Thyroid Tests

Thyroid hormones T_4 and T_3 circulate throughout the bloodstream bound to proteins or unbound, in which case they are metabolically active by themselves. Thyroxine-binding globulin (TBG) is one of the major thyroid transport proteins.[9] Serum levels of T_4 and T_3 are usually measured by RIA. Table 10-2 describes the tests used to measure thyroid hormones, and Table 10-3 summarizes other tests used to measure thyroid function.

> ✎ **CLINICAL TIP**
>
> Low levels of thyroid hormones T_3 or T_4 may result in weakness, muscle aching, and stiffness. Based on this information, the physical therapist may decide to alter treatment parameters by decreasing the treatment intensity to optimize activity tolerance, minimize patient discomfort, or both. Radionuclide testing may also affect a patient's mobility: patients may be on bed rest or precautions after radionuclide studies. The physical therapist should refer to the physician's orders after testing to clarify the patient's mobility status.

Thyroid Disorders

Disorders of the thyroid gland result from a variety of causes and can be classified as hyperthyroidism or hypothyroidism.

TABLE 10-2 Thyroid Hormone Tests

Hormone	Test Description	Normal Value (adults)
Serum thyroxine (T_4)	Radioimmunoassay (RIA) measurement.	4-12 mcg/dl
Serum triiodothyronine (T_3)	RIA measurement.	40-204 ng/dl
Free thyroxine index	Direct RIA measurement or indirect calculated measurement.	0.93-1.71 ng/ml
Thyroid-stimulating hormone (TSH)	Radioisotope and chemical labeling measurement.	0.4-4.5 μU/ml
Thyrotropin-releasing hormone (TRH)	Intravenous administration of TRH to patients. TRH augments the function of TSH in patients with hypothyroidism. Only performed in difficult diagnostic cases. The expected response is a rise in TSH levels.	Normal rise in men and women is 6 μU/ml above baseline TSH levels. Normal rise in men older than 40 years is 2 μU/ml above baseline. Hypothyroidism is indicated by increased response to TRH. Hyperthyroidism is indicated by no response to TRH.

Data from Sacher RA, McPherson RA, Campos JM, editors: Widman's clinical interpretation of laboratory tests, ed 11, Philadelphia, 2000, FA Davis, pp 741-823; Cohee L: Endocrinology. In Johns Hopkins Hospital, Arcara K, Tschudy M, editors: The Harriet Lane handbook, ed 19, St Louis, 2011, Mosby.

TABLE 10-3 Thyroid Function Tests

Test	Description
Triiodothyronine resin uptake (RT_3U)	RT_3U qualifies levels of bound versus unbound T_4 and T_3 and helps to distinguish protein-binding disorders from true thyroid disease. Thyroid hormone uptake is high with hyperthyroidism and low with hypothyroidism.
Thyroidal 24-hour radioactive iodine uptake (RAIU)	Used to determine metabolic activity of the thyroid gland. Radioactive iodine is administered, and the percentage of total administered radioactive iodine taken up by the thyroid in 24 hours is then calculated. Normal radioactive iodine uptake is 10% to 25%. Hypothyroidism results in reduced uptake.
Thyroid imaging or scan	Intravenous administration of radionuclides allows imaging or scanning of particular areas of the thyroid gland. Increased or decreased uptake of the radionuclide can help diagnose dysfunction.
Ultrasound	Nodules of the thyroid gland that are palpable or detected by other imaging modalities are indications for ultrasound to help diagnose possible malignancy.
Needle biopsy	Fine-needle aspiration of thyroid cells may help diagnose a suspected neoplasm.

Data from Sacher RA, McPherson RA, Campos JM, editors: Widman's clinical interpretation of laboratory tests, ed 11, Philadelphia, 2000, FA Davis, pp 786-793; Bastin S, Bolland MJ, Croxson MS: Role of ultrasound in the assessment of nodular thyroid disease, J Med Imaging Radiat Oncol 53;177-187, 2009; McDermott M: Endocrine secrets, ed 5, St Louis, 2009, Mosby, pp 279-282.

Hyperthyroidism

Hyperthyroidism, or thyrotoxicosis, is primarily characterized by excessive sympathomimetic and catabolic activity resulting from overexposure of tissues to thyroid hormones. In addition, it has been reported that hyperthyroidism results in both an increased sympathetic activity with concurrent decreased vagal (parasympathetic) tone.[11] Spectral analysis of heart rate variability has been shown to detect these changes and is helpful in determining the severity of hyperthyroidism.[11] Heart rate variability is discussed further in Chapter 3. Patients may also present with *subclinical hyperthyroidism*, which may or may not lead to overt hyperthyroidism. Subclinical hyperthyroidism is defined by low TSH levels and normal T_3 and T_4 levels.[12] The most common causes of hyperthyroidism are outlined in Table 10-4.

Signs and symptoms of hyperthyroidism include the following[8,10,13]:

- Nervousness, irritation, emotional lability, tremors, insomnia
- Fatigue, weakness, increased reflexes
- Palpitations, atrial fibrillation, tachycardia
- Moist and warm skin, or smooth and velvety skin
- Increased perspiration, heat intolerance
- Diarrhea, thirst, weight loss despite increased appetite
- Reduced menstruation
- Lid lag, retraction, or both
- Finger nails that grow away from the nail bed, thinning or loss of hair
- Thyroid bruit, presence of goiter
- Patients may also present with subclinical hyperthyroidism

TABLE 10-4 Common Causes of Hyperthyroidism

Cause	Description
Graves' disease	A familial, autoimmune disorder responsible for approximately 80% to 90% of hyperthyroid cases. Occurs more commonly in women than men. Distinguishing features include diffuse thyroid enlargement, ophthalmopathy (double vision and sensitivity to light), exophthalmos (excessive prominence of the eyes), pretibial myxedema (thickening, redness, and puckering of skin in the front of the tibia), atrial fibrillation, fine hand tremors, and weakness of the quadriceps muscle.
Thyroiditis	Inflammation of the thyroid gland can result from an acute bacterial infection, a subacute viral infection, or chronic inflammation with unknown etiology. Pain may or may not be present on palpation of the gland.
Toxic nodular and multinodular goiter	Areas of the enlarged thyroid gland (goiter) become autonomous and produce excessive amounts of thyroid hormones.
Thyroid adenoma	Solitary, benign follicular adenomas that function autonomously result in hyperthyroidism if the adenoma nodule is larger than 4 cm in diameter. May present as a painless lump in the throat.
Thyroid carcinoma	Four types of malignancies in the thyroid gland: papillary carcinoma (most common), follicular carcinoma, anaplastic carcinoma, and medullary carcinoma.
Exogenous hyperthyroidism	Ingestion of excessive amounts of thyroid hormone or iodine preparation. Can be classified as iatrogenic hyperthyroidism, factitious hyperthyroidism, or iodine-induced hyperthyroidism.

Data from Woolf N, editor: Pathology, basic and systemic, London, 1998, Saunders, pp 863-873; Mitrou P, Raptis SA, Dimitriadis G: Thyroid disease in older people, Maturitas 70:5-9, 2011.

Management of hyperthyroidism primarily includes pharmacologic therapy, which is summarized in Chapter 19, Table 19-42. Surgical management is indicated for patients with large goiters, large "hot" nodules or where other options have been ruled out.[14] Surgical options include six different procedures that remove portions or all of the thyroid gland.[15]

Hypothyroidism

Hypothyroidism is the insufficient exposure of peripheral tissues to thyroid hormones. It affects growth and development, as well as many cellular processes. *Primary hypothyroidism* is caused by decreased thyroid hormone production by the thyroid gland and accounts for the majority of thyroid disease. *Secondary hypothyroidism* is caused by either pituitary or hypothalamic disease resulting in reduced TSH levels.[13]

The following are the causes of primary and secondary hypothyroidism[13,14]:

- Congenital maldevelopment, hypoplasia, or aplasia of the thyroid gland
- Hashimoto's thyroiditis (autoimmune inflammation)
- Hypopituitarism or hypothalamic disease
- Severe iodine deficiency
- Thyroid ablation from surgery, radiation of cervical neoplasms, or radioiodine therapy for hyperthyroidism
- Drug toxicity (from amiodarone or lithium)

General signs and symptoms of hypothyroidism vary according to the degree of thyroid deficiency. Signs and symptoms include the following[8,10,13]:

- Lethargy, somnolence, and reduced cognitive function
- Constipation and ileus (decreased motility)
- Rough, scaly, dry, and cool skin, decreased perspiration, yellowish complexion
- Delayed deep tendon reflexes
- Cold intolerance
- Weakness, muscle cramps, and aching and stiffness
- Slow speech, decreased hearing
- Paresthesia
- Nonpitting edema of eyelids, hands, and feet
- Bradycardia with elevated systolic and diastolic blood pressure
- Cardiac failure, pericardial effusion
- Coma and respiratory failure in severe cases

Additional laboratory findings that are associated with hypothyroidism include the following[16]:

- Low glucose and serum sodium levels
- Anemia
- Elevated levels of cholesterol, creatinine phosphokinase (CK-MM), serum myoglobin, lactate dehydrogenase, liver enzymes, homocysteine, and prolactin
- Proteinuria

Management of hypothyroidism typically includes lifelong thyroid hormone replacement, primarily consisting of generic and brand-name variations of levothyroxine.[10,13] A complete list of medications is provided in Chapter 19, Table 19-42.

✎ **CLINICAL TIP**

Properly managed hyperthyroidism or hypothyroidism should not affect physical therapy intervention or activity tolerance. If the signs or symptoms just mentioned are present during physical therapy evaluation, treatment, or both, then consultation with the medical team is indicated to help differentiate the etiology of the physical findings.

TABLE 10-5 Target Sites and Actions of Pituitary Gland Hormones

Hormone(s)	Target Site(s)	Action(s)
Anterior Lobe		
Growth hormone	Systemic	Stimulates body growth, lipolysis, inhibits insulin action on carbohydrates and lipids
Thyrotropin (thyroid-stimulating hormone)	Thyroid	Stimulates production of thyroid hormones
Adrenocorticotropic hormone (ACTH)	Adrenal cortex	Stimulates production of androgens and glucocorticoids by adrenal cortex
Follicle-stimulating hormone	Ovaries	Development of follicles and secretion of estrogen
	Testes	Development of seminiferous tubules and spermatogenesis
Luteinizing or interstitial cell–stimulating hormone	Ovaries	Ovulation, formation of corpus luteum, and secretion of progesterone
	Testes	Secretion of testosterone
Prolactin or lactogenic hormone	Mammary glands	Stimulates milk production and secretion
Posterior Lobe		
Antidiuretic hormone* (also called vasopressin)	Kidney	Controls rate of water excretion into the urine
		Fluid and electrolyte balance
Oxytocin*	Uterus	Contraction
	Breast	Expression of milk

From Hall JE: Pituitary hormones and their control by the hypothalamus. In Guyton and Hall textbook of medical physiology, ed 12, St Louis, 2010, Saunders Elsevier, pp 895-906.

*Actually produced in the hypothalamus but stored in the pituitary gland.

Pituitary Gland

Body Structure and Function

Hormones secreted by the pituitary gland are responsible for a variety of functions that are summarized in Table 10-5. Secretions of hormones from the pituitary gland are closely regulated by the hypothalamus and by negative feedback from the hormones that are secreted from the pituitary gland.[8]

Pituitary Tests

Individual pituitary hormone levels can be measured (1) by random blood samples; (2) by blood samples before and after the administration of specific releasing substances, such as serum TSH, during a thyrotropin-releasing hormone test (see Table 10-2); or (3) by blood samples before and after the administration of specific stimuli acting directly on the pituitary or via the hypothalamus, such as serum growth hormone (GH), serum cortisol, and plasma adrenocorticotropic hormone (ACTH). Table 10-6 describes common tests of pituitary function.

Pituitary function can also be evaluated by (1) thyroid function tests, which are an indirect assessment of TSH secretion from the pituitary, and (2) plain x-rays or computed tomography with contrast to highlight a pituitary tumor.[17]

Pituitary Disorders

Dysfunction of the pituitary-hypothalamic system generally results from hypersecretion or hyposecretion of tropic hormones. Hypersecretion of pituitary hormones (hyperpituitarism) is most commonly due to adenoma in the anterior lobe (benign tumors).[18] Hyposecretion of pituitary hormones (pituitary insufficiency) can result from pituitary disease, diseases affecting the hypothalamus or surrounding structures, or disturbance of blood flow around the hypothalamus and pituitary.[19,20]

Hyperpituitarism

The overproduction of the pituitary hormones GH, ACTH, and antidiuretic hormone (ADH) is discussed next.

Growth Hormone Overproduction. Excessive GH secretion is referred to as acromegaly in adults or gigantism in children. Excessive GH secretion has been linked primarily to anterior pituitary adenomas and not necessarily to excessive hypothalamic stimulation of the pituitary.[20]

Clinical manifestations for children with gigantism are characterized by disproportionately long limbs.[18]

Signs and symptoms of adults with acromegaly include the following[20,21]:

- Enlargement of hands and feet, coarse facial features with furrowed brows
- Oligomenorrhea or amenorrhea in women
- Paresthesia of hands, carpal tunnel syndrome
- Sweating
- Headaches
- Impotence in men
- Diabetes mellitus
- Hypertension
- Joint pains, osteoarthritis

Management of acromegaly may include the following: transsphenoidal surgical resection for microadenoma (treatment of choice in both Europe and the United States) and neurosurgery for macroadenomas.[22] Medical therapy consists of GH

> ✎ **CLINICAL TIP**
>
> Given the multisystem effects in patients with acromegaly, activity progression should proceed cautiously, with a focus on energy conservation, joint protection techniques, and fall-prevention strategies.

TABLE 10-6 Pituitary Hormone Tests

Hormone(s)	Test Description
Growth hormone (GH)	Serum level measurement by radioimmunoassay (RIA); normal values for men are 0 to 5 ng/ml; normal values for women are 0 to 10 ng/ml. *Growth hormone–stimulation test* (arginine test or insulin tolerance test). A baseline level of GH is established, then arginine or insulin is administered to the patient, and serial blood draws are performed to measure GH levels. GH should normally rise. Failure of GH levels to rise significantly may indicate growth hormone deficiency. *Growth hormone suppression test* (glucose load test). A baseline level of GH is established, followed by patient ingestion of a glucose solution. Levels of GH are redrawn at timed intervals. Normally, glucose inhibits the secretion of GH. If GH levels remain high despite the glucose load, then the likelihood of gigantism or acromegaly is increased.
Adrenocorticotropic hormone (ACTH)	Plasma ACTH levels are measured by RIA. Normal values are 25-100 pg/ml in the morning and 0-50 pg/ml in the evening. *ACTH-stimulation test* (Cortrosyn stimulating test). Indicated for evaluating primary or secondary adrenal insufficiency. Cosyntropin (Cortrosyn, a synthetic form of ACTH) is administered to the patient after a baseline level of cortisol is measured. ACTH acts to increase cortisol secretion from the adrenal gland. Normal results show an increased plasma cortisol level to >20 pg/dl after 30-60 minutes. *ACTH-suppression test* (dexamethasone suppression test). Dexamethasone is administered to the patient to determine ACTH response, which should be a reduction in ACTH levels in non-obese individuals. May be used in the diagnosis of Cushing's syndrome.
Antidiuretic hormone (ADH or vasopressin)	Normal plasma levels of ADH are 2-12 pg/ml if serum osmolality is > 290 mOsm/kg and <2 if serum osmolality is <290 mOsm/kg. *Water deprivation test* (dehydration test or concentration test). Indicated to aid in the diagnosis of diabetes insipidus (DI), either central or nephrogenic DI, or primary polydipsia. *Water loading test.* Indicated to aid in the diagnosis of syndrome of inappropriate antidiuretic hormone (SIADH). During the test, the patient ingests 20 to 25 ml/kg of fluid, with hourly serum and urine osmolality levels being measured for 4 hours.

Data from Malarkey LM, McMorrow ME, editors: Nurse's manual of laboratory tests and diagnostic procedures, Philadelphia, 2000, Saunders, pp 580-584, 552-555, 613-614, 616-619; and Wilson G, Mooradian A, Alexandraki I, Samrai G: Endocrinology. In Rakel RE, Rakel DP, editors: Textbook of family medicine, ed 8, Philadelphia, 2011, Elsevier Saunders, pp 756-784.

suppression with somatostatin receptor ligands (SRLs), dopamine agonists (DAs), and GH receptor antagonists (GHRA). Radiation therapy is considered third-line treatment.[23]

Adrenocorticotropic Hormone Overproduction. An increase in ACTH production by the pituitary gland results in increased levels of serum cortisol, which is a glucocorticoid secreted by the adrenal glands. Glucocorticoids are involved with carbohydrate, protein, and fat metabolism; therefore excess cortisol levels affect these cellular processes. Cushing's syndrome results from glucocorticoid excess (hypercortisolism). Cushing's disease, however, is specific to ACTH-producing microadenomas in the pituitary gland.[24] Pituitary hypersecretion of ACTH occurs in approximately 70% of patients with Cushing's syndrome. The hypersecretion of ACTH may originate either from a tumor in the pituitary gland or from ectopic neuroendocrine tumors elsewhere in the body.[8,25]

Signs and symptoms of Cushing's syndrome include the following[8,17,20,25]:

- Truncal obesity with thin extremities (loss of type II muscle fibers)[18]
- Redness and rounding of the face (moon face)
- Easy bruising, thinning of the skin, and presence of striae and darker pigmentation
- Hirsutism, oligomenorrhea, or amenorrhea
- Hypertension

- Osteoporosis (radiographically confirmed)
- Peripheral muscle wasting
- Backache
- Glucose intolerance, glycosuria, and polydipsia resulting in diabetes mellitus

Diagnosis of Cushing's syndrome is established by increased levels of urinary cortisol in a 24-hour period.[18] Management of Cushing's syndrome may include the following: surgical resection of pituitary lesion, radiation, or gamma-knife surgery.[25] Medical management may consist of steroidogenic inhibitors (ketoconazole) or neuromodulators of ACTH release with somatostatin analogs and dopamine agonists.[25]

Management of weakness, pain, edema, and osteoporosis should be the focus of physical therapy intervention and should be complementary to the medical management of the patient.

✎ CLINICAL TIP

Blood pressure changes during activity should be monitored, given the possibility of hypertension. Caution should also be taken to avoid bruising during mobility. Refer to the Diabetes Mellitus section for further activity considerations.

Antidiuretic Hormone Overproduction. The syndrome of inappropriate ADH (SIADH) secretion is a condition of fluid and electrolyte imbalance resulting in hyponatremia (reduced sodium levels) from excessive water reabsorption. In this condition, ADH is secreted from the posterior pituitary gland when it should be inhibited. Hyponatremia is fairly common in hospitalized patients and can result in significant morbidity and mortality.[26] Numerous etiologies of SIADH exist, with the most frequent cause being small cell or oat cell carcinomas of the lung. Other etiologies include the following[27,28]:

- Bacterial pneumonias, chronic obstructive pulmonary disease, tuberculosis, lung abscesses
- Malignancies of the pancreas, duodenum, colon, lymphoid tissue, and thymus
- Medication side effects from antipsychotics, sedative-hypnotics, antidepressants, diuretics, antihypertensives, analgesics, cardiac drugs, nonsteroidal antiinflammatory drugs, and antibiotics[29]
- Head trauma, central nervous system neoplasms

Mild SIADH is usually asymptomatic. More severe cases, however, can result in fluid and electrolyte imbalances, resulting in interstitial edema from a lack of serum sodium. Many systems will be affected by this edema, with the nervous system being most severely involved. Manifestations may include the following: headaches, nausea, confusion, gait disturbances, falls, and cerebral edema that leads to seizures and coma (in severe cases).[18,26,27]

Management of SIADH may include the following: treatment of the underlying cause, fluid restriction, or administration of select agents such as demeclocycline, lithium, and urea. Intravenous administration of sodium chloride (saline) solution, or administration of diuretics (furosemide) may also be used as initial therapies but not for long-term management.[26,27,29]

The developing use of vaptans or vasopressin-2 receptor antagonists for mild to moderate cases of SIADH has resulted in good outcomes.[26,30]

✎ **CLINICAL TIP**

The physical therapist should be aware of fluid restriction guidelines for patients with SIADH, especially because activity during physical therapy may increase the patient's thirst. These guidelines are often posted at the patient's bedside.

Hypopituitarism

Decreased secretion of pituitary hormones can result from either pituitary or hypothalamic dysfunction. Complete anterior pituitary hormone deficiency is referred to as panhypopituitarism.[31] Most cases of pituitary hypofunction arise from destructive processes involving the anterior pituitary, such as ischemic necrosis occurring during the late stages of pregnancy (Sheehan's syndrome). Additional causes may include pituitary adenomas, traumatic brain injury, pituitary surgery, or radiation.[31]

Symptoms and physical findings depend on the extent of the disorder and the specific hormone (GH, TSH, or ACTH) and target cells involved, such as[32]:

- Decreased libido, impotence with loss of pubic and axillary hair in men
- Amenorrhea and infertility in women
- Pallor
- Short stature (in children)
- Hypothyroidism
- Hypoadrenalism

Management of panhypopituitarism may include the following: replacement therapy or pituitary hormones, such as thyroxine, glucocorticoids, and GH for children; desmopressin for DI; androgen therapy for men; or estrogen therapy for women younger than 50 years of age. Management of other clinical sequelae of hypopituitarism is specific to the involved areas.[17,33]

Diabetes Insipidus

DI involves the excretion of a large volume (i.e., greater than 50 ml/kg per day) of dilute urine (hypotonic polyuria). DI may result from an absence of vasopressin or an inadequate response to vasopressin. Four categories of DI exist: primary polydipsia, central (hypothalamic) DI, gestational DI, and nephrogenic DI.[34]

Signs and symptoms of DI may be transient or permanent, and include the following[28,33,35,36]:

- Polyuria, nocturia with resultant hypernatremia (increased sodium)
- Thirst (especially for cold or iced drinks), polydipsia
- Dehydration
- Weight loss
- Dry skin with decreased turgor
- Central nervous system manifestations (e.g., irritability, mental dullness, ataxia, hyperthermia, and coma) if access to water is interrupted

Management of DI may include pharmacologic treatment, such as the following: deamino-8-D-arginine vasopressin (desmopressin), chlorpropamide (Diabinase), clofibrate (Atromid-S), carbamazepine (Tegretol), and thiazide diuretics in combination with a sodium-restricted diet.[37]

Adrenal Gland

Body Structure and Function

The adrenal gland has two distinct areas, the outer cortex and the inner medulla, that differ in their function and embryologic origin.[8] Table 10-7 summarizes the target sites and actions of the adrenal gland hormones.

Adrenal and Metabolic Tests

Adrenal Tests

Evaluation of the adrenal cortical (glucocorticoids, androgens, and mineralocorticoids) and medullary (epinephrine and norepinephrine) hormones is typically performed by measuring plasma and/or urinary levels of the hormone in question. Reference values for adults for each hormone are listed in Table 10-7. The primary method for evaluating adrenal activity is by measuring plasma cortisol levels. Levels are usually drawn at 8 AM and then

TABLE 10-7 Target Sites and Actions of Adrenal Gland Hormones

Hormone(s)	Target Site(s)	Action(s)	Reference Values*
Cortex			
Mineralocorticoids (aldosterone)	Kidney	Reabsorption of sodium and water Elimination of potassium	Upright position†: 5-30 ng/dl (females) 6-22 ng/dl (males) Urine: 2-26 mcg/24 hr
Glucocorticoids (cortisol)	Systemic	Metabolism of carbohydrate, protein, and fat Response to stress Suppresses immune responses Anti-inflammation	5 to 23 mcg/dl (8 to 10 AM) 3 to 13 mcg/dl (4 to 6 PM)[39] Urine: <100 mcg/dl in 24 hours
Sex hormones (androgens, progesterone, and estrogen)	Systemic	Preadolescent growth spurt, affects secondary sex characteristics	Testosterone: 280-180 ng/dl (males) <70 ng/dl (females) Estrogen: 10-50 pg/ml (males) 20-750 pg/ml (females, menstrual phase dependent) <20 pg/ml (postmenopausal female)
Medulla			
Epinephrine	Cardiac and smooth muscle, glands	Emergency functions Stimulates the action of the sympathetic system	Epinephrine: 1.7-22.4 mcg/24 hr
Norepinephrine	Organs innervated by sympathetic nervous system	Chemical transmitter substance Increases peripheral resistance	Norepinephrine: 12.1 to 85.5 mcg per 24 hours

Data from Fuller BF: Anatomy and physiology of the endocrine system. In Hudak CM, Gallo BM, editors: Critical care nursing: a holistic approach, ed 6, Philadelphia, 1994, Lippincott, p 875; Corbett JV, editor: Laboratory tests and diagnostic procedures with nursing diagnoses, ed 5, Upper Saddle River, NJ, 2000, Prentice Hall Health, p 391; Pagana KD, Pagana TJ: Mosby's diagnostic and laboratory test reference, ed 9, St Louis, 2009, Mosby.

*Blood levels unless otherwise specified.

†Aldosterone levels vary from supine to upright positions.

4 PM to evaluate whether there is any deviation from the expected diurnal variation. Cortisol levels peak in the morning and taper during the rest of the day. Increased levels indicate Cushing's syndrome, decreased levels suggest Addison's disease. Normal serum levels are 5 to 23 mcg/dl (8 to 10 AM) and 3 to 13 mcg/dl (4 to 6 PM).[38,39]

Analysis of urine over a 24-hour period is used to determine the urinary levels of free cortisol. Normal levels are less than 100 mcg/dl for a 24-hour period.[38,39] ACTH levels are usually examined concomitantly with cortisol levels, as ACTH secretion from the pituitary gland is necessary for cortisol secretion from the adrenal glands. Refer to Table 10-6 for details on ACTH measurement.

Anatomic investigation of the adrenal glands may also be performed to diagnose possible adrenal dysfunction. Common methods to accomplish this are computed tomography scan (to identify adrenal tumors), radioisotope scan using selenocholesterol, ultrasound, arteriogram, adrenal venogram (allows measurements of hormone levels), and intravenous pyelogram (see the Diagnostic Tests section in Chapter 9).[38]

Metabolic Tests

Metabolic tests are described in this section, as glucocorticoids (cortisol) affect carbohydrate, protein, and fat metabolism.

Glucose Tolerance Test. One of the criteria of the National Diabetes Data Group is to have a glucose tolerance test (GTT) result that presents with normal fasting blood glucose and a peak GTT and a 2-hour value of greater than 200 mg/dl on more than one occasion.[39] To perform the test, a 75-g or 100-g glucose load is given to the subject in the morning after a 12-hour fast. Blood glucose levels are then measured at variable time periods, ranging from every half hour to every hour for the next 2 to 4 hours after the glucose administration. The subject must remain inactive and refrain from smoking throughout the duration of the test. Normally, the blood glucose levels should fall back to baseline values in a 2-hour period. Normal glucose value for a fasting blood sugar (BS) is less than approximately 110 mg/dl. After 1 hour of ingesting the glucose load, expected levels of glucose are less than 200 mg/dl and 70 to 115 mg/dl after 4 hours.[39]

Adrenal Disorders

Adrenal Hyperfunction

Increased secretion of glucocorticoids (hypercortisolism) results in Cushing's syndrome, which is discussed in detail earlier in this chapter.

Adrenal Insufficiency

Autoimmune dysfunction can lead to destruction of the adrenal cortex (i.e., primary adrenal insufficiency or Addison's disease). Additionally, ACTH deficiency from the pituitary gland can lead to atrophy of the adrenal cortex (secondary adrenal insufficiency). The net result is an impaired adrenal system with decreased levels of glucocorticoids (cortisols), mineralocorticoids (aldosterone), and androgens. Given the systemic functions of these hormones, Addison's disease can have severe consequences if left untreated. Fortunately, the incidence of Addison's disease is rare.[40]

Cortisol deficiency results in decreased gluconeogenesis (glucose production), which in turn alters cellular metabolism. Decreased gluconeogenesis also results in hypoglycemia and decreased ability to respond to stress. Aldosterone deficiency causes fluid and electrolyte imbalance, primarily as a result of increased water excretion that leads to dehydration.[41,42]

Symptoms and physical findings common to adrenal insufficiency include the following[40,43]:

- Weakness, fatigue
- Weight loss, nausea, vomiting, vague abdominal pain
- Muscle and joint pain
- Salt craving in fewer than 20% of patients
- Hyperpigmentation
- Hypotension

Management of adrenal insufficiency typically includes pharmacologic intervention with any of the following steroids: hydrocortisone, prednisone, dexamethasone fludrocortisone, or cortisone.[36,40]

Pheochromocytoma

Pheochromocytoma is a rare adrenomedullary disorder caused by a tumor of the chromaffin cells in the adrenal medulla, which results in excess secretion of the catecholamines, epinephrine, and norepinephrine. Disease presentation can occur either in childhood or early adulthood with sporadic pheochromocytomas occurring between 40 and 50 years of age.[44] Given the rare occurrence of this tumor, it often goes undiagnosed. Proper diagnosis is essential, as the sustained release of catecholamines can be life threatening.[43,45,46]

Signs and symptoms of pheochromocytoma include the following[41,43,45,46]:

- Classic triad of palpitations, headaches, and sweating lasting minutes to hours
- Flushing, nausea, tiredness, or weight loss
- Abdominal pain, constipation, or chest pain
- Elevated blood glucose levels and glucosuria

Management of pheochromocytoma generally includes surgical excision of the tumor with preoperative pharmacologic management to block the effects of circulating catecholamine in all patients with catecholamine-producing tumors with alpha-adrenergic blockers and/or calcium channel blockers: nifedipine, diltiazem, phenoxybenzamine, or doxazosin. Low-dose beta-blockade with metoprolol, bisoprolol, or atenolol may also be implemented preoperatively.[46]

Pancreatic Disorders

Insulin Resistance

Insulin resistance is an important link to the development of metabolic syndrome, type 2 diabetes, cardiovascular disease, and possibly some cancers. Patients who are overweight or obese are more likely to develop insulin resistance over time; however, patients who are not obese may also have insulin resistance. Patients who have insulin resistance also present with compensatory hyperinsulinemia and hyperglycemia. Furthermore, insulin resistance in the absence of metabolic syndrome criteria (see the next section) has also been shown to be independently related to developing cardiovascular disease. Insulin resistance has been detected 10 to 20 years before developing diabetes in individuals who are offspring of patients with type 2 diabetes.[47-50]

Metabolic Syndrome

According to an international, multiassociation statement, "metabolic syndrome is a complex of interrelated risk factors for cardiovascular disease (CVD) and diabetes mellitus. Patients with the metabolic syndrome have twice the risk of developing CVD over the next 5 to 10 years as compared to individuals without the syndrome. Additionally, metabolic syndrome confers a fivefold increase in risk for developing type 2 diabetes mellitus."[51]

Metabolic syndrome is defined as the cluster of clinical manifestations that are present just before the onset of type 2 diabetes.[52] Patients with metabolic syndrome have a high likelihood of having concurrent insulin resistance. However, the difference between metabolic syndrome and insulin resistance syndrome is that metabolic syndrome focuses on establishing a diagnosis for patients who are at higher risk for type 2 diabetes and cardiovascular disease and prescribing timely intervention to offset the development of these diseases and their complications. Currently, there are no defined diagnostic criteria for insulin resistance syndrome.[47,53]

The diagnosis of metabolic syndrome is established when patients have at least three of the criteria outlined in Table 10-8.

The cornerstone of management of this syndrome is weight loss, with a modest reduction in initial weight of 7% to 10% demonstrating significant reduction in the development of diabetes and cardiovascular disease.[52] In addition to this therapeutic lifestyle change, participation in an exercise program has

> ✎ **CLINICAL TIP**
>
> In the acute care setting, physical therapists unfortunately will not have a significant role in exercise prescription to create the long-term changes necessary to modify metabolic syndrome. However, if working with patients who have metabolic syndrome, physical therapists should either ensure that patients can continue with a current exercise program or strongly recommend follow-up services for patients to begin an exercise program.

TABLE 10-8 Criteria for Diagnosis of Metabolic Syndrome

Sign	Diagnostic Range
Elevated waist circumference*	Population- and country-specific definitions USA: >102 cm in men; > 88 cm in women
Elevated triglycerides#	≥150 mg/dl (1.7 mmol/L)
Reduced HDL-C†#	<40 mg/dl (1.0 mmol/L) in males <50 mg/dl (1.3 mmol/L) in females
Elevated blood pressure#	Systolic ≥ 130 and/or diastolic 85 mm Hg
Elevated fasting glucose#	≥100 mg/dl

Data from Alberti KGMM et al: Harmonizing the metabolic syndrome: a joint interim statement of the International Diabetes Federation Task Force on Epidemiology and Prevention; National Heart, Lung, and Blood Institute; American Heart Association; World Heart Federation; International Atherosclerosis Society; and International Association for the Study of Obesity, Circulation 120:1640-1645, 2009.

*Waist circumferences vary depending on specific country definitions.

†HDL-C indicates high-density lipoprotein cholesterol.

#If values are not available, then presence of drug therapy is an alternate indicator.

been shown to either delay or prevent the development of type 2 diabetes as well as improve the cardiovascular risk profile of patients by increasing HDL levels and lowering blood pressure.[53]

Diabetes Mellitus

Diabetes mellitus is a syndrome with metabolic, vascular, and neural components that originates from glucose intolerance, which in turn leads to hyperglycemic states (increased plasma glucose levels). Hyperglycemia can result from insufficient insulin production, insulin action, or both. Insulin promotes storage of glucose as glycogen in muscle tissue and the liver. Deficiency of insulin leads to increased levels of plasma glucose.[54,55]

The diagnosis of diabetes is based on the presence of any one of the following four factors[8,56]:

1. Presence of polyuria, polydipsia, weight loss, blurred vision, and random plasma glucose (regardless of last meal) ≥ 200 mg/dl (11.1 mmol/L)
2. Fasting plasma glucose (FPG) ≥ 126 mg/dl (7.0 mmol/L). Fasting involves no caloric intake for at least 8 hours.
3. Two-hour postload glucose ≥ 200 mg/dl, during an oral glucose tolerance test (OGTT) using a 75-g oral glucose load dissolved in water, as described by the World Health Organization.
4. A1C ≥ 6.5%, measured with a standardized assay. A1C is a widely used marker for chronic glycemia and glycemic management.

The diagnosis is confirmed when one of the listed factors is also found on a subsequent day or in situations when hyperglycemia is unclear.[8,55,56]

The two primary types of diabetes mellitus are type 1 (insulin-dependent or juvenile-onset diabetes) and type 2 (non–insulin-dependent or adult-onset diabetes). After much debate on the classification of diabetes, the current terminology for diabetes uses type 1 and type 2 diabetes to distinguish between the two primary types.[54,56] Other forms of glucose intolerance disorders exist but are not discussed in this book.

Recent studies indicate a bidirectional association between diabetes and depression with increased risk among individuals who are being treated for type 2 diabetes.[57-59] Routine screening for depression should be considered if clinicians note increased risk of elevated symptoms in those with diabetes. If patient is found to be at risk for depression, referral may be appropriate.[57-59] Outcome measure tools that are useful to assess depression include the Center for Epidemiologic Studies Depression Scale (CES-D), Mini Mental State Exam (MMSE), and Patient Health Questionaire.[59-61]

Type 1 Diabetes

Type 1 diabetes is an autoimmune disorder with a genetic-environmental etiology that leads to the selective destruction of beta cells in the pancreas. This destruction results in decreased or absent insulin secretion. Type 1 diabetes represents 5% to 10% of the population with diabetes and generally occurs in individuals under the age of 40 years.[54,56,62-64] Other etiologies for type 1 diabetes exist but are not discussed in this book.

Classic signs and symptoms of type 1 diabetes are described in the previous section with the diagnostic criteria for diabetes.[62]

Management of type 1 diabetes may include the following[63-65]:

- Close self- or medical monitoring of blood glucose levels (Table 10-9).
- Insulin administration through oral medications, intramuscular injection, or continuous subcutaneous insulin infusion (CSII) pump. CSII therapy has been shown to be as effective as multiple daily injections of insulin, while also providing the ability to mimic a more natural glycemic response in fasting and postprandial states (Table 10-10). A medication summary is provided in Chapter 19, Table 19-39.
- New options for insulin routes of administration have been in various stages of investigation and development, including oral spray, insulin pill, insulin patch, artificial pancreas, and inhaled insulin.[66] These routes of administration are further described later, after the type 2 diabetes section.
- Diet modification based on caloric content, proportion of basic nutrients and optimal sources, and distribution of nutrients in daily meals.
- Meal planning.
- Exercise on a regular basis.

Research directed at curing type 1 diabetes is aimed at specifically identifying the causative genes, permanent replacement of lost beta-cell function (which could involve islet cell transplantation), regeneration of beta cells, or development of an immortalized insulin-secreting cell line.[54] These therapies are administered directly after diagnosis to increase beta-cell function. Currently stem cells from donor bone marrow and a patient's own umbilical cord blood are being investigated. Drug studies are also being investigated in an attempt to prevent this autoimmune attack by reeducating the immune system.[67,68]

TABLE 10-9 Tests to Monitor Control of Diabetes

Test	Description
Self-monitoring	
Blood glucose finger stick samples Reference, 60-110 mg/dl (fasting) ≤200 mg/dl (non-fasting)	Monitors immediate control of diabetes. Very effective in establishing the correct insulin dosages and preventing complications from diabetes. Capillary blood is obtained by a needle stick of a finger or an earlobe and placed on a reagent strip. The reagent strip is compared to a color chart or placed in a portable glucometer to read the glucose level. Patients in the hospital can also have blood drawn from an indwelling arterial line, for ease of use, without compromising accuracy of measurement.
Urine testing Random specimen: negative	A reagent strip is dipped in the patient's urine, and the strip is compared to a color chart to measure glucose levels in the urine. Provides satisfactory results only for patients who have stable diabetes; otherwise, results can be insensitive for truly delineating hyperglycemia.
Medical Monitoring	
Glycosylated hemoglobin (GHB), HbA1C Reference, 4%-5.9% of total hemoglobin for a patient with controlled diabetes	Hyperglycemia results in saturation of hemoglobin molecules during the life span of a red blood cell (approximately 120 days). Measuring the amount of GHB in the blood provides a weighted average of the glucose level over a period of time and is a good indicator of long-term control of diabetes, without confounding factors such as a recent meal or insulin injection. Measurements are performed every 3 to 6 months.

Data from Pagana KD, Pagana TJ: Mosby's diagnostic and laboratory test reference, ed 9, St Louis, 2009, Mosby.

TABLE 10-10 Summary of Insulin Pump Therapy

Parameter	Description
Patient candidacy	Demonstrated ability to self-monitor glucose and adjust insulin doses based on preprandial blood glucose levels and anticipated future activity level. Motivated to achieve and maintain improved glycemic control using intensive insulin therapy. Pregnant patients with type 1 diabetes. Patients unaware of hypoglycemic episodes with insulin therapy. Patients who experience wide glycemic variations on a day-to-day basis. Patients with a significant rise in hyperglycemia in the morning ("dawn phenomenon"). Patients who need flexibility in their insulin regimen (e.g., erratic work schedules, travel frequently). Adolescents who experience frequent diabetic ketoacidosis. Nighttime use for children under 10 years of age who may not be able to adjust their own insulin requirements.
Pump description	Approximately the size of an electronic pager, weighing only 4 oz. Patients are instructed on how to insert and change (every 2 to 3 days) infusion catheters into the subcutaneous space of their abdomen. The catheter can be detached from the insulin pump for bathing or intimate contact. Two settings: basal rate and bolus doses, both adjustable by the patient depending on needs (e.g., preprandial bolus or decreased basal rate with exercise). Battery life is approximately 6 weeks.
Types of insulin	Regular human buffered insulin (short acting). Insulin analog (rapid acting).
Pump complications	Hyperglycemia and diabetic ketoacidosis. Hypoglycemia and hypoglycemic unawareness. Skin infections. Weight gain.

Data from Unger J: A primary care approach to continuous subcutaneous insulin infusion, Clin Diabetes 17(3):113, 1999; Continuous subcutaneous insulin, Diabetes Care 26(1):S125 2003; Kaufman FR, Halvorson M, Kim C, et al: Use of insulin pump therapy at nighttime only for children 7-10 years of age with type 1 diabetes, Diabetes Care 123(5):579, 2000.

Type 2 Diabetes

Type 2 diabetes is more common in the United States than type 1 diabetes and generally occurs after 40 years of age. Type 2 diabetes is significantly linked to obesity, a sedentary lifestyle, and aging. Genetic predisposition has also been established.[54,56,64]

The mechanism of type 2 diabetes involves increasing cellular resistance to insulin, which results in a compensatory hypersecretion of insulin from the pancreatic beta cells that ultimately leads to a failure in insulin production.[54,56,62-64] Other etiologies for type 2 diabetes exist but are not discussed in this text. A growing epidemic of concern in recent years is the number of children in the United States who are being diagnosed with type 2 diabetes. Of all new diagnoses of type 2 diabetes in the United States, 8% to 45% are children and adolescents. The onset generally occurs between ages 12 and 16 and has higher prevalence in girls and minorities. According to the CDC, between 2002 and 2005, 3600 youth were newly diagnosed with type 2 diabetes annually.[69-73]

Signs and symptoms of type 2 diabetes may be similar to those of type 1 diabetes but can also include the following:

- Recurrent infections and prolonged wound healing
- Genital pruritus
- Visual changes
- Paresthesias

Management of type 2 diabetes is similar to that of type 1 diabetes, with an emphasis on medical nutritional therapy (MNT) and exercise to control hyperglycemia. Monitoring carbohydrate intake, by carbohydrate counting, exchanges, or experience-based estimation, is a component of MNT.[74] Oral hypoglycemic agents and insulin administration may also be used.[63,65,75,76] CSII has been shown to be as effective as multiple dose injections of insulin in patients with type 2 diabetes.[77] Clinical studies are also investigating the use of inhaled insulin for these patients, with preliminary findings demonstrating promising results.[78,79]

Chapter 19 provides a summary of medications used to manage type 2 diabetes (see Table 19-39).

Research trends for type 2 diabetes includes identifying the gene(s) responsible for the predisposition to type 2 diabetes and the mechanisms by which environmental factors trigger this predisposition. Also, identification of the cellular defects responsible for insulin resistance and impaired insulin secretion in type 2 diabetes will, it is hoped, lead to the development of new medications that will be specific and relatively free of unwanted adverse effects.[54]

✎ CLINICAL TIP

Blood sugar or glucose levels are denoted in the medical record as BS or BG levels, respectively.

Physical Therapy Considerations

- Glycemic control for patients with type 1 or type 2 diabetes may be altered significantly with the onset of new illnesses, such as systemic infection, because these new processes require added glucose metabolism. It is important for the therapist to carefully monitor the patient's blood glucose levels during therapeutic interventions, because the symptoms of diabetes may be exacerbated in a patient with significant comorbidities.
- Patients with diabetes present with a wide range of their individual "normal" values. Therefore establishing the tolerable high or low value for each patient during the initial evaluation is very important in determining the parameters for physical therapy intervention.
- Patients with poor glycemic control can have wide fluctuations in the BS levels on a daily basis. Therefore be sure to always verify their BS level before physical therapy intervention.
- Consult with the nurse or physician to determine if therapy should be deferred for patients who were recently placed on

intravenous insulin to stabilize their glucose levels. A pre-exercise glucose level less than 100 mg/dl may require added carbohydrate ingestion before starting the activity.[74] Patients who are hyperglycemic before exercise should be monitored for ketosis (ketone bodies in blood or urine). If the patient feels well and there is an absence of ketosis, then monitored exercise can proceed.[74]

- Patients who were following a regular exercise program for glycemic control before hospital admission will require education about how to modify their exercise parameters during the hospitalization and on discharge. Modification of exercise parameters will be dependent on the nature of concurrent illnesses.
- Hypoglycemia may occur during exercise or up to 24 hours after exercise because of an inability to regulate insulin levels. To help prevent this, the patient should consume extra carbohydrates before and during exercise (e.g., 10 g of carbohydrates per 30 minutes of activity), and the nurse or patient may also decrease the dose or rate of insulin infusion, especially with CSII.
- The physical therapist should be aware of catheter placement on the patient for CSII therapy so the catheter will not be disrupted during intervention.
- Circulation of insulin that is injected into an exercising limb is enhanced as a result of increased blood flow and temperature. Insulin injection into the exercising limb may therefore lead to hypoglycemia. Insulin can be injected into the abdomen to help prevent this process.
- Insulin is necessary to modulate lipolysis and hepatic (liver) glucose production during exercise. Performing exercise without adequate insulin can lead to hyperglycemia and ketogenesis.
- Coordinating physical therapy sessions with meals and insulin injections may help optimize exercise tolerance.
- Keeping glucose sources, such as graham crackers, close by is helpful in case hypoglycemia does occur with activity.

Insulin Routes of Administration

Subcutaneous injection of insulin has been the only effective self-insulin delivery option available until recent years. Complicated equipment and the need for self-injections contribute to noncompliance with medication and treatment. Subcutaneous injections tend to have slow absorption and can result in peripheral hyperinsulinemia as well as stress, pain, burden of daily injections, high cost, infection, inability to handle insulin, and localized subcutaneous deposits of insulin. These localized deposits of insulin can lead to local hypertrophy and fat deposits, which can contribute to diabetic microangiography and macroangiopathy.[80-85]

Alternative routes of insulin administration currently include the continuous subcutaneous insulin infusion (CSII) pump (see Table 10-10), an implanted pump, an insulin pen, and an insulin patch pump. Under ongoing investigation and development is a fully artificial pancreas. In addition there has been interest in developing new noninvasive routes of insulin administration, including buccal, transdermal, pulmonary, oral, and nasal delivery.

Implanted Pump. An implanted pump provides continuous subcutaneous insulin and eliminates multiple daily injections for individuals with type 1 diabetes while delivering a continuous basal rate for 24 hours. It also allows for manual adjustments due to changes in glucose levels. A catheter is surgically inserted into the peritoneal cavity, and the pump is implanted into the abdominal wall, which can then be programmed by an external handheld device. Reduced frequency of hypoglycemic episodes and better glucose regulation compared to subcutaneous injections have been demonstrated, resulting in fewer instability-related diabetic hospitalizations. Current use has been limited to select patients.[80,81]

Artificial Pancreas. The fully artificial pancreas for type 1 diabetes has made steady progress toward development. This system functions as a "closed-loop system" because insulin release is controlled through feedback in response to glucose level changes, essentially mimicking the body's regulation of glucose. It consists of an insulin pump and a device that continuously monitors glucose levels, which then regulates the pump based on current levels.[86,87] One study concluded that the closed-loop system was superior to open-loop systems in controlling type 1 diabetes; however, improvements were needed to account for post-breakfast glucose changes.[87]

Insulin Pen. Currently approved for use, the insulin pen is advantageous because it is easy to use, portable, and discreet. It can be used for either type 1 or 2 diabetes and has a premeasured amount of insulin. This form of subcutaneous insulin administration has been shown to be most accurate with doses of less than 5 IU. Improved health-related quality of life has been reported when compared to using a subcutaneous insulin syringe.[88]

Patch Pump. A patch pump consists of an insulin reservoir, delivery system, and cannula integrated into a small, wearable, and disposable/semidisposable device. It is convenient because it eliminates tubing, is easy to use with simplified training, and

is discreet. OmniPod is an example of the insulin patch pump currently approved for use, which attaches to skin by adhesive. It communicates wirelessly to a personal data manager and needs to be changed every 3 days. It is waterproof to allow for showering/swimming.[81,88,89]

Buccal Insulin Spray. Research reports indicate that buccal insulin spray can provide a constant, predictable drug concentration to the blood as the insulin is absorbed by the buccal mucosa in the mouth cavity and cheek.[66,84,88] Buccal insulin spray is short acting; therefore it may need to be used more frequently. It has also been found to irritate the buccal mucosa and leave a bitter taste in the mouth.[66,88,90]

Transdermal Patch, Iontophoresis, Ultrasound, and Microneedles. Transdermal delivery via patch, iontophoresis, ultrasound, and microneedles is still being investigated. These methods of delivery are expensive because they require equipment to aid insulin in crossing the skin barrier. Investigation is also complicated by the increased length of time required to transmit a therapeutic level of insulin across the skin and into the bloodstream via these methods.[66,88]

Pulmonary Inhaled Insulin. Inhaled insulin has been in various stages of use and research for patients with either type 1 or 2 diabetes. It is an inhaler, making it easy to transport. It can be in a dry powder or solution form. Inhaled insulin goes directly to the lungs, which offer a large surface area for absorption. Mild to moderate cough was reported as a side effect, as well as more episodes of hypoglycemia compared to oral agents. Important to note is that different doses are needed for smokers and asthmatics. It is also not clear how inhaled insulin absorption will affect different types of lung disease.[66,88,91]

Oral Insulin Pill. The oral insulin pill has been an area of investigation for noninvasive insulin delivery. Researchers are currently trying to identify a polymeric matrix to carry insulin and protect it from the gastrointestinal tract. Insulin delivery by pill is potentially the most acceptable route of administration.[66,92] Should this mode be approved, then possible physical therapy considerations are listed in Table 10-11.

Oral Pill plus Mucoadhesive. The oral pill plus mucoadhesive form of insulin delivery is currently in the research phase. It consists of a pill that encapsulates a patch that attaches to the intestines, promoting unidirectional diffusion into the mucosa lining of the intestines. Although animal trials are still being conducted, the plasma insulin levels are said to be comparable to that of injected insulin. Toxicity of mucoadhesive polymeric delivery over a long period of time is unknown and therefore a concern.[66,93]

Nasal Spray. Nasal spray is currently in the research stage. This route of delivery would access a large and highly vascularized area, allowing for quicker onset. Unfortunately, long-term use of spray is known to damage the nasal mucosa, resulting in bleeding. Also, repeated doses are likely needed to achieve adequate glucose control.[66,88].

Complications of Diabetes Mellitus

Patients with diabetes mellitus, despite management, can still develop organ and organ-system damage linked to lesions of the small and large blood vessels. Complications can manifest 2 to

15 years after diagnosis. They can be classified as (1) microangiopathy (microvascular disease), which causes retinopathy (occurs in 60% to 80% of patients), nephropathy, and foot ischemia; (2) macroangiopathy (macrovascular disease), which accelerates widespread atherosclerosis; or (3) neuropathy.[49,63] Another complication from diabetes that is not directly linked to vascular damage is diabetic ketoacidosis (DKA).

Diabetic Ketoacidosis. Patients with type 1 diabetes have the potential to develop this complication as a result of unusual metabolic stress (e.g., changes in diet, infection) and can progress from mild to moderate glucose intolerance, to fasting hyperglycemia, to ketosis, and, finally, to ketoacidosis. Most patients do not progress to the ketotic state but have the potential to do so if proper treatment is not administered.[19]

Patients who progress to DKA usually present with a plasma glucose level between 500 and 700 mg/dl.[49]

DKA is the end result of ineffective levels of circulating insulin, which lead to elevated levels of ketone bodies in the tissues, a state referred to as ketosis. Decreased insulin levels lead to uncontrolled lipolysis (fat breakdown), which increases the levels of free fatty acids released from the liver and ultimately leads to an overproduction of ketone bodies. Ketone bodies are acids, and if they are not buffered properly by bases, a state of ketoacidosis occurs. Ketoacidosis almost always results from uncontrolled diabetes mellitus; however, it may also result from alcohol abuse.[8,19,64]

Signs and symptoms of DKA include the following[19]:
- Polyuria, polydipsia, dehydration
- Weakness and lethargy
- Myalgia, hypotonia
- Headache, difficulty paying attention, and confusion
- Anorexia
- Nausea, vomiting, abdominal pain, acute abdomen
- Dyspnea, deep and sighing respirations (Kussmaul's respiration)

- Acetone-smelling ("fruity") breath
- Hypothermia
- Stupor (coma), fixed, dilated pupils
- Uncoordinated movements
- Hyporeflexia

Management of DKA may include the following: insulin administration, hydration, electrolyte (sodium, potassium, and phosphorus) replacement, supplemental oxygen, and mechanical ventilation.[8,62,64]

Hyperosmolar Hyperglycemic Nonketotic Syndrome/ Coma. Similar to ketoacidosis, it is experienced by older individuals with type 2 diabetes. The most common symptom is increased sugar in the urine.[94]

Diabetic Dermopathy. Skin lesions in patients with diabetes, particularly on their feet, are common and multifactorial in nature. Diabetic dermopathy will often look like circular, scaly, light brown patches. It is most commonly seen on the anterior aspect of the bilateral lower extremities.[94]

Lesions may result from any combination of the following[20,63,95]:
- Loss of sensation from sensory neuropathy
- Skin atrophy from microangiopathy
- Decreased blood flow from macroangiopathy
- Sensory and autonomic neuropathy, resulting in abnormal blood distribution that may cause bone demineralization and Charcot's joint (disruption of the midfoot)[96]

Proper foot care in diabetic individuals helps prevent complications, such as poor wound healing, which can progress to tissue necrosis and ultimately lead to amputation.[95] Box 10-1 describes patient information regarding foot care for patients with diabetes. Refer to Chapter 12 for more details on diabetic ulcers.

Infection. Individuals with diabetes are at a higher risk for infection because of (1) decreased sensation (vision and touch); (2) poor blood supply, which leads to tissue hypoxia; (3) hyperglycemic states, which promote rapid proliferation of pathogens

---

BOX 10-1 Foot Care for Patients with Diabetes

Don't	Do
Smoke.	Encourage the patient to have regular medical or podiatric examinations to determine integrity of his or her feet.
Wash feet in cold or hot water. The water temperature should be lukewarm (approximately 85° to 95°F).	Inspect feet daily for abrasions, blisters, and cuts. Use a mirror if soles cannot be seen. If vision is poor, another person should check feet.
Use a heating pad, heating lamp, or hot water bottles to warm the feet.	Wash feet daily with lukewarm water and soap.
Use razor blades or scissors to cut corns or calluses. Have a podiatrist perform this procedure.	Dry feet carefully, especially between the toes.
Use over-the-counter medications on corns or calluses.	Apply hand cream or lanolin to feet (dry areas).
Cross legs when sitting.	Be careful not to leave cream between the toes.
Wear girdles or garters.	Wear clean socks or stockings daily.
Walk barefoot.	Cut nails straight across and file down edges with an emery board.
Wear shoes without socks or stockings.	Wear comfortable shoes that fit and don't rub.
Wear sandals with thongs between the toes.	Wear wide toe-box or custom-made shoes if foot deformities exist.
Wear socks or stocking with raised seams.	Inspect the inside of shoes for any objects, tacks, or torn linings before putting on the shoes.
Place hands in shoes for inspection, if sensory neuropathy is present in the hands. Instead shake out the shoes for any objects.	

Data from Mayfield JA, Reiber GE, Sanders LJ: Preventive foot care in people with diabetes, Diabetes Care 24(1):S56, 2001.

that enter the body; (4) decreased immune response from reduced circulation, which leaves white blood cells unable to get to the affected area; (5) impaired white blood cell function, which leads to abnormal phagocytosis; and (6) chemotaxis.[62,97]

Bacterial infections are most commonly caused by *Staphylococcus* bacteria. Presentation includes boils, folliculitis, carbuncles, and infections around the nails. Fungal infections are also commonly caused by *Candida albicans* in individuals with diabetes. These infections are often found in folds of the skin, including under the breasts, around nails, and between fingers and toes. Other areas of the body where it can be found are at the corners of the mouth, axillae, and groin.[94]

> ✎ **CLINICAL TIP**
>
> Skin checks are an especially important part of a physical therapists screening process for those with diabetes due to increased likelihood of infections, particularly in less active or bed-bound patients.

Diabetic Neuropathy. Of people with diabetes, 60% to 70% have mild to severe nerve damage, including impaired sensation or pain in the feet or hands. Diabetic neuropathy can also cause slow digestion of food in the stomach, carpal tunnel syndrome, erectile dysfunction, or other nerve problems.[98] The exact link between neural dysfunction and diabetes is unknown; however, the vascular, metabolic, and immunologic changes that occur with diabetes can promote destruction of myelin sheaths and therefore interfere with normal nerve conduction.[99]

Neuropathies can be manifested as (1) focal mononeuropathy and radiculopathy (disorder of single nerve or nerve root);

(2) symmetric sensorimotor neuropathy, associated with disabling pain and depression; or (3) autonomic neuropathy.

The most common diabetic neuropathy is peripheral symmetric polyneuropathy. Sensory deficits are greater than motor deficits and occur in a glove-and-stocking pattern, resulting in a loss of pinprick and light-touch sensations in these areas. However, patients will commonly present with a mixture of these three primary types of neuropathies. Foot ulcers and footdrop are common manifestations of diabetic neuropathies.[17,62-64,99]

Table 10-11 outlines the signs and symptoms of the different types of diabetic neuropathy. Management of diabetic neuropathy may include the following[99]:

- Strict glycemic control (primary method)
- Pain relief with:
  - Tricyclic antidepressants, such as amitriptyline, nortriptyline, and desipramine
  - Anticonvulsants, such as carbamazepine, phenytoin, gabapentin, and clonazepam
  - Topical agents, such as capsaicin cream (0.025% to 0.075%) or lidocaine ointment
  - Opioids (used as a last resort)
  - Transcutaneous electrical nerve stimulation
- Aldose reductase inhibitors aimed at slowing the progression of nerve damage
- Exogenous nerve growth factors
- Immunotherapy
- Pancreatic transplant

Additional complications from diabetes include coronary artery disease, stroke, peripheral vascular disease, and nephropathy. These are described in other chapters as listed next.

TABLE 10-11   Signs and Symptoms of Diabetic Neuropathy

Classification of Diabetic Neuropathy	Symptoms	Signs
Symmetric Polyneuropathies		
Peripheral sensory polyneuropathy	Paresthesias, numbness, coldness, tingling pins and needles (mainly in feet) Pain, often disabling, worse at night	Absent ankle jerk Impairment of vibration sense in feet Foot ulcers (often over metatarsal heads)
Peripheral motor neuropathy	Weakness	Bilateral interosseous muscle atrophy, claw or hammer toes, decreased grip strength, decreased manual muscle test grades
Autonomic neuropathy	Constipation or diarrhea, nausea or vomiting, tremulousness, impotence, dysphagia	Incontinence, orthostatic hypotension, tachycardia, peripheral edema, gustatory sweating
Focal and Multifocal Neuropathies		
Cranial neuropathy	Pain behind or above the eye, headaches, facial or forehead pain	Palpebral ptosis Inward deviation of one eye
Trunk and limb mononeuropathy	Abrupt onset of cramping or lancinating pain Constricting band-like pain in trunk or abdomen Cutaneous hyperesthesia of the trunk	Peripheral nerve-specific motor loss Abdominal wall weakness
Proximal motor neuropathy or diabetic amyotrophy	Pain in lower back, hips, and thighs that is worse at night; loss of appetite, depression	Asymmetric proximal weakness Atrophy in lower limbs Absent or diminished knee jerk

Data from Boissonault JS, Madlon-Kay D: Screening for endocrine system disease. In Boissonault WG, editor: Examination in physical therapy: screening for medical disease, New York, 1991, Churchill Livingstone, p 159; Melvin-Sater PA: Diabetic neuropathy, Physician Assist 24(7):63, 2000; Saudek CD: Diabetes mellitus. In Stobo JD, Hellmann DB, Ladenson PW et al: editors: The principles and practice of medicine, ed 23, Stamford, CT, 1996, Appleton & Lange, p 330.

Coronary Artery Disease. See Acute Coronary Syndrome in Chapter 3 for a discussion of coronary artery disease.

Stroke. See the Cerebrovascular Accident section in Chapter 6 for a discussion of stroke.

Peripheral Vascular Disease. See the Atherosclerosis section in Chapter 7 for a discussion of peripheral vascular disease.

Nephropathy. See Chapter 9 for a discussion on nephropathy.

Hypoglycemia (Hyperinsulinism). Hypoglycemia is a state of decreased BS levels (<50 mg/dl serum glucose). Excess serum insulin results in decreased BS levels, which leads to symptoms of hypoglycemia. Causes for this imbalance of insulin and sugar levels can be grouped as (1) fasting, (2) postprandial, or (3) induced.[28,49]

Fasting hypoglycemia occurs before eating and can be caused by insulin-producing beta-cell tumors (insulinomas), liver failure, chronic alcohol ingestion, GH deficiency, or extrapancreatic neoplasm, or it can be leucine induced. It can also occur in infants whose mothers have diabetes.[49]

Postprandial hypoglycemia occurs after eating and can be caused by reactive hypoglycemia (inappropriate insulin release after a meal), early diabetes mellitus, or rapid gastric emptying.[28]

Hypoglycemia can also be induced by external causes, such as exogenous insulin or oral hypoglycemic overdose.[8,28,100]

Signs and symptoms of hypoglycemia may include:
- Tachycardia and hypertension
- Tremor, irritability, pallor, and sweating
- Hunger
- Weight changes
- Headache
- Mental dullness, confusion, and amnesia
- Seizures
- Paralysis and paresthesias
- Dizziness
- Visual disturbance
- Loss of consciousness

Management of hypoglycemia may include the following: glucose administration (fruit juice or honey); strict monitoring of insulin and oral hypoglycemic administration; dietary modifications; pharmacologic agents, such as glucagon, which is the first agent used in emergency cases of hypoglycemia; diazoxide (Hyperstat) or streptozocin (Zanosar); surgery (e.g., subtotal pancreatectomy, insulinoma resection); or a combination of these.[28,101]

Parathyroid Gland

Body Structure and Function

Parathyroid hormone (PTH) is the primary hormone secreted from the parathyroid gland. The target sites are the kidneys, small intestine, and bone. The primary function of PTH is to raise blood calcium levels by mobilizing calcium that is stored in bone, increasing calcium reabsorption from the kidneys, and increasing calcium absorption from the small intestine.[8,102]

TABLE 10-12 Primary Tests Used to Evaluate Parathyroid (PTH) Function

Test	Description
Serum calcium	Measurement of blood calcium levels indirectly examines parathyroid function. Normally, low calcium levels stimulate parathyroid hormone secretion, whereas high calcium levels could be reflective of high PTH levels. Reference value for serum calcium is 9.0 to 10.5 mg/dl in adults. Calcium levels can also be measured in the urine. Reference value for urinary calcium is 50 to 300 mg/dl.
Parathyroid hormone	Radioimmunoassays and urinalysis are used to measure parathyroid hormone levels. Reference value for blood is 10 to 65 pg/ml.

Data from Corbett JV, editor: Laboratory tests and diagnostic procedures with nursing diagnoses, ed 5, Upper Saddle River, NJ, 2000, Prentice Hall Health, pp 167-176; and Sacher RA, McPherson RA, Campos JM, editors: Widman's clinical interpretation of laboratory tests, ed 11, Philadelphia, 2000, FA Davis, pp 803-804; Pagana KD, Pagana TJ: Mosby's diagnostic and laboratory test reference, ed 9, St Louis, 2009, Mosby.

Parathyroid Tests

The primary measurements of parathryoid hormone are summarized in Table 10-12. However, because PTH exerts its effects on the intestines and kidneys, calcium metabolism can also be evaluated by testing gastrointestinal and renal function. Refer to Chapters 8 and 9, respectively, for a summary of diagnostic tests for the gastrointestinal and renal systems.

Parathyroid Disorders

Hyperparathyroidism

Hyperparathyroidism is a disorder caused by overactivity of one or more of the parathyroid glands that leads to increased PTH levels, resulting in increased blood calcium level, decreased bone mineralization, and decreased kidney function. This disorder occurs more frequently in women than in men. Radiation therapy is also a risk factor for developing this disorder.[103,104]

Hyperparathyroidism can be classified as primary, secondary, or tertiary. Primary hyperparathyroidism represents the most cases and usually results from hyperplasia or an adenoma in the parathyroid gland(s). Secondary hyperparathyroidism results from another organ system disorder, such as renal failure, osteogenesis imperfecta, Paget's disease, multiple myeloma, lymphoma, or bone metastases from primary breast, lung, or kidney tumors. Tertiary hyperparathyroidism occurs when PTH secretion is autonomous despite normal or low serum calcium levels.[8,41,105]

The primary clinical manifestations of hyperparathyroidism are hypercalcemia and hypercalciuria (calcium in urine). Hypercalcemia may then result in the following cascade of signs and symptoms[41,103-105]:

- Fatigue, weakness, bony pain
- Depression, memory loss, decreased concentration, sleep disturbances
- Osteopenia, osteoporosis and increased fracture risk
- Kidney stone formation (nephrolithiasis)
- Hypertension, left ventricular hypertrophy

Management of hyperparathyroidism may include the following[28,41,105]:

- Minimally invasive surgery is the current standard.[104]
- Pharmacologic intervention is summarized in Chapter 19, Table 19-40.
- Fluid replacement.
- Dietary modification (a diet low in calcium and high in vitamin D).

Hypoparathyroidism

Hypoparathyroidism is a disorder caused by underactivity of one or more of the parathyroid glands that leads to decreased PTH levels, and thus to low serum calcium levels. Decreased levels of PTH occur most commonly as a result of damage to the parathyroid glands during thyroid or parathyroid surgery (postoperative hypoparathyroidism). Less common causes may include radiation-induced damage, infiltration by metastatic cells, congenital defects in parathyroid glands, and autoimmune dysfunction.[41,105,106]

Signs and symptoms of hypoparathyroidism include the following[41,106]:

- Osteomalacia in adults, rickets in children
- Increased neuromuscular irritability (tetany); painful muscle spasms
- Paresthesias
- Laryngospasm
- Dysrhythmias, QRS & ST segment changes on electrocardiogram
- Thin, patchy hair; brittle nails; dry, scaly skin
- Seizures
- Visual impairment from cataracts

Management of hypoparathyroidism may include the following[28,41,105,106]:

- Pharmacologic intervention with the following:
  - PTH replacement
  - Vitamin D supplements: calcitriol
  - Calcium carbonate
  - Magnesium sulfate
  - Thiazide diuretics
- Parathyroid autotransplantation: for patients who are at risk for hypoparathyroidism from neck surgery, the parathyroid glands are autotransplanted into the forearm or sternocleidomastoid muscle before the neck surgery.

Metabolic Bone Disorders

Osteoporosis

Osteoporosis is a multifactorial skeletal disorder that leads to decreased bone density and organization, which ultimately reduces bone strength.[107]

> ✎ **CLINICAL TIP**
> Always consult with the physician to determine if there are any weight-bearing precautions in patients with osteoporosis.

Bone strength is often measured by bone mineral density studies, which are used in the diagnosis of osteoporosis, as well as monitoring tools for therapeutic improvements. Dual-energy x-ray absorptiometry (DEXA) measurement is currently the gold standard for determining bone mineral density, which is reported as T- and Z-scores. The Z-score for bone density is used in premenopausal women, young men, and children. According to the World Health Organization (WHO), the T-score is to be used for postmenopausal white women.[98,108] Investigations[109] are ongoing regarding the use of biochemical markers in blood and urine to help detect bone loss and possibly to predict risk of fracture in patients. The FRAX tool is a fracture risk assessment tool developed by WHO. It integrates information on fracture risk from clinical risk factors and can be used to target individuals at high risk for fracture.[110]

Osteoporosis can be classified as primary or secondary. Primary osteoporosis is the deterioration of bone mass not associated with other illnesses.[98,108] It can occur in both genders at all ages, but often follows menopause in women and occurs later in life in men. Secondary osteoporosis is a result of medications (e.g., glucocorticoids or anticonvulsants), alcoholism, other chronic conditions (e.g., hypogonadism or hypoestrogenism), or diseases (e.g., hyperthyroidism).[107]

There is no clear etiology for osteoporosis. However, many risk factors for women have been elucidated. These risk factors include Caucasian or Asian race, petite frame, inadequate dietary intake of calcium, positive family history of osteoporosis, alcohol abuse, cigarette smoking, high caffeine intake, sedentary lifestyle, reduced bone mineral content (most predictive factor), and early menopause or oophorectomy (ovary removal).[105,107]

Signs and symptoms of osteoporosis may include the following[98,105,108]:

- Back pain (aggravated by movement or weight bearing, relieved by rest).
- Low body weight.
- Renal disease.
- Vertebral deformity (kyphosis and anterior wedging).
- Presence of vertebral compression fractures, Colles' fracture, hip and pelvic fractures.
- Pulmonary embolism and pneumonia are complications that can occur secondary to these fractures.[111]

Management of osteoporosis may include the following[7,107,112,113]:

- Daily supplementation with calcium and vitamin D for all women with low bone mineral density. According to the Institute of Medicine it is recommended to have 600 international units (IU) of vitamin D daily for healthy adults less than 71 years of age and 800 IU for healthy people older than 71.[114]
- Hormone replacement therapy with estrogen or estrogen combined with progesterone (considered only for women with significant osteoporosis risk).

- Selective estrogen receptor modulation (SERM) therapy with raloxifene.
- Bisphosphonate supplementation (inhibits bone resorption) with alendronate, ibandronate, and risedronate.
- Calcitonin supplementation (increases total body calcium).
- Administration of PTH (teriparatide) in patients who cannot tolerate estrogen therapy.[111]
- Physical therapy for exercise prescription. In a recent systematic review, resistance exercises have been found to increase physical function in older adults with osteoporosis and osteopenia.[115]
  - An abdominal corset can provide additional support for stable vertebral compression fracture(s). A rolling walker that is adjusted higher than normal can promote a more upright posture. Both of these techniques may also help to decrease back pain in patients with osteoporosis.
- Fracture management (if indicated; refer to Chapter 5).

✎ CLINICAL TIP

Although evidence supports resistive exercises, caution should still be taken with resistive exercises and manual contacts during therapeutic activities in patients with severe osteoporosis to avoid risk of microtrauma or fracture to osteoporotic bones.

Osteomalacia

Osteomalacia, or rickets in children, is a disorder characterized by decreased bone mineralization, reduced calcium absorption from the gut, and compensatory hyperparathyroidism. The etiology of osteomalacia stems from any disorder that lowers serum levels of phosphate, calcium, or vitamin D.[17,105] Osteoporosis is often a previously existing condition.[98]

Signs and symptoms of osteomalacia include the following[17,98,105]:

- Bone pain and tenderness
- Softening of cranial vault (in children)
- Swelling of costochondral joints (in children)
- Predisposition to femoral neck fractures (in adults)
- Pathologic fractures
- Proximal myopathy
- Waddling gait

Medical management of osteomalacia may include treating the underlying or predisposing condition or supplementation with calcium and vitamin D.[17,116]

Paget's Disease

Paget's disease is a bone disease of unknown etiology that usually presents after the age of 55 years. It may affect one bone (monostotic) or more than one bone (polyostotic); only 27% of individuals are symptomatic at diagnosis.[98] The primary feature is thick, spongy bone that is unorganized and brittle as a result of excessive osteoclastic and subsequent osteoblastic activity. Some evidence points to an inflammatory or viral origin. The axial skeleton and femur are involved in 80% of cases, with the tibia, ilium, skull, and humerus having less involvement.[111] Fractures and compression of the cranial nerves (especially the eighth nerve) and spinal cord are complications of Paget's disease.[105,117]

Paget's disease is generally asymptomatic; however, the following clinical manifestations may present[98,105,117]:
- Bone pain that is unrelieved by rest and persists at night
- Bone deformity (e.g., skull enlargement, bowing of leg and thigh, increased density and width)
- Increased warmth of overlying skin of affected areas
- Headaches or hearing loss
- Chalk-stick fractures from softening of bone
- Kyphosis

Management of Paget's disease primarily includes bisphosphonate and calcitonin administration. Bisphosphonates include etidronate, alendronate, risedronate, pamidronate, and ibandronate.[117,118]

Other interventions may include the following[105,117]:
- Calcium supplementation (if necessary)
- Promotion of mobility
- Adequate hydration
- Symptomatic relief with nonsteroidal antiinflammatory agents or acetaminophen

---

Physical Therapy Management

Clinical management of endocrine dysfunction is discussed earlier in sections on specific endocrine-gland and metabolic disorders. This section focuses on goals and guidelines for physical therapy intervention. The following are general physical therapy goals and guidelines for working with patients who have endocrine or metabolic dysfunction. These guidelines should be adapted to a patient's specific needs. Clinical tips have been provided earlier to address specific situations in which the tips may be most helpful.

Goals

The primary physical therapy goals in this patient population are the following: (1) to optimize functional mobility, (2) to maximize activity tolerance and endurance, (3) to prevent skin breakdown in the patient with altered sensation (e.g., diabetic neuropathy), (4) to decrease pain (e.g., in patients with osteoporosis or hyperparathyroidism), and (5) to maximize safety for prevention of falls, especially in patients with altered sensation or muscle function.

Guidelines

Patients with diabetes or osteoporosis represent the primary patient population with which the physical therapist intervenes. Physical therapy considerations for these patients are discussed in earlier sections, Diabetes Mellitus and Osteoporosis, respectively.

For other patients with endocrine or metabolic dysfunction, the primary physical therapy treatment guidelines are the following:

1. To improve activity tolerance, it may be necessary to decrease exercise intensity when the patient's medication regimen is being adjusted. For example, a patient with insufficient

thyroid hormone replacement will fatigue more quickly than will a patient with adequate thyroid hormone replacement. In this example, knowing the normal values of thyroid hormone and reviewing the laboratory tests helps the therapist gauge the appropriate treatment intensity.

2. Consult with the clinical nutritionist to help determine the appropriate activity level based on the patient's caloric intake, because caloric intake and metabolic processes are affected by endocrine and metabolic disorders.

References

1. Saguil A: Evaluation of the patient with muscle weakness, Am Fam Physician 71:1327-1336, 2005.
2. Golden SH, Robinson KA, Saldanha I et al: Prevalence and incidence of endocrine and metabolic disorders in the United States: a comprehensive review, J Clin Endocrinol Metab 94:1853-1878, 2009.
3. Centers for Disease Control and Prevention: National Hospital Ambulatory Medical Care Survey: 2008 Emergency Department Summary Tables. http://www.cdc.gov/nchs/data/ahcd/nhamcs_emergency/2008_ed_web_tables.pdf. Accessed March 26, 2013.
4. Schappert SM, Rechtsteiner EA: Ambulatory medical care utilization estimates for 2007. National Center for Health Statistics, Vital Health Stat 13(169):1-38, 2011.
5. Hall MJ, DeFrances CJ, Williams SN et al: National Hospital Discharge Survey: 2007 summary, in Centers for Disease Control and Prevention: National health statistics report, 2010, p 29.
6. Bullock, BL, editor: Pathophysiology: adaptations and alterations in function, ed 4, Philadelphia, 1996, Lippincott.
7. Diagnostic procedures. In Thompson JM, McFarland GK, Hirsch JE et al: editors: Mosby's manual of clinical nursing practice, ed 2, St Louis, 1989, Mosby, p 1594.
8. Sacher RA, McPherson RA, Campos JM, editors: Widman's clinical interpretation of laboratory tests, ed 11, Philadelphia, 2000, FA Davis, pp 741-823.
9. Brashers VL, Jones RE: Mechanisms of hormonal regulation. In McCance KL, Huether SE, Brashers VL et al, editors: Pathophysiology: the biologic basis for disease in adults and children, ed 6, St Louis, 2010, Mosby, pp 697-726.
10. Hall S; Prescribing in thyroid disease, Nurse Prescribing 8(8):382-387, 2010.
11. Chen JL, Chiu HW, Tseng YJ et al: Hyperthyroidism is characterized by both increased sympathetic and decreased vagal modulation of heart rate: evidence from spectral analysis of heart rate variability, Clin Endocrinol 64(6):611-616, 2006.
12. Donangelo I, Braunstein GD: Update on subclinical hyperthyroidism, Am Fam Physician 83(8):933-938, 2011.
13. Jones RE, Brashers VL, Huether SE: Alterations of hormonal regulation. In McCance KL, Huether SE, Brashers VL et al, editors: Pathophysiology: the biologic basis for disease in adults and children, ed 6, St Louis, 2010, Mosby, pp 727-780.
14. Raisbeck E: Understanding thyroid disease, Pract Nurse 37(1):34-36, 2009.
15. Furtado L: Thyroidectomy: post-operative care and common complications. Nurs Stand [serial online] 25(34):43-52, 2011.
16. Guha B, Krishnaswamy G, Peiris A: The diagnosis and management of hypothyroidism, South Med J 95(5):475-480, 2002.
17. Hartog M, editor: Endocrinology. Oxford, UK, 1987, Blackwell Scientific.
18. Maitra A, Kumar V: The endocrine system. In Kumar V, Cotran RS, Robbins SL, editors: Robbins basic pathology, ed 7, Philadelphia, 2003, Saunders, pp 720-754.
19. Hershman JM, editor: Endocrine pathophysiology: a patient-oriented approach, ed 3, Philadelphia, 1988, Lea & Febiger, p 225.
20. Woolf N: In Pathology, basic and systemic, London, 1998, Saunders, pp 820-873.
21. Burch WM, editor: Endocrinology for the house officer, ed 2, Baltimore, 1988, Williams & Wilkins.
22. Giustina A, Bronstein MD, Casanueva FF et al: Current management practices for acromegaly: an international survey, Pituitary 14:125-133, 2011.
23. Melmed S, Colao A, Barkan A et al: Guidelines for acromegaly management: an update, J Clin Endocrinol Metab 94:1509-1517, 2009.
24. Orth DN: Cushing's syndrome, N Engl J Med 332(12):791-803, 1995.
25. Bertagna X, Guignat L: Approach to the Cushing's disease patient with persistent/recurrent hypercortisolism after pituitary surgery, J Clin Endocrinol Metab 98(4):1307-1318, 2013.
26. Sherlock M, Thompson CJ: The syndrome of inappropriate antidiuretic hormone: current and future management options, Eur J Endocrinol 162:S13-S18, 2010.
27. Terpstra TL, Terpstra TL: Syndrome of inappropriate antidiuretic hormone secretion: recognition and management, MedSurg Nurs 9(2):61, 2000.
28. Allen MA, Boykin PC, Drass JA et al: Endocrine and metabolic systems. In Thompson JM, McFarland GK, Hirsch JE et al, editors: Mosby's manual of clinical nursing practice, ed 2, St Louis, 1989, Mosby, p 876.
29. Gross P: Clinical management of SIADH, Ther Adv Endocrinol 3(2):61-73, 2012.
30. Hoorn EJ, Bouloux PM, Burst V: Perspectives on the management of hyponatremia secondary to SIADH across Europe, Best Pract Res Clin Endocrinol Metab 26(S1):S27-32, 2012.
31. Pituitary. In Stevens, editor: Core pathology, ed 3, St Louis, 2009, Elsevier.
32. Hypopituitarism. In Robbins and Cotran pathologic basis of disease, professional edition, ed 8, Elsevier,2009.
33. Beers MH, Berkow R, editors: Merck manual of diagnosis and therapy, ed 17, Whitehouse Station, NJ, 1999, Merck.
34. Verbalis JG: Posterior pituitary. In Cecil medicine, ed 24, Philadelphia, 2011, Elsevier Saunders, e57-e64.
35. Lavin N, editor: Manual of endocrinology and metabolism, ed 2, Boston, 1994, Little, Brown.
36. Wand GS: Pituitary disorders. In Stobo JD, Hellmann DB, Ladenson PW et al: editors: The principles and practice of medicine, ed 23, Stamford, CT, 1996, Appleton & Lange, pp 274-281.
37. Ozer K, Balasubramanyam A: Diabetes insipidus. In Bope ET, Kellerman RD: Conn's current therapy, ed 1, Philadelphia, 2012, Saunders, pp 686-689.
38. Tolbutamide stimulation test. In Malarkey LM, McMorrow ME, editors: Nurse's manual of laboratory tests and diagnostic procedures, Philadelphia, 2000, Saunders, pp 619-620.
39. Pagana KD, Pagana TJ: Mosby's diagnostic and laboratory test reference, ed 9, St Louis, 2009, Mosby, p 303.
40. Chakera AJ, Vaidya B: Addison disease in adults: diagnosis and management, Am J Med 123:409-413, 2010.
41. Malarkey LM, McMorrow ME, editors: Nurse's manual of laboratory tests and diagnostic procedures, Philadelphia, 2000, Saunders, pp 555-556.

42. Baker JR Jr: Autoimmune endocrine disease, JAMA 278(22):1931-1937, 1997.

43. Wand GS, Cooper DS: Adrenal disorders. In Stobo JD, Hellmann DB, Ladenson PW et al: editors: The principles and practice of medicine, ed 23, Stamford, CT, 1996, Appleton & Lange, pp 282-292.

44. Subramamiam R: Pheochromocytoma—current concepts in diagnosis and management, Trends Anaesth Crit Care 1:104-110, 2011.

45. Kizer JR, Koniaris JS, Edelman JD et al: Pheochromocytoma crisis, cardiomyopathy, and hemodynamic collapse, Chest 118(4):1221, 2000.

46. Darr R, Lenders JWM, Hofbauer LC et al: Pheochromocytoma—update on disease management, Ther Adv Endocrinol Metab 3:11-26, 2012.

47. Reaven G: The metabolic syndrome or the insulin resistance syndrome? Different names, different concepts, and different goals, Endocrinol Metab Clin North Am 33(2):283-303, 2004.

48. Jeppesen J, Hansen TW, Rasmussen S et al: Insulin resistance, the metabolic syndrome, and risk of incident cardiovascular disease, J Am Coll Cardiol 49(21):2112-2119, 2007.

49. Maitra A: The endocrine system. In Kumar V, Abbas AK, Fausto N et al: editors: Robbins basic pathology, ed 8, Philadelphia, 2007, Saunders, pp 778-788.

50. Utzschneider KM, Lagemaat AV, Faulenbach MV et al: Insulin resistance is the best predictor of the metabolic syndrome in subjects with a first-degree relative with type 2 diabetes, Obesity 18:1781-1787, 2010.

51. Alberti KGMM et al: Harmonizing the metabolic syndrome a joint interim statement of the International Diabetes Federation Task Force on Epidemiology and Prevention; National Heart, Lung, and Blood Institute; American Heart Association; World Heart Federation; International Atherosclerosis Society; and International Association for the Study of Obesity, Circulation 120:1640-1645, 2009.

52. Fernandez ML: The metabolic syndrome, Nutr Rev 65(6 Pt 2):S30-S34, 2007.

53. Carroll S: What is the relationship between exercise and metabolic abnormalities? A review of the metabolic syndrome, Sports Med 34(6):371-418, 2004.

54. Olefsky JM: Prospects for research in diabetes mellitus, JAMA 285(5):628, 2001.

55. American Diabetes Association: Position statement: diagnosis and classification of diabetes mellitus, Diabetes Care 34(S1):S62-S69, 2011.

56. Report of the Expert Committee on the Diagnosis and Classification of Diabetes Mellitus, Diabetes Care 24(1):S5, 2001.

57. Musselman DL, Betan E, Larsen H et al: Relationship of depression to diabetes types 1 and 2: epidemiology, biology and treatment, Biol Psychiatry 54:317-329, 2003.

58. Saydah SH, Brancati FL, Hill Golden S et al: Depressive symptoms and the risk of type 2 diabetes mellitus in a U.S. sample, Diabetes Metab Res Rev 19:202-208, 2003.

59. Hill Golden S, Lazo M, Carnethon M et al: Examining a bidirectional association between depressive symptoms and diabetes, JAMA 299(23):2751-2759, 2008.

60. Wellens NI, Flamaing J, Tournoy J et al: Convergent validity of the cognitive performance scale of the interRAI Acute Care and the Mini-Mental State Examination, Am J Geriatr Psychiatry, April 2012. doi: 10.1097/JGP.0b013e31824afaa3. Accessed March 26, 2013.

61. Kroenke K, Spitzer RL, Williams JB et al: The Patient Health Questionnaire somatic, anxiety and depressive symptom scales: a systematic review, Gen Hosp Psychiatry 32(4):345-359, 2010.

62. McCance KL, Huether SE, editors: Pathophysiology: the biologic basis for disease in adults and children, ed 2, St Louis, 1994, Mosby, p 674.

63. Lorenzi M: Diabetes mellitus. In Fitzgerald PA, editor: Handbook of clinical endocrinology, ed 2, East Norwalk, CT, 1992, Appleton & Lange, p 463.

64. Saudek CD: Diabetes mellitus. In Stobo JD, Hellmann DB, Ladenson PW et al: editors: The principles and practice of medicine, ed 23, Stamford, CT, 1996, Appleton & Lange, pp 321-331.

65. American Diabetes Association clinical practice recommendations 2001: Standards of medical care for patients with diabetes mellitus, Diabetes Care 24(1), S1-S133, 2001.

66. Khafagy S, Morishita M, Onuki Y et al: Current challenges in non-invasive insulin delivery systems: a comparative review, Adv Drug Deliv Rev 59:1521-1546, 2007.

67. Rewers M, Gottlieb P: Immunotherapy for the prevention and treatment of type 1 diabetes human trials and a look into the future, Diabetes Care 32(10):1769-1782, 2009.

68. Voltarelli JC, Couri C, Stracieri A et al: Autologous hematopoietic stem cell transplantation for type 1 diabetes. Ann N Y Acad Sci 1150:220-229, 2008.

69. Centers for Disease Control and Prevention: National Diabetes fact sheet: national estimates and general information on diabetes and prediabetes in the United States, 2011. Atlanta, GA, 2011, U.S. Department of Health and Human Services, Centers for Disease Control and Prevention.

70. Type 2 diabetes in children and adolescents, Am Diabetes Assoc Pediatr 105:671-680, 2000.

71. Dabelea D, Bell RA, D'Agostino RB et al: Incidence of diabetes in youth in the United States, JAMA 297(24):2716-2724, 2007.

72. 2011 National Diabetes Fact Sheet: www.diabetes.org/diabetes-basics/diabetes-statistics.

73. Fagot-Campagna A, Pettitt DJ, Engelgau MM et al: Type 2 diabetes among North American children and adolescents: an epidemiologic review and a public health perspective. J Pediatr 136(5):664-672, 2000.

74. Position statement: standards of medical care in diabetes—2011, American Diabetes Association, Diabetes Care 34(S1):S11-S61, 2009.

75. Nutrition recommendations and principles for people with diabetes mellitus, Diabetes Care 24(1):S44, 2001.

76. Zinran B, Ruderman N, Phil O et al: Diabetes mellitus and exercise, Diabetes Care 24(1):S51, 2001.

77. Saudek CD, Duckworth WC, Giobbie-Hurder A et al: Implantable insulin pump vs multiple-dose insulin for non-insulin dependent diabetes mellitus: a randomized clinical trial. Department of Veterans Affairs Implantable Insulin Pump Study Group, JAMA 276(16):1322-1327, 1997.

78. Cefalu, WT: Inhaled human insulin treatment in patients with type 2 diabetes mellitus [Abstract], JAMA 285(12):1559, 2001.

79. Skyler JS, Cefalu WT, Kourides IA et al: Efficacy of inhaled human insulin in type 1 diabetes mellitus: a randomised proof-of-concept study, Lancet 357(9253):331, 2001.

80. Pancreatic hormones and antidiabetic drugs. In P Panus, editor: Pharmacology for the physical therapist, New York, 2009, McGraw-Hill, pp 331-342.

81. Schaepelynck P, Darmon P, Molines L et al: Advances in pump technology: insulin patch pumps, combined pumps and glucose sensors, and implanted pumps, Diabetes Metab 37:S85-S93, 2011.

82. Davis SN: Insulin, oral hypoglycemic agents, and the pharmacology of the endocrine pancreas. In Brunton LL et al: editors: The pharmacological basis of therapeutics, ed 11, New York, 2006, McGraw-Hill.

83. Oiknine R, Bernbaum M, Mocradian AD: A critical appraisal of the role of insulin analogues in the management of diabetes mellitus, Drugs 65:325-340, 2005.

84. Ciccone CD: Pancreatic hormones and the treatment of diabetes mellitus. In Pharmacology in rehabilitation, ed 4, Philadelphia, 2007, FA Davis.

85. Guerci B, Sauvanet JP: Subcutaneous insulin: pharmacokinetic variability and glycemic variability, Diabetes Metab 31:4S7-4S24, 2005.

86. Cefalu WT: Concept, strategies and feasibility of non-invasive insulin delivery, Diabetes Care 27(1):239-246, 2004.

87. Bruttomesso D, Farret A, Costa S et al: Closed-loop artificial pancreas using subcutaneous glucose sensing and insulin delivery and a model predictive control algorithm: preliminary studies in Padova and Montpellier, J Diabetes Sci Technol 3(5):1014-1021, 2009.

88. Heinemann L: Advanced technologies and treatments for diabetes: new ways of insulin delivery, Int J Clin Pract 65(170):31-46, 2011.

89. Skladany MJ, Miller M, Guthermann JS et al: Patch-pump technology to manage type 2 diabetes: hurdles to market acceptance, J Diabetes Sci Technol 2(6):1147-1150, 2008.

90. Guevara-Aguirre J, Guevara M, Saavedra J et al: Oral spray insulin in treatment of type 2 diabetes: a comparison of efficacy of the oral spray insulin (Oralin) with subcutaneous insulin injection, a proof of concept study, Diabetes Metab Re 20(6):472-478, 2004.

91. Petersen AH, Korsatko S, Kohler G et al: The effect of terbutaline on the absorption of pulmonary administered insulin in subjects with asthma, J Clin Pharm 69(3):271-278, 2010.

92. Sonia TA, Sharma CP: An overview of natural polymers for oral insulin delivery, Drug Discov Today 17(13-14):784-792, 2012. Doi:10.1016/j.drudis.2012.03.019.

93. Whitehead K, Shen Z, Mitragotri S: Oral delivery of macromolecules using intestinal patches: applications for insulin delivery, J Control Release 98(1):37-45, 2004.

94. American Diabetes Association: Living with diabetes: www.diabetes.org/living-with-diabetes/complications/.html. Accessed March 26, 2013.

95. Mayfield JA, Reiber GE, Saunders LJ et al: Preventive foot care in people with diabetes, Diabetes Care 24(1):S56, 2001.

96. Houston DS, Curran J: Charcot foot, Orthop Nurs 20(1):11, 2001.

97. Frykberg RG: Diabetic foot infections: evaluation and management. Advances in wound care, J Prev Healing 11(7):329, 1998.

98. Fitzgerald PA: Endocrine disorders. In McPhee SJ, Papadakis MA, editors: 2011 current medical diagnosis and treatment, New York, 2011, McGraw-Hill, pp 1098-1105.

99. Melvin-Sater PA: Diabetic neuropathy, Physician Assist 24(7):63, 2000.

100. Cryer P: Defining and reporting hypoglycemia in diabetes: a report from the American Diabetes Association Work Group on Hypoglycemia, Diabetes Care 28(5):1245-1249, 2005.

101. Cooper PG: Insulin-reaction hypoglycemia, Clin Reference Syst Ann, 919, 2000.

102. Hudak CM, Gallo BM, editors: Critical care nursing: a holistic approach, ed 6, Philadelphia, 1994, Lippincott, p 874.

103. Trotto NE, Cobin RH, Wiesen M: Hypothyroidism, hyperthyroidism, hyperparathyroidism, Patient Care 33(14):186, 1999.

104. Felger EA, Kandil E: Primary hyperparathyroidism, Otolaryngol Clin North Am 43(2):417-432, 2010.

105. Levine MA: Disorders of mineral and bone metabolism. In Stobo JD, Hellmann DB, Ladenson PW et al: editors: The principles and practice of medicine, ed 23, Stamford, CT, 1996, Appleton & Lange, pp 312-320.

106. Cheng V, Gopalakrishnan G: Hypoparathyroidism. In Ferri's clinical advisor, Philadelphia, 2012, Saunders Elsevier.

107. NIH Consensus Development Panel: Osteoporosis prevention, diagnosis, and therapy, JAMA 285(6):785, 2001.

108. Jeannette E: Osteoporosis: part 1. Evaluation and assessment. Am Fam Physician 63(5):897-905, 2001.

109. Srivastava AK, Vliet EL, Lewiecki EM et al: Clinical use of serum and urine bone markers in the management of osteoporosis, Curr Med Res Opin 21(7):1015-1026, 2005.

110. Kanis JA, McCloskey EV, Johansson H et al: Development and use of FRAX in osteoporosis, Osteoporos Int 21:S407-S413, 2010.

111. Burns DK: The musculoskeletal system. In Kumar V, Abbas AK, Fausto N et al: editors: Robbins basic pathology, ed 8, Philadelphia, 2007, Saunders, pp 806-807.

112. Altkorn D, Voke T: Treatment of postmenopausal osteoporosis, JAMA 285(11):1415, 2001.

113. Mulder JE, Kolatkar NS, LeBoff MS: Drug insight: existing and emerging therapies for osteoporosis, Nat Clin Pract Endocrinol Metab 2(12):670-680, 2006.

114. Dietary reference intakes for calcium and vitamin D. National Osteoporosis Foundation, Institute of Medicine: www.iom.edu/vitamind. Accessed March 26, 2013.

115. Wilhelm M, Roskovensky G, Emery K et al: Effect of resistance exercises on function in older adults with osteoporosis or osteopenia: a systematic review, Physiother Can 64(4):386-394, 2012. doi:10.3138/ptc.2011-31BH.

116. Vieth R: Vitamin D supplementation, 25-hydroxyvitamin D concentrations, and safety, Am J Clin Nutr 69(5):842, 1999.

117. Hines SE: Paget's disease of bone: a new philosophy of treatment, Patient Care 33(20):40, 1999.

118. Ciccone CD: Thyroid and parathyroid drugs: agents affecting bone mineralization. In Ciccone CD, editor: Pharmacology in rehabilitation, ed 4, Philadelphia, 2007, FA Davis, p 468.

CHAPTER 11

Oncology

Jaime C. Paz

CHAPTER OBJECTIVES

The objectives for this chapter are to provide the following:

1. An understanding of the medical assessment and diagnosis of a patient with cancer, including staging and classification
2. An understanding of the various medical and surgical methods of cancer management
3. An overview of a variety of the different body system cancers, including common sites of metastases
4. Examination, evaluation, and intervention considerations for the physical therapist

PREFERRED PRACTICE PATTERNS

The most relevant practice patterns for the diagnoses discussed in this chapter, based on the American Physical Therapy Association's *Guide to Physical Therapist Practice*, second edition, are as follows:

- Cancer (Including but Not Limited to Cancer of the Breast, Prostate, Lung, Colon, Oral, Uterine, Stomach): 4A, 4B, 4C, 5A, 6A, 6B, 6E
- Skin Cancer: 7C
- Kaposi's Sarcoma: 6H, 7B, 7C, 7E
- CNS-Related Cancers: 6E
- Connective Tissue–Related Cancers: 7E

Please refer to Appendix A for a complete list of the preferred practice patterns, as individual patient conditions are highly variable and other practice patterns may be applicable.

Cancer is a term that applies to a group of diseases characterized by the abnormal growth of cells. The physical therapist requires a foundational understanding of underlying cancer disease processes, as well as the side effects, considerations, and precautions related to cancer care, to enhance clinical decision making to safely and effectively treat the patient with cancer. This knowledge will also assist the physical therapist with the early detection of previously undiagnosed cancer. Do note that the field of oncology is vast; this chapter only highlights specific information pertinent to physical therapy management.

Terminology

Several terms are used in oncology to describe cancer or cancer-related processes, which are outlined in Table 11-1. Neoplasms, or persistent abnormal dysplastic cell growth, are classified by cell type, growth pattern, anatomic location, degree of dysplasia, tissue of origin, and their ability to spread or remain in the original location. Two general classifications for neoplasm

TABLE 11-1 Cancer Terminology

Term	Definition
Neoplasm	"New growth" pertaining to an abnormal mass of tissue that is excessive, persistent, and unregulated by physiological stimuli.
Tumor	Common medical language for a neoplasm.
Cancer	A term for diseases in which abnormal cells divide without control and can invade nearby tissues. Malignant tumors are referred to as cancers.
Dysplasia	Variability of cell size and shape with an increased rate of cell division (mitosis). This situation may be a precancerous change or result from chronic infection.
Metaplasia	Replacement of one mature cell type by a different mature cell type, resulting from certain stimuli such as cigarette smoking.
Hyperplasia	An increased *number* of cells resulting in an enlarged tissue mass. It may be a mechanism to compensate for increased demands, or it may be pathological when there is a hormonal imbalance.
Differentiation	The extent to which a cell resembles mature morphology and function. A cell that is well differentiated is physiological and functions as intended. A poorly differentiated cell does not resemble a mature cell in both morphology and function.

Data from Stricker TP, Kumar V: Neoplasia. In Kumar V, Abbas AK, Fausto N et al, editors: Robbins basic pathology, ed 8, Philadelphia, 2007, Saunders, pp 174-175; National Cancer Institute: http://www.cancer.gov/dctionary. Accessed June 27, 2012; Gould B, Dyer R: Pathophysiology for the health professions, ed 4, Philadelphia, 2010, Saunders, p. 8.

are benign and malignant. *Benign tumors* generally consist of differentiated cells that reproduce at a higher rate than normal and are often encapsulated, allowing expansion, but do not spread to other tissues.[1] Benign tumors are considered harmless unless their growth become large enough to encroach on surrounding tissues and impair their function. *Malignant neoplasms*, or malignant tumors, consist of undifferentiated cells, are uncapsulated, and grow uncontrollably, invading normal tissues and causing destruction to surrounding tissues and organs. Malignant neoplasms may spread, or metastasize, to distant sites of the body.[1,2] Tumors may also be classified as primary or secondary. Primary tumors are the original tumors in the original location. Secondary tumors or cancers are metastases that have moved from the primary site.[3]

Nomenclature

Benign and malignant tumors are named by their cell of origin (Table 11-2). Benign tumors are customarily named by attaching -*oma* to the cell of origin. Malignant tumors are usually named by adding *carcinoma* to the cell of origin if they originate from epithelium and *sarcoma* if they originate in mesenchymal tissue.[2] Variations to this naming exist, such as melanoma and leukemia.

Risk Factors

There are numerous carcinogens (cancer-causing agents) and risk factors that are thought to predispose a person to cancer. Most cancers probably develop from a combination of genetic and environmental factors. According to the American Cancer Society, cigarette smoking, heavy use of alcohol, physical inactivity, and being overweight or obese contribute to or cause several types of cancers. Infectious agents such as the hepatitis B virus (HBV), human papillomavirus (HPV), human immunodeficiency virus (HIV), and *Helicobacter pylori (H. pylori)* have also been related to certain cancers such as cervical cancer (HPV).[4] A complete overview of risk factors is beyond the scope of this text. As specific cancers are described later in the chapter, relevant etiological agents or risk factors are stated.

Signs and Symptoms

Signs and symptoms of cancer are most often due to the tumor's growth and invasion of surrounding tissues. Specific manifestations will depend on the particular cancer and body system(s) affected and are described later in the chapter in those respective sections. General signs and symptoms that may be indicative of early or progressive cancer include[1,5]:

- Unusual bleeding or discharge
- Unexplained weight loss of 10 pounds or more
- Fever
- Fatigue
- Pain
- Persistent cough or hoarseness without a known cause
- Skin changes
  - Hyperpigmentation (darker-looking skin)
  - Jaundice (yellowish skin and eyes)
  - Erythema (reddened skin)
  - Pruritus (itching)
  - Excessive hair growth

Paraneoplastic syndromes are symptoms that cannot be related directly to the cancer's growth and invasion of tissues. They are thought to be due to abnormal hormonal secretions by the tumor. The syndromes are present in approximately 15% of persons diagnosed with cancer and often are the first sign of malignancy, represent significant clinical problems, and/or mimic metastatic disease. Clinical findings of paraneoplastic syndromes are similar to endocrinopathies (Cushing's syndrome, hypercalcemia), nerve and muscle syndromes (myasthenia), dermatological disorders (dermatomyositis), vascular and hematological disorders (venous thrombosis, anemia), and many others.[2]

Diagnosis

After obtaining a medical history and performing a physical examination, specific medical tests are employed to diagnose cancer. These tests may include medical imaging, blood tests

TABLE 11-2 Classification of Benign and Malignant Tumors

Tissue of Origin	Benign	Malignant
Epithelial Tissue		
Surface epithelium (skin) and mucous membrane	Papilloma	Squamous cell, basal cell, and transitional cell carcinoma
Epithelial lining of glands or ducts	Adenoma	Adenocarcinoma
Pigmented cells (melanocytes of basal layer)	Nevus (mole)	Malignant melanoma
Connective Tissue and Muscle		
Fibrous tissue	Fibroma	Fibrosarcoma
Adipose	Lipoma	Liposarcoma
Cartilage	Chondroma	Chondrosarcoma
Bone	Osteoma	Osteosarcoma
Blood vessels	Hemangioma	Hemangiosarcoma
Smooth muscle	Leiomyoma	Leiomyosarcoma
Striated muscle	Rhabdomyoma	Rhabdomyosarcoma
Nerve Tissue		
Nerve cells	Neuroma	—
Glia	—	Glioma or neuroglioma
Ganglion cells	Ganglioneuroma	Neuroblastoma
Nerve sheaths	Neurilemoma	Neurilemma sarcoma
Meninges	Meningioma	Meningeal sarcoma
Retina	—	Retinoblastoma
Lymphoid Tissue		
Lymph nodes	—	Lymphoma
Spleen	—	—
Intestinal lining	—	—
Hematopoietic Tissue		
Bone marrow	—	Leukemias, myelodysplasia, and myeloproliferative syndromes
Plasma cells	—	Multiple myeloma

From Goodman CC: Pathology: implications for the physical therapist, ed 3, Philadelphia, 2008, Saunders, p. 349.

for cancer markers, and several types of biopsy. Biopsy, or removal and examination of tissue, is the definitive test for cancer identification. Advancements in the technology of positron emission tomography (PET) scans in recent years have improved detection of cancer and subsequent management.[6] Table 11-3 lists common medical tests used to diagnose cancer. Tumor markers that may help to provide a prognosis for patients who are diagnosed with certain cancers, as well possibly monitor response to treatment, are listed in Table 11-4.

Staging and Grading

After the diagnosis of cancer is established, staging is performed to describe the location and size of the primary site of the tumor, the extent of lymph node involvement, and the presence or absence of metastasis. Staging helps to determine treatment options, predict life expectancy, and determine prognosis for complete resolution.

The mostly commonly used method to stage cancer is the TNM system. Tumors are classified according to the American Joint Committee on Cancer, which bases this system on the extent (size and/or number) of the primary tumor (T), lymph nodes involvement (N), and presence or absence of metastasis (M) (Table 11-5).[2,7] Certain types of cancers will have specific staging criteria, and these are identified later in this chapter for the various cancers.

Grading reports the degree of dysplasia, or differentiation, from the original cell type. Cells that are more highly differentiated resemble the original cells more strongly and this is associated with a *lower* grade and a less aggressive tumor. A higher grade is linked to aggressive, fatal tumors (Table 11-6).

Management

Not all cancers are curable. Physicians may therefore focus treatment on quality of life with palliative therapies rather than on curative therapies. Four major treatment options include:

- Surgical removal of the tumor
- Radiation therapy
- Chemotherapy
- Biotherapy (including immunotherapy, hormonal therapy, bone marrow transplantation, and monoclonal antibodies)

Additional treatments may include physical therapy, nutritional support, acupuncture, chiropractic treatment, alternative medicine, and hospice care. Treatment protocols differ from physician to physician and from cancer to cancer. Standard treatment includes some combination of surgery, radiation, and/or chemotherapy.

Surgery

Surgical intervention is determined by the size, location, and type of cancer, as well as the patient's age, general health, and

TABLE 11-3 Diagnostic Tests for Cancer

Test	Description
Biopsy	Tissue is taken via incision, needle, or aspiration procedures. A pathologist examines the tissue to identify the presence or absence of cancer cells; if cancer is present, the tumor is determined to be benign or malignant. The cell or tissue of origin, staging, and grading are also performed.
Stool guaiac	Detects small quantities of blood in stool.
Pap smear	A type of biopsy in which cells from the cervix are removed and examined.
Sputum cytology	A sputum specimen is inspected for cancerous cells.
Sigmoidoscopy	The sigmoid colon is examined with a sigmoidoscope.
Colonoscopy	The upper portion of the rectum is examined with a colonoscope.
Bronchoscopy	A tissue or sputum sample can be taken by rigid or flexible bronchoscopy.
Mammography	A radiographic method is used to look for a mass or calcification in breast tissue.
Radiography	X-ray is used to detect a mass.
Magnetic resonance imaging (MRI) and computed tomography (CT)	These noninvasive imaging techniques are used to localize lesions suspected of being cancerous.
Bone scan	Radionuclide imaging used to detect the presence, amount of metastatic disease, or both in bones.
Positron emission tomography (PET) scan	An imaging technique that uses radionuclides that emit positively charged particles (positrons) injected into the body, followed by imaging, to detect subtle changes in metabolic and chemical activity within the body. Can be combined with CT scanning. Currently used to help detect biopsy location, discern benign versus malignant conditions, stage disease, and diagnose cancer recurrence.

functional status. Successful localization and resection of recurrent and/or metastatic lesions found on PET positive scans may be optimized with the intraoperative use of a hand-held PET probe.[8] The following are indications for invasive surgical management[9]:

- Removal of precancerous lesions or of organs at high risk for cancer
- Establishing a diagnosis by biopsy
- Assisting in staging by sampling lymph nodes
- Definitive treatment by removing the primary tumor
- Reconstruction of a limb or organ with or without skin grafting
- Palliative care such as decompressive or bypass procedures
  Specific surgical procedures relevant to musculoskeletal and neurological cancers are discussed in Chapters 5 and 6,

TABLE 11-4 Tumor Markers

Cancer	Marker
Prostate cancer	Prostate surface antigen (PSA)
Prostate cancer	Prostatic-acid phosphatase
Testicular cancer	Human chorionic gonadotropin (HCG)
Liver cell cancer Testicular cancer	Alpha-fetoprotein (AFP)
Ovarian cancer	CA125
Breast cancer	CA15-3 Estrogen and progesterone receptors
Metastatic melanoma	S-100
Chronic myeloid leukemia	Bcr-abl gene
Bladder cancer	No tumor markers recommended for screening. Bladder tumor antigen (BTA) and NMP22 along with cystoscopy to diagnose patients.
Lung cancer	No tumor markers recommended for screening. Carcinoembryonic antigen (CEA) in non–small-cell lung cancer and neuron-specific enolase (NSE) in small-cell lung cancer may be elevated.
Pancreatic cancer	No tumor markers recommended for screening. CA 19-9 can provide prognosis for people with pancreatic cancer.
Colorectal cancer	Carcinoembryonic antigen (CEA) can provide prognosis for people with colorectal cancer.

CA, Carbohydrate antigen.
From American Cancer Society: Tumor markers. American Cancer Society website. http://www.cancer.org/Treatment/UnderstandingYourDiagnosis/ExamsandTestDescriptions/TumorMarkers/tumor-markers-common-ca-and-t-m. Updated March 24, 2011. Accessed August 10, 2011.

TABLE 11-5 TNM System

Stage	Parameters
T: Primary tumor	TX: Primary tumor cannot be assessed. T0: No evidence of primary tumor. Tis: Carcinoma in situ (site of origin). T1, T2, T3, T4: Progressive increase in tumor size and local involvement.
N: Regional lymph node involvement	NX: Nodes cannot be assessed. N0: No metastasis to local lymph nodes. N1, N2, N3: Progressive involvement of local lymph nodes.
M: Distant metastasis	MX: Presence of distant metastasis cannot be assessed. M0: No distant metastasis. M1: Presence of distant metastasis.

From Stricker TP, Kumar V: Neoplasia. In Kumar V, Abbas AK, Fausto N et al, editors: Robbins basic pathology, ed 8, Philadelphia, 2007, Saunders, pp 174-223.

TABLE 11-6 Grading of Neoplasms

Grade	Description
GX	Undetermined grade, cannot be assessed
G1	Low grade, well-differentiated tumor
G2	Intermediate grade, moderately differentiated tumor
G3	High grade, poorly differentiated tumor
G4	High grade, undifferentiated tumor

From National Cancer Institute: cancer.gov/cancertopics/factsheet/detection/tumor-grade. Accessed June 27, 2012; American Joint Committee on Cancer: AJCC Cancer Staging Manual, ed 6, New York, 2002, Springer.

respectively. Additional surgical procedures for specific cancers are covered later in the chapter.

> ✎ **CLINICAL TIP**
>
> Range of motion and muscle contraction in newly reconstructed limbs or regions should be tailored to physician's orders to help facilitate surgical healing.

Radiation Therapy

The primary objective in administering radiation therapy[10,11] is to eradicate tumor cells, either benign or malignant, while minimizing damage to healthy tissue. This objective can further be divided into six different indications based on the disease presentation and practitioner's intentions:

1. Definitive treatment with the intent to cure
2. Neoadjuvant treatment to improve chances of successful surgical resection
3. Adjuvant treatment to improve local control of cancer growth after chemotherapy or surgery
4. Prophylactic treatment to prevent growth of cancer in asymptomatic, yet high-risk areas for metastasis
5. Control to limit growth of existing cancer cells
6. Palliation to relieve pain, prevent fracture, and enhance mobility when cure is not possible

Before a patient receives radiation therapy, a simulation procedure is performed in order to circumscribe the tumor and adjacent tissues and organs to prepare for delivery of ionizing radiation. Simulation can be performed with computed tomography (CT), virtual simulation software, or magnetic resonance imaging (MRI). Further mapping is then performed to synchronize the radiation energy with the patient's respiratory cycle, and PET scanning is also used to specifically map the tumor.[12]

Radiation therapy is delivered by three different modalities: external beam radiation therapy (EBRT), brachytherapy, or radioimmunotherapy (RIT). EBRT is the primary modality used in most cases. Technological advances have allowed EBRT to be further divided into different modalities that allow better localization of tumor margins along with gradation of radiation dose, both of which can minimize damage to surrounding tissues and maximize therapeutic effect. These different forms of EBRT include intensity-modulated radiation therapy (IMRT),

image-guided radiotherapy (IGRT), stereotactic radiosurgery, and image-guided cyberknife radiosurgery.[10,12]

Brachytherapy involves the placement (temporary or permanent) of selected radioactive sources directly into a body cavity (intracavitary), into tissue (interstitial), into passageways (intraluminal), or onto tissue surfaces (plaque).[12] The following malignancies can be treated with brachytherapy: gynecological, breast, lung, esophageal, head and neck, brain, and prostate tumors, as well as certain types of melanoma. Brachytherapy can be used alone or in combination with EBRT.

Another form of radiation therapy, intraoperative radiation therapy (IORT), consists of delivering a single, large fraction of radiation to an exposed tumor or to a resected tumor bed during a surgical procedure. IORT is generally used in the management of gastrointestinal, genitourinary, gynecological, and breast cancers.[10] Advances in radiation therapy include using high-intensity focused ultrasound with magnetic resonance guidance (MRgFUS) and selective internal radiation therapy (SIRT).[12]

> ✎ **CLINICAL TIP**
>
> A patient may be prescribed antiemetics (see Chapter 19, Table 19-22) after radiation treatment to control nausea and vomiting. Notify the physician if antiemetic therapy is insufficient to control the patient's nausea or vomiting during physical therapy sessions.

General side effects that commonly occur with radiation therapy include skin reactions, fatigue, weight loss, and myelosuppression (bone marrow suppression). Numerous site-specific toxicities may include limb edema, alopecia, cerebral edema, seizures, visual disturbances, cough, pneumonitis, fibrosis, esophagitis, nausea, vomiting, diarrhea, cystitis, and cardiomyopathy. These side effects may occur immediately after radiation therapy and/or reappear at a later time. In addition, radiation-induced malignancies may occur, including breast cancer, leukemia, and sarcoma.[13]

> ✎ **CLINICAL TIP**
>
> Radiation may lead to decreased skin distensibility and resultant decreased range of motion. Special care should be taken with the skin and other tissues in that area because it will be very fragile. Promotion of active or passive range of motion may help to prevent contracture.

Chemotherapy

The overall purpose of chemotherapy is to inhibit various signaling pathways that control cancer cell proliferation, invasion, metastasis, angiogenesis, and cell death. Chemotherapy agents can potentially provide a cure or manage metastatic disease and reduce the size of the tumor for surgical resection or palliative care.[14] Chemotherapy can be performed preoperatively and postoperatively. Chemotherapy is usually delivered systemically, via intravenous or central lines, but may be directly injected in or near a tumor. Refer to Chapter 18, Table 18-7 for information regarding totally implantable intravascular catheters or tunneled central venous catheters often used for chemotherapy. Patients may receive a single or multiple rounds of chemotherapy over time to treat their cancer and to possibly minimize side effects. Side effects of chemotherapy include nausea, vomiting, "cancer pain," and loss of hair and other fast-growing cells, including platelets, red blood cells, and white blood cells. A variety of chemotherapy agents have different mechanisms of action and are described in Chapter 19, Table 19-23.

Physical Therapy Considerations

- Nausea and vomiting after chemotherapy vary on a patient-to-patient basis. The severity of these side effects may be due to the disease stage, chemotherapeutic dose, or number of rounds. Some side effects may be so severe as to limit physical therapy, whereas others allow patients to tolerate activity. Rehabilitation should be delayed or modified until the side effects from chemotherapy are minimized or alleviated.
- Patients may be taking antiemetics, which help to control nausea and vomiting after chemotherapy. The physical therapist should alert the physician when nausea and vomiting limit the patient's ability to participate in physical therapy so that the antiemetic regimen can be modified or enhanced. Antiemetics are listed in Chapter 19, Table 19-22.
- Chemotherapy agents affect the patient's appetite and ability to consume and absorb nutrients. This decline in nutritional status can inhibit the patient's progression in strength and conditioning programs. Proper nutritional support should be provided and directed by a nutritionist. Consulting with the nutritionist may be beneficial when planning the appropriate activity level based on a patient's caloric intake.
- Patients should be aware of the possible side effects and understand the need for modification or delay of rehabilitation efforts. Patients should be given emotional support and encouragement when they are unable to achieve the goals that they have initially set. Intervention may be coordinated around the patient's medication schedule.
- Vital signs should always be monitored, especially when patients are taking the more toxic chemotherapy agents that affect the heart, lungs, and central nervous system.
- Platelet, red blood cell, and white blood cell counts should be monitored with a patient on chemotherapy. The Stem Cell Transplantation section in Chapter 14 suggests therapeutic activities with altered blood cell counts.
- Patients receiving chemotherapy can become neutropenic and are at risk for infections and sepsis.[15] (A neutrophil is a type of leukocyte or white blood cell that is often the first immunological cell at the site of infection; neutropenia is an abnormally low neutrophil count. Absolute neutrophil count [ANC] will determine whether or not a patient is neutropenic and subsequent precautions.) Therefore patients undergoing chemotherapy may be on neutropenic precautions, such as being in isolation. Follow the institution's guidelines for precautions when treating these patients to help reduce the risk of infections. Examples of these

guidelines can be found in the Stem Cell Transplantation section in Chapter 14.

Biotherapy

Biological therapy, also referred to as immunotherapy, uses a patient's native host defense system as mechanisms to treat cancer. This form of therapy can be highly targeted while minimizing toxicity. Agents currently used for biotherapy include cytokines, monoclonal antibodies, and vaccines.[16] Chapter 19, Table 19-23 provides a list of cytokines and monoclonal antibodies used for cancer management as well as their side effects and physical therapy considerations. Vaccines are currently used to prevent viral infections that have been shown to lead to cancer. Human papillomavirus has been linked to cervical cancer, and hepatitis B can lead to liver cancer. Vaccination is available for both of these pathogens.[17]

Gene Therapy

The potential exists for treating many genetic disorders as well as autoimmune disorders, cancer, and infectious diseases by genetically modifying cells that may have defective genetic material. A common therapeutic approach is performed by introducing normal genes into a patient's cell nuclei in order to enhance, repair, or replace altered genetic material. Somatic gene therapy is approved in the United States and involves somatic, nonreproductive cells of the body including skin, muscle, bone, and liver.[18]

Cancers in the Body Systems

Cancers can invade or affect any organ or tissue in the body. The following is an overview of various cancers in each body system.

Respiratory Cancers

Cancer can affect any structure of the respiratory system, including the larynx, lung, and bronchus. There are two major categories of lung cancer, non–small-cell lung cancer (NSCLC) and small-cell lung cancer (SCLC). Approximately 85% of lung cancers are NSCLC, which is composed of three subtypes: squamous cell carcinoma, adenocarcinoma, and large-cell carcinoma.[19,20] The risk of developing lung cancer is 13 to 23 times higher, respectively, in female and male smokers as compared to nonsmokers. Eighty percent of lung cancer deaths are related to smoking.[4] Symptoms associated with lung cancer include chronic cough, dyspnea, hoarseness, chest pain, and hemoptysis. Additional symptoms may also include weakness, weight loss, anorexia, and, rarely, fever.[20] Common sites of metastases for lung cancer include bone, adrenal glands, liver, intraabdominal lymph nodes, brain and spinal cord, and skin (20%).[20,21]

Bronchoscopy, biopsy, and imaging techniques such as radiography, CT, and PET can be used to stage lung cancer.[20-22] In addition to the TNM staging, NSCLC is further staged to help guide interventions and prognosis. Table 11-7 outlines the specific TNM components, and Table 11-8 illustrates the staging components from Ia to IV.

TABLE 11-7 Staging of Non–Small-Cell Lung Cancer

Descriptors	Definitions
T	Primary tumor
T0	No primary tumor
T1	Tumor ≤3 cm in the greatest dimension, surrounded by lung or visceral pleura, not more proximal than the lobar bronchus
T1a	Tumor ≤2 cm in the greatest dimension
T1b	Tumor >2 but ≤3 cm in the greatest dimension
T2	Tumor >3 but ≤7 cm in the greatest dimension or tumor with any of the following*: Invades visceral pleura Involves main bronchus ≥2 cm distal to the carina† Atelectasis/obstructive pneumonia extending to hilum but not involving the entire lung
T2a	Tumor >3 but ≤5 cm in the greatest dimension
T2b	Tumor >5 but ≤7 cm in the greatest dimension
T3	Tumor >7 cm; or directly invading chest wall, diaphragm, phrenic nerve, mediastinal pleura, or parietal pericardium; or tumor in the main bronchus <2 cm distal to the carina†; or atelectasis/obstructive pneumonitis of entire lung; or separate tumor nodules in the same lobe
T4	Tumor of any size with invasion of heart, great vessels, trachea, recurrent laryngeal nerve, esophagus, vertebral body, or carina; or separate tumor nodules in a different ipsilateral lobe
N	Regional lymph nodes
N0	No regional node metastasis
N1	Metastasis in ipsilateral peribronchial and/or perihilar lymph nodes and intrapulmonary nodes, including involvement by direct extension
N2	Metastasis in ipsilateral mediastinal and/or subcarinal lymph nodes
N3	Metastasis in contralateral mediastinal, contralateral hilar, ipsilateral or contralateral scalene, or supraclavicular lymph nodes
M	Distant metastasis
M0	No distant metastasis
M1a	Separate tumor nodules in a contralateral lobe; or tumor with pleural nodules or malignant pleural dissemination‡
M1b	Distant metastasis
Special situations	
TX, NX, MX	T, N, or M status not able to be assessed
Tis	Focus of in situ cancer
T1†	Superficial spreading tumor of any size but confined to the wall of the trachea or mainstem bronchus

From Detterbeck FC, Boffa DJ, Tanoue LT: The new lung cancer staging system, Chest 136(1):260, 2009.

*T2 tumors with these features are classified as T2a if ≤5 cm.

†The uncommon superficial spreading tumor in central airways is classified as T1.

‡Pleural effusions are excluded that are cytologically negative, nonbloody, transudative, and clinically judged not to be due to cancer.

TABLE 11-8 Staging Components of Non–Small-Cell Lung Cancer

T/M	Subgroup	N0	N1	N2	N3
T1	T1a	Ia	IIa	IIIa	IIIb
	T1b	Ia	IIa	IIIa	IIIb
T2	T2a	Ib	IIa	IIIa	IIIb
	T2b	IIa	IIb	IIIa	IIIb
T3	T3>7	IIb	IIIa	IIIa	IIIb
	T3lev	IIb	IIIa	IIIa	IIIb
	T3Satell	IIb	IIIa	IIIa	IIIb
T4	T4lev	IIIa	IIIa	IIIb	IIIb
	T4Ipsi Nod	IIIa	IIIa	IIIb	IIIb
M1	M1aContra Nod	IV	IV	IV	IV
	M1aPl Disem	IV	IV	IV	IV
	M1b	IV	IV	IV	IV

From Detterbeck FC, Boffa DJ, Tanoue LT: The new lung cancer staging system, Chest 136(1):260, 2009. DOI: 10.1378/chest.08-0978

Small-cell lung cancer is defined as either limited-stage or extensive-stage disease according to the Veterans Administration Lung Study Group. Limited-stage disease is restricted to a single hemithorax that may or may not have contralateral mediastinal or supraclavicular lymph node involvement.[23]

Surgery is the treatment of choice for stage I and II NSCLC, with a lobectomy considered as the gold standard for definitive surgery. Wedge resection, segmentectomy, or pneumonectomy can also be performed in patients with NSCLC. Surgical intervention for SCLC is controversial and not standard practice.[23,24]

Bone and Soft-Tissue Cancers

Tumors of bone are most commonly discovered after an injury or fracture or during a medical workup for pain. A majority of tumors in the bone arise from other primary sites. Common primary tumors that metastasize to bone include breast, lung, prostate, kidney, and thyroid tumors.[25]

Pain, a palpable mass, possible bony tenderness, and increasing disability are the main clinical manifestations of primary or

Thoracic surgery involves a large incision on the thoracic wall, the location of which generally results in a very painful incision. Surgical incisions into the pleural space will cause deflation of the lung. Deep-breathing exercises (along with mucus-clearance techniques with incisional splinting and range-of-motion exercises of the upper extremity on the side of the incision) are important to prevent postoperative pulmonary complications and restore shoulder and trunk mobility. Note that patients may have chest tubes in place immediately after surgery (see Chapter 18). Oxygen supplementation may be required in patients who have undergone thoracic surgery. Oxyhemoglobin saturation (Sao$_2$) should be monitored to ensure adequate oxygenation, especially when increasing activity levels.

Patients commonly experience fractures owing to metastatic disease in the vertebrae, proximal humerus, and femur.[26] Therefore patients should be instructed in safety management to avoid falls or trauma to involved areas. A patient with bone metastases must receive clearance from the physician before mobility, along with clarifying the patient's weight-bearing status. This applies to patients who have undergone surgical intervention as well. Assistive devices may be prescribed based on the patient's weight-bearing and functional status.

TABLE 11-9 Malignant Tumors in Bone and Soft Tissue

Sarcoma Subtype	Involved Tissue or Cells
Angiosarcoma Kaposi's sarcoma Lymphangiosarcoma Hemangioendothelioma	Blood and lymph vessels
Chondrosarcoma Ewing's sarcoma Osteosarcoma	Bone and cartilage
Liposarcoma Atypical lipoma	Adipose tissue
Fibrosarcoma Dermatofibrosarcoma protuberans (DFSP) Malignant fibrous histiocytoma (MFH) Myxofibrosarcoma	Fibrous tissue
Gastrointestinal stromal tumor (GIST) Malignant mesenchymoma	Mesenchymal cells (precursor to blood vessels, connective tissue, lymphatic tissue)
Malignant granular cell tumor Malignant peripheral nerve sheath tumor (MPNST) or neurofibrosarcoma	Neural/peripheral nerves
Glomangiosarcoma Malignant hemangiopericytoma	Perivascular tissues
Rhabdomyosarcoma	Skeletal muscle
Leiomyosarcoma	Smooth muscle
Synovial sarcomas	Synovial tissue

Adapted from Table 46-1 of Samuel LC: Bone and soft tissue sarcomas. In Yarboro CH, Wujcik D, Gobel BH, editors: Cancer nursing, ed 7, Sudbury, MA, 2011, Jones & Bartlett, p 1053.

secondary bone cancer as well as soft-tissue cancers.[27] Soft-tissue cancers can be found in tissues that surround, connect, or support body organs and structures. Types of primary bone and soft-tissue cancers, both of which occur less frequently,[25] are described in Table 11-9. Treatment of bone and soft tissue cancers can include radiation, chemotherapy, amputation, and surgery on involved limbs.[25] Although not all metastases to bone cause pathological fractures, surgical intervention can be used for a patient with a bone metastasis because of the risk of pathological fracture. These procedures may include the use of intramedullary rods, plates, and prosthetic devices (e.g., total joint arthroplasty) and are described in Chapter 5.

Breast Cancer

Breast cancer, although more prevalent in women, is also diagnosed in men to a lesser extent. The risk for developing breast cancer in women is related to increasing age, family history, and carrying either of the two breast cancer genes, BRCA1 and BRCA2.[28] The U.S. Preventative Services Task Force recommends "biennial screening with mammography for women aged 50 to 75 years."[29] In contrast, the American College of Radiology and the Society of Breast Imaging recommend annual screening with mammography for women beginning at the age of 40.[30]

Progression of breast cancer is staged according to growth and spread of the tumor (Table 11-10). Areas that are prone to metastases from breast cancer, in order of occurrence, are the lungs, bones, liver, adrenal glands, brain, and meninges. Advancement in the treatment of breast cancer includes inhibition of growth factor receptors, stromal proteases, and angiogenesis by pharmacological agents or specific antibodies.[31] Common surgical procedures for the treatment of breast cancer are described in Table 11-11.

Physical Therapy Considerations

- The physical therapist should clarify the physician's orders regarding upper-extremity range-of-motion restrictions, particularly after surgery involving muscle transfers. The therapist must know what muscles were resected or transferred during the procedure, the location of the incision, and whether there was any nerve involvement before mobilization. Once this information is clarified, the therapist should proceed to examine the range of motion of the shoulder and neck region, as it may be affected during surgical interventions for breast cancer. Shoulder and arm mobility may begin as early as 24 hours after surgery.[32]
- Patients may exhibit postoperative pain, lymphedema, or nerve injury due to trauma or traction during the operative procedure.

TABLE 11-10 Stages of Breast Cancer

Stage	TNM	Description
Stage 0	Tis, N0, M0	Ductal carcinoma in situ (DCIS).
Stage IA	T1, N0, M0	Tumor is 2 cm or less and has not spread to lymph nodes or distant sites.
Stage IB	T0 or T1, N1mi, M0	Tumor is 2 cm or less across (or is not found) with micrometastases in 1 to 3 axillary lymph nodes and no distant metastases.
Stage IIA (two possible situations)	T0 or T1, N1 (but not N1mi), M0	The tumor is 2 cm or less across (or is not found) and either: • It has spread to 1 to 3 axillary lymph nodes, with the cancer in the lymph nodes larger than 2 mm across (N1a), OR • Tiny amounts of cancer are found in internal mammary lymph nodes on sentinel lymph node biopsy (N1b), OR • It has spread to 1 to 3 lymph nodes under the arm and to internal mammary lymph nodes (found on sentinel lymph node biopsy) (N1c).
	T2, N0, M0	The tumor is larger than 2 cm across and less than 5 cm (T2) but has not spread to the lymph nodes (N0) or to distant sites (M0).
Stage IIB (two possible situations)	T2, N1, M0	The tumor is larger than 2 cm and less than 5 cm across (T2). It has spread to 1 to 3 axillary lymph nodes and/or tiny amounts of cancer are found in internal mammary lymph nodes on sentinel lymph node biopsy (N1). The cancer has not spread to distant sites (M0).
	T3, N0, M0	The tumor is larger than 5 cm across but does not grow into the chest wall or skin and has not spread to lymph nodes (T3, N0) or to distant sites (M0).
Stage IIIA (two possible situations)	T0 to T2, N2, M0	The tumor is not more than 5 cm across (or cannot be found) (T0 to T2). It has spread to 4 to 9 axillary lymph nodes, or it has enlarged the internal mammary lymph nodes (N2). The cancer has not spread to distant sites (M0).
	T3, N1 or N2, M0	The tumor is larger than 5 cm across but does not grow into the chest wall or skin (T3). It has spread to 1 to 9 axillary nodes, or to internal mammary nodes (N1 or N2). The cancer has not spread to distant sites (M0).
Stage IIIB	T4, N0 to N2, M0	The tumor has grown into the chest wall or skin (T4), and one of the following applies: • It has not spread to the lymph nodes (N0). • It has spread to 1 to 3 axillary lymph nodes and/or tiny amounts of cancer are found in internal mammary lymph nodes on sentinel lymph node biopsy (N1). • It has spread to 4 to 9 axillary lymph nodes, or it has enlarged the internal mammary lymph nodes (N2). The cancer has not spread to distant sites (M0).
Stage IIIC	Any T, N3, M0	The tumor is any size (or cannot be found), and one of the following applies: • Cancer has spread to 10 or more axillary lymph nodes (N3). • Cancer has spread to the lymph nodes under the clavicle (collar bone) (N3). • Cancer has spread to the lymph nodes above the clavicle (N3). • Cancer involves axillary lymph nodes and has enlarged the internal mammary lymph nodes (N3). • Cancer has spread to 4 or more axillary lymph nodes, and tiny amounts of cancer are found in internal mammary lymph nodes on sentinel lymph node biopsy (N3). The cancer has not spread to distant sites (M0).
Stage IV	Any T, any N, M1	The cancer can be any size (any T) and may or may not have spread to nearby lymph nodes (any N). It has spread to distant organs or to lymph nodes far from the breast (M1). The most common sites of spread are the bone, liver, brain, or lung.

From the American Joint Committee on Cancer TNM system reported by the American Cancer Society. http://www.cancer.org/Cancer/BreastCancer/DetailedGuide/breast-cancer-staging. Accessed June 29, 2012.

• Postoperative drains may be in place immediately after surgery, and the physical therapist should take care to avoid manipulating these drains. Range-of-motion exercises may cause the drain to be displaced.
• Incisions resulting from muscle transfer flaps involving the rectus abdominis, pectoralis, or latissimus dorsi should be supported when the patient coughs.
• The physical therapist should instruct the patient in the log-roll technique, which is used to minimize contraction of the abdominal muscles while the patient is getting out of bed. The therapist should also instruct the patient to minimize contraction of the shoulder musculature during transfers.
• Lymphedema may need to be controlled with lymphedema massage, elevation, exercise while wearing nonelastic wraps, elastic garments, or compression pneumatic pumps, especially when surgery involves lymph nodes that are near the extremities. These techniques have been shown to be of value in decreasing lymphedema.[33-35] Circumferential or water displacement measurements of the involved upper extremity may be taken to record girth changes and to compare with the noninvolved extremity.

TABLE 11-11 Surgical Interventions for Breast Cancer

Surgery	Description
Breast-conserving surgery	Primary goal of minimizing local recurrence while maintaining cosmesis. Types include lumpectomy, segmental mastectomy, partial mastectomy, quadrantectomy, and wide local excision.
Modified radical mastectomy	Removal of all breast tissue and the nipple-areola complex, plus axillary node dissection while preserving the pectoralis muscle.
Axillary and sentinel lymph node mapping and dissection	Performed to help determine prognosis and risk for recurrence. Sentinel node is the first node that receives primary lymphatic flow from the tumor and has been found to predict the histological characteristics of the remaining lymph nodes in the region.
Breast reconstruction	Types include breast implant reconstruction, autogenous breast reconstruction, consisting of pedicle flaps or free flaps. Pedicle flaps consist of the transverse rectus abdominis myocutaneous (TRAM) procedure and the latissimus dorsi procedure. Free flaps include microsurgery consisting of a TRAM, the deep inferior epigastric perforator (DIEP) flap, the superficial inferior epigastric (SIEA) flap, and the superior and inferior gluteal artery flaps.

Data from Foxson SB, Lattimer JG, Felder B: Breast cancer. In Yarboro CH, Wujcik D, Gobel BH, editors: Cancer nursing, ed 7, Sudbury, MA, 2011, Jones & Bartlett, pp 1091-1145.

- The physical therapist should consider the impact of reconstructive breast surgery on the patient's sexuality, body image, and psychological state.[36]

Gastrointestinal and Genitourinary Cancers

Gastrointestinal (GI) cancers can involve the esophagus, stomach, colon, and rectum, with colorectal cancer being the most prevalent type of GI cancer.

> ✎ **CLINICAL TIP**
>
> Patients with genitourinary cancer may experience urinary incontinence. Bladder control training, pelvic floor exercises, and biofeedback or electrical stimulation may be necessary to restore control of urinary flow.[37-39] Patients with gastrointestinal cancer may experience bowel as well as urinary incontinence. Both bowel and bladder incontinence can lead to areas of dampened skin, which are prone to breakdown.[40] Therefore physical therapists should be careful to minimize shearing forces in these areas during mobility.

TABLE 11-12 Surgical Interventions for Genitourinary System Cancers

Area Involved	Surgical Intervention	Excision
Uterus	Hysterectomy	Uterus through abdominal wall or vagina
	Total abdominal hysterectomy	Body of uterus and cervix through abdominal wall
	Subtotal abdominal hysterectomy	Uterus (cervix remains)
Ovary	Oophorectomy	One ovary
Ovaries and oviducts	Bilateral salpingo-oophorectomy	Both ovaries and oviducts
Prostate	Prostatectomy	Entire prostate
Testes	Orchiectomy	One or both testes

The risk of colorectal cancer increases with age (over 50 years), obesity, physical inactivity, a diet rich in processed or red meat, alcohol consumption, and long-term smoking.[4] Common areas for metastases for colorectal cancer include, in order of occurrence, regional lymph nodes, liver, lungs, and bones.[41] Cancers of the liver and pancreas, although considered gastrointestinal, are discussed separately in this chapter. Surgical procedures used to treat gastrointestinal cancers involve resection of the involved region (e.g., gastrectomy or colectomy) with or without accompanying chemotherapy or radiation therapy.[4]

Genitourinary cancers can involve the uterus, ovaries, testicles, prostate, bladder, and kidney. Renal cell carcinoma tends to metastasize widely before symptoms are recognized, which generally leads to a later discovery of the disease. In addition, renal cell carcinoma is usually discovered on unrelated imaging scans of the abdomen.[42]

Surgical interventions for the kidney are described in Chapter 9. Additional surgical procedures used to treat genitourinary cancers are listed in Table 11-12.

> ✎ **CLINICAL TIP**
>
> Patients who have undergone GI surgery may have resultant colostomy placements. Please refer to Chapter 8 for details and guidelines regarding this procedure.

Hepatobiliary Cancers

Hepatocellular carcinoma (HCC) accounts for 80% of primary liver cancers and carries high rates of mortality. Risk factors for developing HCC include hepatitis B virus or hepatitis C virus infection, cirrhosis of any etiology, smoking, obesity, and diabetes.[4,43]

Metastatic cancer to the liver from breast, lung, or colon cancer is a common source of secondary hepatic cancer.[44] Partial hepatectomy is the standard treatment for resectable HCC in patients without cirrhosis. In patients with cirrhosis, liver transplantation becomes the gold standard of surgically managing HCC in appropriate candidates.[43] Chapter 8 describes cirrhosis in further detail, and Chapter 14 reviews liver transplantation.

Cancer of the biliary tract consists of gallbladder cancer and bile duct cancer. Associations exist with gallstones or chronic inflammation in the region. Surgical resection can be curative if the tumor is contained; however, the median survival rate is 3 months for all patients with gallbladder cancer.[45]

> ✎ **CLINICAL TIP**
> Hepatic cancers can result in metabolic complications involving glucose metabolism, which primarily occurs in the liver. The patient therefore may have subsequent energy deficits.

Pancreatic Cancer

The incidence of pancreatic cancer has been increasing by 1.5% each year since 2004 and has a 5-year survival rate of 6%.[4,46] Most pancreatic tumors arise from the pancreatic duct and are found in the head of the pancreas. Symptoms may include weight loss, pain in the upper abdomen with or without radicular pain to the back, and jaundice if bile duct obstruction occurs from the tumor.[4] Risk factors for developing pancreatic cancer include tobacco smoking and smokeless tobacco use, family history and personal history of pancreatitis, obesity, and high levels of alcohol consumption. Treatment usually focuses on slowing tumor growth with chemotherapy and radiation therapy. As a result of tumor spread, fewer than 20% of patients are surgical candidates.[4]

Hematological Cancers

Leukemia

The leukemias are malignancies of hematopoietic stem cells originating in the bone marrow. Hematopoietic stem cells are immature blood cells that have the potential to differentiate into mature blood cells such as red blood cells, platelets, or white blood cells (lymphocytes).[47] Because the malignant cells first occupy the bone marrow, they can occlude the space occupied by normal bone marrow cells. As a result, patients can have anemia, thrombocytopenia, and leukopenia. Often, the clinical manifestations of leukemia are fatigue, easy bruising, weight loss, and infections.[4] (Refer to Chapter 7 for hematological information.)

There are four main groups of leukemia classified according to the cell type involved as well as the rate of growth of the cancer cells[4]:

- Acute lymphocytic leukemia (ALL)
- Chronic lymphocytic leukemia (CLL)
- Acute myeloid leukemia (AML)
- Chronic myeloid leukemia (CML)

These four groups have further subtypes that are determined by numerous factors such as characteristics of bone marrow and clinical presentation. It is beyond the scope of this text to outline all of the different subtypes. Table 11-13 outlines the

TABLE 11-13 Epidemiology of Leukemia in the United States

Type	Median Age at Diagnosis (years)	Survival Rate (5 year)
Acute lymphocytic leukemia	13	64.7%
Acute myeloid leukemia	67	2.19%
Chronic myeloid leukemia	66	50.2%
Chronic lymphocytic leukemia	72	75.9%

Adapted from Kurtin SE: Leukemia and myelodysplastic syndromes. In Yarboro CH, Wujcik D, Gobel BH, editors: Cancer nursing, ed 7, Sudbury, MA, 2011, Jones & Bartlett, p 1371.

median age at diagnosis as well as the 5-year survival rate. Leukemia can be managed by systemic therapies such as chemotherapy, immunotherapy, targeted therapies, or stem cell transplantation (see Chapter 14).[48]

Previous subtypes of leukemia have been established to be a distinct entity called *myelodysplastic syndrome (MDS)*. There is overlap in clinical presentation with leukemia such as anemia, thrombocytopenia, and neutropenia, thus creating difficulties in establishing early diagnosis. MDS occurs commonly in the elderly but can be present at any age.[48,49] Bone marrow transplantation is the primary therapeutic approach with proven potential to cure MDS; however, there is a high morbidity and mortality rate associated with the procedure in this population. Promising reports of several chemotherapy agents have been recently documented in patients with MDS.[50]

> ✎ **CLINICAL TIP**
> Complete blood count should be assessed to determine a safe level of activity or exercise. Refer to the Stem Cell Transplantation section in Chapter 14 for specific guidelines.

Lymphomas

Lymphomas are malignancies of lymphocytes and may be T cell, B cell, or natural killer (NK) cell in origin.[51,52] Unlike leukemic cells that primarily occupy bone marrow, lymphomas occupy lymph tissue (lymph nodes and spleen). Lymphoma results in painless enlargement (lymphadenopathy) of involved lymph nodes, which can also be firm and rubbery. Fever, night sweats, or fatigue may also be reported.[51,53]

> ✎ **CLINICAL TIP**
> Enlarged lymph nodes, discovered on examination, without a known cause may necessitate physician referral.

There are two primary types of lymphoma: Hodgkin's lymphoma (HL) and non-Hodgkin's lymphoma (NHL). More cases of NHL were reported in 2012 (70,130, as compared to 9060 cases of HL). Accounting for this difference is that NHL includes a wide variety of disease subtypes.[4] Characteristics of Hodgkin's and non-Hodgkin's lymphomas can be found in Table 11-14.

TABLE 11-14 Characteristics of Hodgkin's and Non-Hodgkin's Lymphomas

	Hodgkin's Lymphoma	Non-Hodgkin's Lymphoma
Cell characteristics	Presence of Reed-Sternberg cells, which are large, multinucleated cells found in involved lymph nodes	Wide variety of cell types involving B cells, T cells, and natural killer (NK) cells
Extranodal disease	Uncommon	Common
5-year survival rate	84%	67%

Data from Manson SD: Lymphoma. In Yarboro CH, Wujcik D, Gobel BH, editors: Cancer nursing, ed 7, Sudbury, MA, 2011, Jones & Bartlett, pp 1459-1512; American Cancer Society: Cancer facts & figures 2012, Atlanta, 2012, American Cancer Society.

Clinical staging for lymphoma is based on the Cotswolds Modification of the Ann Arbor Staging Classification found in Table 11-15. Treatment for both HL and NHL involves chemotherapy, radiation therapy, and/or stem cell transplantation.[4,51,52]

> ✎ **CLINICAL TIP**
>
> In a patient with diagnosed lymphoma, awareness of the areas of lymphadenopathy is advisable before working with the patient in order take caution with manual techniques and also to monitor any progression of the disease.

Multiple Myeloma

Multiple myeloma is a malignancy of plasma cells, which are derived from B lymphocytes (B cells) and are responsible for creating antibodies. The disease is characterized by infiltration of the myeloma cells into the bone and, eventually, other organs. These malignant cells produce monoclonal (M) proteins that may increase the viscosity of blood. Classically, the disease produces bone pain and a decreased number of normal hematological cells (e.g., red blood cells, white blood cells, and platelets).[54] Staging of the disease has been updated from the Durie-Salmon Classification to the International Staging System (Table 11-16).

> ✎ **CLINICAL TIP**
>
> Patients with advanced stages of multiple myeloma may be dehydrated. Ensure proper hydration before intervention.[55]

The median age of patients diagnosed with multiple myeloma[55] is approximately 70 years, with only 2% being younger than 40 years. Bone pain is usually the first symptom, with lesions by the malignant cells potentially causing osteoporosis and pathological fractures, especially in the vertebral

TABLE 11-15 Cotswolds Modification of Ann Arbor Staging Classification

Stage*	Description
I	Involvement of a single lymph node region or lymphoid structure (e.g., spleen, thymus)
I_E	Involvement of a single extralymphatic site or extranodal organ or site
II	Involvement of two or more lymph node regions on the same side of the diaphragm
II_E	Localized contiguous involvement of only one extranodal organ or side and its regional lymph nodes with or without other lymph node regions on the same side of the diaphragm
III	Involvement of lymph node regions on both sides of the diaphragm
III_S	Involvement of both sides of the diaphragm including the spleen
III_E	Localized contiguous involvement of only one extranodal organ side
III_{ES}	Localized contiguous involvement of only one extranodal organ side and the spleen
IV	Disseminated (multifocal) involvement of one or more extranodal organs or tissues, with or without associated lymph node involvement or isolated extralymphatic organ involvement with distant (nonregional) nodal involvement

Data from Lister TA, Crowther DM, Sutcliffe SB, et al: Report of a committee convened to discuss the evaluation and staging of patients with Hodgkin's disease: Cotswolds meeting, J Clin Oncol 7:1630-1636, 1989; Matasar MJ, Zelenetz AD: Overview of lymphoma diagnosis and management, Radiol Clin North Am 46;75-198, 2008; Manson SD: Lymphoma. In Yarboro CH, Wujcik D, Gobel BH, editors: Cancer nursing, ed 7, Sudbury, MA, 2011, Jones & Bartlett, p 1464.

*Any disease stage can have any of the further designations:

A: No symptoms

B: Fever, drenching night sweats, unexplained weight loss during the previous 6 months

X: Bulky disease, defined as greater than 10 cm in long axis or for a mediastinal mass as measuring greater than one third of the internal transverse thoracic diameter of a standard 5th or 6th thoracic vertebral body

E: Involvement of an extranodal site that is contiguous or proximal to the known nodal site

TABLE 11-16 International Myeloma Working Group Staging System

Stage	Criteria
I	β_2-Microglobulin < 3.5 μg/ml and albumin ≥ 3.5 g/dl
II	β_2-Microglobulin < 3.5 μg/ml and albumin < 3.5 g/dl or β_2-Microglobulin = 3.5-5.5 μg/ml
III	β_2-Microglobulin ≥ 5.5 μg/ml

From Ng AK, Anderson KC, Mahindra A: Multiple myeloma and other plasma cell neoplasms. In Gunderson LL, Tepper JE, editors: Clinical radiation oncology, ed 3, Philadelphia, 2012, Saunders, p 1576.

bodies. As further bone is destroyed, calcium is released, resulting in hypercalcemia. Acute kidney insufficiency is present in approximately 20% of patients with myeloma. Treatment can include chemotherapy, radiation therapy, and stem cell transplantation.[55] The 5-year survival rate is approximately 41%.[4]

> ✎ **CLINICAL TIP**
>
> Activity clearance should be obtained from the physician before mobilizing anyone with bone lesions.

Head and Neck Cancers

Head and neck cancers involve the paranasal sinuses, nasal and oral cavities, salivary glands, pharynx, nasopharynx, oropharynx, hypopharynx, larynx, and upper cervical lymph nodes.[56] Risk factors for developing cancer in the oral cavity and pharynx include all forms of smoked and smokeless tobacco products and excessive consumption of alcohol. An association with HPV infection has also been documented in both men and women.[4]

Symptoms can include a sore throat, a poorly healing sore in the mouth, ear pain, a neck mass, or hemoptysis (coughing up blood). Difficulties in chewing may present as the disease advances. Cancer management includes radiation therapy and/or surgery, along with chemotherapy in advanced stages.[4]

A tumor with clear margins and no lymph node involvement can be successfully resected. However, when lymph node involvement occurs, a radical neck dissection (RND) or modified neck dissection (MND) can be performed.[56] An RND includes removal of the sternocleidomastoid muscle (SCM), cervical lymph nodes, spinal accessory nerve, internal jugular vein, and submaxillary gland. An MND does not include resection of the SCM, spinal accessory nerve, or internal jugular vein.[57] Reconstructive surgery may also be performed including a skin flap, muscle flap, or both to cover resected areas of the neck and face. A facial prosthesis is sometimes used to help the patient attain adequate cosmesis and speech.

> ✎ **CLINICAL TIP**
>
> Proper positioning is important to prevent aspiration and excessive edema that may occur after surgery of the face, neck, and head. Clarify the surgeon's orders regarding head and neck positioning: patients may require a tracheostomy, artificial airway, or both to manage the airway and secretions. (Refer to Chapter 18, Appendix A.)

Physical Therapy Considerations

- Postoperatively, impairment of the respiratory system should be considered in patients with head, neck, and facial tumors because of possible obstruction of the airway or difficulty managing oral secretions. A common associated factor in patients with oral cancer is the use of tobacco (both chewing and smoking); therefore possible underlying lung disease must also be considered. During physical therapy examination, the patient should be assessed for adventitious breath sounds and effectiveness of airway clearance. Oral secretions should be cleared thoroughly before assessing breath sounds.
- After a surgical procedure, the physician should be contacted to determine activity and range-of-motion parameters, especially after skin and muscle flap reconstructions. Physical therapy treatment to restore posture and neck, shoulder, scapulothoracic, and temporomandibular motion is emphasized.
- When treating patients with head, neck, and facial cancers, it is important to consider the potential difficulties with speech, chewing, or swallowing and loss of sensations, including smell, taste, hearing, and sight.
- Because the patient may have difficulty with communicating and swallowing, referring the patient to a speech therapist and registered dietitian may be necessary. If these disciplines are already involved with the patient, be aware of posted guidelines to facilitate communication, including the use of an electronic larynx (electropharynx).

Neurological Cancers

Primary tumors of the central nervous system (CNS) include these types: gliomas, neuronal tumors, poorly differentiated neoplasms, primary central nervous system lymphomas, and meningiomas.[58] Secondary tumors can be the result of another systemic cancer (lung, breast, melanoma, kidney, and gastrointestinal tract) that has metastasized to the CNS.[58] Symptoms related to cancers of the nervous system depend on the size of the tumor and the area of the nervous system involved. Because of the compressive nature of CNS tumors, clinical manifestations can occur whether they are malignant or benign.[59] Neurological symptoms can persist after tumor excision, owing to destruction of neurological tissues. Changes in neurological status due to compression of tissues within the nervous system can indicate further spread of the tumor or may be related to edema of brain tissue. Sequelae include cognitive deficits, skin changes, bowel and bladder control problems, sexual dysfunction, and the need for assistive devices and positioning devices.[59]

After resection of a brain tumor, patients may demonstrate many other neurological sequelae, including hemiplegia and ataxia. Radiation therapy to structures of the nervous system may also cause transient neurological symptoms. Refer to Chapter 6 for more details on neurological examination and intervention.

> ✎ **CLINICAL TIP**
>
> A patient with neurological cancer may have a variety of needs depending on the location and extent of the cancer. Therefore the therapist should evaluate the patient's needs for skin care, splinting, positioning, cognitive training, gait and balance training, assistive devices, special equipment, and assistance with activities of daily living.

Skin Cancer

There are two major groups of skin cancers: melanoma and nonmelanoma. Melanoma encompasses 5% of all diagnosed cancers in the United States with 15% proving to be fatal.[60]

Nonmelanoma skin cancers are divided into the following categories: keratinocytic (including basal cell and squamous cell carcinoma), melanocytic, appendageal, soft tissue, neural, and cutaneous tumors.[60] Risk factors for developing melanoma include a personal or family history of melanoma along with numerous and/or atypical moles. For all skin cancers risk includes sun sensitivity, history of excessive sun exposure including sunburns, use of indoor tanning, presence or history of immunosuppressive diseases, and history of basal cell or squamous cell skin cancers.[4] According to the American Cancer Society, "approximately 2.2 million cases of skin cancer diagnosed annually can be prevented by protecting the skin from intense sun exposure and avoiding indoor tanning."[4]

Basal cell carcinoma is potentially the most common cancer diagnosed in humans.[60] It is usually found in areas exposed to the sun, including the head and neck regions. Lesions caused by basal cell carcinoma are mostly noduloulcerative: appearing as small, reddish and translucent with telangiectasis (small, widened blood vessels on the skin). Diagnosis is made with a biopsy or a tissue sample, and surgical excision is the treatment of choice.[60]

Squamous cell cancer is the second most common cancer in the United States but is more likely than basal cell carcinoma to be fatal.[60] Lesions may be variable in presentation, including small, pink, erythematous, and scaly plaque or large, ulcerated, and indurated plaque. The lesions may also bleed and be painful along with peripheral neural symptoms depending on location of the lesion. Surgical excision is also the treatment of choice for squamous cell cancer.[60]

Malignant melanoma is a neoplasm that arises from the melanocytes. Moles or pigmented spots exhibiting the following signs (called the ABCD rule) may indicate malignant melanoma[4]:

- A = Asymmetry
- B = Irregular border
- C = Varied color, pigmentation
- D = Diameter of more than 6 mm

Management of malignant melanoma can range from surgical excision with or without lymph node dissection, radiation therapy, chemotherapy, immunotherapy, or palliative care.[4] The 5-year survival rate for localized melanoma is 98%, with rates declining as the disease spreads.[4]

✎ CLINICAL TIP

After resection of skin lesions, proper positioning is important to prevent skin breakdown. The use of positioning or splinting devices may be necessary. The physical therapist should determine the location of the lesion and the need for range-of-motion exercises to prevent contractures. If the lesion involves an area that will be stressed (e.g., joints), the physical therapist should clarify the physician's orders for precautions limiting motion.

General Physical Therapy Guidelines for Patients with Cancer

The following are general goals and guidelines for the physical therapist working with the patient who has cancer. These guidelines should be adapted to a patient's specific needs.

The primary goals of physical therapy in this patient population are similar to those of other patients in the acute care setting; however, because of the systemic nature of cancer, the time frames for achieving goals will most likely be longer. These goals are to (1) optimize functional mobility, (2) minimize or prevent cancer-related fatigue (CRF), (3) prevent joint contracture and skin breakdown, (4) prevent or reduce limb edema, and (5) prevent postoperative pulmonary complications.

General guidelines include, but are not limited to, the following:

- Knowing the stage and grade of cancer can help the physical therapist modify a patient's treatment parameters and establish realistic goals and intervention.
- Patients may be placed on bed rest postoperatively and/or while receiving cancer treatment and will be at risk for developing pulmonary complications, deconditioning, and skin breakdown. Deep-breathing exercises,[61] frequent position changes, and an exercise program that can be performed in bed are beneficial in counteracting these complications.
- Patients who have metastatic processes, especially to bone, are at high risk for pathological fracture. Pulmonary hygiene is indicated for most patients who undergo surgical procedures. Care should be taken with patients who have metastatic processes during the performance of manual secretion clearance techniques. Metastatic processes should also be considered when prescribing resistive exercises to patients, as the muscle action on the frail bone may be enough to cause fracture.

According to a literature review by McNeely and Courneya,[62] current research indicates that aerobic and resistive exercise programs can help to minimize the complications of CRF.

In order to minimize the sequelae of cancer related fatigue, the following guidelines are recommended[63]:

- Before prescribing an exercise program, evaluate fatigue level and determine the need for more medical intervention. If the patient is cleared for exercise, then use the following:
  - Begin an exercise program when patients start cancer treatment, and continue until the end of treatment.
  - Before exercise sessions, evaluate the patient to rule out instability and/or decline in medical status.[64]
  - Before, several times during, and after exercise sessions, be sure to monitor vital signs including heart rate, blood pressure, and oxygen saturation.[64]
  - Emphasize the importance of an exercise log or diary to help monitor progress and promote adherence to the exercise program.
  - Refer to Table 11-17[64,65] for specific aerobic, resistive, and flexibility exercise prescription guidelines for cancer survivors with cancer-related fatigue.

TABLE 11-17 Exercise Prescription Guidelines for Cancer-Related Fatigue*

Mode	Duration	Intensity	Frequency
Aerobic	>20 minutes (may perform shorter sessions of 5-10 minutes 2-3×/day)[64]	40%-60% of HRR	3 to 5 days/week[64]
Resistive	1-2 sets of 8-12 repetitions of 8-10 exercises, including all major muscle groups[68] For those more fatigued or deconditioned: 1 set with increased repetitions of 12-15 for muscular endurance[65]	60%-70% of 1 RM[65] For those more fatigued or deconditioned: decreased resistance to 30% of 1 RM	2-3 days/week with 48 hours between sessions for recovery time[65] Increased recovery period between exercises, sets, and sessions during first few weeks of program to avoid fatigue[65]
Flexibility	4 repetitions of 10- to 30-second hold of slow static stretches, focusing on cancer treatment deficits or functional needs of the patient[64]		>2 days/week[64]

Please refer to Chapter 3 for a description of heart rate reserve (HRR).

RM, Repetition maximum.

*These guidelines are documented in literature regarding cancer survivors with cancer-related fatigue. Thus use caution or seek medical clarification for patients who do not fall into this category, as these guidelines may not be applicable for all cancer patients.

- Provide patient and family education regarding safety management, energy conservation, postural awareness, and body mechanics during activities of daily living. An assessment of the appropriate assistive devices, prosthetics, and required orthotics should also be performed. Decreased sensation requires special attention when prescribing and fitting adaptive devices.
- If a patient is placed on isolation precautions, place exercise equipment, such as stationary bicycles or upper-extremity ergometers (after being thoroughly cleaned or disinfected with facility-approved solutions), in his or her room. Assessment is necessary for the appropriateness of this equipment, along with the safety of independent use.
- When performing mobility or exercise treatments, care should be taken to avoid bruising or bleeding into joint spaces when patients have low platelet counts.
- Emotional support for both the patient and family is at times the most appreciated and effective method in helping to accomplish the physical therapy goals.
- Timely communication with the entire health care team is essential for safe and effective care. Communication should minimally include the patient's current functional status, progress toward the patient's goals, and any factors that are interfering with the patient's progress.

- Laboratory values, especially hemoglobin/hematocrit, white blood cell count, platelet count, and international normalized ratio (INR) should be monitored daily. The term *nadir* is sometimes used to denote when the patient's blood count is at its lowest point.

Because the cause of CRF is multifactorial and patient dependent, there is no distinct etiology. Therefore using several instruments to monitor CRF is essential.[66] There are unidimensional measures, single-question scales that focus on the presence or absence and severity of the symptom, and multidimensional measures that emphasize the effect of CRF on cognitive, physical, and emotional domains. Single-question assessments are the most regularly used assessment tools. Refer to Jean-Pierre and colleagues for a review of CRF assessments.[67]

A commonly used tool used for CRF is the Brief Fatigue Inventory (BFI).[68] This unidimensional, self-reported patient tool includes measuring nine items on severity and impact of fatigue during the previous 24 hours. The BFI is short and simple to complete, taking less than 5 minutes, and is able to include psychological and physical aspects. It is useful for screening and outcome assessments and had been validated in male and female cancer patients.[68] In the acute care physical therapy setting, the tool enables a quick assessment of fatigue levels in patients with cancer and recognizes patients with severe fatigue.

References

1. Gould B, Dyer R: Pathophysiology for the health professions, ed 4, Philadelphia, 2010, Saunders.
2. Stricker TP, Kumar V: Neoplasia. In Kumar V, Abbas AK, Fausto N et al, editors: Robbins basic pathology, ed 8, Philadelphia, 2007, Saunders, pp 174-175.
3. National Cancer Institute. http://www.cancer.gov/dictionary. Accessed June 27, 2012.
4. American Cancer Society: Cancer facts & figures 2012, Atlanta, 2012, American Cancer Society.
5. American Cancer Society: http://www.cancer.org/Cancer/CancerBasics/signs-and-symptoms-of-cancer. Accessed June 27, 2012.
6. Lobrano MB, Singha P: Positron emission tomography in oncology, Clin J Oncol Nurs 7(4):379-385, 2003.
7. National Cancer Institute: http://www.cancer.gov/cancertopics/factsheet/detection/staging. Accessed June 27, 2012.
8. Gulec SA, Hoenie E, Hostetter R et al: PET Probe-guided surgery: applications and clinical protocol, World J Surg Oncol 5:65, 2007.

9. Khorana AK, Burtness BA: Principles of cancer therapy. In Andreoli TE, Benjamin IJ, Griggs RC, Wing EJ, editors: Andreoli and Carpenter's Cecil essentials of medicine, ed 8, Philadelphia, 2010, Saunders.

10. Hogle WP: The state of the art in radiation therapy, Semin Oncol Nurs 22(4):212-220, 2006.

11. Gosselin TK: Principles of radiation therapy. In Yarboro CH, Wujcik D, Gobel BH, editors: Cancer nursing, ed 7, Sudbury, MA, 2011, Jones & Bartlett, pp 249-268.

12. Behrend SW: Radiation treatment planning. In Yarboro CH, Wujcik D, Gobel BH, editors: Cancer nursing, ed 7, Sudbury, MA, 2011, Jones & Bartlett, pp 269-311.

13. Haas ML: Radiation therapy: toxicities and management. In Yarboro CH, Wujcik D, Gobel BH, editors: Cancer nursing, ed 7, Sudbury, MA, 2011, Jones & Bartlett, pp 312-351.

14. Baskowsky LS, Supko JG, Chabner BA: Principles of chemotherapy. In Gunderson LL, Tepper JE, editors: Clinical radiation oncology, ed 3, Philadelphia, 2011, Saunders, pp 165-179.

15. Tierney LM, McPhee SJ, Papadakis MA, editors: Current medical diagnosis and treatment, New York, 2000, McGraw-Hill.

16. Adjuvant antineoplastic drugs. In Wecker L, Crespo LM, Dunaway G et al, editors: Brody's human pharmacology, ed 5, Philadelphia, 2009, Mosby Elsevier.

17. Muehlbauer PM: Biotherapy. In Yarboro CH, Wujcik D, Gobel BH, editors: Cancer nursing, ed 7, Sudbury, MA, 2011, Jones & Bartlett, pp 531-560.

18. Lea DH: Gene therapy. In Yarboro CH, Wujcik D, Gobel BH, editors: Cancer nursing, ed 7, Sudbury, MA, 2011, Jones & Bartlett, p 585-586.

19. Wagner H: Image-guided conformal radiation therapy planning and delivery for non-small-cell lung cancer, Cancer Control 10(4):277-288, 2003.

20. Johnson DH, Blot WJ, Carbone DP, et al: Cancer of the lung: non-small cell lung cancer and small cell lung cancer. In Abeloff MD, Armitage JO, Neiderhuber JE et al, editors: Abeloff's clinical oncology, ed 4, Philadelphia, 2008, Churchill Livingstone, pp 1307-1366.

21. Husain AN, Kumar V: The lung. In V Kumar, AK Abbas, N Fausto, editors: Robbins and Cotran pathologic basis of disease, ed 7, Philadelphia, 2005, Saunders, p 760.

22. Lewis RJ, Caccavale RJ, Bocage JP, et al: Video-assisted thoracic surgical non-rib spreading simultaneously stapled lobectomy; a more patient-friendly oncologic resection, Chest 116(4):1119-1124, 1999.

23. Eaby-Sandy B: Lung cancer. In Yarboro CH, Wujcik D, Gobel BH, editors: Cancer nursing, ed 7, Sudbury, MA, 2011, Jones & Bartlett, pp 1425-1457.

24. Silvestri GA, Tanoue LT, Margolis ML et al: The noninvasive staging of non-small cell lung cancer: the guidelines, Chest 123:147S-156S, 2003.

25. Coleman RE, Holen I: Bone metastases. In Abeloff MD, Armitage JO, Neiderhuber JE et al, editors: Abeloff's clinical oncology, ed 4, Philadelphia, 2008, Churchill Livingstone, pp 845-872.

26. Norris J, editor: Professional guide to diseases, ed 5, Springhouse, PA, 1995, Springhouse.

27. Samuel LC: Bone and soft tissue sarcomas. In Yarboro CH, Wujcik D, Gobel BH, editors: Cancer nursing, ed 7, Sudbury, MA, 2011, Jones & Bartlett, pp 1053-1079.

28. Nadella PC, Godette K, Rizzo M et al: Breast carcinoma. In Beiber EJ, Sanfilippo JS, Horowitz IR, editors: Clinical gynecology, Philadelphia, 2006, Churchill Livingstone, pp 597-606.

29. U.S. Preventative Task Force: http://www.uspreventiveservicestaskforce.org/uspstf/uspsbrca.htm. Accessed June 29, 2012.

30. Lee CH, Dershaw D, Kopans D et al: Recommendations from the Society of Breast Imaging and the ACR on the use of mammography, breast MRI, breast ultrasound, and other technologies for the detection of clinically occult breast cancer, J Am Coll Radiol 7:18-27, 2010.

31. Lester SC: The breast. In Kumar V, Abbas AK, Fausto N, editors: Robbins and Cotran pathologic basis of disease, ed 7, Philadelphia, 2005, Saunders, pp 1129-1151.

32. Foxson SB, Lattimer JG, Felder B: Breast cancer. In Yarboro CH, Wujcik D, Gobel BH, editors: Cancer nursing, ed 7, Sudbury, MA, 2011, Jones & Bartlett, pp 1091-1145.

33. Badger CM, Peacock JL, Mortimer PS: A randomized, controlled, parallel-group clinical trial comparing multilayer bandaging followed by hosiery versus hosiery alone in the treatment of patients with lymphedema of the limb, Cancer 88(12):2832-2837, 2000.

34. Berlin E, Gjores JE, Ivarsson C, et al: Postmastectomy lymphoedema. Treatment and a five-year follow-up study, Int Angiol 18(4):294-298, 1999.

35. Johansson K, Albertsson M, Ingvar C et al: Effects of compression bandaging with or without manual lymph drainage treatment in patients with postoperative arm lymphedema, Lymphology 32(3):103-110, 1999.

36. Matin TA, Goldberg M: Surgical staging of lung cancer, Oncology 13(5):679-685, 1999.

37. Mattiasson A: Discussion: bladder and pelvic floor muscle training for overactive bladder, Urology 55(Suppl 5A):12-16, 2000.

38. Lewey J, Lilas L: Electrical stimulation of the overactive bladder, Prof Nurse 15(3):211-214, 1999.

39. Cammu H, Van Nylen M, Amy JJ: A 10-year follow-up after Kegel pelvic floor muscle exercises for genuine stress incontinence, BJU Int 85(6):655-658, 2000.

40. Gibbons G: Skin care and incontinence, Community Nurse 2(7):37, 1996.

41. Liu C, Crawford JM: The gastrointestinal tract. In Kumar V, Abbas AK, Fausto N, editors: Robbins and Cotran pathologic basis of disease, ed 7, Philadelphia, 2005, Saunders, pp 856-868.

42. Alpers CE: The kidney. In V Kumar, AK Abbas, N Fausto, editors: Robbins and Cotran pathologic basis of disease, ed 7, Philadelphia, 2005, Saunders, pp 1018-1019.

43. Abrams P, Marsh JW: Current approach to hepatocellular carcinoma, Surg Clin North Am 90(4):803-816, 2010.

44. Crawford JM: Liver and biliary tract. In Kumar V, Abbas AK, Fausto N, editors: Robbins and Cotran pathologic basis of disease, ed 7, Philadelphia, 2005, Saunders, p 928.

45. Afdha NH: Diseases of the gallbladder and bile ducts. In Goldman L, Schafer AI, editors: Goldman's Cecil medicine, ed 24, Philadelphia, 2011, Saunders, pp 1011-1020.

46. Hruban RH, Wilentz RE: The pancreas. In Kumar V, Abbas AK, Fausto N, editors: Robbins and Cotran pathologic basis of disease, ed 7, Philadelphia, 2005, Saunders, pp 948-952.

47. Patton KT: Anatomy & physiology (with media), ed 7, St Louis, 2010, Mosby, p 586.

48. Kurtin SE: Leukemia and myelodysplastic syndromes. In Yarboro CH, Wujcik D, Gobel BH, editors: Cancer nursing, ed 7, Sudbury, MA, 2011, Jones & Bartlett, pp 1369-1398.

49. Head DR, Hamilton KS: The myelodysplastic syndromes. In Jaffe ES, Harris NL, Vardiman JW et al, editors: Hemopathology, Philadelphia, 2010, Saunders, pp 656-672.

50. Ebert BL: The biology and treatment of myelodysplastic syndrome, Hematol Oncol Clin North Am 24(2):xiii-xvi, 2010.

51. Manson SD: Lymphoma. In Yarboro CH, Wujcik D, Gobel BH, editors: Cancer nursing, ed 7, Sudbury, MA, 2011, Jones & Bartlett, pp 1459-1512.

52. Matasar MJ, Zelenetz AD: Overview of lymphoma diagnosis and management, Radiol Clin North Am 46:75-198, 2008.

53. Cheson BD: Staging and evaluation of the patient with lymphoma, Hematol Oncol Clin North Am 22:825-837, 2008.

54. Nau KC, Lewis WD: Multiple myeloma: diagnosis and treatment, Am Fam Physician 78(7):853-859, 2008.

55. Kyle RA, Rajkumar SV: Multiple myeloma. In Conn's current therapy 2012, Philadelphia, 2012, Saunders, pp 818-822.

56. Carr E: Head and neck malignancies. In Yarboro CH, Wujcik D, Gobel BH, editors: Cancer nursing, ed 7, Sudbury, MA, 2011, Jones & Bartlett, pp 1335-1368.

57. Lester SC: Manual of surgical pathology, ed 3, Philadelphia, 2010, Saunders, pp 475-478.

58. Frosch MP: The nervous system. In Kumar V, Abbas AK, Fausto N et al, editors: Robbins basic pathology, ed 8, Philadelphia, 2007, Saunders, pp 882-887.

59. Frosch MP, Anthony DC, Girolami UD: The central nervous system. In Kumar V, Abbas AK, Fausto N, editors: Robbins and Cotran pathologic basis of disease, ed 7, Philadelphia, 2005, Saunders, p 1401.

60. Ricotti C, Bouzari N, Agadi A et al: Malignant skin neoplasms, Med Clin North Am 93(6):1241-1264, 2009.

61. Restrepo R, Wettstein R, Wittnebel L et al: Incentive spirometry: 2011. Respir Care [serial online] 56(10):1600-1604, 2011.

62. McNeely ML, Courneya KS: Exercise programs for cancer-related fatigue: evidence and clinical guidelines, JNCCN 8(8):945-953, 2010.

63. Watson T, Mock V: Exercise as an intervention for cancer-related fatigue, Phys Ther 84:736-743, 2004.

64. McNeely ML, Peddle CJ, Parliament M et al: Cancer rehabilitation: recommendations for integrating exercise programming in the clinical practice setting, Curr Cancer Ther Rev 2:351-360, 2006.

65. ACSM: ACSM's guidelines for exercise testing and prescription, ed 7, Baltimore, 2006, Lippincott Williams & Wilkins.

66. Schwartz AH. Validity of cancer-related fatigue instruments, Pharmacotherapy 22(11):1433-1441, 2002.

67. Jean-Pierre P, Figueroa-Moseley CD, Kohli S et al: Assessment of cancer-related fatigue: implications for clinical diagnosis and treatment, Oncologist 12(suppl 1):11-21, 2007.

68. Mendoza TR, Wang XS, Cleeland CS et al: The rapid assessment of fatigue severity in cancer patients: use of the Brief Fatigue Inventory, Cancer 85(5):1186-1196, 1999.

CHAPTER OBJECTIVES

The objectives of this chapter are to provide a fundamental review of the following:

1. The structure and function of the skin (integument)
2. The evaluation and physiologic sequelae of burn injury, including medical-surgical management and physical therapy intervention
3. The etiology of common types of wounds and the process of wound healing
4. The evaluation and management of wounds, including physical therapy intervention

PREFERRED PRACTICE PATTERNS

The most relevant practice patterns for the diagnoses discussed in this chapter, based on the American Physical Therapy Association's *Guide to Physical Therapist Practice*, second edition, are as follows:

- Burns: Thermal, Electrical, Chemical, Ultraviolet, Ionizing, Radiation: 6C, 6E, 7B, 7C, 7D, 7E
- Trauma Wounds: 4I, 4J, 7C, 7D, 7E
- Surgical Wounds: 4I, 7A, 7C, 7D, 7E
- Vascular Wounds (Arterial, Venous, Diabetic): 5G, 7A, 7B, 7C, 7D, 7E
- Pressure Wounds: 7A, 7B, 7C, 7D, 7E
- Neuropathic or Neurotrophic Ulcers: 7A, 7C, 7D, 7E

Please refer to Appendix A for a complete list of the preferred practice patterns, as individual patient conditions are highly variable and other practice patterns may be applicable.

Treating a patient with a major burn injury or other skin wound is often a specialized area of physical therapy.* All physical therapists should, however, have a basic understanding of normal and abnormal skin integrity, including the etiology of skin breakdown and the factors that influence wound healing.

Body Structure and Function: Normal Integument

Structure

The integumentary system consists of the skin and its appendages (hair and hair shafts, nails, and sebaceous and sudoriferous [sweat] glands), which are located throughout the skin, as shown in Figure 12-1. Skin is 0.5 to 6.0 mm thick[1,2] and is composed of two major layers: the epidermis and the dermis. These layers are supported by subcutaneous tissue and fat that connect the skin to muscle and bone. The thin, avascular epidermis is composed mainly of cells containing keratin. The epidermal cells are in different stages of maturity and degeneration and are therefore seen as five distinct layers within the epidermis. The thick, highly vascularized dermis is divided into two layers and is composed mainly of collagen and elastin. The epidermis and dermis are connected at the dermal-epidermal junction by a basement membrane. Table 12-1 reviews the cellular composition and function of each skin layer.

---

*For the purpose of this chapter, an alteration in skin integrity secondary to a burn injury is referred to as a *burn*. Alteration in skin integrity from any other etiology is referred to as a *wound*.

The skin has a number of clinically significant variations: (1) men have thicker skin than women; (2) the young and elderly have thinner skin than adults[3]; and (3) the skin on different parts of the body varies in thickness, number of appendages, and blood flow.[4] These variations affect the severity of a burn injury or skin breakdown, as well as the process of tissue healing.

Function

The integument has seven major functions[5]:

1. Temperature regulation. Body temperature is regulated by increasing or decreasing sweat production and superficial blood flow.
2. Protection. The skin provides a physical, chemical, and biological barrier to protect the body from microorganism invasion, ultraviolet (UV) radiation, abrasion, chemicals, and dehydration.

3. Sensation. Multiple sensory cells within the skin detect pain, temperature, and touch.
4. Excretion. Heat, sweat, and water can be excreted from the skin.
5. Immunity. Normal periodic loss of epidermal cells removes microorganisms from the body surface, and immune cells in the skin transport antigens from outside the body to the antibody cells of the immune system. An intact integumentum also creates a physical barrier, and the relatively acidic pH of the skin's surface provides chemical protection from microorganism invasion.[6]
6. Blood reservoir. Large volumes of blood can be shunted from the skin to central organs or muscles as needed.
7. Vitamin D synthesis. Modified cholesterol molecules are converted to vitamin D when exposed to UV radiation.

BURNS

Pathophysiology of Burns

Skin and body tissue destruction occurs from the absorption of heat energy and results in tissue coagulation. This coagulation is depicted in zones (Figure 12-2). The zone of coagulation, located in the center of the burn, is the area of greatest damage and contains nonviable tissue referred to as *eschar*. Although eschar covers the surface and may appear to take the place of skin, it does not have any of the characteristics or functions of normal skin. Instead, eschar is constrictive, attracts microorganisms, houses toxins that may circulate throughout the body, and prevents progression through the normal phases of healing.[3] The zone of stasis, which surrounds the zone of coagulation, contains marginally viable tissue which can easily be further damaged from processes such as hypoperfusion, edema, or infection. Proper wound care can minimize this conversion and preserve the integrity of the viable tissue in this zone. The zone

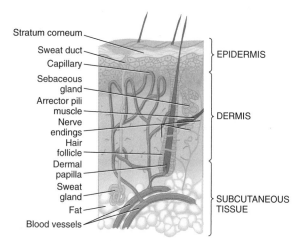

FIGURE 12-1
Three-dimensional representation of the skin and subcutaneous connective tissue layer showing the arrangement of hair, glands, and blood vessels. (From Black JM: Medical-surgical nursing: clinical management for positive outcomes, ed 8, St Louis, 2009, Saunders.)

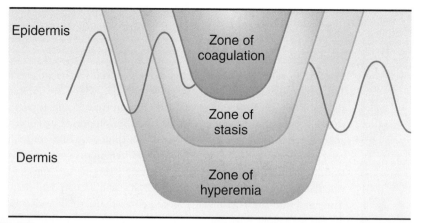

FIGURE 12-2
Zones of injury after a burn. The zone of coagulation is the portion irreversibly injured. The zones of stasis and hyperemia are defined in response to the injury. (From Townsend Jr CM, Beauchamp RD, Evers BM, Mattox KL: Sabiston textbook of surgery: the biological basis of modern surgical practice, ed 19, Philadelphia, 2012, Saunders.)

TABLE 12-1 Normal Skin Layers: Structure and Function

Layer	Cellular/Structural Composition	Function
Epidermis		
Stratum corneum	Dead, flattened keratinocytes	Tough outer layer that protects deeper layers of epidermis.
Stratum lucidum	Dead keratinocytes	Only present in areas with "thick skin" (i.e., palms, soles).
Stratum granulosum	Mature keratinocytes	Slowly dying as they migrate farther from vascularized dermis.
	Langerhans' cells	Involved in immunoregulation.
Stratum spinosum	Keratinocytes	Maturing as they move superficially.
	Langerhans' cells	See above.
	Melanocytes	Produce melanin, which protects from ultraviolet absorption. These cells may be present in more superficial layers in darker-skinned individuals.
Stratum basale or germinativum	Keratinocytes	Primary epidermal cell, undergoes mitosis and moves superficially. Produces keratin, a structural protein providing structural and waterproofing properties.
	Melanocytes	See above.
	Merkel cells	Mechanoreceptors involved in light touch.
Basement membrane		Irregular surface anchoring the epidermis to the dermis, which flattens with age, decreasing contact between the layers of skin.
Dermis		
Papillary layer	Collagen, elastin, and ground substance	Thin, superficial, dermal layer produced by fibroblasts; conforms into overlying basement membrane.
	Vasculature and lymph network	Provides blood supply and drainage to deeper layers of the avascular epidermis.
Reticular layer	Collagen, elastin, and reticular fibers	Produced by fibroblast cells, provides tensile strength and resilience.
	Macrophages, mast cells	Immunoregulation.
	Meissner's corpuscles	Detect light touch.
	Pacinian cells	Detect pressure.
	Free nerve endings	Detect temperature, pain, and mechanical stimulation.
	Vasculature and lymph vessels	Circulation and drainage.
	Hair follicles	Sensation, temperature regulation.
	Sweat glands	Thermoregulation.
	Sebaceous glands	Sebum production, lubricates skin.
Hypodermis		
		Attaches dermis to underlying structures.
	Subcutaneous fat (adipose)	Provides insulation and shock absorption.
	Fascia	Fibrous connective tissue separating and facilitating movement between adjacent structures.

Data from Myers BA: Wound management: principles and practice, ed 3, Upper Saddle River, NJ, 2012, Pearson Education, p 4; Baronoski S: Integumentary anatomy: skin—the largest organ. In McCulloch JM, Kloth LC, editors: Wound healing: evidence-based management, ed 4, Philadelphia, 2010, FA Davis, p 1; Sussman C, Bates-Jensen B: Wound care: a collaborative practice manual for health professionals, ed 3, Baltimore, 2007, Lippincott Williams & Wilkins, p 87; Wolff K et al: Development and structure of skin. In Fitzpatrick's dermatology in general medicine, ed 7, Columbus, 2008, McGraw-Hill; Bryant RA, Nix DP: Acute and chronic wounds: current management concepts, ed 4, St Louis, 2012, Mosby.

of hyperemia, the outermost area, is the least damaged and heals rapidly unless additional tissue injury occurs.[7-9]

The depth of a burn can be described as superficial, moderate partial thickness, deep partial thickness, or full thickness (Figure 12-3). Each type has its own appearance, sensation, healing time, and level of pain, as described in Table 12-2. First-degree burns have no significant structural damage and therefore no zone of stasis or coagulation. Differentiation between moderate and deep second-degree burns can be made based on the presence of the zones of coagulation, stasis, and hyperemia in the deeper burns while moderate second-degree burns will only have zones of stasis and hyperemia. Third-degree burns contain a significant and easily identifiable zone of coagulation as well.[10]

Physiologic Sequelae of Burn Injury

A series of physiologic events occurs after a burn (Figure 12-4). The physical therapist must appreciate the multisystem effects of a burn injury—namely, that the metabolic demands of the body increase dramatically. Tissue damage or organ dysfunction can be immediate or delayed, minor or severe, and local or systemic.[11] A summary of the most common complications of burns is listed in Table 12-3. The amount of total body surface area involved in the burn and the presence of inhalation injury are the primary risk factors for mortality after burn injury.[12]

Types of Burns

Thermal Burns

Thermal burns are the result of conduction or convection, as in contact with a hot object, liquid, chemical, flame, or steam. In order of frequency, the common types of thermal burns are scalds, flame burns, flash burns, and contact burns

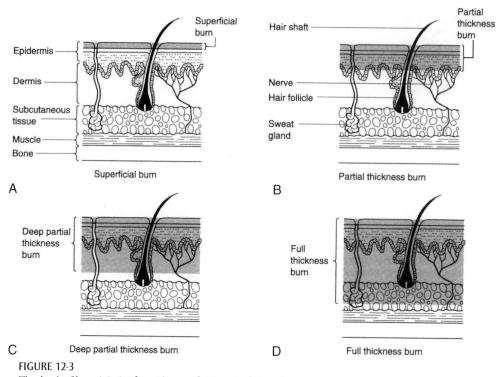

FIGURE 12-3

The depth of burn injuries from (**A**) superficial to (**D**) full thickness. (From Walsh M, editor: Nurse practitioners: clinical skills and professional issues, Oxford, England, 1999, Butterworth-Heinemann.)

TABLE 12-2 Burn Depth Characteristics

Depth	Appearance	Healing	Pain
Superficial (first-degree): Epidermis injured	Pink to red With or without edema Dry appearance without blisters Blanches Sensation intact Skin intact when rubbed	3-5 days by epidermal resurfacing through regenerating and migrating keratinocytes	Tenderness to touch or painful
Moderate partial-thickness (second degree): Superficial dermis injured	Pink to mottled red or red with edema Moist appearance with blisters Blanches with brisk capillary refill Sensation intact	1-2 weeks by epithelialization Pigmentation changes likely	Very painful
Deep partial-thickness (second degree): Deep dermis injured with hair follicles and sweat glands intact	Pink to pale ivory Dry appearance with blisters May blanch with slow capillary refill Decreased sensation to pinprick Hair readily removed	2-3 weeks by epithelialization[8] Will likely be grafted if healing time expected to be greater than 3 weeks Scar formation likely	Pain present but decreasing with depth of destruction[11]
Full-thickness: Entire dermis injured (third degree) or fat, muscle, and bone injured (fourth degree)	White, red, brown, or black (charred if fourth degree) Dry appearance without blanching May be blistered Insensate to pinprick Depressed wound	>3 weeks and requires granulation followed by epithelialization Often undergoes early surgical intervention	Insensate

Data from Wiebelhaus P, Hansen SL: Burns: handle with care, RN 62:52-75, 1999; Gomez R, Cancio LC: Management of burn wounds in the emergency department, Emerg Med Clin North Am 25:135-146, 2007; Arnoldo B, Klein M, Gibran MS: Practice guidelines for the management of electrical injuries, J Burn Care Res 27(4):439-447, 2006; Pham TN, Gibran NS, Heimbach DM: Evaluation of the burn wound: management decisions. In Herndon DN, editor: Total burn care, ed 3, Philadelphia, 2007, Saunders, p 119.

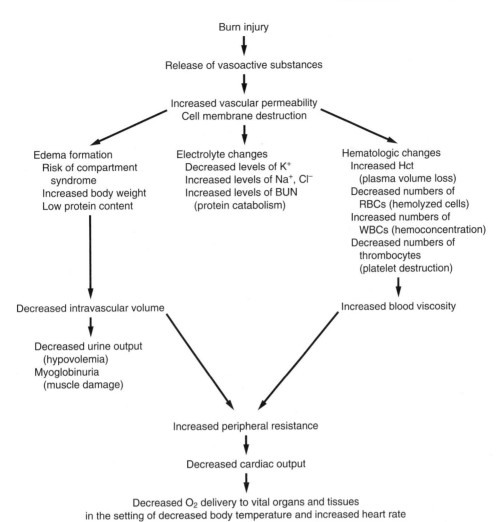

Burn injury

↓

Release of vasoactive substances

↓

Increased vascular permeability
Cell membrane destruction

Edema formation
  Risk of compartment
    syndrome
  Increased body weight
  Low protein content

Electrolyte changes
  Decreased levels of K⁺
  Increased levels of Na⁺, Cl⁻
  Increased levels of BUN
    (protein catabolism)

Hematologic changes
  Increased Hct
    (plasma volume loss)
  Decreased numbers of
    RBCs (hemolyzed cells)
  Increased numbers of
    WBCs (hemoconcentration)
  Decreased numbers of
    thrombocytes
    (platelet destruction)

Decreased intravascular volume

Increased blood viscosity

Decreased urine output
  (hypovolemia)
Myoglobinuria
  (muscle damage)

Increased peripheral resistance

↓

Decreased cardiac output

↓

Decreased O₂ delivery to vital organs and tissues
in the setting of decreased body temperature and increased heart rate

FIGURE 12-4

The physiologic sequelae of major burn injury. *BUN*, Blood urea nitrogen; *Cl⁻*, chlorine; *Hct*, hematocrit; *K⁺*, potassium; *Na⁺*, sodium; *O₂*, oxygen; *RBC*, red blood cell; *WBC*, white blood cell. (Modified from Marvin J: Thermal injuries. In Cardona VD, Hurn PD, Bastnagel Mason PJ, et al, editors: Trauma nursing from resuscitation through rehabilitation, ed 2, Philadelphia, 1994, Saunders; Demling RH, LaLonde C: Burn trauma, New York, 1989, Thieme, p 99.)

TABLE 12-3 Systemic Complications of Burn Injury

Body System	Complications
Respiratory	Inhalation injury, restrictive pulmonary pattern (which may occur with a burn on the trunk), atelectasis, pneumonia, microthrombi, and adult respiratory distress syndrome
Cardiovascular	Hypovolemia/hypotension, pulmonary hypertension, subendocardial ischemia, arrhythmias, anemia, deep venous thrombosis, and disseminated intravascular coagulopathy
Gastrointestinal/ genitourinary	Stress ulceration, hemorrhage, ileus, ischemic colitis, cholestasis, liver failure, and urinary tract infection
Renal	Edema, hemorrhage, acute tubular necrosis, and acute renal failure

Data from Linares HA: The burn problem: a pathologist's perspective. In Herndon DN, editor: Total burn care, London, 1996, Saunders.

(Table 12-4).[13] The severity of the burn depends on the location of the burn, the temperature of the source, and the duration of contact.[14]

Electrical Burns

An electrical burn is caused by exposure to a low- or high-voltage current and results in varied degrees of visible cutaneous tissue destruction at the contact points, as well as less visible but massive damage of subcutaneous tissue, muscle, nerve, and bone.[15] Tissue necrosis of these deeper structures occurs from the high heat intensity of the current and the electrical disruption of cell membranes.[13] Tissue damage occurs along the path of the current, with smaller distal areas of the body damaged most severely. This pattern of tissue damage accounts for the high incidence of amputation associated with electrical injury.[13,16] The severity of an electrical burn depends primarily on the duration of contact with the source, the voltage of the source, the type and pathway current, and the amperage and resistance through the body tissues.[16]

TABLE 12-4 Thermal Burns: Types and Characteristics

Burn Type	Description	Characteristics
Scald burn	Spill of or immersion in a hot liquid, such as boiling water, grease, or tar	Often causes deep partial- or full-thickness burns. Exposure to thicker liquids or immersion causes a deeper burn from increased contact time. Immersion burns commonly cover a larger total body surface area than do spills.
Flame burn	Flame exposure from fire or flammable liquids, or ignition of clothing	Often causes superficial and deep partial-thickness burns. Associated with carbon monoxide poisoning and inhalation injuries.
Flash burn	Explosion of flammable liquid, such as gasoline or propane	Often causes partial-thickness burns. Burns may be distributed over all exposed skin. Associated with upper airway thermal damage. Most common in the summer and associated with the consumption of alcohol.
Contact burn	Exposure to hot objects	Often causes deep partial- or full-thickness burns. Most common cause of serious burns in the elderly.

Data from Warden GD, Heimbach DM: Burns. In Schwartz SI, editor: Principles of surgery, vol 1, ed 7, New York, 1999, McGraw-Hill; Edlich RF, Moghtader JC: Thermal burns. In Rosen P, editor: Emergency medicine concepts and clinical practice, vol 1, ed 4, St Louis, 1998, Mosby.

Electrical burns are characterized by deep entrance and exit wounds and arc wounds. The entrance wound is usually an obvious necrotic and depressed area, whereas the exit wound varies in presentation. The exit wound can be a single wound or multiple wounds located where the patient was grounded during injury.[14] An arc wound is caused by the passage of current directly between joints in close opposition. For example, if the elbow is fully flexed and an electrical current passes through the arm, burns may be located at the volar aspect of the wrist, antecubital space, and axilla.[13]

Complications specific to electrical injury include[13,17]:

- Cardiovascular: Cardiac arrest (ventricular fibrillation for electric current or systole for lightning), arrhythmia (usually sinus tachycardia or nonspecific ST segment changes) secondary to alterations in electrical conductivity of the heart, myocardial contusion or infarction, or heart wall or papillary muscle rupture.
  - As a result of the high risk of fatal arrhythmias in this population, the American Burn Association (ABA) recommends an electrocardiogram (ECG) be performed on all patients who sustain electrical injuries, and those with a documented loss of consciousness or presence of arrhythmia following injury should be admitted for telemetry monitoring.[18]
- Neurologic: Headache, seizure, brief loss of consciousness or coma, peripheral nerve injury (resulting from ischemia), spinal cord paralysis (from demyelination), herniated nucleus pulposus, or decreased attention and concentration.
- Orthopedic: Dislocations or fractures secondary to sustained muscular contraction or from a fall during the electrical injury.
- Other: Visceral perforation or necrosis, cataracts, tympanic membrane rupture, anxiety, depression, or posttraumatic stress disorder.

Lightning. Lightning, considered a form of very high electrical current, causes injury via four mechanisms[19]:

1. Direct strike, in which the person is the grounding site
2. Flash discharge, in which an object deviates the course of the lightning current before striking the person
3. Ground current, in which lightning strikes the ground and a person within the grounding area creates a pathway for the current
4. Shock wave, in which lightning travels outside the person and static electricity vaporizes moisture in the skin

Chemical Burns

Chemical burns can be the result of reduction, oxidation, corrosion, or desecration of body tissue with or without an associated thermal injury.[20] The severity of the burn depends on the type and concentration of the chemical, duration of contact, and mechanism of action. Unlike thermal burns, chemical burns significantly alter systemic tissue pH and metabolism. These changes can cause serious pulmonary complications (e.g., airway obstruction from bronchospasm, edema, or epithelial sloughing) and metabolic complications (e.g., liver necrosis or renal dysfunction from prolonged chemical exposure).

Ultraviolet and Ionizing Radiation Burns

A nonblistering sunburn is a first-degree burn from the overexposure of the skin to UV radiation.[8] More severe burns can also occur due to UV exposure and would appear as described in Table 12-2. Ionizing radiation burns with or without thermal injury occur when electromagnetic or particulate radiation energy is transferred to body tissues, resulting in the formation of chemical free radicals.[21] Ionizing radiation burns usually occur in laboratory or industrial settings, but can also be seen in the medical setting following radiation treatment, most often for cancer. The severity of the ionizing radiation burn depends on the dose, the dose rate, and the tissue sensitivity of exposed cells. Often referred to as acute radiation syndrome, complications of ionizing radiation burns include[21]:

- Gastrointestinal: Cramps, nausea, vomiting, diarrhea, and bowel ischemia
- Hematologic: Pancytopenia (decreased number of red blood cells, white blood cells, and platelets), granulocytopenia (decreased number of granular leukocytes), thrombocytopenia (decreased number of platelets), and hemorrhage
- Vascular: Endothelium destruction

Burn Assessment and Acute Care Management of Burn Injury

Classification of a Burn

The extent and depth of the burn determine its severity and dictate acute care management.

Assessing the Extent of a Burn

Accurate assessment of the extent of a burn is necessary to calculate fluid volume therapy and is a predictor of morbidity.[22] The extent of a burn injury is referred to as total body surface area (TBSA) and can be calculated by using the rule of nines, the Lund and Browder formula, or the palmar method.

Rule of Nines

The rule of nines divides the adult body into sections, seven of which are assigned 9% of TBSA. The anterior and posterior trunks are each assigned 18%, and the genitalia are assigned 1% (Figure 12-5). This formula is quick and easy to use, especially when a rapid initial estimation of TBSA is needed in the field or the emergency room. To use the rule of nines, the burned area is drawn in on the diagram and the percentages are added for a TBSA. Modifications can be made if an entire body section is not burned. For example, if only the posterior left arm is burned, the TBSA is 4.5%. A modified version is available for use in children.

Lund and Browder Formula

The Lund and Browder formula divides the body into 19 sections, each of which is assigned a different percentage of TBSA (Table 12-5). These percentages vary with age from infant to adult to accommodate for relative changes in TBSA with normal growth. The Lund and Browder formula is a more accurate predictor of TBSA than the rule of nines because of the inclusion of a greater number of body divisions along with the adjustments for age and growth.

Estimating the Extent of Irregularly Shaped Burns

To estimate TBSA of irregularly shaped burns, ABA Practice Guidelines recommend preferential use of the Lund and Browder supplemented with the palmar method, in which size of the patient's palm is used to estimate the size of the burn. The palm represents approximately 1% of TBSA.[22,23]

Assessing the Depth of a Burn

The assessment of burn depth provides a clinical basis in the decision of appropriate burn care or surgery and the expected

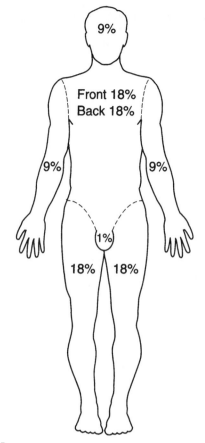

FIGURE 12-5
The rule of nines method of assessing the extent of a burn injury. (From Walsh M, editor: Nurse practitioners: clinical skills and professional issues, Oxford, England, 1999, Butterworth-Heinemann.)

functional outcome and cosmesis.[24] Refer to Figure 12-3 and Table 12-2 to review the depth of tissue destruction in burn injuries. Although clinical observation remains the standard for burn depth estimation, there is often error or underestimation. Experimental technologies for more precise burn depth estimation include cell biopsy, vital dyes, fluorescein fluorometry, laser Doppler flowmetry, thermography, ultrasound, and nuclear magnetic resonance.[13]

A burn is considered to be a dynamic wound in that it can change in appearance, especially during the first few days following injury. Therefore exact classification of depth of injury cannot be made until the burn has fully developed.[9] In addition, later conversion of a burn from a superficial to a deeper injury can occur as a result of inadequate burn management, edema, infection, inadequate fluid resuscitation, impaired perfusion, or excessive pressure from dressings or splints.[1,25]

Acute Care Management of Burn Injury

This section discusses the admission guidelines and resuscitative and reparative phases of burn care.

Admission Guidelines

In addition to the burn's extent and depth, the presence of other associated injuries and premorbid medical conditions

TABLE 12-5 Lund and Browder Method of Assessing the Extent of Burns*

	Birth	1-4 yr	5-9 yr	10-14 yr	15 yr	Adult
Head and Trunk						
Head	19	17	13	11	9	7
Neck	2	2	2	2	2	2
Anterior trunk	13	13	13	13	13	13
Posterior trunk	13	13	13	13	13	13
Right buttock	2.5	2.5	2.5	2.5	2.5	2.5
Left buttock	2.5	2.5	2.5	2.5	2.5	2.5
Genitalia	1	1	1	1	1	1
Upper Extremity						
Right upper arm	4	4	4	4	4	4
Left upper arm	4	4	4	4	4	4
Right forearm	3	3	3	3	3	3
Left forearm	3	3	3	3	3	3
Right hand	2.5	2.5	2.5	2.5	2.5	2.5
Left hand	2.5	2.5	2.5	2.5	2.5	2.5
Lower Extremity						
Right thigh	5.5	6.5	8	8.5	9	9.5
Left thigh	5.5	6.5	8	8.5	9	9.5
Right lower leg	5	5	5.5	6	6.5	7
Left lower leg	5	5	5.5	6	6.5	7
Right foot	3.5	3.5	3.5	3.5	3.5	3.5
Left foot	3.5	3.5	3.5	3.5	3.5	3.5

Adapted from McManus WF, Pruitt BA: Thermal injuries. In Feliciano DV, Moore EE, Mattox KL, editors: Trauma, Stamford, CT, 1996, Appleton & Lange, p 941; Lund CC, Browder NC: The estimation of areas of burns, Surg Gynecol Obstet 79:355, 1944.
*Values represent percentage of total body surface area.

determines what level of care is optimal for the patient. The American Burn Association recommends medical care at a burn center if the patient has any of the following[26]:

- Partial-thickness burns greater than 10% TBSA
- Burns that involve the face, hands, feet, genitalia, perineum, or major joints
- Third-degree burns in any age group
- Electrical burns, including lightning injury
- Chemical burns
- Inhalation injury
- Burn injury in patients who have preexisting medical disorders that could complicate management, prolong recovery, or affect mortality
- Burns and concomitant trauma (such as fractures) in which the burn injury poses the greatest risk of morbidity or mortality. In such cases, if the trauma poses the greater immediate risk, patients may be stabilized initially in a trauma center before being transferred to a burn unit. Physician judgment is necessary in such situations and should be in concert with the regional medical control plan and triage protocols.
- Burns in children who are in hospitals without qualified personnel or equipment for the care of children
- Burn injury in patients who require special social, emotional, or long-term rehabilitative intervention

Resuscitative Phase. The objectives of emergency room management of the patient who has a major burn injury include simultaneous general systemic stabilization and burn care. The prioritization of care and precautions during this initial time period has a great impact on survival and illustrates some key concepts of burn care. General systemic stabilization involves:

- The assessment of inhalation injury and carbon monoxide (CO) poisoning and the maintenance of the airway and ventilation with supplemental oxygen or mechanical ventilation (see Chapter 18)
- Fluid resuscitation
- The use of analgesia (see Chapter 21)
- The treatment of secondary injuries[27]

Inhalation Injury and Carbon Monoxide Poisoning. ABA Practice Guidelines define an inhalation injury as aspiration of superheated gases, steam, hot liquids, or noxious products of incomplete combustion.[23] This inhalation, which may be related to burn injuries, can cause asphyxia, direct cellular injury, or both. The severity of inhalation injury is dependent on the inhalant and exposure time and significantly increases mortality. Inhalation injury is suspected based on a combination of history and physical exam and is confirmed with diagnostic studies such as a bronchoscopy.[28] Injury can be suspected if the patient had a known exposure to noxious inhalants, especially in an enclosed space, or if the patient demonstrates any of the following:

- Altered mental status
- Burns on the face, neck, or upper chest
- Singed eyebrows or nose hair
- Laryngeal or mucosal edema with possible loss of airway patency
- Arterial blood gas levels consistent with hypoxia
- Abnormal breath sounds
- The presence of soot in the mouth or sputum
- Positive blood test results for chemicals[23,29]

The oropharynx and tracheobronchial tree are usually damaged by thermal injury, whereas the lung parenchyma is damaged by the chemical effects of the inhalant. Thermal airway injury is characterized by immediate upper-airway mucosal edema, erythema, hemorrhage, and ulceration.[13] Elective endotracheal intubation is often indicated with this type of injury, as progressive edema can readily lead to airway obstruction.[30] The pathophysiology of inhalation injury generally occurs in three stages: (1) inhalation injury (0 to 36 hours after injury), (2) pulmonary edema (6 to 72 hours after injury), and (3) bronchopneumonia (3 to 10 days after injury). Pulmonary edema occurs from increased lung capillary permeability, increased bronchial blood flow, and impaired lymph function.[31] De-epithelialization and exudate formation occurs throughout the airways, as well as decreased alveolar surfactant.[13] Decreased lung compliance (functional residual capacity and vital capacity) and hypoxia are the primary effects of inhalation injury, each of which is dependent on the location and severity of the injury. Supplemental oxygen, elective intubation, bronchodilators, and fluid resuscitation are initiated to maximize gas exchange and reverse hypoxia.[32-34]

The inhalation of carbon monoxide (CO), which is a colorless, odorless, tasteless, combustible, nonirritating gas produced by the incomplete combustion of organic material, results in asphyxia. CO molecules displace oxygen molecules from hemoglobin to form carboxyhemoglobin and shift the oxyhemoglobin curve to the left, thereby decreasing the release of oxygen. In addition, CO molecules increase pulmonary secretions and decrease the effectiveness of the mucociliary elevator.[35] Elevated carboxyhemoglobin levels can cause headache, disorientation, nausea, visual changes, syncope, coma, or death depending on the concentration and exposure time. CO poisoning is usually reversible with the use of 100% oxygen if the patient has not lost consciousness.[13]

Burn Care in the Resuscitative Phase.
During the first 72 hours after a burn injury, medical stabilization is a priority. The medical team will also initiate burn management, which consists of continued fluid resuscitation, infection control, body temperature maintenance, pain and anxiety management, and initial burn care, which may include escharotomy or fasciotomy.

Fluid Resuscitation. After a burn, fluid shifts from vascular to interstitial and intracellular spaces because of increased capillary pressure, increased capillary and venular permeability, decreased interstitial hydrostatic pressure, chemical inflammatory mediators, and increased interstitial protein retention.[36] This is compounded by evaporative water loss from a disruption of the skin.[37] In burns of more than 20% TBSA, this fluid shift becomes massive and requires immediate fluid repletion.[24] This fluid shift, referred to as *burn shock*, is a life-threatening condition because of hypovolemia and the potential for shock-induced renal failure (see Figure 12-4). Plasma, sodium-rich solutions, and other fluids are infused according to a formula derived from individual TBSA and body weight. The specific formula used varies according to hospital preference.

During and after fluid administration, the patient is monitored closely for adequacy of fluid resuscitation. Heart rate, blood pressure, cardiac output, base deficit, urine output, and bowel sounds provide valuable information about the effectiveness of fluid resuscitation, as do peripheral body temperature, capillary refill, and mental status.[36,38]

Infection Control. Prevention of infection at the burn site(s) is crucial in the resuscitative and reparative phases of burn care. The patient with a major burn is considered immunocompromised because of the loss of skin and the inability to prevent microorganisms from entering the body. Infection control is achieved by the following[24]:

- Observation of the patient for signs and symptoms of sepsis (see the Sepsis section in Chapter 13)
- Minimization of the presence of microorganisms in the patient's internal and external environment
- Use of aseptic techniques in all interactions with the patient
- Use of topical antimicrobial agents or systemic antibiotics, as needed
- Tetanus prophylaxis

✎ CLINICAL TIP

To minimize the risk of infection, the physical therapist must follow burn unit isolation procedures when entering a patient's room or approaching the patient's bedside. The physical therapist should be familiar with the institution's policies regarding the use and disposal of protective barriers, such as gloves, gowns, caps, and masks. Family and visitors should be encouraged to comply with these policies when visiting the patient as well.

Body Temperature Maintenance. The patient with a major burn injury is at risk for hypothermia from skin loss and the inability to thermoregulate. Body heat is lost through conduction to the surrounding atmosphere and to the surface of the bed. Initially, dry dressings may be placed on the patient to minimize heat loss. The patient should be placed in a warm environment to maintain body temperature, which may include warming blankets, heat lamps, and warmed IV fluids. The patient's room and the burn unit may have overhead radiant heat panels and may be humidified in an effort to preserve the patient's body heat.

Pain Management. A patient with a burn injury can experience pain as a result of any of the following:

- Free nerve ending exposure
- Edema
- Exudate accumulation
- Burn debridement and dressing changes
- Mobility
- Secondary injury, such as fracture

Patients may also experience fear from the injury and burn treatment, which can exacerbate pain. Analgesia, given intravenously, is therefore started as soon as possible. Opioids are the mainstays in pain management, supplemented by nonsteroidal antiinflammatory drugs (NSAIDs), mild analgesics, parenteral and inhaled anesthetic agents, and anxiolytics. Initial doses of opioids may exceed the standard weight-based recommendations in order to achieve adequate pain control. No evidence exists for any increased risk of addiction in this population as compared to others who require opioids for pain management.[39] Refer to Chapters 19 and 21 for more information about pharmacologic agents.

Initial Burn Care. To neutralize the burn source, the patient's clothing and jewelry are removed, and the burn is rinsed or lavaged. Once the patient is medically stable, the burn is debrided, cleaned, and dressed with the hospital's or burn unit's topical agent of choice. Topical antimicrobial agents may be used in an attempt to prevent or minimize bacterial growth. There are a variety of antimicrobial agents, each with their own application procedures, advantages, and disadvantages. Ideally, the antimicrobial agent of choice should penetrate eschar, work against a wide variety of microorganisms, have minimal systemic absorption, and not impede healing.[40] The physician determines whether to cover the burn or leave it open, estimates the time frame for burn repair, and determines the need for surgical intervention.

Escharotomy and Fasciotomy. Circumferential burns of the extremities or trunk can create neurovascular and respiratory complications. Inelastic eschar paired with edema can cause increased tissue swelling in all directions with the result of decreased blood flow, nerve compression, impaired chest expansion, and increased compartment pressures. In the extremities, tissue ischemia and loss of limb can ensue if these conditions are not treated with escharotomy or fasciotomy. *Escharotomy* is the surgical incision through eschar to decompress tissue below the burn. *Fasciotomy* is the surgical incision through fascia to decompress tissue within a fascial compartment. Both procedures are typically performed at the bedside. Clinical indications for escharotomy or fasciotomy are decreased arterial blood flow, as determined by loss of Doppler flowmetry signal, or increased compartment pressure measurements ($\geq$30 mm Hg).[40]

Burn Management in the Reparative Phase.
Tissue healing occurs over days to months according to the depth of the burn and is described in the Process of Wound Healing section. For a discussion of variables that can slow the process of healing, see the Factors That Can Delay Wound Healing section. After the burn has closed, a scar forms. A burn scar may be normotrophic, with a normal appearance when dermal collagen fibers are arranged in an organized parallel formation, or hypertrophic, with an abnormal raised appearance as a result of the disorganized alignment of dermal collagen fibers.[41] Another form of abnormal appearance or pathologic scar is a keloid scar, which tends to extend beyond the boundaries of the primary wound (whereas a hypertrophic scar will stay within the boundaries of the wound).[42] A keloid scar is more prevalent in people of color and presents as a prominent, raised scar as a result of excessive collagen accummulation.[43]

Burn management can be divided into two major categories: (1) surgical management and (2) nonsurgical management including routine burn cleaning and debridement. It is beyond the scope of this book to discuss in great detail the indications, advantages, and disadvantages of surgical interventions to facilitate burn closure. A brief discussion and description of procedures is presented next.

Surgical Procedures. The cornerstone of present surgical management is early excision and grafting in burns that are unlikely to heal in a reasonable time frame through conservative treatment.[44] Excision is the surgical removal of eschar and exposure of viable tissue to minimize infection and promote burn closure. Grafting is the implantation or transplantation of skin onto a prepared wound bed.[45] Early burn closure minimizes scarring, infection, the incidence of multisystem organ failure, and morbidity. Table 12-6 describes the various types of excision and grafting. Table 12-7 describes the different artificial and biological skin substitutes available for use when there is a lack of viable autograft sites. Many of these are used in the management of other wound etiologies as well.

Surgical excision and grafting are completed at any site if patient survival will improve. If morbidity is greater than 50%, the priority is for the excision and grafting of large flat areas to

TABLE 12-6 Types of Excision and Grafting

Procedure	Description
Tangential excision	Removal of eschar in successive layers down to the dermis
Full-thickness excision	Removal of eschar as a single layer down to the subcutaneous tissue
Split-thickness skin graft (STSG)	Graft consisting of epidermis and a portion of dermis
Full-thickness skin graft (FTSG)	Graft consisting of epidermis and the entire dermis
Mesh graft	Graft placed through a mesher to expand the size approximately 3-4 times prior to placement on the recipient site
Sheet graft	Graft placed on the recipient site as a single piece without meshing
Autograft	Surgical harvesting of a patient's own skin from another part of the body (donor site) and placing it permanently on the burn (recipient site)
Cultured epidermal autograft (CEA)	Autograft of unburned epidermal cells cultured in the laboratory, which provides epidermal replacement only
Composite skin graft	Autograft of unburned epidermal and dermal cells cultured in the laboratory with the intention of immediate replacement of both the dermis and epidermis
Allogenic graft/allograft	Temporary graft from donated human cadaver skin
Heterograft/xenograft	Temporary graft from another animal species, typically of porcine skin
Amnion graft	Temporary graft from placental membrane

Data from Miller SF, Staley MJ, Richard RL: Surgical management of the burn patient. In Richard RL, Staley MJ, editors: Burn care and rehabilitation: principles and practice, Philadelphia, 1994, FA Davis; Sheridan RL, Tompkins RG: Alternative wound coverings. In Herndon DN, editor: Total burn care, ed 3, Philadelphia, 2007, Saunders, p 239; Muller M, Gahankari D, Herndon DN: Operative wound management. In Herndon DN, editor: Total burn care, ed 3, Philadelphia, 2007, Saunders, p 117.

TABLE 12-7 Skin Substitutes for the Treatment of Burns and Wounds

Product	Description	Use
Biobrane (UDL Laboratories, Rockford, IL)	Temporary skin substitute. Two-layered graft composed of nylon mesh impregnated with porcine collagen and silicone; the outer silicone layer is permeable to gases but not to fluid or bacteria. Spontaneously separates from a healed wound in 7-14 days.	Clean, freshly debrided partial-thickness burns Donor sites Protect a meshed autograft Limited success on full-thickness burns because of infection with residual necrotic tissue
Dermagraft (Advanced BioHealing, San Diego, CA)	Dermal substitute composed of human fibroblasts, extracellular matrix, and a bioreabsorbable scaffold. Derived from newborn foreskin tissue. Remains in wound, assisting in restoration of the dermal bed in preparation for re-epithelialization.	Full-thickness diabetic foot ulcers without underlying structure exposure
TransCyte (Advanced BioHealing, San Diego, CA)	Temporary skin substitute composed of a polymer membrane and newborn human fibroblast cells cultured on a porcine collagen-coated nylon mesh. The fibroblasts secrete human dermal collagen, matrix proteins, and growth factors.	Surgically excised full-thickness and deep partial-thickness thermal burns before autograft placement Partial-thickness burns that require debridement but are expected to heal without formal grafting
AlloDerm (LifeCell, Branchburg, NJ)	Composed of chemically treated cadaver dermis with the epidermal antigenic cellular components removed so that it is immunologically inert. Provides dermal and basement layer replacement.	Repair or replacement of damaged integument, no specific limitations to wound type Can be applied to a debrided burn with an ultrathin split-thickness autograft immediately applied over it
Integra (Integra Life Sciences, Plainsboro, NJ)	Two-layered material composed of a disposable outer silicone film that acts as a barrier to evaporative water loss and bacteria, and an inner layer of bovine collagen and chondroitin 6-sulfate that becomes incorporated into the burn to form a neodermis. When the neodermis becomes vascularized, the silicone covering is removed and replaced with thin autografts.	Full-thickness burns or deep partial-thickness burns Also used in the repair of scar contractures
GRAFTJACKET (LifeCell, Branchburg, NJ)	Acellular dermal matrix from donated human cadaver skin.	Superficial and deep integumentary defects
Apligraf (Graftskin) (Organogenesis, Canton, MA)	Bilayered skin substitute containing bovine collagen and human fibroblasts (which produce additional growth factors and proteins for dermal regrowth) and keratinocytes (which reproduce to replace the epithelial surface). Human cellular components are derived from neonatal foreskin.	Chronic venous leg ulcers and diabetic foot ulcers
OASIS Wound Matrix (Cook Biotech, West Lafayette, IN)	Bioresorbable matrix derived from porcine small intestinal submucosa.	Partial- and full-thickness wounds of most etiologies (including donor sites and grafts) Not indicated for use in third-degree burns

Data from Muller M, Gahankari D, Herndon DN: Operative wound management. In Herndon DN, editor: Total burn care, ed 3, 2007, p 117; Greenhalgh DB: Wound healing. In Herndon DN, editor: Total burn care, ed 3, Philadelphia, 2007, Saunders, p 578; udllabs.com; transcyte.com/index.html; dermagraft.com; lifecell.com/health-care-professionals; ilstraining.com/imwd/imwd/imwd_it_02.html; apligraf.com; oasiswoundmatrix.com; kci1.com/KCI1/tissue-regeneration.

rapidly reduce the burn wound area.[40] Grafting is otherwise performed to maximize functional outcome and cosmesis, with the hands, arms, face, feet, and joint surfaces grafted before other areas of the body.[46] Permanent grafting is ideal; however, grafting may be temporary in order to provide short-term closure to assist in pain control, drainage management, and protection of the underlying wound tissue. Temporary grafting may be indicated in small wounds expected to heal secondarily or in large wounds for which an autograft would not last, or if permanent coverage is not available.[47]

Grafts, which typically adhere in 2 to 7 days, may not adhere or "take" in the presence of any of the following[45,46]:
- Incomplete eschar excision
- Movement or shear of the graft on the recipient site
- Infection, inadequate blood flow, or hematoma formation at the recipient site
- Poor nutritional status

Physical Therapy Considerations
- To promote grafting success, restrictions on weight bearing and movement of a specific joint or entire limb may be

present postoperatively. The therapist should become familiar with the surgeon's procedures and protocols and alter positioning, range of motion (ROM), therapeutic exercise, and functional mobility accordingly.

- The therapist should check with the physician to determine whether the graft crosses a joint or how closely the graft borders the joint.
- If possible, observe the graft during dressing changes to get a visual understanding of its exact location.
- The donor site is often more painful than the burn itself.
- Donor sites are oriented longitudinally and are commonly located on the thigh, buttocks, low back, or outer arm and may be reharvested in approximately 2 weeks.

Nonsurgical Procedures. Burn cleaning and debridement may be performed multiple times a day to minimize infection and promote tissue healing.[44] These procedures, as described in the Wound Cleaning and Debridement section, may be performed by a physician, nurse, or physical therapist depending on the hospital's or burn unit's protocol. Dressings for the burn are dependent on wound characteristics (i.e., depth of destruction, drainage, infection, presence of nonviable tissue, edema management), patient comfort, clinician preference, and product availability. The priority is maintaining a moist healing environment while maximizing granulation and epithelialization and minimizing tissue trauma and infection. Examples of dressing types are found later in the chapter, in Table 12-12.

> ✎ **CLINICAL TIP**
>
> The use of immersion hydrotherapy for wound cleaning carries a risk of hypothermia in patients with burn injury secondary to lack of thermoregulation from loss of dermal tissue and associated vascular components.

Physical Therapy Examination in Burn Care

Physical therapy intervention for the patient with a burn injury is often initiated within 48 hours of hospital admission.

History

In addition to the general chart review (see Chapter 2), the following information is especially relevant in the evaluation, treatment planning, and understanding of the physiological status of a patient with a burn.

- How, when, where, and why did the burn occur?
- Did the patient get thrown (as in an explosion) or fall during the burn incident?
- Is there an inhalation injury or CO poisoning?
- What are the secondary injuries?
- What are the extent, depth, and location of the burn?
- Does the patient have a condition(s) that might impair tissue healing?
- Was the burn self-inflicted? If so, is there a history of self-injury or attempted suicide?
- Were friends or family members also injured?

Inspection and Palpation

To assist with treatment planning, pertinent data that can be gathered from the direct observation of a patient or palpation include the following:

- Level of consciousness
- Presence of agitation, pain, and stress
- Location of the burn or graft, including the proximity of the burn to a joint
- Presence and location of dressings, splints, or pressure garments
- Presence of lines, tubes, or other equipment
- Presence and location of edema
- Posture
- Position of head, trunk, and extremities
- Heart rate and blood pressure, respiratory rate and pattern, and oxygen saturation

---

> ✎ **CLINICAL TIP**
>
> When examining a patient with burn injuries:
> Avoid popping any blisters on the skin during palpation or with manual contacts.
> Do not place a blood pressure cuff over a burn or graft site or an area of edema.
> Be cautious with gait belt placement where trunk burns are present. Nylon belts are preferable for easier cleaning and infection management.

Pain Assessment

Adequate pain control increases patient participation and activity tolerance; therefore pain assessment occurs daily. For the conscious patient, the physical therapist should note the presence, quality, and grade of (1) resting pain; (2) pain with passive, active-assisted, or active ROM; (3) pain at the burn and the donor sites; and (4) pain before, during, and after physical therapy intervention.

The physical therapist should become familiar with the patient's pain medication schedule and arrange for physical therapy treatment when pain medication is most effective and when the patient is as comfortable as possible. Restlessness and vital sign monitoring (i.e., heart rate, blood pressure, and respiratory rate increases) may be the best indicators of pain in sedated or unconscious patients who cannot verbally report pain. Refer to Chapter 21—for information on various pain assessment scales. The Visual Analog Scale and the Faces Pain Rating Scale are most commonly used by burn centers for pain assessment.[39]

Range of Motion

ROM of the involved joints typically requires goniometric measurements. ROM can be difficult to perform and exact goniometric values difficult to obtain when the patient has bulky dressings in place; therefore some estimation of ROM may be necessary. If possible, the therapist should coordinate with the nursing or physical therapy wound care team to evaluate ROM when the dressings are temporarily off or down. This will also allow the physical therapist to visualize the extremity during ROM exercise and to observe for banding, or areas of tissue that appear white when stretched, which is an initial sign of scar contracture. This observation may not be possible if dressings are in place. The uninvolved joints or extremities can be grossly addressed actively or passively, depending on the patient's level of alertness or participation.

The physical therapist should pay attention to the position of adjacent joints when measuring ROM to account for any length-tension deficits of healing tissues. The physical therapist should also be aware of the presence of tendon damage before ROM assessment; ROM should not be performed on joints with exposed tendons.

> ### ✎ CLINICAL TIP
>
> The physical therapist should appreciate the fact that a major burn injury is usually characterized by areas of different depths. The therapist must also be aware of the various qualities of combination burns when performing ROM or functional activities.

Strength

Strength on an uninvolved extremity is usually assessed grossly by function. More formal strength testing, such as resisted isometrics or manual muscle testing, is often indicated on the involved side and may be appropriate on the uninvolved side if there is severe edema, extended period of immobility following injury, or secondary injuries.[48]

Functional Mobility

Functional mobility may be limited depending on state of illness, medication, need for warm or sterile environment, and pain. The physical therapist should evaluate functional mobility as much as possible, according to medical stability and precautions.

> ### ✎ CLINICAL TIP
>
> The skin at grafted areas, as well as at donor site areas, is more fragile than normal skin. These areas should be wrapped in Ace bandages figure-of-eight style to provide support against venous pooling when the patient is being mobilized out of bed. Without this extra support, the skin is more prone to shearing at graft sites and subcutaneous bleeding.

Physical Therapy Intervention

Goals

The primary goal of physical therapy intervention for patients with burn injuries is to maximize function through ROM exercise, stretching, positioning, strengthening, and functional activity. Significant improvements in functional outcomes, as measured by the cognitive and motor components of the functional independence measure (FIM), have been demonstrated following inpatient rehabilitation for patient's status post burn injury.[49] General considerations for physical therapy intervention by impairment are listed in Table 12-8.

Basic Concepts for the Treatment of Patients with Burn Injury

- The patient with a burn can have multisystem organ involvement and be in a hypermetabolic state; thus the physical therapist needs to be aware of cardiac, respiratory, and neurologic status, as well as musculoskeletal and integumentary issues.
- Fluid resuscitation and pain medications can affect blood pressure, heart rate, and respiratory pattern and rate, as well as level of alertness. Monitoring these variables will help the therapist gauge pain level and determine how aggressively to intervene during the therapy session.
- The patient with a burn requires more frequent reevaluations than other patient populations, because the patient's status and therapy intervention can change dramatically as swelling decreases, wound debridement and closure occur, hemodynamic and respiratory stability are achieved, and mental status improves. The goals and plan of care need to be updated throughout the patient's admission because activity may be temporarily restricted after surgical grafting.
- A portion(s) of the plan of care is often held for 2 to 7 days after skin grafting to prevent shearing forces on the new graft. Shearing can disrupt the circulation to the graft and cause it to fail. Grafts over joints or areas with bony prominences, as well as grafts on the posterior surfaces of the body, are at greater risk for shear injury.
- Time frames for physical therapy goals vary widely and are based heavily on TBSA, the location of the burn, age, and preexisting functional status.
- The joints at risk for contracture formation need to be properly positioned (Table 12-9). The positioning needs to be consistently carried out by all caregivers and documented in the patient care plan. Proper positioning will decrease edema and prevent contracture formation to facilitate the best recovery.
- The therapist should be creative in treating the patient with a burn. Traditional exercise works well; however, incorporating recreational activities and other modalities into the plan of care can often increase functional gains and compliance with less pain.
- The plan of care must be comprehensive and address all areas with burns. For example, burns of the face, neck, and trunk require intervention specifically directed to these areas.
- The therapist should attend bedside rounds with the burn team to be involved in multidisciplinary planning and to inform the team of therapy progression.

TABLE 12-8 Physical Therapy Considerations for Burn Injury

Variable	Considerations
Decreased ROM and altered limb position	Most patients have full ROM on admission but may readily begin to exhibit decreased ROM due to edema (localized or systemic), pain, and immobility. Devices that help to properly position the patient include splints, abduction wedges, arm boards attached to the bed, pillows, and blanket rolls. Incorporate the use of a modality (i.e., pulley) into stretching activities.
Decreased strength	Active exercise is preferred unless sedation or the patient's level of consciousness or cognition prevents it. Active exercise (i.e., proprioceptive neuromuscular facilitation) provides muscle conditioning, increased blood flow, edema reduction, and contraction prevention and helps reduce hypertrophic scar formation.
Decreased endurance and functional mobility	Prolonged bed rest (see Chapter 1) may be necessary for weeks or months secondary to medical status or to accommodate grafting, especially of the lower extremity. The use of a tilt table for progressive mobilization from bed rest may be necessary if orthostatic hypotension or decreased lower-extremity ROM exists. Assistive devices may need adaptations (i.e., platform walker) to accommodate for ROM and strength deficits or weight-bearing restrictions. Consider the use of active exercise (i.e., restorator) that addresses cardiovascular conditioning while increasing ROM and strength.
Risk for scar development	Healing of deeper burns and skin grafts is accompanied by scarring. Hypertrophic scarring can be decreased through the use of pressure garments, silicone gel sheets, ROM, and scar massage.
Patient/family knowledge deficit related to burns and physical therapy	Patient/family education emphasizes information about the role of physical therapy, exercise, positioning, pain and edema control, and skin care. Education before discharge is of the utmost importance to improve compliance, confidence, and independence.

Data from Trees DW, Ketelsen CA, Hobbs JA: Use of a modified tilt table for preambulation strength training as an adjunct to burn rehabilitation: a case series, J Burn Care Rehabil 24(2):97-103, 2003; Ward RS: Burns. In Cameron MH, Monroe LG, editors: Physical rehabilitation: evidence-based examination, evaluation, and intervention, St Louis, 2007, Saunders.
    ROM, Range of motion.

TABLE 12-9 Preferred Positions for Patients with Burn Injury

Area of Body	Position
Neck	Extension, no rotation
Shoulder	Abduction (90 degrees) External rotation Horizontal flexion (10 degrees)
Elbow and forearm	Extension with supination
Wrist	Neutral or slight extension
Hand	Functional position (dorsal burn) Finger and thumb extension (palmar burn)
Trunk	Straight postural alignment
Hip	Neutral extension/flexion Neutral rotation Slight abduction
Knee	Extension
Ankle	Neutral or slight dorsiflexion No inversion Neutral toe extension/flexion

Adapted from Ward RS: Splinting, orthotics, and prosthetics in the management of burns. In Lusardi MM, Nielson CC, editors: Orthotics and prosthetics in rehabilitation, Boston, 2000, Butterworth-Heinemann, p 315.

WOUNDS

Pathophysiology of Wounds

The different types of wounds, their etiologies, and the factors that contribute to or delay wound healing are discussed in the following sections.

Types of Wounds

Traumatic Wounds

A traumatic wound is an injury caused by an external force, such as a laceration from broken glass, a cut from a knife, or penetration from a bullet.

Surgical Wounds

A surgical wound is the residual skin defect after a surgical incision. For individuals who do not have problems healing, these wounds are sutured or stapled, and they heal without special intervention. As the benefits of moist wound healing become more widely accepted, gels and ointments are now more frequently applied to surgical wounds. When complications such as infection, arterial insufficiency, diabetes, or venous insufficiency are present, surgical wound healing can be delayed and require additional care.

Arterial Insufficiency Wounds

A wound resulting from arterial insufficiency occurs secondary to ischemia of the tissue, frequently caused by atherosclerosis, which can cause irreversible damage. Arterial insufficiency wounds, described in Table 12-10, occur most commonly in the distal and anterolateral lower leg because of a lack of collateral circulation to this area. Clinically, arterial ulcers frequently occur in the pretibial areas and the dorsum of the toes and feet, but they may be present proximally if the ulcers were caused by trauma on an already ischemic limb.[50-52] They show minimal signs of healing and are often gangrenous.

Venous Insufficiency Wounds

A wound resulting from venous insufficiency is caused by the improper functioning of the venous system, which impairs nutrition and oxygen delivery to the tissues. This lack of nutrition causes tissue damage, and ultimately tissue death, resulting in ulceration. The exact mechanism by which this occurs has not been established, although some theories do exist. The *fibrin cuff theory* states that venous hypertension is transmitted to the superficial veins in the subcutaneous tissue and overlying skin, which causes widening of the capillary pores.[53,54] Clinically, this would result in the first sign of venous disease, which is the presence of a dilated long saphenous vein on the medial aspect of the calf. This dilation allows the escape of large macromolecules, including fibrinogen, into the interstitial space. This results in the development of edema because of the pooling of fluid in the dermis. In long-standing venous disease, fibrin accumulates in the dermis, creating a fibrin cuff that presents as hard, nonpitting edema, and the surface skin is rigid and fixed. This fibrin cuff forms a mechanical barrier to the transfer of oxygen and other nutrients, which progressively leads to cellular dysfunction, cell death, and skin ulceration.[53,54]

Another hypothesis is called the *white blood cell–trapping hypothesis*. This theory states that transient elevations in venous pressures decrease capillary blood flow, resulting in trapping of white blood cells at the capillary level, which in turn plugs capillary loops, resulting in areas of localized ischemia.[54] These white blood cells may also become activated at this level, causing the release of various proteolytic enzymes, superoxide free radicals, and chemotactic substances, which can lead to direct tissue damage, death, and ulceration.[54,55] Venous stasis ulcers, described in Table 12-10, are frequently present on the medial malleolus, where the long saphenous vein is most superficial and has its greatest curvature. Venous ulcers may be present on the foot or above the midcalf but are more likely to

---

TABLE 12-10 Clinical Indicators of Common Lower Extremity Wounds

Wound Etiology	Clinical Indicators
Arterial insufficiency	Intermittent claudication Extreme pain, decreased with rest and increased with exercise and elevation Decreased or absent pedal pulses Decreased temperature of the distal limb Distinct, well-defined wound edges Deep wound bed with pale granulation (if any) and minimal drainage Cyanosis, anhydrous skin
Venous insufficiency	Localized limb pain, decreased with elevation and increased with dependency Pain with deep pressure or palpation Pedal pulses present Increased temperature around the wound Indistinct, irregular edges Lower extremity edema Shallow, fibrous covered wound bed, substantial drainage Hemosiderin staining and lipodermatosclerotic changes
Diabetic ulcer (neuropathic)	Painless ulcer; however, general lower-limb pain is present Absent pedal pulses if vascular disease is present, otherwise may be normal May be decreased temperature, or hyperperfused because of autonomic neuropathy component or in areas of repetitive trauma Deep wound bed frequently located at pressure points (e.g., metatarsal heads) often surrounded by areas of callus Shiny skin with trophic changes of skin, hair, and nails due to autonomic neuropathy
Pressure wound	Pain generally present if sensation intact Present over areas of pressure, most commonly bony prominences Vary significantly in depth and appearance Periwound may be intact/normal in appearance or characterized by nonblanchable erythema or induration Pulses intact unless vascular compromise is also present

Data from Myers BA: Wound management: principles and practice, ed 3. Upper Saddle River, NJ, 2012, Pearson, p 4; Jordan BS, Harrington DT: Management of the burn wound, Nurs Clin North Am 32(2):251-271, 1997; McCulloch JM: Evaluation of patients with open wounds. In Kloth LC, Miller KH, editors: Wound healing: alternatives in management, Philadelphia, 1995, FA Davis, p 118; Sibbald RG: An approach to leg and foot ulcers: a brief overview, Ostomy Wound Manage 44(9):28-32, 34-35, 1998; Laing P: Diabetic foot ulcers, Am J Surg 167(1A):31, 1994; Levin ML, O'Neal LW, Bowker JH, editors: The diabetic foot, ed 5, St Louis, 1993, Mosby; Sussman C, Bates-Jensen B: Wound care: a collaborative practice manual for health professionals, ed 3, Baltimore, 2007, Lippincott Williams & Wilkins, p 87; Mahoney E: Diabetic foot ulcerations. In McCulloch, JM, Kloth, LC, editors: Wound healing: evidence-based management, ed 4, Philadelphia, 2010, FA Davis, p 213.

have another primary etiology, such as trauma or infection. The leakage of red blood cells over time results in the deposit of hemosiderin and stimulated melanin, causing the characteristic hyperpigmentation around the medial ankle. Lipodermatosclerosis is the result of inflammation of the subcutaneous adipose tissue, which becomes sclerotic over time. The skin appears thickened, hard, and contracted with an inverted champagne-bottle appearance. Other characteristics may include a thin skin surface with a loss of hair follicles and sweat glands.[53]

Neuropathic or Neurotrophic Ulcers

A neuropathic or neurotrophic ulcer (see Table 12-10) is a secondary complication that occurs from a triad of disorders, including peripheral vascular disease, peripheral neuropathy, and infection.[56] Although neuropathic ulcers can occur in individuals with spina bifida, neurologic diseases and injury, muscular degenerative disease, alcoholism, and tertiary syphilis because of similar risk factors, they are most commonly associated with diabetes.[52] The development of ulcers and foot injuries is the leading cause of lower-extremity amputation in people with diabetes.[57] In addition, there is an increased incidence of atherosclerosis, which appears earlier and progresses more rapidly than in patients without diabetes. However, many people with diabetes who develop foot ulcers have palpable pulses and adequate peripheral blood flow.[58]

Individuals with diabetes may also have changes in the mechanical properties of the skin. Insulin is essential for fibroblastic and collagen synthesis. A lack of insulin in type 1 diabetes can lead to diminished collagen synthesis, which can cause stiffness and decreased tensile strength of tissue, both of which increase the susceptibility of wound development and decrease healing potential.[59]

The peripheral and central nervous systems can be adversely affected in diabetes. Peripheral neuropathy is common, and sensation and strength can be impaired. Diminished light touch, proprioception, and temperature and pain perception decrease the ability of the patient with diabetes to identify areas that are being subjected to trauma, shearing forces, excessive pressure, and warm temperatures, all of which can cause ulcers.[58-62]

Loss of protective sensation can be examined by several methods including vibration testing with a 128-Hz tuning fork, vibration perception threshold testing, and pressure assessment with Semmes-Weinstein monofilaments.[63]

Structural deformities and contractures can occur as the result of the peripheral motor neuropathies that may be present secondary to diabetes. An equinus contracture may develop at the ankle as stronger plantarflexors overcome the weaker dorsiflexors. Weakness of the small intrinsic muscles of the foot can result in clawing of the toes. These and other structural deformities, such as "hammer toes" and excessive pronation or supination, can lead to altered weight distribution, creating areas of increased pressure and leading to ischemia and subsequent ulceration.[60-62] These abnormal mechanical and intermittent forces can also stimulate callus formation.[58] Excessive plantar callus formation in itself can increase pressure to the affected area.[58] The minor repetitive pressure that occurs every time the patient bears weight on the callus causes an increase in ischemia to the underlying tissue with eventual tissue failure and ulcer formation.[62]

A neuropathy of the autonomic nervous system is present in the majority of individuals with diabetes and neuropathic ulcers. The autonomic nervous system regulates skin perspiration and blood flow to the microvascular system. Arteriovenous shunting and altered regulation of moisture result in trophic changes of the skin and toenails, such as dry, cracked, calloused skin and frequent toenail infections. Lack of sweat production also contributes to the development of a callus. Altered cross-linkage between collagen and keratin results in predisposal to hyperkeratosis and callus formation. Beneath the callus, a cavity often forms as a response to the increased pressure and shear forces and fills with serous fluid, causing a seroma. If the deep skin fissure comes in contact with an underlying seroma, it can become colonized with bacteria and result in ulcer formation.[58]

The immune system is also affected by elevated glucose levels and their resultant problems. Edematous tissues and decreased vascularity, which contribute to lack of blood flow, decrease the body's ability to fight infection because of its inability to deliver oxygen, nutrients, and antibiotics to the area.[64-70]

> ### ✎ CLINICAL TIP
> In patients with diabetes, evaluation of their footwear, if available, is essential to help determine appropriateness of use, wear pattern, and fit, all of which can contribute to ulcer formation, particularly in the presence of foot deformities.

Pressure Wounds

A pressure ulcer, sometimes referred to as a decubitus ulcer, is caused by ischemia that develops as a result of sustained pressure on tissues. The pressure usually originates from prolonged weight bearing on a bony prominence, causing internal ischemia at the point of contact. This initial point of pressure is where tissue death first occurs. The tissue continues to necrotize externally until a wound is created at the skin surface. By this time, there is significant internal tissue damage. Tissue ulceration is caused by the effect of mechanical forces acting on localized areas of skin and subcutaneous tissue, whether the forces are of low intensity over long periods or are higher forces applied intermittently.[71,72] The relationships between the amount of force applied, the duration of force, and the direction of the force contribute to the occurrence and severity of a pressure ulcer. Not only can direct pressure create tissue ischemia, but friction and shearing forces, along with moisture, contribute as well.[71,73-76] Refer to the Wound Staging and Classification section for the pressure ulcer grading system (Table 12-11).

All bed- or chair-bound patients, patients with an impaired ability to reposition themselves or weight shift, and patients with altered cognition who are unable to report areas of pressure to their caregivers are at risk of developing pressure ulcers. Common pressure ulcer sites for prolonged supine positioning

TABLE 12-11 Pressure Ulcer Staging

Stage	Definition
Suspected deep tissue injury	Localized area of discoloration (purple or maroon) under intact skin or blood-filled blister due to damage of underlying soft tissue from pressure and/or shear.
Stage I	Usually over a bony prominence, presents as intact, reddened skin that does not blanch. Skin with darker pigmentation may present as a differing color from surrounding areas.
Stage II	A shallow open ulcer with a red pink wound bed, denoting partial-thickness loss of dermis, without slough. Can present as an intact or open/ruptured serum-filled blister.
Stage III	Subcutaneous fat may be visible, denoting full-thickness loss; however, muscle, tendon, or bone is not exposed. May include tunneling and undermining. Slough may be present but does not obscure the depth of tissue loss.
Stage IV	Muscle, tendon, or bone is exposed with this full-thickness loss. Often includes tunneling and undermining as well as slough or eschar on some parts of the wound bed. Slough or eschar cannot obscure the depth of tissue loss in order to be staged.
Unstageable	Slough and/or eschar is covering full-thickness loss in the wound bed. True depth cannot be determined until eschar has been debrided and wound base is exposed.

Adapted from National Pressure Ulcer Advisory Panel and European Pressure Ulcer Advisory Panel: Prevention and treatment of pressure ulcers: clinical practice guideline, Washington, DC, 2009, National Pressure Ulcer Advisory Panel, pp 19-20. In Baronski S, Ayello EA, editors: Wound care essentials: practice principles, ed 3, Philadelphia, 2012, Wolters Kluwer Health/Lippincott Williams & Wilkins, pp 325-326.

include the back of the head, scapular spines, spinous processes, elbows, sacrum, and heels. While side-lying, a patient may experience increased pressure on the ear, acromion process, rib, iliac crest, greater trochanter, medial and lateral condyles, and malleoli.[73,77] In sitting, sites of pressure include spinous processes, greater trochanter, ischial tuberosity, sacrum/coccyx, and heels. The prone position, such as after an extended period in the operating room, may lead to pressure wounds on the chin, anterior iliac crest, patella, and tibial crests.[1] A person's body weight also plays a role in pressure ulcer development. A person who is too thin has more prominent bony prominences, whereas a person who is overweight has increased pressure on weight-bearing surfaces.[74-77]

Process of Wound Healing

Wounds limited to epidermal and dermal damage (superficial and partial-thickness wounds) close through re-epithelialization. Within 24 to 48 hours after an injury, new epithelial cells begin to proliferate and migrate across the surface of the wound. Full-thickness wounds undergo a rather complex and lengthy

sequence of (1) an inflammatory response, (2) a proliferation phase, and (3) a remodeling phase.[72-76]

In the inflammatory phase, platelets aggregate and form clots to minimize blood and fluid loss at the site of the wound. Neutrophils, followed by macrophages and lymphocytes, migrate to the area, and phagocytosis begins. These cells also secrete the growth factors and cellular mediators that are needed for wound repair and stimulation of the proliferation phase. Angiogenesis is part of the proliferation phase in which capillary buds begin growing into the wound bed. Concurrently, fibrocytes and other undifferentiated cells multiply and migrate to the area. These cells network to transform into fibroblasts, which begin to secrete strands of collagen, forming immature pink/red scar tissue referred to as granulation. Granulation will continue to fill the depth of the wound while wound contracture occurs to pull the edges closer together. Wound closure is completed when re-epithelialization naturally occurs over the granulation or a skin graft is placed for more immediate coverage. A closed wound is one in which the integumentum has been replaced. Wound healing continues into the remodeling phase, in which the scar tissue matures. New scar tissue is characterized by its pink color, as it is composed of white collagen fibers and a large number of capillaries. The amount of time the entire healing process takes depends on the size and type of wound.[64-70]

Factors That Can Delay Wound Healing

In addition to the problems indigenous to the wound, many other factors can delay wound healing. Age, lifestyle, nutrition, cognitive and self-care ability, vascular status, medical complications, and medications can all affect wound healing. These factors may also be risk factors for the development of new wounds and should therefore be included in the physical therapy assessment and considered when determining goals, interventions, and time frames.

Age

Skin, just like other tissues and organs, changes with age. Decreased cellular activity during the aging process leads to decreased collagen production, which results in less collagen organization in older individuals. Reduced collagen organization results in decreased tensile strength of the skin that could result in greater damage after trauma in the older individual. Other examples of skin changes with age include delayed wound contraction, decreased epithelialization, and delayed cellular migration and proliferation.[78] Comorbidities that delay wound healing, such as diabetes, peripheral neuropathies, and related vascular problems, occur with greater frequency in older individuals.

Lifestyle

A patient's lifestyle can have a great impact on the prognosis for healing, decision making regarding wound management, and preventive care. For example, occupations and hobbies that require prolonged standing may predispose some individuals to varicosities and other venous problems. Patients exposed to traumatic situations, such as construction workers, are also more likely to reinjure healing wounds. Behaviors such as cigarette smoking can impede wound healing significantly because of the vasoconstriction that nicotine creates.

Nutrition

Good nutrition is necessary for the growth and maintenance of all body tissues. Macronutrients (such as carbohydrates, fats, and proteins) and micronutrients (such as vitamins) are necessary for cell metabolism, division, and growth. Therefore nutrition is closely linked with all phases of healing.[79] Generally, poor nutrition decreases the body's ability to heal. In addition, patients with burns, wounds, or infection who are adequately nourished at the time of their injury or the development of their wound may also develop protein-calorie malnutrition.

There are major metabolic abnormalities associated with injury that can deplete nutritional stores, including increased output of catabolic hormones, decreased output of anabolic hormones, a marked increase in metabolic rate, a sustained increase in body temperature, a marked increase in glucose demands, rapid skeletal muscle breakdown with amino acids used as an energy source, lack of ketosis, and unresponsiveness to catabolism to nutrient intake.[80] Protein-calorie malnutrition can delay wound healing and cause serious health consequences in patients with wounds, especially if infection exists. Poor nutritional status, whether due to decreased intake or the stress response, can set off a series of metabolic events leading to weight loss, deterioration of lean tissues, increased risk of infection, edema, and breathing difficulty.[80] These events can lead to severe debilitation and even death.

Inadequate diet control in patients with diabetes exacerbates all symptoms of diabetes, including impaired circulation, sensation, altered metabolic processes, and delayed healing. A nutritional assessment by a registered dietitian, nutritional supplements, and careful monitoring of the patient's nutritional status and weight are important components of a comprehensive assessment and treatment program for the patient with a wound.

In addition, therapists should work with other health care professionals to curb the systemic stress response. Removing necrotic tissues, treating infections, and ensuring adequate hydration and blood volumes will help to limit physiologic stressors. Premedication before painful procedures and avoiding extreme temperatures help minimize stress. Exercise serves as an anabolic stimulus for muscle, facilitating a reduction of the catabolic state.[80]

✎ CLINICAL TIP

Measurement of blood glucose levels (<110 mg/dl fasting), serum albumin (3.2 to 4.5 g/dl) and prealbumin (15 to 35 mg/dl) help to determine metabolic and nutritional status of the patient.[76]

Cognition and Self-Care Ability

There is an increased risk of infection and other wound-healing complications if neither the patient nor the caregiver has the cognitive or physical ability to properly care for a wound, including wound cleaning and dressing removal and application. The patient's and caregiver's abilities have a great influence on the choice of dressing(s) and on discharge planning. Certain dressings require more skill than others to maintain. Complex wound care can justify a stay at a rehabilitation hospital or skilled nursing facility or recommendations for home health or outpatient wound care services.

Vascular Status

Any compromised vascular status may contribute to the development of delayed wound healing owing to a lack of oxygenation and nutrition to the tissues.

Medical Status

Generally, compromised health causes a decrease in the body's ability to progress through the healing process. Preexisting infection or a history of cancer, chemotherapy, radiation, acquired immunodeficiency syndrome, or other immunodeficiency disorders can decrease the patient's ability to heal. Congestive heart failure, hypertension, diabetes, and renal dysfunction can also slow wound healing.

Medications

Steroids, antihistamines, NSAIDs, and oral contraceptives may delay wound healing, as can chemotherapy and radiation. These medications can decrease the tensile strength of connective tissue, reduce blood supply, inhibit collagen synthesis, and increase the susceptibility to infection.[81] Anticoagulants thin the blood and decrease its ability to clot; therefore the health care provider needs to diligently monitor bleeding during dressing removal and consider debridement methods that will not cause bleeding. Antibiotics can create hypersensitivity skin reactions as well as cause gastrointestinal disturbances including diarrhea, which is a contributing factor to skin ulceration.[76]

Chronic Wounds

In healthy patients without comorbidities, an acute wound should close within 3 to 6 weeks, with remodeling occurring over the next year. If a wound remains in one of the stages of healing without progression, it becomes a chronic wound.[82] Chronic wounds are defined as wounds that have "failed to proceed through an orderly and timely process to produce anatomic and functional integrity, or proceeded through the repair process without establishing a sustained anatomic and functional result."[83] The acute care therapist should be inclined to search for underlying causes of delayed wound healing, especially when treating a wound that has not healed in more than 6 weeks.

Wound Assessment and Acute Care Management of Wounds

The evaluation of a patient with a wound includes a general history (identification of factors that can delay healing), a physical examination (of sensation, pain, ROM, strength, and functional mobility), and a specific examination of the wound itself.

History

In addition to the general chart and medical history review (see Chapter 2), the following information is especially relevant for determining wound etiology and risk factors, an intervention plan, and potential outcomes.

Wound History

- How and when did the wound occur?
- What diagnostic tests have been performed?
- What laboratory studies have been ordered?
- What interventions have been administered to the wound thus far? What were the results?
- Is there a previous history of wounds? If so, what were the etiology, intervention, and time frame of healing?

Risk Factors

- How old is the patient?
- Is the patient cognitively intact?
- Where and for how long is the patient weight bearing on areas involving the wound site?
- What is the patient's occupation or hobby? How many hours does the patient spend on his or her feet per day? In what positions and postures is the patient throughout the day?
- Does the patient smoke?
- Is the patient generally well nourished? Is the patient taking any supplements?
- Has the patient experienced any weight loss or gain lately?
- If the patient has diabetes, is it well controlled?
- Does the patient have an immunodeficiency disorder or a medical condition that increases his or her risk of infection?
- Does the patient have a medical condition that causes altered sensation?
- What medications (including anticoagulants) is the patient taking? What are their effects on wound healing?

Psychosocial Factors

- Does the patient have a good support system, including physical assistance if necessary?
- What are the patient's mobility needs?

A review of vascular tests, radiographic studies, and tissue biopsy results also lends valuable information about the integrity of the vascular and orthopedic systems and the presence of underlying disease.

Physical Examination

Sensation

Sensation to light touch, pressure, pinprick, temperature, and proprioception should be examined. Impaired or absent sensation should be addressed through instruction in the appropriate prevention techniques, such as modifications to shoes, weight bearing, and water temperatures in bathing.

Pain

The evaluation of pain in the patient with a wound is not unlike the evaluation of pain in any other type of patient. The therapist should evaluate the nature of the pain, including the location, onset, severity (using a pain-rating scale), duration, aggravating and alleviating factors, and the impact on activities of daily living. Understanding the nature of the pain will ultimately allow the physical therapist to provide or recommend the appropriate intervention.

The pain experience associated with wounds has been described as having one of three components: a noncyclic acute component, a cyclic acute component, or a chronic wound pain component.

Noncyclic acute wound pain is a single episode of pain that is likely to occur with treatment (e.g., the pain felt during sharp debridement). Cyclic acute pain is wound pain that recurs predictably because of repeated events such as positioning or daily dressing changes. For example, a patient may experience pain after several days of dressing changes, which creates repetitive trauma to the wound. Chronic or consistent wound pain is persistent wound pain that occurs intrinsically, not as a result of external intervention (e.g., a patient with a neuropathic ulcer who has a constant, dull ache in the foot).[84]

> ### ✎ CLINICAL TIP
> The American Geriatric Society promotes the use of "persistent" pain rather than "chronic" pain to help lessen negative connotations that accompany the term *chronic*. Additionally, this society advocates stating that patients "report pain," rather than "complain of pain," again to maximize the positive interactions with patients.[85]

Range of Motion

Specific measurement of ROM may not be necessary in a patient with a wound. However, specific goniometric measurements are necessary if a wound crosses a joint line, if edema is present at a joint, or if decreased ROM inhibits mobility. Decreased ROM that inhibits mobility or increases weight bearing or pressure may contribute to wound development. Therefore passive or active ROM exercise, or both, should be included, as necessary, in the treatment plan.

Strength

Strength should be evaluated for its impact on the patient's function. The therapist should keep in mind that the patient may have different functional demands secondary to the wound. For example, a patient who needs to be non–weight bearing because of a wound on his or her foot requires sufficient upper-extremity strength to use an assistive device to maintain this precaution while ambulating. If the patient does not have adequate upper-extremity strength, then he or she may be nonambulatory until the weight-bearing status is changed.

Functional Mobility

Functional mobility, including bed mobility, transfers, and ambulation or wheelchair mobility, should be evaluated. The therapist should consider that the patient's function may have changed simply because of the consequences of the presence of the wound. For example, balance may be compromised if the patient requires orthotics or shoe modifications because of a wound. Gait training with an assistive device is often necessary to decrease weight bearing on an affected lower extremity.

Edema and Circulation

The evaluation of edema is important because it is frequently an indicator of an underlying pathology. Edema is also a critical factor in lowering tissue perfusion of oxygen and increasing susceptibility to infection. In fact, edema is almost equivalent to insufficient blood supply in lowering the oxygen tension in the area of the wound. Ultimately, the presence of edema must be addressed to heal the wound. Refer to Table 3-5 for the scale on how to grade pitting edema.

Therapists should also consider that lymphedema and chronic wounds can be closely linked. Lymphedema is commonly associated with individuals who have undergone a mastectomy; however, it can also occur secondary to venous insufficiency (phlebolymphedema) as well as after surgeries and traumas that affect the integrity of the lymphatic system. Cellulitis may actually be due to a compromised lymphatic system that creates small, weeping blisters from fluids being literally pushed through the skin. Refer to Chapter 7 for a description of lymphedema.

Circulation can be grossly evaluated and monitored by examining skin temperature, distal limb color, capillary refill, and the presence of pulses. Transcutaneous oxygen monitoring (TCOM, Tco_2, $Tcpo_2$) assesses arterial circulation through the use of surface electrodes that measure oxygen content in periwound tissues. Values greater than 35 mm Hg are considered adequate for healing, whereas those less than 30 mm Hg likely indicate a need for surgical intervention.[1,6] Measurement of ankle-brachial index will help determine healing potential in patients with diabetes or vascular disease. Refer to Table 7-5 in Chapter 7 for more information on the evaluation of circulation. The therapist should notify the physician when any significant changes in these indicators occur. The therapist should be aware of any arterial compromise before using compression bandages.

Wound Inspection and Evaluation

Wound observation and measurements create an objective record of the baseline status of a wound and can help to determine the best intervention to facilitate wound healing.

> ✎ **CLINICAL TIP**
>
> During any interaction with the patient, the clinician should screen the wound for any overt changes as well as determine the stability of the wound before performing examination and intervention techniques.

Location, Orientation, Size, and Depth

The location of the wound should be documented in relation to anatomic landmarks. Wound orientation, length, width, depth,

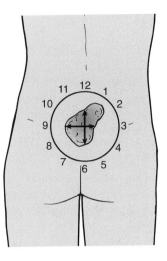

FIGURE 12-6
Clockwise method of measuring pressure ulcer size. (From Hamm RL: Tissue healing and pressure ulcers. In Cameron MH, Monroe LG, editors: Physical rehabilitation: evidence-based examination, evaluation, and intervention, St Louis, 2007, Saunders.)

and presence of undermining or tunneling are essential measurements in wound assessment.

The orientation of the wound must be determined to ensure consistent length and width measurements, particularly for a wound with an abstract shape or odd location. One method of determining wound orientation is to consider the wound in terms of a clock, with the patient's head being 12 o'clock (Figure 12-6).

When documenting length, the measurement is the vertical distance of the wound (measured in the direction from the patient's head to toe), and the width is the horizontal measurement. There are a variety of methods for measuring wounds. Tape measurements are a common method, but a calibrated grid on an acetate sheet on which the wound can be traced is optimal, especially for irregularly shaped wounds. Digital photography and volumetric methods of measurement can also be used.

> ✎ **CLINICAL TIP**
>
> To ensure consistency and accuracy in wound assessments, use a consistent unit of measure among all individuals measuring the wound. Centimeters, rather than inches, are more universally used in the literature. Multiple wounds can be documented relative to each other if the wounds are numbered—for example, "Wound #1: left lower extremity, 3 cm proximal to the medial malleolus. Wound #2: 2 cm proximal to wound #1." When taking a photograph of a wound, create or follow a consistent procedure, as changes in the distance of the camera from the wound as well as the position of the patient can affect the appearance of the wound.

Depth can be measured by placing a sterile cotton-tipped applicator or wound probe perpendicular to the wound bed. The applicator is then grasped or marked at the point of the wound edge and measured. If the wound has varying depths, this measurement is repeated.

Undermining describes wound erosion underneath intact skin resulting in a large wound with a small opening. This is evaluated by probing underneath the skin parallel to the wound bed and grasping or marking the applicator at the point of the wound edge. Assessment of undermining should be done circumferentially around the wound edge and can be documented using the clock orientation (e.g., "Undermining: 2 cm at 12 o'clock, 5 cm at 4 o'clock"; Figure 12-7). *Tunneling* is a single linear channel that should be measured by probing the depth and marking the applicator at the point of the wound edge. Caution must be taken when measuring extent of undermining and tunneling to avoid traumatic separation of tissues or increasing areas of depth.

Color

The color of the wound should be documented because it is an indicator of the general condition and vascularity of the wound. Granulation tissue can vary in coloration from beefy red to pale pink depending on the amount of vasculature associated with it. Pink may also indicate recently epithelized tissue. Yellow may indicate infection or necrotic material being sloughed off from the wound. However, adipose, fascia, tendons and other viable tissues may also be yellow in coloration. Brown and black indicate necrotic tissue and eschar.

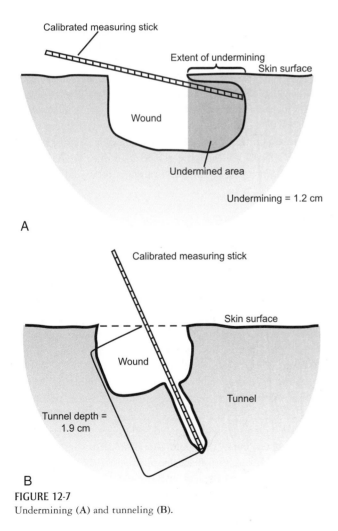

FIGURE 12-7
Undermining (**A**) and tunneling (**B**).

It is important to document the percentage of each color in the wound bed. An increase in the amount of pink and red tissue or a decrease in the amount of yellow, brown, and black tissue is indicative of progress. An increase in the amount of yellow, brown, or black tissue is indicative of regression.

Drainage

Wound drainage is described by type, color, amount, and odor. Drainage can be (1) serous (clear and thin; may be present in a healthy, healing wound), (2) serosanguineous (containing blood; may also be present in a healthy, healing wound), (3) sanguineous (primarily blood), or (4) purulent (thick, white, and pus-like; may be indicative of infection and should be cultured). Color is generally clear to pale yellow (normal), red (fresh blood), brown (dried or old blood), white (see above), or blue-green (usually indicative of *Pseudomonas* infection and should be cultured). The amount of drainage is generally documented as absent, scant, minimal, moderate, large, or copious. (Note: there is no consistent objective measurement that correlates to these descriptions.) A large amount of drainage can indicate infection, whereas a reduction in the amount of drainage can indicate an infection that is resolving or inadequate arterial circulation. The presence and degree of odor can be documented as absent, mild, or foul. Foul odors can be indicative of an infection.

Wound Culture

A wound culture is a sampling of microorganisms from the wound bed that is subsequently grown in a nutrient medium for the purpose of identifying the type and number of organisms present. A wound culture is indicated if there are clinical signs of infection, such as purulent drainage, large amounts of drainage, increased local or systemic temperature, inflammation, abnormal granulation tissue, local erythema, edema, cellulitis, increased pain, foul odor, and delayed healing.[86] Results of aerobic and anaerobic cultures can determine whether antibiotic therapy is indicated.[87] Methods of culturing include tissue biopsy, needle aspiration, and swab cultures. Physical therapists may administer swab cultures. Tissue biopsy and needle aspirations are performed by the nurse or physician, depending on the protocol of the institution.

All wounds are contaminated, which does not necessarily mean they are infected. Contamination is the presence of non-replicating organisms on the wound surface. Colonization is the presence and multiplication of surface microbes without impact on wound healing. Infection is the invasion, multiplication, and penetration of microorganisms in body tissues resulting in local cellular injury.[86,88]

> ✎ **CLINICAL TIP**
>
> Unless specifically prescribed otherwise, cultures should be taken after debridement of eschar and necrotic material and wound cleaning; otherwise, the culture will reflect the growth of the microorganisms of the external wound environment rather than the internal environment.

Wound Staging and Classification

Superficial wounds involve only the epidermis. *Partial-thickness* wounds involve varying degrees of the dermis, whereas *full-thickness* wounds continue through to subcutaneous tissues and structures. This terminology should be used to describe and classify wounds that are not pressure ulcers. Pressure ulcers have their own classification system because of their unique characteristic of developing from the "inside out," including injury to the deeper subcutaneous tissues under intact skin (see Table 12-11). As stage III and IV pressure ulcers heal to a more shallow depth, lost muscle, subcutaneous fat, or dermis is not replaced; rather, granulation tissue fills in this space. Therefore avoid "reverse staging" when documenting improvement in a pressure ulcer (e.g., a stage III ulcer does not improve to a stage II ulcer). It is more advisable to use descriptive terms to denote improved wound characteristics or use available tools to monitor progress over time such as the Pressure Ulcer Scale for Healing (PUSH) tool or the Bates-Jensen Wound Status Tool (formerly known as the Pressure Score Status Tool [PSST]).[76,89]

Periwound Assessment

The area surrounding the wound should also be evaluated and compared to noninvolved areas. Skin color, temperature, and integrity, the absence of hair, shiny or flaky skin, the presence of reddened or darkened areas or old scars, edema, and changes in nail beds should all be examined and documented accordingly.

> ✎ **CLINICAL TIP**
>
> Increased localized temperature can indicate local infection; decreased temperature can indicate decreased blood supply. Increased temperature, erythema, and edema can occur with both inflammation and infection processes, and the therapist should be aware of other clinical signs to determine appropriate course of action. Darker underlying skin tones may make coloration changes more difficult to observe.

Wound Cleaning and Debridement

It is beyond the scope of this book to discuss in detail the methods of wound cleaning and debridement. Instead, general descriptions and indications of each are provided. Wound cleaning and debridement can be performed by physical therapists, nurses, or physicians, depending on the policy of an individual facility. Physical therapists should also verify state practice acts regarding their ability to perform sharp debridement. Specific management considerations for physical therapists who work with patients who have wounds are described in the Physical Therapy Intervention section at the end of this chapter.

Wound Cleaning

Wound cleaning is not synonymous with wound debridement or wound decontamination. The purpose of cleaning a wound is to remove loosely attached cellular debris and bacteria from the wound bed in order to both prepare the wound bed for healing and help prevent infection. In most cases, the use of

---

> ✎ **CLINICAL TIP**
>
> Sterile saline expires 24 hours after opening the bottle and must be discarded. A saline solution can be made by adding 2 tablespoons of salt to 1 quart of boiling water.[90,92] This recipe may be an inexpensive alternative to purchasing saline for the patient who will be cleaning wounds at home. If the water source is known or suspected to be contaminated, it should not be used for wound cleaning.[90] If the physical therapist is unsure, the water can be cultured in the hospital laboratory.

---

sterile saline is effective and safe for cleaning the wound surface.[90,91] Many studies indicate that using unsterile tap water does not increase the rate of infection and is safe to use to cleanse wounds.[90]

There are many commercial wound cleansers that contain surfactants. Surfactants help to break the bonds between contaminants and debris and the wound surface.[90] The use of antiseptics may be appropriate in the early management of acute traumatic wounds and in some infected wounds but is of little benefit in healthy healing wounds, as these solutions may be cytotoxic to living cells and tissues and can delay healing.[90,92,93] Wound cleaning can be achieved by a variety of devices such as scrubbing cloths, sponges, and brushes, as well as irrigation devices.[94]

The most neutral solution that will meet the needs of the patient should be used. Whirlpool, although commonly and perhaps habitually used, is not indicated for use as a wound cleanser. The use of whirlpool jets is actually mechanical debridement and therefore should be used only if mechanical debridement is indicated. Use aggressive agents only when indicated. For example, a bleaching agent may help to dry a heavily exudating wound. To avoid damaging new tissue, discontinue cleansing when the majority of the wound bed is granulating or when re-epithelialization is occurring.

> ✎ **CLINICAL TIP**
>
> It is best to use cleaning materials at body temperature. The application of a cold solution will reduce the temperature of the wound and may affect blood flow.[93]

Clean versus Sterile Technique. Although clean versus sterile technique remains somewhat controversial, clean technique is sufficient for local wound care to most wounds and is generally accepted in the medical community. This is because the wound is already contaminated and far from sterile. Sterile technique is typically reserved for surgical and acute traumatic wounds.[95]

Sterile technique, which includes the use of sterile instruments and sterile gloves, should always be used when invading the bloodstream, as with sharp debridement. Otherwise, the use of clean gloves is sufficient. Additionally, originally sterile dressings, once opened, can still be used as long as they are kept in a clean, controlled area.[95]

Wound Debridement

Debridement has three primary purposes. The first is to remove necrotic tissue or foreign matter from the wound bed, optimizing healing potential. The presence of devitalized tissue and debris prevents re-epithelialization and can splint the wound open, preventing contraction and closure. The second purpose is to prevent infection. The necrotic tissue itself can be the source of the pathogenic organisms. Removal of nonviable tissue is especially important in the patient who is immunocompromised, because its presence can provide a medium for bacterial growth. The debridement of the slough and eschar also increases the effectiveness of topical agents. The third purpose is to correct abnormal wound repair. Debridement is generally indicated for any necrotic tissue present in a wound, although occasionally it is advantageous to leave eschar in place. For example, eschar on heel ulcers that is firmly adherent to surrounding tissue (without inflammation of surrounding tissue and without drainage and tenderness on palpation) may not need to be removed.[96]

There are two types of debridement: selective and nonselective. Selective debridement removes nonviable tissue only and is indicated for wounds with necrotic tissue adjacent to viable tissue. Methods of selective debridement include sharp, autolytic, and enzymatic debridement. Nonselective debridement removes both viable and nonviable tissues. It is indicated in necrotic wounds with minimal to no healthy tissue. Mechanical debridement is a method of nonselective debridement.[96,97] Surgical debridement is also a form of nonselective debridement; however, this is not within the scope of practice for a physical therapist and will not be discussed here.

Selective Debridement

Sharp Debridement. Sharp debridement involves the use of scalpels, scissors, and forceps to remove necrotic tissue. It is a highly skilled technique best performed by or under the direct supervision of an experienced clinician. Because the true selectivity of sharp debridement depends on the skill of the clinician, sharp debridement can also result in damage to healthy tissues, which can cause bleeding and a risk of infection. Sharp debridement is especially expedient in the removal of large amounts of thick, leathery eschar. Sharp debridement has been shown to increase the degree of wound healing when combined with the use of a topical growth factor.[98,99]

Sharp debridement can be painful; it is therefore recommended that pain medications or topical analgesics be administered before treatment. When debriding, the clinician should spare as much tissue as possible and be careful to have the technique remain selective by not removing viable tissue. Because of the potential for excessive bleeding, extra care should be taken with patients who are taking anticoagulants.

Autolytic Debridement. Autolytic debridement is naturally occurring and the most selective form of debridement. The body uses its own enzymes to lyse necrotic tissue, a normal process that occurs in any wound. It is painless and does not harm healthy tissues. Applying a moisture-retentive dressing, such as films, hydrocolloids, hydrogels, and calcium alginates, facilitates autolytic debridement in a pain-free manner for patients with adequate tissue perfusion.[96,98,99] When using autolytic debridement, it is important to cleanse the wound to remove partially degraded tissue.[98] Because it takes time for autolytic debridement to occur, sharp debridement of eschar is recommended before autolytic debridement to expedite the removal of the necrotic tissue. Owing to their risk of infection, autolytic debridement is contraindicated as the primary method of debridement in patients who are immunosuppressed or otherwise require quick elimination of necrotic material. Additionally, the occlusive multiday dressings required for autolytic debridement are contraindicated in the presence of an active infection.

Enzymatic Debridement. Enzymatic debridement is achieved through the topical application of enzymes that lyse collagen, fibrin, and elastin. Enzymatic debridement agents are available only by prescription and should be discontinued as soon as the wound is clean. Sharp debridement of the wound can be performed before the use of enzymes to facilitate tissue healing. When applying an enzymatic debriding agent to eschar that cannot be immediately sharp debrided, crosshatch the eschar to allow better penetration of the enzymes.

> ### ✎ CLINICAL TIP
> Certain metals, such as silver and zinc oxide, which are present in some cleansing agents and dressings, can inactivate enzymes and interfere with enzymatic debridement.[98]

Nonselective Debridement

Mechanical Debridement. Mechanical debridement removes dead tissue by agitating the necrotic tissue of the wound or adhering it to a dressing and removing it. Dry gauze dressings, whirlpool, pulsed lavage, and irrigation are all examples of mechanical debridement.

Wet-to-dry dressings mechanically debride the wound by removing the dressing along with the necrotic tissue embedded in it. If mechanical debridement is indicated and gauze is used, the sponge or gauze with the largest pores is the most effective for debridement.[98] This technique involves applying a moistened gauze dressing to the wound, allowing it to dry, and then removing the dressing. The dried dressing will adhere to any growing tissue in the wound bed and remove it.[96] The Centers for Medicare and Medicaid Services (CMS) has stated that wet-to-dry dressings should not be used on clean, granulating wound beds, regardless of the type of wound.[99]

Whirlpool may be used to debride loosely adherent tissue and exudate and deodorize the wound. It may also help to prepare a wound for sharp debridement by softening necrotic tissue and separating desiccated tissues from the wound bed, or it can be used to soak off adhered dressings. If the intention of the therapist is to use a wet-to-dry technique for mechanical debridement, the dressings should not be soaked off, as necrotic tissue will not be removed.[75,97,100]

There are many precautions and contraindications for the therapist to consider before using whirlpool. For example, it may be inappropriate to place the lower extremity of a patient with venous insufficiency in a dependent position with warm water, or perhaps the treatment may need to be modified by decreasing the temperature or length of a treatment. Treatment duration can range between 10 and 20 minutes, and water temperature can range from tepid (80° to 92° F [26.7° to 33.3° C]) to close to body temperature (92° to 96° F [33.3° to 35.5° C]).[99] As with wound cleaning, the therapist should carefully weigh the benefits of antibacterial agents that can be added to the whirlpool versus their cytotoxic effects and use a solution that is most neutral and least damaging to viable tissue. Infected wounds that have foul odors, copious amounts of drainage, and a great deal of exudate and necrotic tissue require more aggressive additives.

Whirlpool should be limited to wounds with greater than 50% of necrotic tissue, because, as with gauze debridement, granulating tissue may be damaged. Whirlpool should be discontinued once the objectives of the intervention have been achieved.[75,96,100]

Pulsed lavage uses a pressurized, pulsed solution (usually saline) to irrigate and debride wounds of necrotic tissue. Suction may also be used to remove wound debris and the irrigation solution.[101] The pulsatile action is thought to facilitate growth of granulation tissue because of its effective debridement, and the negative pressure created by the suction may also stimulate granulation.[102] Pulsed lavage may be a more appropriate option than whirlpool for patients who are incontinent, have venous insufficiency, should not be in a dependent position, have an intravenous line, or are mechanically ventilated. Pulsed lavage can access narrow wound tunnels that may not be reached with whirlpool as various flexible tunneling tips are available from manufacturers. One must also consider risk of contamination from aerosolization of droplets during both pulsed lavage and whirlpool treatments.

Dressings and Topical Agents

Wound dressings are identified as either primary or secondary. Primary dressings are applied directly to the wound bed, whereas secondary dressings are used to contain or anchor a primary dressing. Custom dressings, which may contain more than one type of primary or secondary dressing, can also be used.[76] When applying dressings, the therapist should always follow universal precautions and use a clean technique to prevent cross-contamination. When choosing a dressing for a wound, four factors related to the wound itself should be considered: (1) the color of the wound (tissue composition), (2) the amount of drainage, (3) the wound depth, and (4) the periwound. Other significant factors include the patient's and caregiver's cognitive and physical ability to apply the dressing and the accessibility of physical therapy or nursing services to the patient. Cost is also a consideration.

A large number of wound care products are available, and it is virtually impossible to be aware of the purpose and application instructions of every available dressing. It is the responsibility of the therapist to read the manufacturer's instructions for application, to know the purpose of the dressing, and to make educated decisions when choosing the appropriate dressing for a given wound at each stage of the healing process. Although it is not possible to identify every dressing, it is possible to catalog most dressings into some basic categories: gauze, transparent film, hydrocolloids, hydrogels, foams, calcium alginates,

collagen matrix, and topical ointments. Table 12-12 is a summary of the indications, advantages, and disadvantages of various dressings.[61,102-104]

Advanced Therapies

Chronic wounds fail to progress through the phases of healing in an orderly and timely manner despite standard wound care practices. Adjunctive therapies are often used in addition to standard wound practices in the care of chronic and nonhealing wounds. These include negative-pressure wound therapy, ultrasound, electrical stimulation, UV light therapy, laser therapy, and hyperbaric oxygen. It is beyond the scope of this text to discuss each of these at length. Table 12-13 is a brief summary of their method of action, indications, and contraindications. Reimbursement for the use of adjunctive therapies varies, and therapists should be aware of third-party payer regulations.

Physical Therapy Intervention in Wound Care

The responsibility and autonomy of the physical therapist in the treatment of wounds varies greatly among facilities. The physical therapist can and should play a key role in the patient's clinical course of preventing a wound, initiating wound care, and recommending activity and footwear modifications and positioning aids. The physical therapist in the acute care setting can also make recommendations regarding ongoing wound care on discharge from the hospital. Unless the wound is superficial, wound closure is not likely to occur during the acute care phase. Therefore the ultimate long-term goal of complete wound closure, which may occur over many months, occurs at a different level of care, usually outpatient or home care.

The following are the primary goals of physical therapy for wound treatment in the acute care setting:

- To promote wound healing through wound assessment, dressing choice and application, wound cleaning, and debridement
- To educate patients and families about wound care and the prevention of further breakdown and future wounds
- To maximize patient mobility and function while accommodating needs for wound healing (e.g., maintaining non–weight-bearing status)
- To minimize pain
- To provide recommendations for interdisciplinary care
- To provide recommendations and referrals for follow-up care

To fulfill these responsibilities, the therapist must consider all information gathered during the evaluation process and establish appropriate goals and time frames. The etiology of the wound, risk factors, and other data guide the therapist toward the proper intervention. Objective, measurable, and functional goals are as important in wound care as in any other aspect of physical therapy.

Patients with wounds typically have many other medical complications and needs that a physical therapist cannot address alone. To provide optimal care, the physical therapist should be part of an interdisciplinary team that may include a physician, a nurse, a specialized skin and wound care nurse (enterostomal therapist), a dietitian, and others. The physical therapist should be aware of and make proper recommendations to the appropriate personnel for all of the patient's needs for healing.

Specific considerations for physical therapy intervention with a patient who has a wound include pain management, ROM, strengthening, functional mobility, edema management, and wound prevention (Table 12-14).

TABLE 12-12 Indications and Uses of Basic Types of Dressings

Type of Dressing	Description	Indication(s)	Advantages/Disadvantages
Gauze	Highly porous. Applied dry, wet-to-dry (i.e., the dressing is put on wet but will dry before removal), or wet-to-wet (i.e., the dressing is put on wet and removed when wet).	May be used for any type of wound if properly applied and removed (although other dressings may be more effective). Some come impregnated with petroleum, hydrogel, bismuth, or zinc.	Readily available. Inexpensive. Impregnated gauzes used as a contact layer can minimize adherence to granulation tissue. Topical ointments can be added as well.
Transparent film	Polymer sheet with an adhesive layer on one side.	Autolytic debridement, to reduce friction, superficial wounds with minimal drainage, secondary dressing over foam or gauze.	Conforms and adheres well to surfaces, waterproof, allows visualization of the wound with dressing in place, impermeable to bacteria, cost-effective. Minimal to no absorptive qualities.
Hydrocolloids	Dressings that contain absorptive particles that interact with moisture to form a gelatinous mass. Cause the pH of the wound surface to decrease, thereby inhibiting bacterial growth.	Partial- or full-thickness wounds with low to moderate drainage, including partially necrotic wounds. Provide a moist wound environment and promote autolysis.	Prevent secondary wound infection. Impermeable to water, oxygen, and bacteria. Available in many forms (pastes, powders, and sheets). Changed infrequently. May not be able to manage copiously draining wounds.
Hydrogels	Water- or glycerin-based dressings available in sheets, amorphous gels, or impregnated gauzes.	Any wound with minimal drainage; can be beneficial in rehydrating desiccated nonviable tissue for debridement or maintaining moisture content and viability of exposed structures.	Highly conformable. Safe for fragile skin.
Foams	Polyurethane foam with two surfaces: a hydrophilic inner surface and a hydrophobic outer surface.	Partial- or full-thickness wounds with minimal to moderate drainage.	Nonadherent to skin surface. Highly absorbable and conformable. Permeable to oxygen (reduce risk of anaerobic infection).
Calcium alginates	Fibrous sheets and rope derived from brown seaweed. The main component, alginic acid, is converted to calcium and sodium salts, which in turn convert to a viscous gel after contact with wound exudates.	Partial- and full-thickness wounds with large amounts of drainage, infected or noninfected wounds. Provide a moist wound environment and facilitate autolysis.	Highly conformable. Hemostatic properties.
Collagen matrix	Collagen derived from bovine material, processed and shaped into sheets, particles, or gels.	Any recalcitrant wound to facilitate migration of collagen.	Conforms to wound bed, promotes granulation and epithelialization.
Topical ointments	Water- or petrolatum-based gels and ointments (antimicrobials, growth factors, silver, enzymes, anesthetics).	Wounds requiring topical medications.	Allow local application of antimicrobials, bypassing systemic administration. May assist in maintaining moist environment.

Data from Lawrence JC: Dressings and wound infection, Am J Surg 167(1A):21, 1994; Hess CT: When to use hydrocolloid dressings, Adv Skin Wound Care 13:63, 2000; Bolander VP, editor: Sorensen and Luckmann's basic nursing, Philadelphia, 1994, Saunders, p 742; Levin ML, O'Neal LW, Bowker JH: The diabetic foot, ed 5, St Louis, 1993, Mosby; Cuzell J, Krasner D: Wound dressings. In Gogia PP, editor: Clinical wound management, Thorofare, NJ, 1995, Slack, pp 131-144; Feedar JS: Clinical management of chronic wounds. In Kloth LC, Miller KH, editors: Wound healing: alternatives in management, Philadelphia, 1995, FA Davis, pp 156-169; Myers BA: Wound management: principles and practice, ed 3, Upper Saddle River, NJ, 2012, Pearson Education, p 4.

TABLE 12-13 Adjunctive Therapies in Wound Care

Intervention	Method of Action	Indications	Contraindications
Negative-pressure wound therapy (NPWT)	Application of continuous or intermittent localized subatmospheric pressure via a specialized porous dressing and mechanical vacuum pump Removal of exudate, reduction in edema and bioburden, maintenance of moist wound environment, increase in blood flow; produces a mechanical deformation of cells, stimulating all phases of wound healing	Chronic, acute, traumatic, subacute, and dehisced wounds, partial-thickness burns, ulcers (neuropathic, pressure, or venous), flaps, and grafts	Presence of eschar, untreated osteomyelitis, malignancy in the wound, exposed vasculature, nerves, anastomotic sites, or organs, and nonenteric and unexplored fistulas Precaution: High risk of bleeding or hemorrhage including concurrent use of anticoagulants, weakened blood vessels or organs in the vicinity of the wound
Ultrasound	Transmission of acoustic energy to tissues Stimulates growth factor release and cellular activity in all phases of healing, increase in capillary perfusion, improved collagen deposition and scar tensile strength, debridement, and reduction in pain, edema, and bioburden	Adjunct intervention for chronic wounds—not dependent on wound etiology	Over reproductive organs, active epiphyseal plates, eyes, and central nervous system (CNS) tissues; near cardiac pacemaker, active bleeding, untreated osteomyelitis, malignancy, deep venous thrombosis, and thrombophlebitis Precaution: Implanted metal or plastic components, sensory neuropathy, arterial insufficiency, acute infection
Electrical stimulation	Transfer of electrical current into tissues Stimulation of cellular migration and proliferation, increase in localized blood flow and tissue oxygenation, debridement, and reduction in pain, edema and bioburden	Adjunct intervention for chronic wounds—not dependent on wound etiology	In region of malignancy, active osteomyelitis, or known peripheral vascular disease; over electrical implants, eyes, reproductive organs, or CNS structures such as carotid bodies and phrenic nerve In combination with topical agents containing metal ions Precaution: CA, cardiac dysfunction, seizure disorders
Ultraviolet (UV) light therapy	Exposure to UV radiation for bactericidal effects. UVC most effective with 99.99% eradication of common pathogens	Acute, chronic or necrotic wounds with high levels of bioburden	Tuberculosis, systemic lupus erythematosus, cardiac, renal, or liver disease, acute eczema or psoriasis, hyperthyroid, herpes simplex
Low-level laser therapy (LLLT)	Exposure to infrared light in the 600-900 nm range Stimulation of growth factor release and cellular activity in all phases of healing, enhanced rates of healing, and improved tensile strength of scar tissue	Acute, chronic, and nonhealing wounds, infected or colonized wounds	Over reproductive organs, active epiphyseal plates, vagus nerve, sympathetic ganglia, mediastinum, open fontanelles, malignancy, endocrine glands, and hemorrhaging lesions. Avoid direct exposure to eyes
Hyperbaric oxygen therapy (HBOT, HBO)	Inhalation of 100% O_2 at greater than 1.4 atmospheres absolute pressure (ATA). Typically at 2-2.5 ATA Tissue hyperoxygenation, edema reduction, angiogenesis and granulation formation, and reestablishment of normal cellular metabolism	Specific to wound care includes diabetic foot ulcers, chronic osteomyelitis, necrotizing fasciitis, peripheral arterial insufficiency, acute, traumatic ischemia, and preservation of compromised skin grafts	Untreated pneumothorax, concurrent use of certain chemotherapeutic agents Precaution: Seizures, claustrophobia, chronic obstructive pulmonary disease, congestive heart failure, any condition impairing ability to equalize ear pressure, pregnancy, malignancy

Data from McCallon SK: Negative-pressure wound therapy. In McCulloch JM, Kloth LC, editors: Wound healing: evidence-based management, Philadelphia, 2010, FA Davis, pp 602-620; Food and Drug Administration. http://www.accessdata.fda.gov/scripts/cdrh/cfdocs/cfpcd/classification.cfm?ID=5258; Sussman C, Dyson M: Therapeutic and diagnostic ultrasound. In Sussman C, Bates-Jensen B, editors: Wound care: a collaborative practice manual for health professionals, Baltimore, 2007, Lippincott Williams & Wilkins, pp 505-553, 612-643; Myers BA: Wound management: principles and practice, ed 3, Upper Saddle River, NJ, 2012, Pearson Education, p 8; Michlovitz SL, Sparrow KJ: Therapeutic ultrasound. In Michlovitz SL, Bellow JW, Nolan TP, editors: Modalities for therapeutic intervention, Philadelphia, 2012, FA Davis, pp 85-108; Bellow JW: Clinical electrical stimulation: application and techniques. In Michlovitz SL, Bellow JW, Nolan TP, editors: Modalities for therapeutic intervention, Philadelphia, 2012, FA Davis, pp 241-277; Conner-Kerr T: Light therapies. In McCulloch JM, Kloth LC, editors: Wound healing: evidence-based management., Philadelphia, 2010, FA Davis, pp 576-593; Centers for Medicare and Medicaid Services, National Coverage Determination for Hyperbaric Oxygen Therapy (20.29), www.cms.gov; Broussard CL: Hyperbaric oxygen. In Bryant RA, Nix DP, editors: Acute and chronic wounds: current management concepts, St Louis, 2012, Elsevier, pp 345-352.

TABLE 12-14 Physical Therapy Considerations for Wound Care

Physical Therapy Intervention	Consideration
Pain management	Coordinate physical therapy session with pain premedication to reduce acute cyclic and noncyclic pain.
	Consider the use of positioning, relaxation techniques, deep breathing, exercise, or modalities to relieve pain.
	Modify wound treatment techniques as able to eliminate the source of pain.
Range of motion, strength, and functional mobility	Adequate range of motion is necessary for proper positioning and minimizing the risk of pressure ulcer formation.
	Care should be taken with manual contacts over fragile skin and to not disturb dressings during exercise.
	Adequate strength is necessary for weight shifting and functional mobility with the maintenance of weight-bearing precautions.
Edema management	Depending on the etiology, intervention options to manage edema include exercise, compression therapy, lymphatic drainage, limb elevation, or a combination of these. The therapist should be aware of any medically related contraindications for these interventions.
Prevention	Education (e.g., dressing application, infection control, wound inspection, the etiology of wounds).
	Positioning (e.g., splints, turning schedule).
	Skin care and hygiene (e.g., dressing removal, management of incontinence).
	Pressure reduction surfaces (e.g., air mattress, wheelchair cushion).
	Footwear adaptations (e.g., orthotics, inserts, extra-depth shoes).

References

1. Myers BA: Wound management: principles and practice, ed 3, Upper Saddle River, NJ, 2012, Pearson Education, p 4.
2. Bryant RA, Nix DP: Acute and chronic wounds: current management concepts, ed 4, St Louis, 2012, Mosby.
3. Williams WAG, Phillips LG: Pathophysiology of the burn wound. In Herndon DN, editor: Total burn care, London, 1996, Saunders, p 63.
4. Falkel JE: Anatomy and physiology of the skin. In Richard RI, Staley MH, editors: Burn care rehabilitation principles and practice, Philadelphia, 1994, FA Davis, p 10.
5. Totora GJ, Grabowski SR, editors: Principles of anatomy and physiology, ed 7, New York, 1989, Harper-Collins College, p 126.
6. Baronoski S: Integumentary anatomy: skin—the largest organ. In McCulloch JM, Kloth LC, editors: Wound healing: evidence-based management, ed 4, Philadelphia, 2010, FA Davis, p 1.
7. Hettiaratchy S, Dziewulski P: Pathophysiology and types of burns, BMJ 328(7453):1427-1429, 2004.
8. Gomez R, Cancio LC: Management of burn wounds in the emergency department, Emerg Med Clin North Am 25:135-146, 2007.
9. Pham TN, Gibran NS, Heimbach DM: Evaluation of the burn wound: management decisions. In Herndon DN, editor: Total burn care, ed 3, Philadelphia, 2007, Saunders, p 119.
10. Xu RX: Burns: regenerative medicine and therapy, Basel, 2004, Karger, p 20.
11. Shupp JW et al: A review of local pathophysiologic bases of burn wound progression, J Burn Care Res 31(6):849-873, 2010.
12. Lionelli GT, et al: A three decade analysis of factors affecting burn mortality in the elderly, Burns 31(8):958-963, 2005.
13. Warden GD, Heimback DM: Burns. In Schwartz SI, editor: Principles of surgery, vol 1, ed 7, New York, 1999, McGraw-Hill, pp 223-262.
14. Johnson C: Pathologic manifestations of burn injury. In Richard RI, Staley MH, editors: Burn care rehabilitation principles and practice, Philadelphia, 1994, FA Davis, p 29.
15. Faucher LD: Electrical injury: acute care in electrical, chemical and non-thermal burns. American Burn Association Education Symposium, 38th Annual Meeting, Las Vegas. April 4, 2006.
16. Rai J, Jeschke MG, Barrow RE, et al: Electrical injuries: a 30-year review, J Trauma 46(5):933-936, 1999.
17. Winfree J, Barillo DJ: Burn management. Nonthermal injuries, Nurs Clin North Am 32(2):275-296, 1997.
18. Arnoldo B, Klein M, Gibran MS: Practice guidelines for the management of electrical injuries, J Burn Care Res 27(4):439-447, 2006.
19. Demling RH, LaLonde C: Lightning. In Demling RH, LaLonde C, editors: Burn trauma, New York, 1989, Thieme, p 242.
20. Milner SM, Rylah LTA, Nguyen TT, et al: Chemical injury. In Herndon DN, editor: Total burn care, London, 1996, Saunders, p 424.
21. Milner SM, Nguyen TT, Herndon DN, et al: Radiation injuries and mass casualties. In Herndon DN, editor: Total Burn Care, London, 1996, Saunders, p 425.
22. McManus WF, Pruitt BA: Thermal injuries. In Feliciano DV, Moore EE, Mattox KL, editors: Trauma, Stamford, CT, 1996, Appleton & Lange, p 937.
23. Evidence-based guidelines group: practice guidelines for burn care, 2001, American Burn Association.
24. Marvin J: Thermal injuries. In Cardona VD, Hurn PD, Bastnagel Mason PJ, et al, editors: Trauma nursing: from resuscitation through rehabilitation, Philadelphia, 1994, Saunders, p 736.
25. Richard R: Assessment and diagnosis of burn wounds, Adv Wound Care 12(9):468-471, 1999.
26. American College of Surgeons Committee on Trauma: Guidelines for the operations of burn units. resources for optimal care of the injured patient, Chicago, 1999, American College of Surgeons, pp 55-62.
27. Gordon M, Goodwin CW: Burn management. Initial assessment, management, and stabilization, Nurs Clin North Am 32(2):237-249, 1997.
28. Woodson LC: Diagnosis and grading of inhalation injury, J Burn Care Res 30(1):143-145, 2009.
29. Miller K, Chang A: Acute inhalation injury, Emerg Med Clin North Am 21:533-557, 2003.
30. Kao CC, Garner WL: Acute burns, Plast Reconstr Surg 101(7):2482-2493, 2000.

31. Schiller WR: Burn care and inhalation injury. In Grenvik A, editor: Textbook of critical care, ed 4, Philadelphia, 2000, Saunders, pp 365-377.

32. Desai MH, Herndon DN: Burns. In Trunkey DD, Lewis FR, Decker BC, editors: Current therapy of trauma, ed 3, Philadelphia, 1991, Mosby, p 315.

33. Abraham E: Toxic gas and inhalation injury. In Brenner BE, editor: Comprehensive management of respiratory emergencies, Rockville, MD, 1995, Aspen, p 241.

34. Traber DL, Herndon DN: Pathophysiology of smoke inhalation. In Haponik EF, Munster AM, editors: Respiratory injury: smoke inhalation and burns, New York, 1990, McGraw-Hill, p 61.

35. Crapo RO: Causes of respiratory injury. In Haponik EF, Munster AM, editors: Respiratory injury: smoke inhalation and burns, New York, 1990, McGraw-Hill, p 47.

36. Ahrns KS, Harkins DR: Initial resuscitation after burn injury: therapies, strategies, and controversies, AACN Clin Issues 10:46-60, 1999.

37. Edlich RF, Moghtader JC: Thermal burns, ed 4. In Rosen P, editor: Emergency medicine concepts and clinical practice, vol 1, St Louis, 1998, Mosby, pp 941-953.

38. Gomez R, Cancio LC: Management of burn wounds in the emergency department, Emerg Med Clin North Am 25(1):135-146, 2007.

39. Faucher L, Furukawa K: Practice guidelines for the management of pain, J Burn Care Res 27(5):659-668, 2006.

40. Jordan BS, Harrington DT: Management of the burn wound, Nurs Clin North Am 32(2):251-271, 1997.

41. Linares HA: Pathophysiology of burn scar. In Herndon DN, editor: Total burn care, London, 1996, Saunders, p 383.

42. Ward RS: Burns. In Cameron MH, Monroe LG, editors: Physical rehabilitation: evidence-based examination, evaluation, and intervention, St Louis, 2007, Saunders.

43. Kumar V, Abbas AK, Fausto N, et al: Robbins basic pathology, ed 8, Philadelphia, 2007, Saunders, p 77.

44. Pham TN, Gibran NS: Thermal and electrical injuries, Surg Clin North Am 87(1):185-206, 2007.

45. Wild B, Kemp H: Skin cultures in burns care nursing, Nurs Times 95(36):46-49, 1999.

46. Miller SF, Staley MJ, Richard RL: Surgical management of the burn patient. In Richard RI, Staley MH, editors: Burn care rehabilitation principles and practice, Philadelphia, 1994, FA Davis, p 177.

47. Kagan RJ: Skin substitutes: implications for burns and chronic wounds, Adv Wound Care 12(2):94-95, 1999.

48. Richard RL, Staley MJ: Burn patient evaluation and treatment planning. In Richard RI, Staley MH, editors: Burn care rehabilitation principles and practice, Philadelphia, 1994, FA Davis, p 201.

49. Sliwa JA, Heinemann A, Semik P: Inpatient rehabilitation following burn injury: patient demographics and functional outcomes, Arch Phys Med Rehabil 86:1920-1923, 2005.

50. Micheletti G: Ulcers of the lower extremity. In Gogia PP, editor: Clinical wound management, Thorofare, NJ, 1995, Slack, pp 105-106.

51. McCulloch JM: Evaluation of patients with open wounds. In Kloth LC, Miller KH, editors: Wound healing: alternatives in management, Philadelphia, 1995, FA Davis, p 118.

52. Sibbald RG: An approach to leg and foot ulcers: a brief overview, Ostomy Wound Manage 44(9):28-32, 34-35, 1998.

53. Sibbald RG: Venous leg ulcers, Ostomy Wound Manage 44(9):52-64, 1998.

54. Donayre CE: Diagnosis and management of vascular ulcers. In Sussman C, Bates-Jensen B, editors: Wound care: a collaborative practice manual for physical therapists and nurses, Gaithersburg, MD, 1998, Aspen, p 310.

55. Sparks-DeFriese BJ: Vascular ulcers. In Cameron MH, Monroe LG, editors: Physical rehabilitation: evidence-based examination, evaluation, and intervention, St Louis, 2007, Saunders.

56. Brown AC, Sibbald RG: The diabetic neuropathic ulcer: an overview, Ostomy Wound Manage 45(Suppl 1A):6, 1999.

57. Levin ME: Preventing amputation in the patient with diabetes, Diabetes Care 18(10):1383-1394, 1995.

58. Daniels TR: Diabetic foot ulcerations: an overview, Ostomy Wound Manage 44(9):77, 1999.

59. Weiss EL: Connective tissue in wound healing. In Kloth LC, Miller KH, editors: Wound healing: alternatives in management, Philadelphia, 1995, FA Davis, p 26.

60. Laing P: Diabetic foot ulcers, Am J Surg 167(1A):31, 1994.

61. Levin ML, O'Neal LW, Bowker JH: The diabetic foot, ed 5, St Louis, 1993, Mosby.

62. Catanzariti AR, Haverstock BD, Grossman JP et al: Off loading techniques in the treatment of diabetic plantar neuropathic foot ulceration, Adv Wound Care 12(9):452, 1999.

63. Lavery LA, McGuire J, Baronski S, et al: Diabetic foot ulcers, In Baronski S, Ayello EA, editors: Wound care essentials: practice principles, Philadelphia, 2008, Lippincott Williams & Wilkins.

64. Kloth LC, McCulloch JM: The inflammatory response to wounding. In Kloth LC, Miller KH, editors: Wound healing: alternatives in management, Philadelphia, 1995, FA Davis, pp 3-15.

65. Weiss EL: Connective tissue in wound healing. In Kloth LC, Miller KH, editors: Wound healing: alternatives in management, Philadelphia, 1995, FA Davis, pp 16-31.

66. Daly TJ: Contraction and re-epithelialization. In Kloth LC, Miller KH, editors: Wound healing: alternatives in management, Philadelphia, 1995, FA Davis, pp 32-46.

67. Gogia PP: Physiology of wound healing. In Gogia PP, editor: Clinical wound management, Thorofare, NJ, 1995, Slack, pp 1-12.

68. Sussman C: Wound healing biology and chronic wound healing. In Sussman C, Bates-Jensen B, editors: Wound care: a collaborative practice manual for physical therapists and nurses, Gaithersburg, MD, 1998, Aspen, pp 31-47.

69. Keast DH, Orsted H: The basic principles of wound care, Ostomy Wound Manage 44(8):24-31, 1998.

70. Kernstein MD: The scientific basis of healing, Adv Wound Care 10(3):30-36, 1997.

71. Kosiak M: Etiology and pathology of ischemic ulcers, Arch Phys Med Rehabil 40(2):62-69, 1959.

72. Feedar JA: Prevention and management of pressure ulcers. In Kloth LC, Miller KH, editors: Wound healing: alternatives in management, Philadelphia, 1995, FA Davis, pp 187-193.

73. Leigh IH: Pressure ulcers: prevalence, etiology, and treatment modalities. A review, Am J Surg 167(1A):25S-30S, 1994.

74. Feedar JA: Prevention and management of pressure ulcers. In Kloth LC, Miller KH, editors: Wound healing: alternatives in management, Philadelphia, 1995, FA Davis, pp 193-195.

75. The National Pressure Ulcer Advisory Panel's Summary of the AHCPR Clinical Practice Guideline: Pressure ulcers in adults: prediction and prevention (AHCPR Publication No. 92-0047), Rockville, MD, May 1992, AHCPR.

76. Hamm RL: Tissue healing and pressure ulcers. In Cameron MH, Monroe LG, editors: Physical rehabilitation: evidence-based examination, evaluation, and intervention, St Louis, 2007, Saunders.

77. Bolander VP, editor: Sorensen and Luckmann's basic nursing, Philadelphia, 1994, Saunders, p 742.

78. Mulder GD, Brazinsky BA, Seeley JE: Factors complicating wound repair. In Kloth LC, Miller KH, editors: Wound healing: alternatives in management, Philadelphia, 1995, FA Davis, pp 48-49.

79. Bahl SM: Nutritional considerations in wound management. In Gogia PP, editor: Clinical wound management, Thorofare, NJ, 1995, Slack, p 73.
80. DeSanti L: Involuntary weight loss and the nonhealing wound, Adv Skin Wound Care 13(Suppl 1):11-20, 2000.
81. Mulder, GD, Brazinsky, BA, Seeley, JE: Factors complicating wound repair. In Kloth LC, Miller KH, editors: Wound healing: alternatives in management, Philadelphia, 1995, FA Davis, pp 50-51.
82. Keast DH, Orsted H: The basic principles of wound care, Ostomy Wound Manage 44(8):28, 1998.
83. Lazarus G, Cooper DM, Knighton DR, et al: Definitions and guidelines for assessment of wounds and evaluation of healing, Arch Dermatol 130:489-493, 1994.
84. Gallagher SM: Ethical dilemmas in pain management, Ostomy Wound Manage 44(9):20, 1998.
85. Dallam LE, Barkauskas C, Ayello EA, et al: Pain management and wounds. In Baronski S, Ayello EA, editors: Wound care essentials: practice principles, Philadelphia, 2008, Lippincott William & Wilkins.
86. Thomson PD, Smith DJ: What is infection? Am J Surg 167(1A):7S-11S, 1994.
87. Fowler E: Wound infection: a nurse's perspective, Ostomy Wound Manage 44(8):45, 1995.
88. Icrow S: Infection control perspectives. In Krasner D, Kan D, editors: Chronic wound care: a clinical source book for healthcare professionals, Wayne, PA, 1997, Health Management Publications, pp 90-96.
89. Ayello EA, Baronski S, Lyder CH, et al: Pressure ulcers. In Baronoski S, Ayello EA, editors: Wound care essentials: practice principles, ed 2, Philadelphia, 2007, Lippincott Williams & Wilkins.
90. Fowler E: Wound infection: a nurse's perspective, Ostomy Wound Manage 44(8):47, 1995.
91. Gilchrist B: Infection and culturing. In Krasner D, Kane D, editors: Chronic wound care: a clinical source book for healthcare professionals, ed 2, Wayne, PA, 1997, Health Management Publications, pp 109-114.
92. Rodheaver GT: Wound cleaning, wound irrigation and wound disinfection. In Krasner D, Kane D, editors: Chronic wound care: a clinical source book for healthcare professionals, ed 2, Wayne, PA, 1997, Health Management Publications, pp 97-106.
93. Sussman G: Management of the wound environment. In Sussman C, Bates-Jensen B, editors: Wound care: a collaborative practice manual for physical therapists and nurses, Gaithersburg, MD, 1998, Aspen, p 212.
94. Gardner SE, Frantz RA: Wound bioburden. In Baronoski S, Ayello EA, editors: Wound care essentials: practice principles, ed 2, Philadelphia, 2007, Lippincott Williams & Wilkins.
95. Fowler E: Wound infection: a nurse's perspective, Ostomy Wound Manage 44(8):19, 1995.
96. Sieggreen MY, Maklebust JM: Debridement: choices and challenges, Adv Wound Care 10(2):32-37, 1997.
97. Feedar JS: Clinical management of chronic wounds. In Kloth LC, Miller KH, editors: Wound healing: alternatives in management, Philadelphia, 1995, FA Davis, pp 151-156.
98. Rodeheaver GT: Pressure ulcer debridement and cleaning: a review of current literature, Ostomy Wound Manage 45(1A Suppl):80S-87S, 1999.
99. Ayello EA, Baronoski S, et al: Wound debridement. In Baronoski S, Ayello EA, editors: Wound care essentials: practice principles, ed 2, Philadelphia, 2007, Lippincott Williams & Wilkins.
100. Scott RG, Loehne HB: Five questions-and answers-about pulsed lavage, Adv Skin Wound Care 13(3):133-134, 2000.
101. Loehne HB: Pulsatile lavage with concurrent suction. In Sussman C, Bates-Jensen B, editors: Wound care: a collaborative practice manual for physical therapists and nurses, Gaithersburg, MD, 1998, Aspen, pp 389-403.
102. Sussman C: Whirlpool. In Sussman C, Bates-Jensen B, editors: Wound care: a collaborative practice manual for physical therapists and nurses, Gaithersburg, MD, 1998, Aspen, pp 447-454.
103. Cuzell, J, Krasner, D: Wound dressings. In Gogia PP, editor: Clinical wound management, Thorofare, NJ, 1995, Slack, pp 131-144.
104. Feedar JS: Clinical management of chronic wounds. In Kloth LC, Miller KH, editors: Wound healing: alternatives in management, Philadelphia, 1995, FA Davis, pp 156-169.

Infectious Diseases

Harold Merriman

CHAPTER OBJECTIVES

The objectives of this chapter are to provide a brief understanding of the following:

1. Clinical evaluation of infectious diseases and altered immune disorders, including physical examination and laboratory studies
2. Various infectious disease processes, including etiology, pathogenesis, clinical presentation, and management
3. Commonly encountered altered immune disorders, including etiology, clinical presentation, and management
4. Precautions and guidelines that a physical therapist should implement when treating a patient with an infectious disease process or altered immunity

PREFERRED PRACTICE PATTERNS

The most relevant practice patterns for the diagnoses discussed in this chapter, based on the American Physical Therapy Association's *Guide to Physical Therapist Practice*, second edition, are as follows:

- Health Care–Associated or Nosocomial Infections (*Escherichia coli*, *Staphylococcus aureus*, *Enterococcus faecalis*, *Pseudomonas aeruginosa*, *Candida albicans*, and Coagulase-Negative Staphylococci): 6B, 7A
- Antibiotic-Resistant Infections: Methicillin-Resistant *Staphylococcus aureus*, Vancomycin-Resistant Enterococci, Multi-Drug Resistant *Acinetobacter baumannii*: 6B, 7A
- Upper Respiratory Tract Infections (Rhinitis, Sinusitis, Influenza, Pertussis): 6B, 6F, 6G
- Lower Respiratory Tract Infections (Tuberculosis, Histoplasmosis, Legionellosis, Severe Acute Respiratory Syndrome [SARS]): 6B, 7C, 7D
- Cardiac Infections: Pericarditis, Myocarditis, Left-Sided Endocarditis, Acute Rheumatic Fever, Rheumatic Heart Disease. See Chapter 3: 6B, 6D
- Neurological Diseases: Poliomyelitis, Postpoliomyelitis Syndrome, Meningitis, and Encephalitis: 4A, 5C, 5D, 5G, 6E, 5H, 7A
- Musculoskeletal Infections: Osteomyelitis and Its Variations: 4G, 4H, 5H
- Skin Infections: Cellulitis, groups A and G Streptococcus, and *Staphylococcus aureus*: 4E, 6H, 7B, 7C, 7D, 7E
- Gastrointestinal Infections: Gastroenteritis, *Escherichia coli*, *Shigella*, *Clostridium difficile*, *Salmonella*, Rotavirus, Norovirus, Adenovirus, and Astrovirus: Please refer to Chapter 8
- Immune System Infections: HIV, Mononucleosis, Cytomegalovirus Infection, and Toxoplasmosis: 4C, 6B
- Sepsis: Bacteremia, Septicemia, and Shock Syndrome (or Septic Shock): 5C, 6F, 6H

Please refer to Appendix A for a complete list of the preferred practice patterns, as individual patient conditions are highly variable and other practice patterns may be applicable.

A patient may be admitted to the hospital setting with an infectious disease process acquired in the community or may develop one as a complication from the hospital environment. The current terminology is to call this type of infection a health care–associated infection (HAI). In 2002, the estimated number of HAIs in U.S. hospitals was 1.7 million, resulting in about 99,000 deaths.[1] The major source of HAI is likely the patient's endogenous flora, but up to 40% of HAIs can be caused by cross infection via the hands of health care workers.[2] An infectious disease process generally has a primary site of origin; however, it may result in diffuse systemic effects that may limit the patient's functional mobility and activity tolerance. Therefore a basic understanding of these infectious disease processes is useful in designing, implementing, and modifying physical therapy treatment programs. The physical therapist may also provide treatment for patients who have disorders resulting from altered immunity. These disorders are mentioned in this chapter because immune system reactions can be similar to those of infectious disease processes (see Appendix 13-A for a discussion of four common disorders of altered immunity: systemic lupus erythematosus, sarcoidosis, amyloidosis, and rheumatoid arthritis).

Definition of Terms

To facilitate the understanding of infectious disease processes, terminology that is commonly used when referring to these processes is presented in Table 13-1.[3-6]

Body Structure and Function

A person's immune system is composed of many complex, yet synergistic, components that defend against pathogens (Table 13-2).[3] Any defect in this system may lead to the development of active infection. Patients in the acute care setting often present with acquired factors that can create some or most of

these defects, which can ultimately affect their immune system (Box 13-1).[4] Congenital factors such as lymphocyte deficiency occur rarely.

Evaluation

When an infectious disease process is suspected, a thorough patient interview (history) and physical examination are performed to serve as a screening tool for the differential diagnosis and to help determine which laboratory tests are further required to identify a specific pathogen.[7]

History

Potential contributing factors of the infection are sought out, such as immunocompromise, immunosuppression, recent exposure to infectious individuals, or recent travel to foreign countries. Also, a qualitative description of the symptomatology is discerned, such as onset or nature of symptoms (e.g., a nonproductive versus productive cough over the past days or weeks).

Physical Examination

Observation

Clinical presentation of infectious diseases is highly variable according to the specific system that is involved. However,

TABLE 13-1 Terminology Associated with Infectious Disease Processes

Term	Definition
Antibody	A highly specific protein that is manufactured in response to antigens and defends against subsequent infection.
Antigen (immunogen)	An agent that is capable of producing antibodies when introduced into the body of a susceptible person.
Carrier	A person who harbors an infectious agent that can cause a specific disease but who demonstrates no evidence of the disease.
Colonization	The process of a group of organisms living together; the host can carry the microorganism without being symptomatic (no signs of infection).
Communicable	The ability of an infective organism to be transmitted from person to person, either directly or indirectly.
Disseminated host	Distributed over a considerable area. The person whom the infectious agent invades and from whom it gathers its nourishment.
Health care–associated infection (HAI)	Localized or systemic condition resulting from an adverse reaction to the presence of an infectious agents(s) or its toxin(s); there must be no evidence that the infection was present or incubating at the time of admission to the acute care setting.
Immunocompromised	An immune system that is incapable of a normal response to pathogenic organisms and tissue damage.
Immunodeficiency	Decreased or compromised ability to respond to antigenic stimuli by appropriate cellular immunity reaction.
Immunosuppression	The prevention or diminution of the immune response, as by drugs or radiation.
Nosocomial infection	Infection acquired in the hospital setting; note that this has been replaced by HAI (see above).
Opportunistic	An infectious process that develops in immunosuppressed individuals. (Opportunistic infections normally do not develop in individuals with intact immune systems.)
Pathogen	An organism capable of producing a disease.
Subclinical infection	A disease or condition that does not produce clinical symptoms, or the time period before the appearance of disease-specific symptoms.

TABLE 13-2 Components of the Immune System

Lines of Defense	Components	Description
First line of defense	Skin, conjunctivae, mucous membranes	Physical barriers to pathogens.
Second line of defense	Inflammatory response	Inflammatory response acts to (1) contain pathogens and (2) bring immune cells to antigens by releasing histamine, kinins, and prostaglandins that cause vasodilation and vascular permeability.
Third line of defense	Immune response Humoral immunity (B cells)* Cellular immunity (T cells)*	Specific immune response to pathogens. B cells produce antibodies. T cells: (1) Augment production of antibodies. (2) Directly kill antigens. (3) Turn off immune system.

Data from NS Rote: Immunity. In SE Heuther, KL McCance, editors: Understanding pathophysiology, ed 2, St Louis, 2000, Mosby, pp 125-150; Marieb EN, editor: Human anatomy and physiology, ed 2, Redwood City, CA, 1992, Benjamin Cummings, pp 690-723; Guyton AC, Hall JE: Textbook of medical physiology, ed 9, Philadelphia, 1996, Saunders, pp 445-455.

*B cells and T cells can also be referred to as B lymphocytes and T lymphocytes, respectively.

BOX 13-1 Factors Affecting the Immune System

- Pregnancy
- Preexisting infections
- Malignancies (Hodgkin's disease, acute or chronic leukemia, nonlymphoid malignancy, or myeloma)
- Stress (emotional or surgical—anesthesia)
- Malnutrition (insufficiency of calories, protein, iron, and zinc)
- Age
- Chronic diseases (diabetes, alcoholic cirrhosis, sickle cell anemia)
- Lymph node dissection
- Immunosuppressive treatment (corticosteroids, chemotherapy, or radiation therapy)
- Indwelling lines and tubes

Data from Rote NS, Heuther SE, McCance KL: Hypersensitivities, infection, and immunodeficiencies. In Heuther SE, McCance KL, editors: Understanding pathophysiology, ed 2, St Louis, 2000, Mosby, pp 204-208.

---

common physical findings that occur with infection include sweating and inflammation, both of which are related to the metabolic response of the body to the antigen. The classic signs of inflammation (redness [rubor], and swelling [tumor]) in certain areas of the body can help delineate the source, location(s), or both of infection. Delineating the source of infection is crucial to the diagnostic process.

Palpation

The presence of warmth (calor) and possible pain (dolor) or tenderness is another typical classic sign of inflammation that may be consistent with active infection. Lymphoid organs (lymph nodes and spleen) can also be swollen and tender with infection, because lymphocytes (processed in these organs) are multiplying in response to the antigen. Inflammation and tenderness in these or other areas of the body can further help to delineate the infectious process.

Vital Signs

Heart Rate, Blood Pressure, and Respiratory Rate. Measurement of vital signs helps in determining whether an infectious process is occurring. (Infections result in an increased metabolic rate, which presents as an increased heart rate and

respiratory rate.) Blood pressure may also be elevated when metabolism is increased, or blood pressure can be decreased secondary to vasodilation from inflammatory responses in the body.

Temperature. Monitoring the patient's temperature over time (both throughout the day and daily) provides information regarding the progression (a rise in temperature) or a regression (a fall in temperature) of the infectious process. With an infectious process, some of the bacteria and extracts from normal leukocytes are pyrogenic, causing the thermostat in the hypothalamus to rise, resulting in an elevated body temperature.[8] A fall in body temperature from a relatively elevated temperature may also signify a response to a medication.

> ✎ **CLINICAL TIP**
>
> An afebrile status is not always indicative of the absence of infection. If a patient is on antipyretics, the fever symptoms may be controlled. Check the medication list and ask about the administration schedule. A patient must be afebrile for at least 24 hours before being discharged from an inpatient setting.

Auscultation

Heart and lung sounds determine whether infectious processes are a direct result from these areas or are indirectly affecting these areas. Refer to Chapters 3 and 4, respectively, for more information on heart and lung auscultation.

Laboratory Studies

Most of the evaluation process for diagnosing an infectious disease is based on laboratory studies. These studies are performed to (1) isolate the microorganisms from various body fluids or sites; (2) directly examine specimens by microscopic, immunologic, or genetic techniques; or (3) assess specific antibody responses to the pathogen.[9] This diagnostic process is essential to prescribing the most specific medical regimen possible for the patient.

Hematology

During hematologic studies, a sample of blood is taken and analyzed to assist in determining the presence of an infectious process or organism. Hematologic procedures used to diagnose infection include leukocyte count, differential white blood cell (WBC) count, and antibody measurement.[10]

Leukocyte Count. Leukocyte, or WBC, count is measured to determine whether an infectious process is present and should range between 5000 and 10,000 cells/mm[3].[3] An increase in the number of WBCs, termed *leukocytosis*, is required for phagocytosis (cellular destruction of microorganisms) and can indicate the presence of an acute infectious process.[11] Leukocytosis can also be present with inflammation and may occur after a surgery with postoperative inflammation.[8] A decreased WBC count from baseline, termed *leukopenia*, can indicate altered immunity or the presence of an infection that exhausts supplies of certain WBCs.[11] A decreased WBC count relative to a previously high count (i.e., becoming more within normal limits) may indicate the resolution of an infectious process.[11]

Differential White Blood Cell Count. Five types of WBCs exist: lymphocytes, monocytes, neutrophils, basophils, and eosinophils. Specific types of infectious processes can trigger alterations in the values of one or more of these cells. Detection of these changes can assist in identification of the type of infection present. For example, an infection caused by bacteria can result in a higher percentage of neutrophils, which have a normal range of 2.0 to 7.5×10^9/liter. In contrast, a parasitic infection will result in increased eosinophils, which have a normal count of 0.0 to 0.45×10^9/liter.[11]

Antibody Measurement. Antibodies develop in response to the invasion of antigens from new infectious agents. Identifying the presence and concentration of specific antibodies helps in determining past and present exposure to infectious organisms.[12]

Microbiology

In microbiology studies, specimens from suspected sources of infection (e.g., sputum, urine, feces, wounds, and cerebrospinal fluid) are collected by sterile technique and analyzed by staining, culture, or sensitivity or resistance testing, or a combination of all of these.

Staining. Staining allows for morphologic examination of organisms under a microscope. Two types of staining techniques are available: simple staining and the more advanced differential staining. Many types of each technique exist, but the differential Gram's stain is the most common.[12]

Gram's stain is used to differentiate similar organisms by categorizing them as gram-positive or gram-negative. This separation assists in determining subsequent measures to be taken for eventual identification of the organism. A specimen is placed on a microscope slide, and a series of steps are performed.[13] A red specimen at completion indicates a gram-negative organism, whereas a violet specimen indicates a gram-positive organism.[13]

Culture. The purpose of a culture is to identify and produce isolated colonies of organisms found within a collected specimen. Cells of the organism are isolated and mixed with specific media that provide the proper nourishment and environment (e.g., pH level, oxygen content) needed for the organism to reproduce into colonies. Once this has taken place, the resultant

infectious agent is observed for size, shape, elevation, texture, marginal appearance, and color to assist with identification.[13]

Sensitivity and Resistance. When an organism has been isolated from a specimen, its sensitivity (susceptibility) to antimicrobial agents or antibiotics is tested. An infectious agent is sensitive to an antibiotic when the organism's growth is inhibited under safe dose concentrations. Conversely, an agent is resistant to an antibiotic when its growth is not inhibited by safe dose concentrations. Because of a number of factors, such as mutations, an organism's sensitivity, resistance, or both to antibiotics are constantly changing.[14]

Cytology

Cytology is a complex method of studying cellular structures, functions, origins, and formations. Cytology assists in differentiating between an infectious process and a malignancy and in determining the type and severity of a present infectious process by examining cellular characteristics.[12,15] It is beyond the scope of this book, however, to describe all of the processes involved in studying cellular structure dysfunction.

Body Fluid Examination

Pleural Tap. A pleural tap, or thoracentesis, is the process by which a needle is inserted through the chest wall into the pleural cavity to collect pleural fluid for examination of possible malignancy, infection, inflammation, or any combination of these. A thoracentesis may also be performed to drain excessive pleural fluid in large pleural effusions.[16]

Pericardiocentesis. Pericardiocentesis is a procedure that involves accessing the pericardial space around the heart with a needle or cannula to aspirate fluid for drainage, analysis, or both. It is primarily used to assist in diagnosing infections, inflammation, and malignancies and to relieve effusions built up by these disorders.[17]

Synovial Fluid Analysis. Synovial fluid analysis, or arthrocentesis, involves aspirating synovial fluid from a joint capsule. The fluid is then analyzed and used to assist in diagnosing infections, rheumatic diseases, and osteoarthritis, all of which can produce increased fluid production within the joint.[18]

Gastric Lavage. A gastric lavage is the suctioning of gastric contents through a nasogastric tube to examine the contents for the presence of sputum in patients suspected of having tuberculosis. The assumption is that patients swallow sputum while they sleep. If sputum is found in the gastric contents, the appropriate sputum analysis should be performed to help confirm the diagnosis of tuberculosis.[16,19] Historically, gastric lavage has also been administered as a medical intervention to prevent absorption of ingested toxins in the acutely poisoned patient, although its use for this purpose is now rarely recommended.[20]

Peritoneal Fluid Analysis. Peritoneal fluid analysis, or paracentesis, is the aspiration of peritoneal fluid with a needle. It is performed to (1) drain excess fluid, or ascites, from the peritoneal cavity, which can be caused by infectious diseases, such as tuberculosis; (2) assist in the diagnosis of hepatic or systemic malfunctions, diseases, infection such as spontaneous bacterial peritonitis (SBP), or malignancies; and (3) help detect the presence of abdominal trauma.[16,19,21]

Other Studies

Imaging with plain x-rays, computed tomography scans, positron emission tomography, and magnetic resonance imaging scans can also help identify areas with infectious lesions.[22,23] Minuscule amounts of pathogens can be detected by using the molecular biology techniques of enzyme-linked immunosorbent assay (ELISA), radioimmunoassay (RIA), and polymerase chain reaction (PCR).[24,25] In addition, the following diagnostic studies can also be performed to help with the differential diagnosis of the infectious process. For a description of these studies, refer to the sections and chapters indicated below:

- Sputum analysis (see Chapter 4)
- Cerebrospinal fluid (see Chapter 6)
- Urinalysis (see Chapter 9)
- Wound cultures (Chapter 12)

Health Conditions

Various infectious disease processes, which are commonly encountered in the acute care setting, are described in the following sections. Certain disease processes that are not included in this section are described in other chapters. Please consult the index for assistance.

Health Care–Associated or Nosocomial Infections

Nosocomial infection is an older general term that refers to an infection that is acquired in the hospital setting. Since 2008 the Centers for Disease Control and Prevention (CDC) has used the generic term *health care–associated infections* instead of *nosocomial*.[6] Many pathogens can cause an HAI, but the most commonly reported bacteria in past years have been *Escherichia coli*, *Staphylococcus aureus*, *Enterococcus faecalis*, *Pseudomonas aeruginosa*, *Candida albicans*, and coagulase-negative staphylococci.[26,27] Patients who are at risk for developing HAIs are those who present with[28]:

1. Age: the very young or the very old
2. Immunodeficiency: chronic diseases (cancer, chronic renal disease, chronic obstructive pulmonary disease, diabetes, or acquired immunodeficiency syndrome [AIDS])
3. Immunosuppression: chemotherapy, radiation therapy, or corticosteroids
4. Misuse of antibiotics: overprescription of antibiotics or use of broad-spectrum antibiotics, leading to the elimination of a patient's normal flora, which allows for the colonization of pathogens and development of drug-resistant organisms
5. Use of invasive diagnostic and therapeutic procedures: indwelling urinary catheters, monitoring devices, intravenous (IV) catheters, and mechanical ventilation with intubation
6. Agitation: Resulting in removal of medical equipment such as central venous catheters or self-extubation of artificial airways
7. Surgery: incisions provide access to pathogens
8. Burns: disrupt the first line of defense
9. Length of hospitalization: increases the exposure to pathogens and medical intervention

The mode of transmission for pathogens that cause HAIs can vary from contact to airborne. Pathogens can also become opportunistic in patients who are immunocompromised or immunosuppressed. Common sites for HAIs are in the urinary tract, surgical wounds, joints, and the lower respiratory tract (e.g., pneumonia). Clinical manifestations and management of HAIs vary according to the type of pathogen and the organ system involved. However, the primary management strategy for HAIs is prevention by following the standard and specific precautions outlined in Table 13-3.[9,26,29,30]

> ### ✎ CLINICAL TIP
>
> Prevention or minimizing the risk of developing a pneumonia in patients who have been on bed rest and/or on mechanical intervention can be achieved through chest physical therapy and increased mobility. (Refer to Table 4-12, Dean's Hierarchy for Treatment of Patients with Impaired Oxygen Transport.)

TABLE 13-3   Summary of Precautions to Prevent Infection

Precaution	Description
Standard	Treat all patient situations as potentially infectious. Wash hands before and after each patient contact. Wear a different set of gloves with each patient. If splashing of body fluids is likely, wear a mask or face shield, or both, and a gown.
Airborne*	A mask is required in situations where contagious pathogens can be transmitted by airborne droplet nuclei, as in the case of measles, varicella (chickenpox), or tuberculosis.
Droplet*	A mask or face shield, or both, are required when large-particle droplet transmission (usually 3 ft or less) is likely. Droplet transmission involves contact of the conjunctivae or the mucous membranes of the nose or mouth with large-particle droplets (larger than 5 μm in size) generated from coughing, sneezing, talking, and certain procedures, such as suctioning and bronchoscopy. Examples of pathogens requiring droplet precautions are *Haemophilus influenzae*, *Neisseria meningitidis*, mycoplasmal pneumonia, streptococcal pneumonia, mumps, and rubella.
Contact*	Gown and gloves are required when pathogens are transmitted by direct person-to-person contact or person-to-object contact. Examples of these pathogens include *Acinetobacter baumannii*, *Clostridium difficile*, *Escherichia coli*, herpes simplex virus, herpes zoster, methicillin-resistant *Staphylococcus aureus*, and vancomycin-resistant *Enterococcus*.

Data from Rice D, Eckstein EC: Inflammation and infection. In Phipps WJ, Sands JK, Marek JF, editors: Medical-surgical nursing, concepts and clinical practice, ed 6, St Louis, 1999, Mosby, pp 237-245; Anderson KN, editor: Mosby's medical, nursing, and allied health dictionary, ed 5, St Louis, 1998, Mosby, p 2BA5.

*These precautions are in addition to practicing Standard Precautions.

Antibiotic-Resistant Infections

The number of antibiotic-resistance infections is growing in health care facilities. Approximately 50% of antibiotic use in hospitals is unnecessary or inappropriate. In response to this problem, the CDC has launched a program called "Get Smart for Healthcare" whose goals include reducing unnecessary antibiotic use (resulting in less antimicrobial resistance), decreasing health care costs, and improving patient outcomes in hospitals and long-term care facilities.[31]

Microbial experts from the European Centre for Disease Prevention and Control and in the United States from the CDC have recently developed interim standard terminology to describe this resistance.[32] They developed three major definitions for resistance: multidrug-resistant (MDR), extensively drug-resistant (XDR), and pandrug-resistant (PDR) bacteria. The agreed-on definitions are MDR as acquired nonsusceptibility to at least one agent in three or more antimicrobial categories, XDR as nonsusceptibility to at least one agent in all but two or fewer antimicrobial categories (i.e., remaining susceptible to only one or two categories), and PDR as nonsusceptibility to all agents in all antimicrobial categories.

Methicillin-Resistant *Staphylococcus aureus* Infection.

Methicillin-resistant *S. aureus* (MRSA) is a strain of *Staphylococcus* that is resistant to methicillin or similar agents, such as oxacillin and nafcillin. Methicillin is a synthetic form of penicillin and was developed because *S. aureus* developed resistance to penicillin, which was originally the treatment choice for *S. aureus* infection. However, since the early 1980s, this particular strain of *S. aureus* has become increasingly resistant to methicillin. The contributing factor that is suggested to have a primary role in the increased incidence of this HAI is the indiscriminate use of antibiotic therapy.[30,33]

In addition, patients who are at risk for developing MRSA infection in the hospital are patients who[33-35]:

- Are debilitated, elderly, or both
- Are hospitalized for prolonged time periods
- Have multiple surgical or invasive procedures, an indwelling cannula, or both
- Are taking multiple antibiotics, antimicrobial treatments, or both
- Are undergoing treatment in critical care units

MRSA is generally transmitted by person-to-person contact or person-to-object-to-person contact. MRSA can survive for prolonged periods of time on inanimate objects, such as telephones, bed rails, and tray tables, unless such objects are properly sanitized. Hospital personnel can be primary carriers of MRSA, as the bacterium can be colonized in healthy adults. MRSA infections can be diagnosed via nasal swabs.[36]

Management of MRSA is difficult and may consist of combining local and systemic antibiotics, increasing antibiotic dosages, and applying whole-body antiseptic solutions. In recent years, vancomycin has become the treatment of choice for MRSA; however, evidence has shown that patients with this strain of *S. aureus* are also developing resistance to vancomycin (vancomycin intermediate *S. aureus*—VISA).[30] Therefore prevention of MRSA infection is the primary treatment strategy and includes the following[26,33-35]:

- Placing patients with MRSA infection on isolation or contact precautions
- Strict hand-washing regulations before and after patient care using proper disinfecting agent
- Use of gloves, gowns (if soiling is likely), or both
- Disinfection of all contaminated objects

Vancomycin-Resistant Enterococci Infection.

Vancomycin-resistant enterococci (VRE) infection is another HAI that has become resistant to vancomycin, aminoglycosides, and ampicillin. The infection can develop as endogenous enterococci (normally found in the gastrointestinal or the female reproductive tract) become opportunistic in patient populations similar to those mentioned earlier with MRSA. VRE infections can be diagnosed via rectal swab.[26,30,37,38]

Transmission of the infection can also occur by (1) direct patient-to-patient contact, (2) indirect contact through asymptomatic hospital personnel who can carry the opportunistic strain of the microorganism, or (3) contact with contaminated equipment or environmental surfaces.

Management of VRE infection is difficult, as the enterococcus can withstand harsh environments and easily survive on the hands of health care workers and on hospital objects. Treatment options are very limited for patients with VRE, and the best intervention plan is to prevent the spread of the infectious process.[30] Strategies for preventing VRE infections include the following[37]:

- The controlled use of vancomycin
- Timely communication between the microbiology laboratory and appropriate personnel to initiate contact precautions as soon as VRE is detected
- Implementation of screening procedures to detect VRE infection in hospitals where VRE has not yet been detected (i.e., randomly culturing potentially infected items or patients)
- Preventing the transmission of VRE by placing patients in isolation or grouping patients with VRE together, wearing gown and gloves (which need to be removed inside the patient's room), and washing hands immediately after working with an infected patient
- Designating commonly used items, such as stethoscopes and rectal thermometers, to be used only with VRE patients
- Disinfecting any item that has been in contact with VRE patients with the hospital's approved cleaning agent

Multidrug-Resistant *Acinetobacter baumannii*.

Over the past decade *Acinetobacter baumannii* (AB) has become one of the most difficult pathogens to effectively treat because it easily acquires a wide spectrum of antimicrobial resistance, resulting in the commonly found MDR and the much more serious but fortunately rarer PDR forms. It is a gram-negative coccobacillus that has become one of the most important pathogens, particularly in the intensive care unit (ICU). AB infections in the hospital can cause serious complications such as ventilator-associated pneumonia (VAP), bloodstream infection, wound infections, and nosocomial meningitis.[39,40]

AB is remarkable in that it is ubiquitous, exists in diverse habitats (e.g., human skin), can survive for long periods of time on dry inanimate surfaces (e.g., hospital bed rails) and as already mentioned can acquire antimicrobial resistance extremely rapidly. These factors combined, especially the latter two, greatly facilitate MDR-AB outbreaks in the ICU, in physical therapy wound clinics and even multi-facility outbreaks.[41,42] Fortunately, strict infection-control measures (e.g., contact isolation precautions outlined in Table 13-3 and in guidelines for physical therapy intervention at the end of the chapter) can decrease health care staff and environmental colonization and/or contamination.[43] MDR-AB and PDR-AB infections can also be prevented by following the previously mentioned guidelines effective against MRSA and VRE.

> ✎ **CLINICAL TIP**
>
> Equipment used during physical therapy treatments for patients with antibiotic-resistant bacteria (e.g., MRSA, VRE, or MDR-AB), such as assistive devices, gait belts, cuff weights, or goniometers, should be left in the patient's room and not be taken out until the infection is resolved. If there is an equipment shortage, thorough cleaning of the equipment is necessary before using the equipment with other patients. Linens, hospital curtains, and laboratory coats also need to be properly cleaned to avoid transmission of infection.

Respiratory Tract Infections

Infections of the respiratory tract can be categorized as upper or lower respiratory tract infections. Upper respiratory tract infections that are discussed in this section consist of allergic and viral rhinitis, sinusitis, influenza, and pertussis. Lower respiratory tract infections that are discussed in this section consist of tuberculosis, histoplasmosis, legionellosis, and severe acute respiratory syndrome. Pneumonia is the most common lower respiratory tract infection and is discussed under Health Conditions in Chapter 4.

Upper Respiratory Tract Infections

Rhinitis. Rhinitis is the inflammation of the nasal mucous membranes and can result from an allergic reaction or viral infection. Allergic rhinitis is commonly a seasonal reaction from allergens, such as pollen, or a perennial reaction from environmental triggers, such as pet dander or smoke. Viral rhinitis, sometimes referred to as the common cold, is caused by a wide variety of viruses that can be transmitted by airborne particles or by contact.

Clinical manifestations of allergic and viral rhinitis include nasal congestion; sneezing; watery, itchy eyes and nose; altered sense of smell; and thin, watery nasal discharge. In addition to these, clinical manifestations of viral rhinitis include fever, malaise, headache, and thicker nasal discharge.

Management of allergic rhinitis includes antihistamines, decongestants, nasal corticosteroid sprays, and allergen avoidance. Management of viral rhinitis includes rest, fluids, antipyretics, and analgesics.[44-46]

Sinusitis. Sinusitis is the inflammation or hypertrophy of the mucosal lining of any or all of the facial sinuses (frontal, ethmoid, sphenoid, and maxillary). This inflammation can result from bacterial, viral, or fungal infection.

Clinical manifestations of sinusitis include pain over the affected sinus, purulent nasal drainage, nasal obstruction, congestion, fever, and malaise.

Management of sinusitis includes antibiotics (as appropriate), decongestants or expectorants, and nasal corticosteroids.[45]

> ✎ **CLINICAL TIP**
>
> Despite the benign nature of rhinitis and sinusitis, the manifestations (especially nasal drainage and sinus pain) of these infections can be very disturbing to the patient and therapist during the therapy session and may lower the tolerance of the patient for a given activity. The therapist should be sympathetic to the patient's symptoms and adjust the activity accordingly.

Influenza. Influenza (the flu) is caused by any of the influenza viruses (A, B, or C and their mutagenic strains) that are transmitted by aerosolized mucous droplets. These viruses have the ability to change over time and are the reason why a great number of patients are at risk for developing this infection. Influenza B is the most likely virus to cause an outbreak within a community. Health care workers should be vaccinated against the influenza virus to decrease the risk of transmission.

Clinical manifestations of influenza include (1) a severe cough, (2) abrupt onset of fever and chills, (3) headache, (4) backache, (5) myalgia, (6) prostration (exhaustion), (7) coryza (nasal inflammation with profuse discharge), and (8) mild sore throat. Gastrointestinal signs and symptoms of nausea, vomiting, abdominal pain, and diarrhea can also present in certain cases. The disease is usually self-limiting in uncomplicated cases, with symptoms resolving in 7 to 10 days. A complication of influenza infection is pneumonia, especially in the elderly and chronically diseased individuals.[3,4,16,45]

> ✎ **CLINICAL TIP**
>
> A rapid flu nasal swab can diagnose influenza. If results have not come back or they are positive, wear a simple face mask to prevent transmission.

If management of influenza is necessary, it may include the following[3,4,16,45]:

- Antiinfective agents
- Antipyretic agents
- Adrenergic agents
- Antitussive agents
- Active immunization by vaccines
- Supportive care with IV fluids and supplemental oxygen, as needed

Pertussis. Pertussis, or whooping cough, is an acute bacterial infection of the mucous membranes of the tracheobronchial tree, and recently the number of cases has been increasing in the United States.[47] It occurs most commonly in children younger than 1 year and in children and adults of lower socioeconomic populations. The defining characteristics are violent cough spasms that end with an inspiratory "whoop," followed by the expulsion of clear tenacious secretions. Symptoms may last 1 to 2 months. Pertussis is transmitted through airborne particles and is highly contagious.[48]

Management of pertussis may include any of the following[16,48]:

- Antiinfective and antiinflammatory medications
- Bronchopulmonary hygiene with endotracheal suctioning, as needed
- Supplemental oxygen, assisted ventilation, or both
- Fluid and electrolyte replacement
- Active immunization by vaccines
- Respiratory isolation for 3 weeks after the onset of coughing spasms or 7 days after antimicrobial therapy

Lower Respiratory Tract Infections

Tuberculosis. Tuberculosis (TB) is a chronic pulmonary and extrapulmonary infectious disease caused by the tubercle bacillus. It is transmitted through airborne *Mycobacterium tuberculosis* particles, which are expelled into the air when an individual with pulmonary or laryngeal TB coughs or sneezes.[49] When *M. tuberculosis* reaches the alveolar surface of a new host, it is attacked by macrophages, and one of two outcomes can result: Macrophages kill the particles, terminating the infectious process, or the particles multiply within the WBCs, eventually causing them to burst. This cycle is then repeated for a variable time frame between 2 and 12 weeks, after which time the individual is considered to be infected with TB and will test positive on tuberculin skin tests, such as the Mantoux test, which uses tuberculin-purified protein derivative,* or the multiple puncture test, which uses tuberculin. At this point, the infection enters a latent period (most common) or develops into active TB.[49,50]

A six-category classification system has been devised by the American Thoracic Society and the Centers for Disease Control and Prevention (CDC) to describe the TB status of an individual.[49,51]

1. No TB exposure, not infected
2. TB exposure, no evidence of infection
3. Latent TB infection, no disease
4. TB, clinically active
5. TB, not clinically active
6. TB suspect (diagnosis pending)

> ✎ **CLINICAL TIP**
>
> Patients with TB are placed, if available, in negative-pressure isolation rooms. This results in air flowing into, but not out of, the isolation room, thus preventing the escape of contaminated air into the rest of the building. Patients who are suspected of TB, but have not been diagnosed with it, are generally placed on "rule-out TB" protocol, in which case respiratory precautions should be observed.

---

*A person who has been exposed to the tubercle bacillus will demonstrate a raised and reddened area 2 to 3 days after being injected with the protein derivative of the bacilli.

Populations at high risk for acquiring TB include (1) the elderly; (2) Native Americans, Eskimos, and African-Americans (in particular if they are homeless or economically disadvantaged); (3) incarcerated individuals; (4) immigrants from Southeast Asia, Ethiopia, Mexico, and Latin America; (5) malnourished individuals; (6) infants and children younger than 5 years of age; (7) those with decreased immunity (e.g., from AIDS or leukemia, or after chemotherapy); (8) those with diabetes mellitus, end-stage renal disease, or both; (9) those with silicosis; and (10) those in close contact with individuals with active TB.[5,49]

Persons with normal immune function do not normally develop active TB after acquisition and are therefore not considered contagious. Risk factors for the development of active TB after infection include age (children younger than 8 years and adolescents are at greatest risk), low weight, and immunosuppression.[52]

When active TB does develop, its associated signs and symptoms include (1) fever, (2) an initial nonproductive cough, (3) mucopurulent secretions that present later, and (4) hemoptysis, dyspnea at rest or with exertion, adventitious breath sounds at lung apices, pleuritic chest pain, hoarseness, and dysphagia, all of which may occur in the later stages. Chest films also show abnormalities, such as atelectasis or cavitation involving the apical and posterior segments of the right upper lobe, the apical-posterior segment of the left upper lobe, or both.[49]

Extrapulmonary TB occurs with less frequency than pulmonary TB but affects up to 70% of human immunodeficiency virus (HIV)-positive individuals diagnosed with TB.[53] Organs affected include the meninges, brain, blood vessels, kidneys, bones, joints, larynx, skin, intestines, lymph nodes, peritoneum, and eyes. When multiple organ systems are affected, the term *disseminated,* or *miliary,* TB is used.[53] Signs and symptoms that manifest are dependent on the particular organ system or systems involved.

Because of the high prevalence of TB in HIV-positive individuals (up to 60% in some states),[53] it should be noted that the areas of involvement and clinical features of the disease in this population differ from those normally seen, particularly in cases of advanced immunosuppression. Brain abscesses, lymph node involvement, lower lung involvement, pericarditis, gastric TB, and scrotal TB are all more common in HIV-positive individuals. HIV also increases the likelihood that TB infection will progress to active TB by impairing the body's ability to suppress new and latent infections.[53]

Management of TB may include the following[3,4,16]:

- Antiinfective agents (see Chapter 19, Table 19-36, Antitubercular Agents)
- Corticosteroids
- Surgical intervention to remove cavitary lesions (rare) and areas of the lung with extensive disease or to correct hemoptysis, spontaneous pneumothorax, abscesses, intestinal obstruction, ureteral stricture, or any combination of these
- Respiratory isolation until antimicrobial therapy is initiated
- Blood and body fluid precautions if extrapulmonary disease is present

- Skin testing (i.e., Mantoux test and multiple puncture test)
- Vaccination for prevention

In recent years, new strains of *M. tuberculosis* that are resistant to antitubercular drugs (e.g., isoniazid, rifampin, and pyrazinamide) have emerged. These multidrug-resistant TB strains are associated with fatality rates as high as 89% and are common in HIV-infected individuals. Treatment includes the use of direct observational therapy (DOT) and direct observational therapy, short-course (DOTS). These programs designate health care workers to observe individuals to ensure that they take their medications for the entire treatment regimen or for a brief period, respectively, in hopes of minimizing resistance.[53]

✎ CLINICAL TIP

Facilities should provide health care workers personal protective equipment (PPE) effective against TB such as either specialized masks (e.g., N-95) or powered air-purifying respirators (PAPR) to wear around patients on respiratory precautions. These types of PPE are protective against the airborne TB mycobacterium. Always verify with the nursing staff or physician before working with these patients to determine which type of PPE to wear.

Histoplasmosis. Histoplasmosis is a pulmonary and systemic infection that is caused by infective spores (fungi), most commonly found in the soil of the central and eastern United States. Histoplasmosis is transmitted by inhalation of dust from the soil or bird and bat feces. The spores form lesions within the lung parenchyma that can be spread to other tissues. The incidence of fungal infection is rising, particularly in immunocompromised, immunosuppressed, and chronically debilitated individuals who may also be receiving corticosteroid, antineoplastic, and multiple antibiotic therapy.[54,55]

Different clinical forms of histoplasmosis are (1) acute, benign respiratory disease, which results in flulike illness and pneumonia; (2) acute disseminated disease, which can result in septic-type fever; (3) chronic disseminated disease, which involves lesions in the bone marrow, spleen, and lungs and can result in immunodeficiency; and (4) chronic pulmonary disease, which manifests as progressive emphysema.

Management of histoplasmosis may include the following[16,54,56,57]:

- Antiinfective agents
- Corticosteroids
- Antihistamines
- Antifungal therapy (see Chapter 19, Table 19-35, Antifungal Agents)
- Supportive care appropriate for affected areas in the various forms of histoplasmosis

Legionellosis. *Legionellosis* is commonly referred to as *Legionnaire's disease* after a pneumonia outbreak in people who attended an American Legion Convention in Philadelphia in 1976. It is an acute bacterial infection primarily resulting in high fever and pneumonia (patchy or confluent consolidation). *Legionella pneumophila* causes more than 80% of all cases of legionellosis. However, organs beside the lungs may also become involved, especially in the immunocompromised patient. Other risk factors include underlying chronic pulmonary disease, smoking history, and age greater than 50 years. Legionellosis is transmitted by inhalation of aerosolized organisms from infected water sources, such as air-conditioning cooling towers for large buildings including hospitals. Additional examples of infected hospital water sources have included shower heads, tap water from respiratory devices, ice machines, decorative fountains, and even distilled water.[3,58-60]

Primary clinical manifestations include high fever, pneumonia, malaise, myalgia, headache, and nonproductive cough. Other manifestations can also include diarrhea, confusion and other gastrointestinal symptoms. The disease is rapidly progressive during the first 4 to 6 days of illness, with complications that may include renal failure, bacteremic shock, and respiratory failure.[3,59]

Management of legionellosis may consist of the following[3]:

- Antiinfective agents
- Supplemental oxygen with or without assisted ventilation
- Temporary renal dialysis
- IV fluid and electrolyte replacement

Severe Acute Respiratory Syndrome. The single-stranded RNA coronavirus is responsible for severe acute respiratory syndrome (SARS), which affects the epithelial cells of the lower respiratory tract. Pathogenesis is not limited to the lungs but often includes mucosal cells of the intestines, tubular epithelial cells of the kidneys, and brain neurons. This new disease was first identified in China in late 2002, and then spread into the rest of the world in the spring and summer of 2003, resulting in the first pandemic of the twenty-first century. Of the approximately 8000 worldwide cases that occurred during this pandemic, about 25% of patients required mechanical ventilation in the ICU and about 10% of infected patients died.

SARS has flulike symptoms of fever, chills, cough, and malaise along with frequent shortness of breath. A common cause of death during this pandemic was diffuse alveolar damage (DAD). In addition, SARS typically compromises the immune response, which increases lung injury.

The 2003-2004 SARS pandemic showed that a prompt, coordinated worldwide response could help contain the disease. Although SARS was rapidly spread throughout the world by international air travelers, the virus itself was not transmitted through the air. Thus adherence to the basic infection control practice of thorough hand washing, implemented with droplet precautions, was able to ultimately stop this particular SARS pandemic.[61,62]

Cardiac Infections

Infections of the cardiac system can involve any layer of the heart (endocardium, myocardium, or pericardium) and generally result in acute or chronic depression of the patient's cardiac output. Infections that result in chronic cardiomyopathy most likely require cardiac transplantation. Refer to Chapters 3 and 14 for a discussion of cardiomyopathy and cardiac transplantation, respectively. This section focuses on rheumatic fever and resultant rheumatic heart disease.

Acute rheumatic fever is a clinical sequela occurring in up to 3% of patients with group A and β-streptococcal infection of the upper respiratory tract. It occurs primarily in children who are between the ages of 6 and 15 years. Rheumatic fever is characterized by nonsuppurative inflammatory lesions occurring in any or all of the connective tissues of the heart, joints, subcutaneous tissues, and central nervous system. An altered immune reaction to the infection is suspected as the cause of resultant damage to these areas, but the definitive etiology is unknown. *Rheumatic heart disease* is the term used to describe the resultant damage to the heart from the inflammatory process of rheumatic fever.[16,34,63,64]

Cardiac manifestations can include pericarditis, myocarditis, left-sided endocarditis, and valvular stenosis and insufficiency with resultant organic heart murmurs, as well as congestive heart failure. If not managed properly, all of these conditions can lead to significant morbidity or death.[16,34,63]

Management of rheumatic fever follows the treatment for streptococcal infection. The secondary complications mentioned previously are then managed specifically. The general intervention scheme may include the following[16,34,63]:

- Prevention of streptococcal infection
- Antiinfective agents
- Antipyretic agents
- Corticosteroids
- Bed rest
- IV fluids (as needed)

Neurologic Infections

Poliomyelitis

Poliomyelitis is an acute systemic viral disease that affects the central nervous system and fortunately is in rapid decline, with global eradication a distinct possibility.[65] Polioviruses are a type of enterovirus that multiply in the oropharynx and intestinal tract.[16,66]

Poliomyelitis is usually transmitted directly by the fecal-oral route from person to person but can also be transmitted indirectly by consumption of contaminated water sources.[66]

Clinical presentation can range from subclinical infection, to afebrile illness (24 to 36 hours), to aseptic meningitis, to paralysis (after 4 days), and, possibly, to death. If paralysis does occur, it is generally associated with fever and muscle pain. The paralysis is usually asymmetric and involves muscles of respiration, swallowing, and the lower extremities. Paralysis can resolve completely, leave residual deficits, or be fatal.[16,66]

Management of poliomyelitis primarily consists of prevention with inactivated poliovirus vaccine (IPV) given as four doses to children from the ages of 2 to 6 years of age.[66] If a patient does develop active poliomyelitis, then other management strategies may include the following[16]:

- Analgesics and antipyretics
- Bronchopulmonary hygiene
- Bed rest with contracture prevention with positioning and range of motion

Postpoliomyelitis Syndrome. Postpoliomyelitis syndrome, also known as postpolio syndrome, occurs 30 to 40 years after an episode of childhood paralytic poliomyelitis. The syndrome results from overuse or premature aging of motor units that were originally affected by the polio virus. It results in muscle fatigue, pain, and decreased endurance. Muscle atrophy and fasciculations may also be present. Patients who are older or critically ill, who have had a previous diagnosis of paralytic poliomyelitis, and who are female are at greater risk for development of this syndrome.[66-68]

Meningitis

Meningitis is an inflammation of the meninges that cover the brain and spinal cord, which results from acute infection by bacteria, viruses, fungi, or parasitic worms, or from chemical irritation. The route of transmission is primarily inhalation of infected airborne mucus droplets released by infected individuals, or through the bloodstream via open wounds or invasive procedures.[69,70]

The more common types of meningitis are (1) meningococcal meningitis, which is bacterial in origin and occurs in epidemic form; (2) *Haemophilus* meningitis, which is the most common form of bacterial meningitis; (3) pneumococcal meningitis, which occurs as an extension of a primary bacterial upper respiratory tract infection; and (4) viral (aseptic or serous) meningitis, which is generally benign and self-limiting.

Bacterial meningitis is more severe than viral meningitis and affects the pia mater, arachnoid and subarachnoid space, ventricular system, and cerebrospinal fluid. The primary complications of bacterial meningitis include an increase in intracranial pressure, resulting in hydrocephalus. This process frequently results in severe headache and nuchal rigidity (resistance to neck flexion). Other complications of meningitis include arthritis, myocarditis, pericarditis, neuromotor and intellectual deficits, and blindness and deafness from cranial nerve (III, IV, VI, VII, or VIII) dysfunction.[69,70]

Management of any form of meningitis may include the following[16,69,71]:

- Antimicrobial therapy, antiinfective agents, or immunologic agents
- Analgesics
- Mechanical ventilation (as needed)
- Blood pressure maintenance with IV fluids and vasopressors (e.g., dopamine)
- Intracranial pressure control

Encephalitis

Encephalitis is an inflammation of the tissues of the brain and spinal cord, commonly resulting from viral or amebic infection. Types of encephalitis include infectious viral encephalitis, mosquito-borne viral encephalitis, and amebic meningoencephalitis.

Infectious viral encephalitis is transmitted by direct contact with droplets from respiratory passages or other infected excretions and is most commonly associated with the herpes simplex type 1 virus. Viral encephalitis can also occur as a complication of systemic viral infections, such as poliomyelitis, rabies, mononucleosis, measles, mumps, rubella, and chickenpox. Manifestations of viral encephalitis can be mild to severe, with herpes simplex virus encephalitis having the highest mortality rate among all types of encephalitides.[16,69,70]

Mosquito-borne viral encephalitis is transmitted by infectious mosquito bites and cannot be transmitted from person to person. The incidence of this type of encephalitis can be epidemic and typically varies according to geographic regions and seasons.[16,69,70]

Amebic meningoencephalitis is transmitted in water and can enter a person's nasal passages while he or she is swimming. Amebic meningoencephalitis cannot be transmitted from person to person.

General clinical presentation of encephalitis may include the following[16,69,70]:

- Fever
- Signs of meningeal irritation from increased intracranial pressure (e.g., severe frontal headache, nausea, vomiting, dizziness, nuchal rigidity)
- Altered level of consciousness, irritability, bizarre behaviors (if the temporal lobe is involved)
- Seizures (mostly in infants)
- Aphasia
- Focal neurologic signs
- Weakness
- Altered deep tendon reflexes
- Ataxia, spasticity, tremors, or flaccidity
- Hyperthermia
- Alteration in antidiuretic hormone secretion
  Management of encephalitis may include the following[16]:
- Antiinfective agents
- Intracranial pressure management
- Mechanical ventilation, with or without tracheostomy (as indicated)
- Sedation
- IV fluids and electrolyte replacement
- Nasogastric tube feedings

Musculoskeletal Infections

Osteomyelitis is an acute infection of the bone that can occur from direct or indirect invasion by a pathogen. Direct invasion is also referred to as exogenous or acute contagious osteomyelitis and can occur any time there is an open wound in the body. Indirect invasion is also referred to as endogenous or acute hematogenous osteomyelitis and usually occurs from the spread of systemic infection. Both of these types can potentially progress to subacute and chronic osteomyelitis. Acute osteomyelitis typically refers to an infection of less than 1 month's duration, whereas chronic osteomyelitis refers to infection that lasts longer than 4 weeks.[72,73]

Acute contagious osteomyelitis is an extension of the concurrent infection in adjacent soft tissues to the bony area. Trauma resulting in compound fractures and tissue infections is a common example. Prolonged orthopedic surgery, wound drainage, and chronic illnesses, such as diabetes or alcoholism, also predispose patients to acute contagious osteomyelitis.[73,74]

Acute hematogenous osteomyelitis is a blood-borne infection that generally results from *S. aureus* infection (80%)[3] and occurs mostly in infants; children (in the metaphysis of growing long

bones); or patients undergoing long-term IV therapy, hyperalimentation, hemodialysis, or corticosteroid or antibiotic therapy. Patients who are malnourished, obese, or diabetic, or who have chronic joint disease, are also susceptible to acute hematogenous osteomyelitis.[72,73]

Clinical presentation of both types of acute osteomyelitis includes (1) delayed onset of pain, (2) tenderness, (3) swelling, and (4) warmth in the affected area. Fever is present with hematogenous osteomyelitis. The general treatment course for acute osteomyelitis is early and aggressive administration of the appropriate antibiotics to prevent or limit bone destruction.[3,56,72,73]

Chronic osteomyelitis is an extension of the acute cases just discussed. It results in marked bone destruction, draining sinus tracts, pain, deformity, and the potential for limb loss. Chronic osteomyelitis can also result from infected surgical prostheses or infected fractures. Debridement of dense formations (sequestra) may be a necessary adjunct to the antibiotic therapy. If the infection has spread to the surrounding soft tissue and skin regions, then grafting, after debridement, may be necessary. Good treatment results have also been shown with hyperbaric oxygen therapy for chronic osteomyelitis.[72,73]

> ✎ **CLINICAL TIP**
>
> Clarify weight-bearing orders with the physician when performing gait training with patients who have any form of osteomyelitis. Both upper and lower extremities can be involved; therefore choosing the appropriate assistive device is essential to preventing pathologic fracture.

Skin Infections

Cellulitis, or erysipelas, is an infection of the dermis and the subcutaneous tissue that can remain localized or be disseminated into the bloodstream, resulting in bacteremia (rare). Cellulitis occurs most commonly on the face, neck, and legs and is associated with an increased incidence of lymphedema.[75]

Groups A and G *Streptococcus* and *Staphylococcus aureus* are the usual causative agents for cellulitis and generally gain entry into the skin layers when there are open wounds (surgical or ulcers). Patients who are at most risk for developing cellulitis include those who are postsurgical and immunocompromised from chronic diseases or medical treatment.

The primary manifestations of cellulitis are fever with an abrupt onset of hot, stinging, and itchy skin and painful, red, thickened lesions that have firm, raised palpable borders in the affected areas. Identifying the causative agent is often difficult through blood cultures; therefore localized cultures, if possible collected from open wounds, may be more sensitive in helping to delineate the appropriate antibiotic treatment.[74,76,77]

Gastrointestinal Infections

Gastroenteritis is a global term used for the inflammation of the digestive tract that is typically a result of infection. Bacterial sources of gastroenteritis are often caused by *Escherichia coli*, *Shigella* (which causes bacterial dysentery), *Clostridium difficile*, or *Salmonella*. However, most cases of gastroenteritis are caused by viruses. Rotavirus and norovirus are by far the most frequent cause of gastroenteritis; adenovirus and astrovirus also commonly cause gastroenteritis, especially in children. Transmission of both bacterial and viral gastroenteritis is usually through the ingestion of contaminated food, water, or both or by direct and indirect fecal-oral transmission.

✎ CLINICAL TIP

Strict contact and enteric precautions should be observed with patients who have a diagnosis of *C. difficile* (whose spores can persist on fomites and environmental surfaces for months) and norovirus infection because these pathogens are relatively resistant to waterless alcohol-based antiseptics, and they have been associated with frequent surface contamination in hospital rooms and the hands of health care workers.

Of these aforementioned organisms, rotavirus (a double-stranded RNA virus) infection is the most important cause of severe diarrheal disease in young children. Historically, rotavirus has caused 500,000 childhood deaths annually in the world in less-developed countries. In the United States, 50% of gastroenteritis pediatric cases requiring hospitalization or emergency room visits are caused by rotavirus, and the total health and societal costs of rotavirus infections are estimated to exceed $1 billion per year. Fortunately, the annual pediatric death rate in the United States is relatively low (20 to 60 deaths). Rotavirus is very contagious in that the virus can survive on dry surfaces for up to 10 days and on human hands for up to 4 hours. It also has a low infectious dose (10 or fewer particles) and the infected stool can contain up to 10^{11} particles per gram that are present before and up to 2 weeks after the onset of symptoms. Because of its highly contagious nature, it is estimated that for every 4 children admitted to the hospital with a rotavirus infection, 1 additional child acquires it as an HAI. Rotavirus infections also may be transmitted to adults who are around infected children, immunocompromised individuals, and older adults in nursing homes. Fortunately, the newly developed second-generation rotavirus vaccines have proven to be effective and have fewer serious side effects (e.g., intussusception [intestinal invagination]).[78-81]

Norovirus (formally known as Norwalk virus, calicivirus, or small round-structured viruses) is a single-stranded positive sense RNA virus and is the most common cause of nonbacterial gastroenteritis worldwide. These outbreaks occur where groups of individuals gather, including nursing homes, hospitals, restaurants, and cruise ships. Like the rotavirus, norovirus is very contagious (<10 particles can cause infection) and can survive for up to 4 weeks in a dried state at room temperature. In hospitals the most common contaminated sites include toilet tops, door handles, and telephone receivers, and contaminated fingers can spread the norovirus to up to seven clean surfaces.

Research has shown that 1 minute of hand washing with soap and water followed by rinsing the hands for 20 seconds, then drying them with a disposable towel completely removes norovirus from hands contaminated with infected stools. Unlike for rotavirus, there is no fully developed vaccine for norovirus, although vaccines for norovirus are in early stages of development.[82-84]

The primary manifestations of any form of gastroenteritis are crampy abdominal pain, nausea, vomiting, and diarrhea, all of which vary in severity and duration according to the type of infection. Gastroenteritis is generally a self-limiting infection, with resolution occurring in 3 to 4 days. However, patients in the hospital setting with reduced immunity can have longer periods of recovery, with dehydration being a primary concern.[16,56,85]

Management of acute gastroenteritis may include the following[16,56]:

- Antiinfective agents
- IV fluid and electrolyte replacement
- Antiemetic agents (if nausea and vomiting occur)

Immune System Infections

Human Immunodeficiency Virus Infection

Two types of HIV exist: HIV-1 and HIV-2, with HIV-1 being the more prevalent and the one discussed here. It is a retrovirus, occurring in pandemic proportions, that primarily affects the function of the immune system. Eventually, however, all systems of the body become affected directly, such as the immune system, or indirectly, as in the cardiac system, or through both methods, as occurs in the nervous system. The virus is transmitted in blood, semen, vaginal secretions, and breast milk through sexual, perinatal, and blood or blood-product contact. Proteins on the surface of the virus attach to CD4+ receptors, found primarily on T4 lymphocytes.[86] Other types of cells found to house the virus include monocytes, macrophages, uterine cervical cells, epithelial cells of the gastrointestinal tract, and microglia cells.[86]

On entering the cell, the viral and cellular DNA combine, making the virus a part of the cell. The exact pathogenesis of cellular destruction caused by HIV is not completely understood, and several methods of destruction may be entailed. It is known that immediately after initial infection, HIV enters a latent period, or asymptomatic stage, in which viral replication is minimal, but CD4+ T cell counts begin to decline.[86] Continued reduction results in decreasing immunity, eventually leading to symptomatic HIV, in which diseases associated with the virus begin to appear.[86] This eventually leads to the onset of AIDS, which the CDC defines as occurring when the CD4+ T-lymphocyte count falls below 200 cells/µl (reference = 1000 cells/µl) or below 14%; when 1 of 26 specific AIDS-defining disorders is contracted, most of which are opportunistic infections; or a combination of these factors.[87,88]

✎ CLINICAL TIP

Norovirus and rotavirus can be transmitted through aerosolization, so health care workers should wear a mask when disposing of infected vomit and feces.

Six laboratory tests are available to detect HIV infection[89-92]:

1. ELISA or enzyme immunoassay test. This procedure tests for the presence of antibodies to HIV proteins in the patient's serum. A sample of the patient's blood is exposed to HIV antigens in the test reagent. If HIV antibodies are identified, it is inferred that the virus is present within the patient.

2. Western blot test. This test detects the presence of antibodies in the blood of two types of HIV viral proteins and is therefore a more specific HIV test. It is an expensive test to perform and is used as a confirmatory tool for a positive ELISA test.

3. Immunofluorescence assay. In this test, the patient's blood is diluted and placed on a slide containing HIV antigens. The slide is then treated with anti-human globulin mixed with a fluorescent dye that will bind to antigen-antibody complexes. If fluorescence is visible when the specimen is placed under a microscope, then HIV antibodies are present in the patient's blood.

4. p24 antigen assay. This test analyzes blood cells for the presence of the p24 antigen located on HIV virions. It can be used to diagnose acute infection, to screen blood for HIV antigens, to determine HIV infection in difficult diagnostic cases, or to evaluate the treatment effects of antiviral agents.

5. PCR for HIV nucleic acid. This highly specific and extremely sensitive test detects viral DNA molecule in lymphocyte nuclei by amplifying the viral DNA. It is used to detect HIV in neonates and when antibody tests are inconclusive.

6. Rapid HIV testing. This highly sensitive and specific test requires a sample of blood, serum, plasma, or oral fluid to detect HIV antibodies. This test can be complete in 20 minutes.

✎ CLINICAL TIP

Any clinician who sustains a needle-stick injury when working with a patient with a suspected HIV infection should have an HIV test. A false-negative HIV test can occur if an individual has not yet developed HIV antibodies. If an individual has had exposure to HIV, he or she should have a repeat HIV test to ensure a true negative result.[93]

Once HIV has been detected, it can be classified in a number of ways. The Walter Reed staging system has six categories grouped according to the quantity of helper T cells and characteristic signs, such as the presence of an HIV antigen or antibody.[94] However, a more commonly used classification system was devised by the CDC and was last updated in 1993. In this system, infection is divided into three categories, depending on CD4+ T-lymphocyte counts:

1. Category 1 consists of CD4+ T-lymphocyte counts greater than or equal to 500 cells/μl.

2. Category 2 consists of counts ranging between 200 and 499 cells/μl.

3. Category 3 contains cell counts less than 200 cells/μl.

These groups are then subdivided into A, B, and C, according to the presence of specific diseases.[87]

A major advancement in the medical treatment of HIV has been antiretroviral therapy. This therapy consists of four classes of medications (see Chapter 19, Table 19-37)[94]:

1. Nucleoside analog reverse transcriptase inhibitors, otherwise known as nucleoside analogs

2. Protease inhibitors

3. Nonnucleoside reverse transcriptase inhibitors

4. Fusion inhibitor

Each of these therapies assists in limiting HIV progression by helping to prevent viral replication. This prevention is further increased when the drugs are used in combination in a treatment technique termed *highly active antiretroviral therapy* or HAART.[94]

There is a significant need for more effective and cost-efficient preventions for HIV. The HIV Vaccine Trials Network (HVTN) is an international collaboration working to develop HIV preventive vaccines.[95]

As HIV progresses and immunity decreases, the risk for and severity of infections not normally seen in healthy immune systems increase. These opportunistic infections, combined with disorders that result directly from the virus, often result in multiple diagnoses and medically complex patients. These manifestations of HIV can affect every system of the body and present with a wide array of signs and symptoms, many of which are appropriate for physical therapy intervention. Table 13-4 lists common manifestations and complications of HIV and AIDS and the medications generally used in their management.

Disorders affecting the nervous system include HIV-associated dementia complex, progressive multifocal leukoencephalopathy, primary central nervous system lymphoma, toxoplasmosis, and neuropathies. These manifestations may cause paresis, decreased sensation, ataxia, aphagia, spasticity, altered mental status, and visual deficits.[96] In the pulmonary system, TB, cytomegalovirus (CMV) and pneumonia can result in cough, dyspnea, sputum production, and wheezing.[97] In the cardiac system, cardiomyopathy, arrhythmias, and congestive heart failure can cause chest pain, dyspnea, tachycardia, tachypnea, hypotension, fatigue, peripheral edema, syncope, dizziness, and palpitations.[98]

Physical therapy intervention can assist in minimizing the effect of these deficits on functional ability, therefore helping to maximize the independence and quality of life of the individual. However, the course of rehabilitation in HIV-affected individuals can often be difficult owing to coinciding opportunistic infections, an often-rapid downhill disease course, low energy states, and frequent hospitalizations.

Mononucleosis

Mononucleosis is an acute viral disease that has been primarily linked to the Epstein-Barr virus and less commonly to CMV. Mononucleosis is transmitted generally through saliva from symptomatic or asymptomatic carriers (the Epstein-Barr virus can remain infective for 18 months in the saliva).[16,99]

The disease is characterized by fever, lymphadenopathy (lymph node hyperplasia), and exudative pharyngitis. Splenomegaly, hepatitis, pneumonitis, and central nervous system

TABLE 13-4 Common Complications from HIV and AIDS, and Associated Medical Treatment

Complication	Medication
Cardiomyopathy	May be reversed with reduction or discontinuation of interleukin-2, adriamycin, α2-interferon, ifosfamide, and foscarnet
Cerebral toxoplasmosis	Trimethoprim-sulfamethoxazole
Coccidioidomycosis	Amphotericin B, fluconazole, or itraconazole
Congestive heart failure	Removal of all nonessential drugs followed by administration of furosemide (Lasix); digoxin; angiotensin-converting enzyme inhibition
Cryptococcal meningitis	Amphotericin B or fluconazole
Cytomegalovirus	Ganciclovir, foscarnet, cidofovir
Distal symmetric polyneuropathy	Pain management using tricyclic antidepressants, gabapentin, and narcotics for severe cases
Herpes simplex	Acyclovir, famciclovir, valacyclovir
Herpes zoster (shingles)	Acyclovir, valacyclovir, famciclovir, foscarnet
HIV-associated dementia complex	Antiretroviral therapy combining at least three drugs, two of which penetrate the blood-brain barrier
Histoplasmosis	Amphotericin B or itraconazole
Kaposi's sarcoma	Radiotherapy, cryotherapy with liquid nitrogen, daunorubicin hydrochloride, or doxorubicin hydrochloride injections
Lymphomas	Chemotherapy: cyclophosphamide, doxorubicin, vincristine, bleomycin, methotrexate, leucovorin
Mycobacterium avium complex	Clarithromycin, rifabutin, ciprofloxacin, ethambutol
Oral hairy leukoplakia	Acyclovir if symptoms present
Pneumocystis jirovecii pneumonia	Trimethoprim-sulfamethoxazole, dapsone, clindamycin, pentamidine isethionate
Progressive multifocal leukoencephalopathy	Antiretroviral therapy, acyclovir, IV cytosine, adenosine-arabinoside, interferon-alphas
Pulmonary hypertension	Low-flow O_2 if hypoxia present, vasodilators, including nitroglycerin, hydralazine, nifedipine, lisinopril, and prostaglandin E
Toxic neuronal neuropathy: neuropathy caused by certain medications	May be reversed with discontinuation or reduction in the following: zalcitabine, didanosine, and stavudine
Tuberculosis	Four-drug regimen: isoniazid, rifampin, pyrazinamide, and ethambutol

Data from Zwolski K: Viral infections. In Kirton CA, Talotta D, Zwolski K, editors: Handbook of HIV/AIDS nursing, St Louis, 2001, Mosby, pp 303, 310-311, 313, 315; Cheitlin MD: Cardiovascular complications of HIV infection. In Sande MA, Volberding PA, editors: The medical management of AIDS, Philadelphia, 1999, Saunders, pp 278, 280; Boss BJ, Farley JA: Alterations in neurologic function. In Heuther SE, McCance KL, editors: Understanding pathophysiology, ed 2, St Louis, 2000, Mosby, pp 403-406; Smith L: Management of bacterial meningitis: new guidelines from the IDSA, Am Fam Physician 71(10), 2005; Rhuda SC: Nursing management, musculoskeletal problems. In Lewis SM, Heitkemper MM, Dirksen SR, editors: Medical-surgical nursing, assessment and management of clinical problems, ed 5, St Louis, 2000, Mosby, pp 1795-1798; McCance KL, Mourad LA: Alterations in musculoskeletal function. In Heuther SE, McCance KL, editors: Understanding pathophysiology, ed 2, St Louis, 2000, Mosby, pp 1046-1048; Rowland BM: Cellulitis. In Boyden K, Olendorf D, editors: Gale encyclopedia of medicine, Farmington Hills, MI, 1999, Gale Group, p 616.

AIDS, Acquired immunodeficiency syndrome; *HIV*, human immunodeficiency virus; *IV*, intravenous.

involvement may occur as rare complications from mononucleosis. The infection is generally self-limiting in healthy individuals, with resolution in approximately 3 weeks without any specific treatment.[16,99]

If management of mononucleosis is necessary, it may include the following[16,99,100]:

- Corticosteroids in cases of severe pharyngitis
- Adequate hydration
- Bed rest during the acute stage
- Saline throat gargle
- Aspirin or acetaminophen for sore throat and fever

Cytomegalovirus Infection

CMV is a member of the herpesvirus group that can be found in all body secretions, including saliva, blood, urine, feces, semen, cervical secretions, and breast milk. CMV

infection is a common viral infection that is asymptomatic or symptomatic. CMV infection can remain latent after the initial introduction into the body and can become opportunistic at a later point.

If CMV infection is symptomatic, clinical presentation may be a relatively benign mononucleosis in adults, or in patients with HIV infection, manifestations such as pneumonia, hepatitis, encephalitis, esophagitis, colitis, and retinitis can occur.

CMV is usually transmitted by prolonged contact with infected body secretions, as well as congenitally or perinatally.[16,101]

Management of CMV infection may include the following[16,101]:

- Antiviral agents
- Corticosteroids

- Immune globulins
- Blood transfusions for anemia or thrombocytopenia
- Antipyretics

Toxoplasmosis

Toxoplasmosis is a systemic protozoan infection caused by the parasite *Toxoplasma gondii*, which is primarily found in cat feces. Transmission can occur from three mechanisms: (1) eating raw or inadequately cooked infected meat or eating uncooked foods that have come in contact with contaminated meat; (2) inadvertently ingesting oocysts that cats have passed in their feces, either in a cat litter box or outdoors in soil (e.g., soil from gardening or unwashed fruits or vegetables); and (3) transmission of the infection from a woman to her unborn fetus. Fetal transmission of *T. gondii* can result in mental retardation, blindness, and epilepsy.[102]

Clinical manifestations can range from subclinical infection to severe generalized infection, particularly in immunocompromised individuals, and to death.

The primary way to treat toxoplasmosis is through prevention by safe eating habits (thoroughly cooking meats, peeling and washing fruits and vegetables) and minimizing contact with cat feces when pregnant, along with keeping the cat indoors to prevent contamination.[102]

Sepsis

Sepsis is a general term that describes three progressive infectious conditions: bacteremia, septicemia, and shock syndrome (or septic shock).[16]

Bacteremia is a generally asymptomatic condition that results from bacterial invasion of blood from contaminated needles, catheters, monitoring transducers, or perfusion fluid. Bacteremia can also occur from a preexisting infection from another body site. Patients with prosthetic heart valves may need to take prophylactic antibiotics for dental surgery because the bacteremia may progress to endocarditis. Bacteremia can resolve spontaneously or progress to septicemia.

Septicemia is a symptomatic extension of bacteremia throughout the body, with clinical presentations that are representative of the infective pathogen and the organ system(s) involved. Sites commonly affected are the brain, endocardium, kidneys, bones, and joints. Renal failure and endocarditis may also occur.

Shock syndrome is a critical condition of systemic tissue hypoperfusion that results from microcirculatory failure (i.e., decreased blood pressure or perfusion). Bacterial damage of the peripheral vascular system is the primary cause of the tissue hypoperfusion.

Management of sepsis may include any of the following[16]:

- Removal of suspected infective sources (e.g., lines or tubes)
- Antiinfective agents
- Blood pressure maintenance with adrenergic agents and corticosteroids
- IV fluids
- Blood transfusions

- Cardiac glycosides
- Supplemental oxygen, mechanical ventilation, or both
- Anticoagulation

Management

Medical Intervention

Management of the various infectious diseases discussed in this chapter is described in the specific sections of respective disorders. Chapter 19 (Table 19-34, Antibiotics; Table 19-35, Antifungal Agents; Table 19-36, Antitubercular Agents; Table 19-37, Antiretroviral Medications; and Table 19-38, Antiviral Medications) also lists common antiinfective agents used in treating infectious diseases.

Lifestyle Management

The critical importance of encouraging healthy lifestyles to combat disease is indicated by the National Prevention and Health Promotion Strategy that was announced in the summer of 2011. The objective of this strategy is to "move the nation away from a health care system focused on sickness and disease to one focused on wellness and prevention."[103] The American Physical Therapy Association's president has encouraged physical therapists to support this national prevention initiative by "expanding quality preventative services in both clinical and community settings, empowering people to make healthful choices, and eliminating health disparities" and to become "leaders in their communities to advance these directions and priorities."[104] Although the physical therapist may have limited treatment options emphasizing prevention and wellness during the acute care stay, he or she has greater opportunities to effect meaningful lifestyle change in other settings such as in nursing homes and home health. At a minimum, the physical therapist can play a key role in all health care settings in helping patients understand the link between lifestyle and infectious disease. These important links, which may be poorly understood by the typical patient, are discussed in this section.

Many of the same lifestyle and nutrition factors that can delay wound healing (see Chapter 12) also affect the immune system and the infection rate. To have an optimally functioning immune system, one should eat plenty of fresh fruits and vegetables as well as foods rich in fiber. Also, it is important to obtain adequate amounts of the micronutrients zinc, selenium, iron, copper, vitamins A, C, E, and B_6, and folic acid. Vitamin D, which is produced by exposure to sunlight, is known to activate one's innate immunity (i.e., regulatory T cells) by the production of antimicrobial peptides. Excess sugar also decreases the ability of white blood cells to destroy bacteria (leukocytic phagocytosis). Moreover, a healthy immune system is promoted by not only eating proper foods, but also by staying well hydrated, which is a key consideration in combating septic shock.[105-111]

Exposure to fresh and unpolluted air benefits the immune system. It is a well-studied fact that the higher the ventilation rate (amount of outdoor air circulated per unit time), the lower the infection rate of airborne diseases such as measles, TB, influenza, and SARS. The cross-infection problem of the 2002-2003 SARS epidemic was particularly evident where people congregated, such as in airplanes, buses, and hospitals. This would imply a strong benefit for exposing patients to as much fresh air as medically prudent, which is reminiscent of the philosophy behind the "open-air treatment" TB hospitals of the last century.[112,113]

When one obtains the proper balance of exercise and rest, it helps the immune system fight off infection. Exercise and adequate rest are key factors in promoting a healthy psychological state, which also reduces the negative effects of stress (e.g., high levels of cortisol) on the immune system. However, it should be mentioned that the beneficial effects of resistive exercise (as opposed to cardiovascular exercise) on immunity are less clear, though excessive cardiovascular exercise may lead to immunosuppression. The key role that the crucial rest-promoting hormone melatonin plays in influencing our circadian rhythm (sleep-wake cycle) and immune system (specifically T cell populations) is still being unraveled. Melatonin's peak production occurs at night, which is the inverse of another key immunoregulatory hormone, vitamin D. In order to maximize melatonin levels, which promote sleep efficiency and restfulness, one should exercise regularly, be exposed to natural light (sunlight) especially early in the day, minimize exposure to artificial light at night, and go to bed 2 to 3 hours before midnight in a completely dark room. It is important to follow this advice every day because melatonin has a short half-life and thus must be produced every 24 hours.[110,114-119]

Alcohol exposure has a well-known immunosuppression effect, which includes negative impacts on lymphocyte activation, cytokine production by macrophages and T cells, and neutrophil function. This results in increased susceptibility to infection and reduces the body's ability to heal after injury. People who smoke and those who are exposed (especially children) to passive or environmental tobacco smoke (ETS) are at greater risk of impairing their immune system, which can cause infections such as influenza and TB for adults and serious respiratory tract infection and pneumonia for children. Caffeine is largely antiinflammatory in nature and thus has an overall negative effect on the immune system. Specifically, caffeine suppresses lymphocyte function, antibody production, and neutrophil and monocyte chemotaxis. Illicit drug users also have well-documented higher infection rates involving bacteria, viruses, fungi, and protozoans. These rates are even higher in injection drug users.[120-123]

Finally, obesity has now been associated with increased infection risk. Increased infection has been observed in obese patients with conditions as diverse as urinary tract infection (UTI), influenza, hepatitis C, and a history of total hip arthroplasty. With obesity rates increasing throughout the world, the exact mechanism of the link between obesity and infection warrants more study.[124-127]

Physical Therapy Intervention

The following are general physical therapy goals and guidelines to be used when working with patients who have infectious

disease processes, as well as disorders of altered immunity. These guidelines should be adapted to a patient's specific needs.

Goals

The primary physical therapy goals in this patient population are similar to those of patient populations in the acute care setting: (1) to optimize the patient's functional mobility, (2) to maximize the patient's tolerance and endurance, (3) to maximize ventilation and gas exchange in the patient who has pulmonary involvement, and, when appropriate, (4) to educate the patient in proper lifestyle management (see previous section).

Guidelines for Physical Therapy Intervention

General physical therapy guidelines include, but are not limited to, the following:

1. The best modes of preventing the transmission of infectious diseases are to adhere to the standard precautions established by the CDC and to follow proper hand-washing techniques (Box 13-2).
   a. Facilities' warning or labeling systems for biohazards and infectious materials may vary slightly.
   b. Be sure to check the patient's medical record or signs posted on doors and doorways for indicated precautions.
   c. Table 13-3 provides an outline of the types of personal protective equipment that should be worn with specific precautions.
2. Personally follow and also educate patients concerning proper coughing and sneezing hygiene etiquette in order to prevent the spread of disease and illness.
   a. Cover the mouth and nose with a tissue when coughing or sneezing.
   b. Put the used tissue in a waste basket.

BOX 13-2   Proper Hand-Washing Technique

Hand washing with soap and water is the best method to remove pathogens, including highly contagious pathogens (e.g., norovirus, *Clostridium difficile* spores), from your hands.

1. Wet your hands with clean running water (warm or cold) and apply soap.
2. Rub your hands together to make a lather and scrub them well. Be sure to scrub the backs of your hands, between your fingers, and under your nails.
3. Continue rubbing your hands for at least 20 seconds (as previously mentioned, some pathogens such as norovirus require a longer time of at least 60 seconds to remove stool contamination from hands).
4. Rinse your hands well under running water (stool-contaminated norovirus hands should be rinsed for at least 20 seconds).
5. Dry your hands using a clean disposable towel or air dry.

If soap and water are not available, use an alcohol-based hand sanitizer that contains at least 60% alcohol (continue to rub the sanitizer over all hand and finger surfaces until dry). Alcohol-based hand sanitizers can quickly reduce the number of pathogens, but do not remove all pathogen types (e.g., norovirus, *Clostridium difficile* spores).

c. If no tissue is available, cough or sneeze into the upper sleeve and not into the hands.

d. Wash the hands after coughing or sneezing (see Box 13-2 on previous page).

3. The danger of pathogen aerosolization during common hygiene activities and physical therapy treatment is often not fully recognized.

a. Flushing the toilet (even with the lid down) causes aerosolization of pathogens that is greatest with the first flush, and then diminishes with each subsequent flush.

b. Aerosolization danger is greatest when the patient has diarrhea (as contrasted to a normal stool) and/or vomits into the toilet.

c. Gastroenteritis viral pathogens are especially easy to spread in the foregoing manner because each gram of feces can contain up to 10^{11} virus particles.

d. Pulsatile lavage is a common wound physical therapy modality that can cause aerosolization of pathogens.

e. In addition to the therapist wearing appropriate PPE during pulsatile lavage, patients receiving treatment should wear surgical masks, and all IV lines and other wounds should be covered during treatment. The procedure should be performed in a private room, with minimal equipment and supplies. The room should be thoroughly cleaned and disinfected after each procedure.

4. Patients who have infectious processes have an elevated metabolic rate, which will most likely manifest itself as a high resting heart rate. As a result, the activity intensity level should be modified, or more frequent rest periods should be incorporated during physical therapy treatment to enhance activity tolerance.

a. Patients with infectious processes will also be prone to orthostatic hypotension, hypotension with functional activities, or both as a result of the vasodilation occurring from the inflammation associated with infection.

b. Therefore slow changes in positions, especially from recumbent to upright positions, and frequent blood pressure monitoring are essential to promoting tolerance for functional activities.

5. Monitoring the temperature curve and WBC count of patients with infectious processes helps to determine the appropriateness of physical therapy intervention.

a. During an exacerbation or progression of an infection process, rest may be indicated.

b. Clarification with the physician or nurse regarding the type of intended physical therapy intervention is helpful in making this decision.

References

1. Klevens RM, Edwards JR, Richards CL Jr, et al: Estimating health care-associated infections and deaths in U.S. hospitals, Public Health Rep 122(2):160-166, 2007.
2. Weber DJ, Rutala WA, Miller MB et al: Role of hospital surfaces in the transmission of emerging health care-associated pathogens: norovirus, *Clostridium difficile*, and *Acinetobacter* species, Am J Infect Control 38(5 Suppl 1):S25-S33, 2010.
3. Smeltzer SC, Bare BG: In Brunner and Suddarth's textbook of medical-surgical nursing, ed 7, Philadelphia, 1992, Lippincott.
4. Thomas CL, editor: Taber's cyclopedic medical dictionary, ed 17, Philadelphia, 1993, FA Davis.
5. Goodman CC, Snyder TEK: In differential diagnosis in physical therapy: musculoskeletal and systemic conditions, Philadelphia, 1995, Saunders.
6. Horan TC, Andrus M, Dudeck MA: CDC/NHSN surveillance definition of health care–associated infection and criteria for specific types of infections in the acute care setting, Am J Infect Control 36(5):309-332, 2008.
7. Kent TH, Hart MN, editors: Introduction to human disease, ed 4, Stamford, CT, 1998, Appleton & Lange, pp 21-30.
8. Goodman CC, Boissonnault WG: Pathology: implications for the physical therapist, Philadelphia, 1998, Saunders.
9. Gorbach SL, Bartlett JG, Blacklow NR, editors: Infectious diseases, Philadelphia, 1992, Saunders.
10. Delost MD: In Introduction to diagnostic microbiology: a text and workbook, St Louis, 1997, Mosby, pp 1-9.
11. Malarkey LM, McMorrow ME, editors: Nurse's manual of laboratory tests and diagnostic procedures, ed 2, Philadelphia, 2000, Saunders, pp 49-81.
12. Linne JJ, Ringsurd KM, editors: Clinical laboratory science: the basics and routine techniques, St Louis, 1999, Mosby, pp 669-699.
13. Linne JJ, Ringsurd KM, editors: Clinical laboratory science: the basics and routine techniques, St Louis, 1999, Mosby, pp 597-667.
14. Isenburg HD: Clinical microbiology. In Borback SL, Bartlett JG, Blacklow NR, editors: Infectious diseases, Philadelphia, 1998, Saunders, pp 123-145.
15. Anderson KN, editor: Mosby's medical, nursing, and allied health dictionary, ed 4, St Louis, 1994, Mosby.
16. Thompson JM, McFarland GK, Hirsch JE et al, editors: Mosby's manual of clinical nursing, ed 2, 1989, Mosby, St Louis.
17. Malarkey LM, McMorrow ME, editors: Nurse's manual of laboratory tests and diagnostic procedures, ed 2, Philadelphia, 2000, Saunders, pp 337-339.
18. Malarkey LM, McMorrow ME, editors: Nurse's manual of laboratory tests and diagnostic procedures, ed 2, Philadelphia, 2000, Saunders, pp 779-782.
19. Malarkey LM, McMorrow ME, editors: Nurse's manual of laboratory tests and diagnostic procedures, ed 2, Philadelphia, 2000, Saunders, pp 457-460.
20. Albertson TE, Owen KP, Sutter ME, Chan AL: Gastrointestinal decontamination in the acutely poisoned patient, Int J Emerg Med 4:65, 2011.
21. Yu AS, Hu KQ: Management of ascites, Clin Liver Dis 5(2):541-568, 2001.
22. Peterson JJ: Postoperative infection, Radiol Clin North Am 44(3):439-450, 2006.
23. Pineda C, Vargas A, Rodriguez AV: Imaging of osteomyelitis: current concepts, Infect Dis Clin North Am 20(4):789-825, 2006.
24. Holland PV: Overview: diagnostic tests for viral infections transmitted by blood, Nucl Med Biol 21(3):407-417, 1994.
25. Hoorfar J: Rapid detection, characterization, and enumeration of foodborne pathogens, APMIS Suppl 133(Nov):1-24, 2011.

26. Rice D, Eckstein EC: Inflammation and infection. In Phipps WJ, Sands JK, Marek JF, editors: Medical-surgical nursing, concepts and clinical practice, ed 6, St Louis, 1999, Mosby, pp 237-245.

27. Nan DN, Fernandez-Ayala M, Farinas-Alvarez C, et al: Nosocomial infection after lung surgery: incidence and risk factors, Chest 128(4):2647-2652, 2005.

28. Jaber S, Chanques G, Altaira C, et al: A prospective study of agitation in a medical-surgical ICU: incidence, risk factors, and outcomes, Chest 128(4):2749-2757, 2005.

29. Harbarth S, Sax H, Fankhauser-Rodriguez C, et al: Evaluating the probability of previously unknown carriage of MRSA at hospital admission, Am J Med 119(3):275, 2006.

30. Donegan NE: Management of patients with infectious diseases. In Smeltzer SC, Bare BG, editors: Brunner and Suddarth's textbook of medical-surgical nursing, ed 9, Philadelphia, 2000, Lippincott, pp 1876-1877.

31. Centers for Disease Control and Prevention: Get Smart for Healthcare. http://www.cdc.gov/getsmart/healthcare. Accessed April 13, 2012.

32. Magiorakos AP, Srinivasan A, Carey RB, et al: Multidrug-resistant, extensively-resistant, and pandrug-resistant bacteria: an international expert proposal for interim standard definitions for acquired resistance, Clin Microbiol Infect 18(3):268-281, 2011.

33. Lewis SM: Nursing management: inflammation and infection. In Lewis SM, Heitkemper MM, Dirksen SR, editors: Medical-surgical nursing, assessment and management of clinical problems, ed 5, St Louis, 2000, Mosby, pp 201-202.

34. Black JM, Matassarin-Jacobs E, editors: Luckmann and Sorenen's medical-surgical nursing: a psychophysiologic approach, ed 4, Philadelphia, 1993, Saunders.

35. Shovein J, Young MS: MRSA: Pandora's box for hospitals, Am J Nurs 2:49, 1992.

36. Mainous AG, Hueston WJ, Everett CJ, et al: Nasal carriage of *Staphylococcus aureus* and methicillin-resistant *S. aureus* in the United States, 2001-2002, Ann Fam Med 4(2):132-137, 2006.

37. The Hospital Infection Control Practices Advisory Committee: Special communication: recommendations for preventing the spread of vancomycin resistance, Am J Infect Control 23:87, 1995.

38. Silverblatt FJ, Tilbert C, Mikolich D, et al: Preventing the spread of vancomycin-resistant enterococci in a long-term care facility, J Am Geriatr Soc 48(10):1211-1215, 2000.

39. Kemp R, Rolain J-M: Emergence of resistance to carbapenems in *Acinetobacter baumannii* in Europe: clinical impact and therapeutic options, Int J Antimicrob Agents 39(2):105-114, 2012.

40. Neonakis IK, Spandidos DA, Petinaki E: Confronting multidrug-resistant *Acinetobacter baumannii*: a review, Int J Antimicrob Agents 37(2):102-109, 2011.

41. Consales G, Gramigni E, Zamidei L et al: A multidrug-resistant *Acinetobacter baumannii* outbreak in intensive care unit: antimicrobial and organizational strategies, J Crit Care 26(5):453-459, 2011.

42. Maragakis LL, Cosgrove SE, Song X et al: An outbreak of multidrug-resistant *Acinetobacter baumannii* associated with pulsatile lavage wound treatment, JAMA 292(24):3006-3011, 2004.

43. Fournier PE, Richet H: The epidemiology and control of *Acinetobacter baumannii* in health care facilities, Clin Infect Dis 42(5):692-699, 2006.

44. Stedman's medical dictionary, ed 27, 1999, Philadelphia, Lippincott Williams & Wilkins.

45. Hickey MM, Hoffman LA: Nursing management, upper respiratory problems. In Lewis SM, Heitkemper MM, Dirksen SR, editors: Medical-surgical nursing, assessment and

management of clinical problems, ed 5, St Louis, 2000, Mosby, pp 582-588.

46. Prenner BM, Schenkel E: Allergic rhinitis: treatment based on patient profiles, Am J Med 119(3):230-237, 2006.

47. Marconi GP, Ross LA, Nager AL: An upsurge in pertussis: epidemiology and trends, Pediatr Emerg Care 28(3):215-219, 2012.

48. CDC: Pertussis—United States, 2001-2003, Morb Mortal Wkly Rep 54(50):1283-1286, 2005.

49. Piessens WF, Nardell EA: Pathogenesis of tuberculosis. In Reichman LB, Hershfield ES, editors: Tuberculosis: a comprehensive international approach, ed 2, New York, 2000, Marcel Dekker, pp 241-260.

50. Comstock GW: Epidemiology of tuberculosis. In Reichman LB, Hershfield ES, editors: Tuberculosis: a comprehensive international approach, ed 2, New York, 2000, Marcel Dekker, pp 129-156.

51. American Thoracic Society, CDC: Diagnostic standards and classification of tuberculosis in adults and children, Am J Resp Crit Care Med 161:1376-1395, 2000.

52. Lobue PA, Perry S, Catanzaro A: Diagnosis of tuberculosis. In Reichman LB, Hershfield ES, editors: Tuberculosis: a comprehensive international approach, ed 2, New York, 2000, Marcel Dekker, pp 341-376.

53. Hopewell PC, Chaisson RE: Tuberculosis and human immunodeficiency syndrome virus infection. In Reichman LB, Hershfield ES, editors: Tuberculosis: a comprehensive international approach, ed 2, New York, 2000, Marcel Dekker, pp 525-552.

54. Lewis SM: Nursing management, lower respiratory problems. In Lewis SM, Heitkemper MM, Dirksen SR, editors: Medical-surgical nursing, assessment and management of clinical problems, ed 5, St Louis, 2000, Mosby, pp 629-630.

55. Puhlman M: Infectious processes. In Copstead LC, Banasik JL, editors: Pathophysiology, biological and behavioral perspectives, ed 2, Philadelphia, 2000, Saunders, pp 172-173.

56. Rytel MW, Mogabgab WJ, editors: Clinical manual of infectious diseases, Chicago, 1984, Year Book.

57. Wheat J, Sarosi G, McKinsey D, et al: Practice guidelines for the management of patients with histoplasmosis. Infectious Diseases Society of America, Clin Infect Dis 30(4):688-695, 2000.

58. Alary M, Joly JR: Factors contributing to the contamination of hospital water distribution systems by legionellae, J Infect Dis 165(3):565-569, 1992.

59. Darby J, Buising K: Could it be *Legionella*? Aust Fam Physician 37(10):812-815, 2008.

60. Palmore TN, Stock F, White M, et al: A cluster of nosocomial Legionnaire's disease linked to a contaminated hospital decorative water fountain, Infect Control Hosp Epidemiol 30(8):764-768, 2009.

61. Chan WF, Wong TK: Preparing for pandemic influenza: revisit the basics, J Clin Nurs 16(10):1858-1864, 2007.

62. Gu J, Korteweg C: Pathology and pathogenesis of severe acute respiratory syndrome, Am J Pathol 170(4):1136-1147, 2007.

63. Kupper NS, Duke ES: Nursing management, inflammatory and valvular heart diseases. In Lewis SM, Heitkemper MM, Dirksen SR, editors: Medical-surgical nursing, assessment and management of clinical problems, ed 5, St Louis, 2000, Mosby, pp 959-964.

64. Banasik JL: Alterations in cardiac function. In Copstead LC, Banasik JL, editors: Pathophysiology, biological and behavioral perspectives, ed 2, Philadelphia, 2000, Saunders, pp 442-443.

65. Centers for Disease Control and Prevention: Global routine vaccination coverage, 2009, MMWR Morb Mortal Wkly Rep 59(42):1367-1371, 2010.

66. Poliomyelitis prevention in the United States: updated recommendations of the Advisory Committee on Immunization

Practices (ACIP), Morb Mortal Wkly Rep 49(RR05):1-22, 2000.

67. Berkow R, Fletcher AJ, editors: Merck manual of diagnosis and therapy, ed 16, Rahway, NJ, 1992, Merck Research Laboratories.

68. Lambert DA, Giannouli E, Schmidt BJ, et al: Postpolio syndrome and anesthesia, Anesthesiology 103(3):638-644, 2005.

69. Kerr ME: Nursing management, intracranial problems. In Lewis SM, Heitkemper MM, Dirksen SR, editors: Medical-surgical nursing, assessment and management of clinical problems, ed 5, St Louis, 2000, Mosby, pp 1638-1643.

70. Boss BJ, Farley JA: Alterations in neurologic function. In Heuther SE, McCance KL, editors: Understanding pathophysiology, ed 2, St Louis, 2000, Mosby, pp 403-406.

71. Smith L: Management of bacterial meningitis: new guidelines from the IDSA, Am Fam Physician 71(10):2003-2008, 2005.

72. Rhuda SC: Nursing management, musculoskeletal problems. In Lewis SM, Heitkemper MM, Dirksen SR, editors: Medical-surgical nursing, assessment and management of clinical problems, ed 5, St Louis, 2000, Mosby, pp 1795-1798.

73. McCance KL, Mourad LA: Alterations in musculoskeletal function. In Heuther SE, McCance KL, editors: Understanding pathophysiology, ed 2, St Louis, 2000, Mosby, pp 1046-1048.

74. Rowland BM: Cellulitis. In Boyden K, Olendorf D, editors: Gale encyclopedia of medicine, Farmington Hills, MI, 1999, Gale Group, p 616.

75. Gethin G, Byrne D, Tierney S et al: Prevalence of lymphoedema and quality of life among patients attending a hospital-based wound management and vascular clinic, Int Wound J 9(2):120-125, 2012.

76. Cellulitis fact sheet. Bethesda, MD, March 1999, National Institute of Allergy and Infectious Diseases, National Institutes of Health.

77. Kirchner JT: Use of blood cultures in patients with cellulitis, Am Fam Physician 61(8):2518, 2000.

78. Edmonson LM, Ebbert JO, Evans JM: Report of a rotavirus outbreak in an adult nursing home population, J Am Med Dir Assoc 1(4):175-179, 2000.

79. Greenberg HB, Estes MK: Rotaviruses: from pathogenesis to vaccination, Gastroenterology 136(6):1939-1951, 2009.

80. Greenberg HB: Rotavirus vaccination and intussusception—act two, N Engl J Med 364(24):2354-2355, 2011.

81. Grimwood K, Lambert SB, Milne RJ: Rotavirus infections and vaccines: burden of illness and potential impact of vaccination, Paediatr Drugs 12(4):235-256, 2010.

82. Barker J, Vipond IB, Bloomfield SF: Effects of cleaning and disinfection in reducing the spread of norovirus contamination via environmental surfaces, J Hospital Infect 58(1):42-49, 2004.

83. Epple HJ, Zeitz M: [Infectious enteritis], [Article in German], Internist (Berl) 52(9):1038, 1040-1044, 1046, 2011.

84. Koo HL, Ajami N, Atmar RL et al: Noroviruses: the leading cause of gastroenteritis worldwide, Discov Med 10(50):61-70, 2010.

85. Barret J: Gastroenteritis. In Boyden K, Olendorf D, editors: Gale encyclopedia of medicine, Farmington Hills, MI, 1999, Gale Group, p 1258.

86. Flaskerud JH, Ungvarski PJ: Overview and update of HIV disease. In Ungvarski PJ, Flaskerud JH, editors: HIV/AIDS: a guide to preliminary care management, Philadelphia, 1999, Saunders.

87. Centers for Disease Control and Prevention: 1993 revised classification system for HIV infection and expanded surveillance case definition for AIDS among adolescents and adults, Morb Mortal Wkly Rep 41(RR-17):1, 1992.

88. HIV infection and AIDs. An overview. National Institute of Allergy and Infectious Diseases. National Institutes of Health. http://www.niaid.nih.gov/topics/HIVAIDS/Understanding/Pages/whatAreHIVAIDS.aspx. Accessed April 13, 2012.

89. Malarkey LM, McMorrow ME, editors: Nurse's manual of laboratory tests and diagnostic procedures, ed 2, Philadelphia, 2000, Saunders.

90. Galantino ML: Clinical assessment and treatment of HIV: rehabilitation of a chronic illness, Thorofare, NJ, 1992, Slack.

91. US OKs new rapid HIV test, approval to be sought in Canada, Can Med Assoc J 168(2):208, 2003.

92. Greenwald JL, Burstein GR, Pincus J, et al: A rapid review of rapid HIV antibody tests, Curr Infect Dis Rep 8:125-131, 2006.

93. Revised guidelines for HIV counseling, testing, and referral, Morb Mortal Wkly Rep 50(RR-19), 2001.

94. Ungvarski PJ, Angell J, Lancaster DJ, et al: Adolescents and adults HIV disease care management. In Ungvarski PJ, Flaskerud JH, editors: HIV/AIDS: a guide to preliminary care management, Philadelphia, 1999, Saunders, pp 131-193.

95. Kublin JG, Morgan CA, Day TA, et al: HIV Vaccine Trials Network: activities and achievements of the first decade and beyond, Clin Investig (Lond) 2(3):245-254, 2012.

96. Price RW: Neurologic complications of HIV infection, Lancet 348:445, 1996.

97. Rosen MJ: Overview of pulmonary complications, Clin Chest Med 17(4):621, 1996.

98. Yunis NA, Stone VE: Cardiac manifestations of HIV/AIDS, J Acquir Immune Defic Syndr Hum Retrovirol 18:145, 1998.

99. Auwaerter PG: Infectious mononucleosis in middle age. (Grand Rounds at the Johns Hopkins Hospital), JAMA 281(5):454, 1999.

100. Ebell MH: Epstein-Barr virus infectious mononucleosis, Am Fam Physician 70(7):1279-1287, 2004.

101. Carson-De Witt RS: Cytomegalovirus infection. In Boyden K, Olendorf D, editors: Gale encyclopedia of medicine, Farmington Hills, MI, 1999, Gale Group, p 892.

102. Hughes JM, Colley DG: Preventing congenital toxoplasmosis, Morb Mortal Wkly Rep 49(RR02):57-75, 2000.

103. The National Prevention Strategy: America's plan for better health and wellness. http://www.healthcare.gov/news/factsheets/2011/06/prevention06162011a.html. Accessed April 13, 2012.

104. Statement by APTA President on national prevention and health promotion strategy. http://www.apta.org/Media/Releases/Legislative/2011/7/21. Accessed April 13, 2012.

105. Anderson JW, Baird P, Davis RH Jr: Health benefits of dietary fiber, Nutr Rev 67(4):188-205, 2009.

106. Chandra RJ: Nutrition and the immune system: an introduction, Am J Clin Nutr 66(2):460S-463S, 1997.

107. Kau AL, Ahern PP, Griffin NW et al: Human nutrition, the gut microbiome and the immune system: envisioning the future, Nature 474(7351):327-336, 2011.

108. Kijak E, Foust G, Steinman RR: Relationship of blood sugar level and leukocytic phagocytosis, South Calif Dent Assoc 32(9):349-351, 1964.

109. Moser AM, Salzer HJ, Krause R: Immunoplasticity—triggers of regulatory function, Med Hypotheses 77(6):1145-1147, 2011.

110. Nedley N: Proof positive: how to reliably combat disease and achieve optimal health through nutrition and lifestyle, Ardmore, OK, 1998, Niel Nedley, MD.

111. Rivers EP, Jaehne AK, Eichhorn-Wharry L et al: Fluid therapy in septic shock, Curr Opin Crit Care 16(4):297-308, 2010.

112. Li Y, Leung GM, Tang JW, et al: Role of ventilation in airborne transmission of infectious agents in the built environment—a multidisciplinary systematic review, Indoor Air 17(1):2-18, 2007.

113. Nielsen PV: Control of airborne infectious diseases in ventilated spaces, J R Soc Interface 6(Suppl 6):S747-S755, 2009.

114. Arendt J: Shift work: coping with the biological clock, Occup Med (Lond) 60(1):10-20, 2010.

115. Cajochen C, Chellappa S, Schmidt C: What keeps us awake? The role of clocks and hourglasses, light, and melatonin, Int Rev Neurobiol 93:57-90, 2010.

116. Laaksi I: Vitamin D and respiratory infection in adults, Proc Nutr Soc 71(1):90-97, 2012.

117. Lundberg U: Stress hormones in health and illness: the roles of work and gender, Psychoneuroendocrinology 30(10):1017-1021, 2005.

118. Walsh NP, Gleeson M, Shephard RJ, et al: Position statement. Part one: immune function and exercise, Exerc Immunol Rev 17:6-63, 2011.

119. Walsh NP, Gleeson M, Pyne DB, et al: Position statement. Part two: maintaining immune health, Exerc Immunol Rev 17:64-103, 2011.

120. Horrigan LA, Kelly JP, Connor TJ: Immunomodulatory effects of caffeine: friend or foe? Pharmacol Ther 111(3):877-892, 2006.

121. Huttunen R, Heikkinen T, Syrjänen J: Smoking and the outcome of infection, J Intern Med 269(3):258-269, 2011.

122. Kaushik KS, Kapila K, Praharaj AK: Shooting up: the interface of microbial infections and drug abuse, J Med Microbiol 60(4):408-422, 2011.

123. Zahs A, Cook RT, Waldschimdt TJ et al: Alcohol and inflammation and infection: clinical and experimental systems—summary of 2010 Alcohol and Immunology Research Interest Group meeting, Alcohol 46(2):147-153, 2012.

124. Falagas ME, Athanasoulia AP, Peppas G et al: Effect of body mass index on the outcome of infections: a systematic review, Obes Rev 10(3):280-289, 2009.

125. Font-Vizcarra L, Tornero E, Bori G et al: Relationship between intraoperative cultures during hip arthroplasty, obesity, and the risk of early prosthetic joint infection: a prospective study of 428 patients, Int J Artif Organs 34(9):870-875, 2011.

126. Huttunen R, Syrjänen J: Obesity and the outcome of infection, Lancet Infect Dis 10(7):442-443, 2010.

127. Semins MJ, Shore AD, Makary MA et al: The impact of obesity on urinary tract infection risk, Urology 79(2):266-269, 2012.

APPENDIX 13A   DISORDERS OF ALTERED IMMUNITY

Systemic Lupus Erythematosus

Systemic lupus erythematosus (SLE) is a chronic, multisystem autoimmune disease with strong genetic predisposition. There is also evidence suggesting risk factors that can trigger the onset of this disease, such as physical or emotional stress, pregnancy, sulfa antibiotics, and environmental factors, such as sun exposure. Women who are African-American, Asian, or Native American, ages 20 to 40 years, are more susceptible than men in acquiring this disease. SLE is characterized by a systemic, remitting-and-relapsing clinical presentation.[1-4]

The primary laboratory test for diagnosis of SLE is as antinuclear antibody titer.[5] Diagnosis of SLE is confirmed if a patient has 4 of the following 11 manifestations of SLE: malar rash, discoid rash (individual round lesions), photosensitivity, oral ulcers, arthritis, serositis, renal disorder, neurologic disorder, hematologic disorder, immunologic disorder, and the presence of antinuclear antibodies.[3]

Prognosis for 10-year survival after diagnosis is 90%. The most common cause of death in SLE is renal failure, and the second most common is central nervous system dysfunction.[1-3]

Clinical presentation of SLE may include the following[1-4]:
- Arthritis or arthralgias (stiffness and pain in hands, feet, and large joints)
- Red, warm, and tender joints
- Butterfly (malar) rash on face
- Fever, fatigue, anorexia, and weight loss
- Pleurisy, pericarditis
- Headache, seizures
- Hemolytic anemia, thrombocytopenia, leukopenia
- Renal disease or failure

Management of SLE may consist of nonsteroidal antiinflammatory drugs; glucocorticoids; immunosuppressive agents (cyclophosphamide); dialysis; and renal transplantation in severe cases.[1,2,4,6]

Sarcoidosis

Sarcoidosis is a systemic granulomatous disorder that primarily affects women and nonwhite adults in the third decade of their life. The definitive etiology is unknown, although an autoimmune process that is environmentally triggered is the generally agreed-on hypothesis. Sarcoidosis may present as acute or chronic and have periods of progression and remission.[6-10]

Multiple body systems may be affected by sarcoidosis. The lungs are the primary organs affected, with dyspnea, dry cough, and chest pain being common symptoms. Pulmonary involvement can be staged according to the following radiographic evidence[7,8]:
- Stage 0: No radiographic abnormalities
- Stage I: Bilateral hilar lymphadenopathy
- Stage II: Bilateral hilar adenopathy and parenchymal infiltration
- Stage III: Parenchymal infiltration without hilar adenopathy
- Stage IV: Advanced fibrosis with evidence of honeycombing, hilar retraction, bullae, cysts, and emphysema

Other systems of the body can be affected as well, with symptoms including the following:
- Eye and skin lesions
- Fever, fatigue, and weight loss
- Hepatosplenomegaly
- Hypercalcemia, anemia, and leukopenia
- Arthralgia, arthritis

Management of sarcoidosis usually consists of corticosteroid therapy, ranging from topical to oral administration. In addition, cytotoxic agents (methotrexate and azathioprine), antimalarial agents (chloroquine and hydroxychloroquine), and nonsteroidal antiinflammatory drugs may be used. In severe cases of pulmonary disease, single and double lung transplantation may be performed.[6-8]

Amyloidosis

Amyloidosis is a group of disorders characterized by deposition of amyloid (a type of protein) in various tissues and organs. Amyloidosis is classified according to protein type and tissue distribution and affects men more than women, between the ages of 60 and 70 years.[11] Clinical signs and symptoms are representative of the affected areas, with common manifestations including[11]:

- Fatigue
- Shortness of breath
- Edema
- Paresthesia
- Weight loss
- Diarrhea
- Peripheral neuropathy

In general, the deposition of protein in these areas will result in firmer, less distensible tissues that compromise organ function. Management of amyloidosis consists of controlling any primary disease process that may promote deposition of amyloid into the tissues.[11]

Rheumatoid Arthritis

Rheumatoid arthritis (RA) is an autoimmune disease characterized by uncontrolled proliferation of synovial tissue.[12] It is a chronic disease involving systemic inflammation, with periods of exacerbation and remission.[13] The etiology is not fully understood, but it is believed there is a correlation between environmental and genetic factors. Females have an increased risk of developing RA, as do individuals with a positive family history, silicate exposure, or smoking history.[12]

There are two forms of RA: juvenile idiopathic arthritis (JIA) and adult RA. JIA occurs most often during the toddler and early adolescent developmental phases, whereas adult RA has a peak onset in the third and fourth decades of life. Both forms of RA have an inflammatory component in disease development and have similar medical management strategies.[13]

With RA, an interaction between autoantibodies (rheumatoid factors) and immunoglobulins initiates the inflammatory process, which involves an increased infiltration of leukocytes from the peripheral circulation into the synovial joint. Pannus—a destructive granulation tissue that dissolves periarticular tissues—can develop, ultimately leading to joint destruction.[13]

Clinical manifestations of RA can include articular and extra-articular symptoms. Most body systems may be involved, including pulmonary, cardiovascular, neurologic, and gastrointestinal.[13] The joints most commonly affected by RA are those with the highest ratio of synovium compared to articular cartilage, including the wrist, proximal interphalangeal, and metacarpophalangeal joints.[12] Common deformities associated with RA are ulnar drift, swan-neck, and boutonniere deformities.[13] Other symptoms include anorexia, low-grade fever, fatigue, and malaise.[12] Osteoarthritis (OA), also called degenerative joint disease, may result in joint changes and deformation. Table 13A-1 compares OA and RA.[13]

Diagnosis of rheumatoid arthritis can be made through the following seven criteria established by the American Rheumatism Association[12]:

1. Morning stiffness
2. Arthritis of three or more joint areas
3. Hand joint involvement
4. Symmetric arthritis
5. Rheumatoid nodules
6. Serum rheumatoid factor positive
7. Radiographic changes of the wrist and hand joints

TABLE 13A-1 Comparison of Osteoarthritis and Rheumatoid Arthritis

	Osteoarthritis	Rheumatoid Arthritis
Onset	Majority of adult age > 65 Gradual onset	Adult: ages 25-50 Sudden onset
Incidence	12% U.S. adults	1%-2% U.S. adults
Gender	Age < 45: predominantly males Age > 45: predominantly females	Female:male ratio 3:1
Etiology	Inflammatory response Genetic, environmental factors	Autoimmune process with multifactorial components
Manifestations	Unilateral joint involvement Affects: spine, hips, knees, feet, hands Inflammation present in 10% of cases Brief morning stiffness	Symmetric, bilateral joint involvement Affects any joint, predominantly upper-extremity joints Inflammation present in most cases Prolonged morning stiffness
Systemic symptoms	None	Fatigue, malaise, weight loss, fever
Lab values	ESR: mildly-moderately increased Rheumatoid factor: absent	ESR: increased during inflammatory process (exacerbation) Rheumatoid factor: present but not diagnostic for disease

ESR, Erythrocyte sedimentation rate.

Laboratory diagnostic tests include a complete blood cell count with differential, rheumatoid factor, and erythrocyte sedimentation rate (ESR) or C-reactive protein (CRP).[11]

Management of RA may include the following[12,13]:

- Nonsteroidal antiinflammatory drugs
- Glucocorticoids
- Disease-modifying antirheumatic drugs (DMARDs) (Chapter 19, Table 19-13)
- Pain management
- Joint protection
- Control of systemic complications

CLINICAL TIP

Modification of an assistive device may be necessary based on the patient's wrist and hand function. For example, a platform walker may more appropriate than a standard walker, and Lofstrand crutches may be more appropriate than axillary crutches.

References

1. Rote NS: Alterations in immunity and inflammation. In McCance KL, Heuther SE, Brashers VL et al, editors: Pathophysiology: the biologic basis for disease in adults and children, ed 6, St Louis, 2010, Mosby, pp 256-272.
2. Kimberly RP: Research advances in systemic lupus erythematosus, JAMA 285(5):650, 2001.
3. McConnell EA: About systemic lupus erythematosus, Nursing 29(9):26, 1999.
4. Wallace DJ: Update on managing lupus erythematosus, J Musculoskelet Med 16(9):531, 1999.
5. Gill JM, Quisel AM, Rocca PV et al: Diagnosis of systemic lupus erythematosus, Am Fam Physician 68(11):2179-2186, 2003.
6. Chandrasoma P, Taylor CR: Concise pathology, ed 2, East Norwalk, CT, 1995, Appleton & Lange.
7. Morey SS: American Thoracic Society Issues consensus statement on sarcoidosis, Am Fam Physician 61(2):553, 2000.
8. Johns CJ, Michele TM: The clinical management of sarcoidosis. A 50-year experience at the Johns Hopkins Hospital, Medicine 78(2):65, 1999.
9. Judson MA, Thompson BW, Rabin DL et al: The diagnostic pathway to sarcoidosis, Chest 123(2):406-412, 2003.
10. Peterson C, Goodman CC: Problems affecting multiple systems. In Goodman CC, Fuller K, editors: Pathology: implications for the physical therapist, ed 3, Philadelphia, 2009, Saunders, p 180.
11. Naqvi BH, Ferri FF: Amyloidosis: In Ferri FF, editor: Ferri's clinical advisor, Philadelphia, 2013, Elsevier.
12. Rindfleisch JA, Muller D: Diagnosis and management of rheumatoid arthritis, Am Fam Physician 72(6):1037-1047, 2005.
13. Goodman CC: Soft tissue, joint, and bone disorders. In Goodman CC, Fuller K, editors: Pathology: implications for the physical therapist, ed 3, Philadelphia, 2009, Saunders, pp 1235-1317.

CHAPTER 12

Organ Transplantation

Karen Vitak

CHAPTER OBJECTIVES

The objectives for this chapter are to provide information on the following:

1. The transplantation process, including criteria for transplantation, organ donation, preoperative care, and postoperative care
2. Complications after organ transplantation, including rejection and infection
3. The various types of organ transplantation procedures
4. Guidelines for physical therapy intervention with the transplant recipient

PREFERRED PRACTICE PATTERNS

The most relevant practice patterns for the diagnoses discussed in this chapter, based on the American Physical Therapy Association's *Guide to Physical Therapist Practice*, second edition, are as follows:

- Impaired Aerobic Capacity/Endurance Associated With Deconditioning: 6B
- Impaired Aerobic Capacity/Endurance Associated With Cardiovascular Pump Dysfunction or Failure: 6D
- Impaired Ventilation and Respiration/Gas Exchange Associated With Ventilatory Pump Dysfunction or Failure: 6E
- Impaired Ventilation and Respiration/Gas Exchange Associated With Respiratory Failure: 6F

Please refer to Appendix A for a complete list of the preferred practice patterns, as individual patient conditions are highly variable and other practice patterns may be applicable.

With advances in technology and immunology, organ and tissue transplantation has become a more standard practice. There were 28,053 organ transplants performed in the United States in 2012.[1] Physical therapists are frequently involved in the rehabilitation process for pretransplant and posttransplant recipients.[2] Owing to limited organ donor availability, physical therapists often treat more potential recipients than posttransplant recipients. Patients awaiting transplants often require admission to an acute care hospital as a result of their end-stage organ disease. They may be very deconditioned and may benefit from physical therapy during their stay. The goal of physical therapy for transplant candidates is conditioning in preparation for the transplant procedure and postoperative course, and increasing functional mobility and endurance in an attempt to return patients to a safe functional level at home. Some transplant candidates may be too acutely sick and may no longer qualify for transplantation during that particular hospital admission. These patients are generally unable to work and may need assistance at home from family members or even require transfer to a rehabilitation facility.

Whether the patient is pretransplantation or posttransplantation, physical therapists focus on conditioning patients to their maximum functional level and should have a basic knowledge of the patient's end-stage organ disease.

Types of Organ Transplants

The kidney, liver, pancreas, heart, lung, and intestine are organs that are procured for transplantation. The most frequent of those are the kidney, liver, and heart.[3] Double transplants, such as liver-kidney, kidney-pancreas, and heart-lung, are performed if the patient has multiorgan failure. Intestinal transplants are not addressed in this text because they are performed in much smaller numbers, with only 106 transplants in 2012.[1] Candidates for this procedure include individuals with various disorders involving poor intestinal function and who are unable to be maintained with other nutritional support. In addition to these solid organ transplants, stem cell transplants that involve the replacement of abnormal cells with healthy cells are discussed.

> ✎ **CLINICAL TIP**
>
> It is recommended that physical therapists who may be involved in care for patients with intestinal transplantation seek additional information from their transplant center as well as the Intestinal Transplant Association.

Criteria for Transplantation

Transplantation is offered to patients who have end-stage organ disease for which alternative medical or surgical management has failed. The patient typically has a life expectancy of less than 1 to 3 years.[4-6] Criteria for organ recipients vary, depending on the type of organ transplant needed and the transplant facility.

The basic criteria for transplantation include the following[7]:

- The presence of end-stage disease in a transplantable organ
- The failure of conventional therapy to treat the condition successfully
- The absence of untreatable malignancy or irreversible infection
- The absence of disease that would attack the transplanted organ or tissue

In addition to these criteria, transplant candidates must demonstrate emotional and psychological stability, have an adequate support system, and be willing to comply with lifelong immunosuppressive drug therapy. Other criteria, such as age limits and absence of drug or alcohol abuse, are specific to the transplant facility. To determine whether transplantation is the best treatment option for the individual, all transplant candidates are evaluated by a team of health care professionals consisting of a transplant surgeon, transplant nurse coordinator, infectious disease physician, psychiatrist, social worker, nutritionist, and sometimes a physical therapist. The patient undergoes many laboratory and diagnostic studies during the evaluation process. Acceptable candidates for organ transplantation are placed on a waiting list. Waiting times for an organ may range from days to years depending on the organ and an individual's medical status.[3] Improvements in the medical management of transplant recipients, including immunosuppressants and postoperative care protocols, have increased survival rates. As a result, organs are now being offered to recipients that were previously considered "high-risk," including older patients with multiple comorbidities and accompanying activity limitations.[8]

Transplant Donation

Cadaveric Donors

Cadaveric donors are generally individuals who have been determined to be dead by neurological criteria following severe trauma, such as from head or spinal cord injury, cerebral hemorrhage, or anoxia.[9,10] Death must occur at a location where cardiopulmonary support is immediately available to maintain the potential organ donor on mechanical ventilation, cardiopulmonary bypass, or both in order to preserve organ viability.[9] To a more limited extent, death can also be determined on the basis of circulatory criteria, and organs can be expeditiously procured after specific criteria have been met (e.g., asystole for generally between 2 and 5 minutes). However, ethical issues remain surrounding the precise determination of death and decisions to withdraw support. In addition, these organs are subject to potentially greater ischemic injury, which in turn increases the risk for delayed graft function and graft failure.[3,11] Both types of cadaveric donors must have no evidence of malignancy, sepsis, or communicable diseases, such as hepatitis B or human immunodeficiency virus.[7,12,13]

Living Donors

Living donor transplantation offers an alternative means of organ donation that helps to expand the donor pool and also allows for greater evaluation of the organs before transplant. Living donors are always used for stem cell transplants, often used for kidney transplants, and sometimes used for liver, lung, and pancreas transplantation. They may be genetically related (i.e., blood relative), emotionally related to the recipient (i.e., spouse or close friend), or perhaps even a stranger in the case of a donor chain. Living donors also are evaluated by the transplant team to determine medical suitability.

The age of a potential donor generally ranges from a term newborn to 65 years, depending on the organ considered for donation and the recipient. Donors do not have a history of drug or alcohol abuse, chronic disease, malignancy, syphilis, tuberculosis, hepatitis B, or human immunodeficiency virus infection. Ideally, the donor's height and weight approximate those of the recipient for the best "fit."

Donor Shortage

As of April 2013, there were more than 117,000 individuals on the transplant waiting list, with more than 75,000 of those listed as medically suitable for transplant. However, there were just over 14,000 donors from January through December 2012.[1] As a result, many patients die waiting for a suitable organ to become available. Numerous efforts have been undertaken to address the organ donor shortage, including educational campaigns and technological advancements.

Increased use of what are termed "expanded criteria" donor (ECD) grafts is occurring with many transplants including kidney. These are organs that may have previously gone un-used due to advanced age or other complicating factors such as hypertension or death from stroke.[8]

Regenerative medicine entails the development of cellular, tissue, and organ substitutes to help restore function.[14] Engineers continue to work on the development of implantable bioartificial organs, including an artificial kidney and lungs; however, none of these devices have yet gained approval for use in humans in the United States. Stem cell research also has the potential to provide an alternative to solid organ transplant. The goal is for immature stem cells to be directed to differentiate into specific cell types and repair or replace tissues that have been damaged because of injury. For example, stem cells have been shown in animal and a few small human studies to repair injured heart tissue and improve cardiac function.[15]

Donor Matching/Allocation

In the United States, organ procurement and distribution for transplantation are administered by the United Network for Organ Sharing (UNOS) under contract with the federal government. UNOS sets standards for transplant centers and teams, tissue typing laboratories, and organ procurement organizations. Organ allocation is a complex process, and UNOS policies attempt to balance justice and medical utility. Factors that are involved with determining allocation and how they are weighted in the decision making vary by organ but generally include the following[1]:

- ABO blood typing
- Tissue (histocompatibility) typing
- Size
- Waiting time
- Severity of illness/degree of medical urgency
- Geographic location (distance between potential recipient and donor)

The donor and recipient must be ABO blood type identical or compatible for all organ transplants.[16] Tissue typing typically involves a series of several tests to determine how likely a potential recipient is to develop a rejection response with transplantation, which include:

- Human leukocyte antigen (HLA) typing attempts to match HLAs, which are the antigens that cause most graft rejection. The better the histocompatibility match and degree of genetic similarity between the donor and the recipient, the less severe the potential rejection response. This may be performed in several ways; however, the most conventional method involves mixing a serologic sample of the potential recipient's lymphocytes with a standard panel of antisera and observing for lymphocytotoxicity.[17]

- White cell cross-matching is performed by mixing the lymphocytes from the donor with the serum from the recipient and then observing for immune responses. A negative cross-match indicates no antibody reaction and that the recipient's antibodies are compatible with the donor. A negative cross-match is required for successful kidney and kidney-pancreas transplants.[18]

Although pretransplant tissue typing is ideal, it is not always performed due to insufficient time. The time that an organ remains viable after it is recovered varies by organ. Average viability times range from 4 to 6 hours for heart and lungs, 24 hours for pancreas, 24 to 30 hours for liver, and 48 to 72 hours for kidneys.[3] When there is insufficient time, the other factors become the major considerations.[17,19] For example, in lung transplant, the Lung Allocation Score (LAS) is used to estimate the severity of illness and chance for survival to assist with allocation.[1]

General Posttransplantation Care and Complications

Postoperative Care for Living Donors

Postoperative care for living donors is similar to that for any patient who has undergone major abdominal or cardiothoracic surgery. These patients are taken off mechanical ventilation in the recovery room and transferred to the general surgery or transplant ward. Vital signs and blood counts are monitored closely for possible postoperative bleeding. Patients are usually out of bed and ambulating by postoperative day 1. On average, the duration of donor hospitalization may range from 1 to 2 days for a kidney donor to 8 days for a simultaneous pancreas-kidney (SPK) donor.[18,20] Physical therapists are rarely involved with donors, but may become involved if complications arise affecting the donors' functional mobility.

Postoperative Care for Transplant Recipients

Once an organ is transplanted, the postoperative care focuses on the monitoring and treatment of the following[21]:

- Allograft function
- Rejection
- Infection
- Adverse effects of immunosuppressive drugs

General postoperative care for transplant recipients is also similar to the care patients receive after major abdominal or cardiothoracic surgery. Kidney and liver transplant recipients are often taken off of mechanical ventilation before leaving the operating room.[22,23] Most other solid organ recipients are transferred from the operating room to the surgical intensive care unit, where they are weaned from mechanical ventilation (extubated) within 24 to 48 hours.[3,16,24,25] Once extubated and hemodynamically stable, recipients are transferred to specialized transplant floors. The nursing staff monitors the recipient closely for signs and symptoms of infection and rejection, which are the leading causes of morbidity and mortality in the first year after transplantation.

Complications from postoperative transplantation may contribute to an increased length of hospital stay or hospital readmissions. They can be grouped to include the following types:

- Surgical
- Medical
- Rejection
- Infection

Surgical complications include vascular problems, such as thrombosis, stenosis, leakage at anastomotic sites, and postoperative bleeding. Medical complications may include fluid overload or dehydration, electrolyte imbalance, or hypotension/hypertension.

Rejection

Rejection, or the tendency of the recipient's body to reject anything that is "nonself," is one of the leading problems with organ transplantation. This is actually a normal immune response to invasion of foreign matter, the transplanted organ or tissue. Some degree of rejection is normal; however, if the patient is not treated with immunosuppressive drugs, the donor organ will be completely rejected and cease to be viable.[3] Transplant recipients must receive immunosuppressants for the rest of their lives to minimize rejection of their transplanted organs. The pharmacologic agents most often used to prevent organ rejection include double or triple drug therapy, which allows use of smaller doses of individual drugs.[26]

These immunosuppressive drugs decrease the body's ability to fight infection. A delicate balance must be reached between suppressing rejection and avoiding infection. Insufficient immunosuppression may result in rejection that threatens the allograft and patient survival, whereas excessive immunosuppression increases the risk of infection and malignancy.[21] If detected early, rejection can be minimized or reversed with an increase in daily doses of immunosuppressive drugs.

Many different factors influence the combination of drugs used posttransplant including the individual patient's condition, organ transplanted, transplant center–specific practices, and recent literature. There are three general approaches to posttransplant immunosuppression[26]:

- Induction immunosuppression: Encompasses high-dose immunosuppressive medications given to prevent acute rejection immediately after transplantation (usually only in the first 30 days)
- Maintenance immunosuppression: Includes all medications used for long-term immunosuppression
- Antirejection immunosuppression: Includes all immunosuppressive medications given for managing a specific acute rejection episode at any point posttransplantation

The main classes of drugs used for transplant immunosuppression include corticosteroids, calcineurin inhibitors, antimetabolites, target of rapamycin inhibitors, monoclonal antibodies, and polyclonal anti-lymphocyte antibodies. Individual drug classes have different mechanisms that include inhibition of gene transcription, DNA and RNA production, T-cell activation and proliferation, and lymphocyte and antibody production.[27] Please refer to Chapter 19 for additional pharmacology information and physical therapy implications for each medication.

> ### ✎ CLINICAL TIP
>
> Immunosuppressants used in the management of organ transplantation have significant side effects. Drug protocols now promote the rapid tapering of steroids after transplantation, which helps to diminish the harsh side effects of those drugs.[28] The most common side effects include hypertension, bone marrow suppression, electrolyte disturbances, decreased bone density, renal dysfunction, and hepatotoxicity. Physical therapists must routinely monitor for these adverse side effects and take these into account when designing treatment plans. Refer to Chapter 19 for more information on immunosuppressive agents.

Types of Graft Rejection

Hyperacute Rejection. Hyperacute rejection is characterized by ischemia and necrosis of the graft that occurs from the time of transplant to 48 hours after transplant.[7] It is believed to be caused by cytotoxic antibodies present in the recipient that respond to tissue antigens on the donor organ. The manifestations of hyperacute rejection include general malaise and high fever. Rejection occurs before vascularization of the graft takes place. Plasmapheresis may be used to attempt to remove circulating antibodies from the blood. However, usually hyperacute rejection is unresponsive to treatment, and removal of the rejected organ with immediate retransplantation is required.[3,17,29]

Acute Rejection. Acute rejection is a treatable and reversible form of rejection that typically occurs within the first 3 months to 1 year after transplantation. However, changes in the immunosuppressive management may also cause later acute rejection episodes.[3] Almost every patient has some degree of acute rejection after transplantation. It may be due to an antibody-mediated immune response and/or a T-cell–mediated immune response. More commonly, T lymphocytes detect foreign antigens from the graft, become sensitized, and set the immune response into action. Phagocytes, which are attracted to the graft site by the T lymphocytes, damage the inner lining of small blood vessels in the organ. This causes thrombosis of the vessels, resulting in tissue ischemia and eventual death of the graft if left untreated.[3,12]

The first signs of acute rejection may be detected within 4 to 10 days postoperatively.[7,12,17] The actual manifestations of rejection vary with the affected organ. General signs and symptoms of acute rejection include the following[1,3,12]:

- Fever, chills, sweating, body aches/pains
- Swelling and/or tenderness at the graft site
- Malaise and/or fatigue
- Nausea, diarrhea, vomiting, loss of appetite
- Peripheral edema
- Dyspnea, irregular heart beat, increased blood pressure
- Sudden weight gain (6 lb in less than 3 days)
- Decreased urine output
- Abnormal laboratory findings (dependent on organ): electrolyte imbalances, increased blood urea nitrogen (BUN) and serum creatinine levels, increased bilirubin and liver enzymes (alanine transaminase [ALT], aspartate transaminase [AST]), increased urine amylase

Early intervention is the key to reversal of acute rejection, and treatment usually includes use of antirejection drugs.

Chronic Rejection. Chronic rejection of the graft occurs after the first few months of transplantation and is characterized by gradual and progressive deterioration of the graft. It is believed to result from a combination of B-cell–mediated and T-cell–mediated immunity, frequent episodes of acute rejection, and also infection. Persistent inflammation leads to graft necrosis and deterioration in function. Increasing immunosuppressive medications may slow the process, but it cannot stop chronic

rejection, and eventually retransplantation is required. Chronic rejection presents differently depending on the transplanted organ. Individuals who have undergone kidney and liver transplants may present with a more gradual rise in lab values (i.e., creatinine, BUN, bilirubin, liver function tests [LFTs]) compared to what is seen in acute rejection.[7,12,30] In patients with cardiac transplants, coronary allograft vasculopathy may occur in which there is accelerated graft atherosclerosis or myocardial fibrosis leading to myocardial ischemia and infarction.[7] Chronic rejection in patients with lung transplants is manifested as bronchiolitis obliterans with symptoms of increasing airflow obstruction.[4,5] In patients with pancreas transplants, the pancreatic vessels thicken, leading to fibrosis, and there is a decrease in insulin secretion with resultant hyperglycemia.[7]

Infection

Suppression of the immune response prevents rejection of the transplanted organ; however, the recipient is more susceptible to bacterial, fungal, and viral infections. Infection is one of the leading causes of critical illness, hospitalization, morbidity, and mortality following organ transplant.[31] The high risk of infections posttransplant requires that recipients be given antiviral, antibacterial, and antifungal medications prophylactically. Active infections are treated with a reduction of immunosuppressants and addition of other medications targeting the pathogen.[3] Please refer to Chapter 19 for information about specific medications used to treat infections. An overview of the timeline for infection after organ transplant is shown in Figure 14-1.

General signs and symptoms of infection include the following[18]:

- Temperature greater than 38° C (100.5° F)
- Fatigue

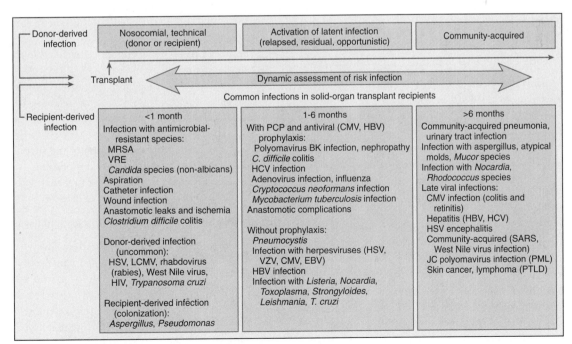

FIGURE 14-1
Changing timeline of infection after organ transplant. (Data from Fishman JA: Infection in solid-organ transplant recipients, N Engl J Med 357:2601, 2007. In Auerbach PS: Wilderness medicine, ed 6, Philadelphia, 2012, Mosby/Elsevier.)

- Shaking, chills, body aches
- Sweating
- Diarrhea lasting longer than 2 days
- Dyspnea
- Cough or sore throat

✎ CLINICAL TIP

Some signs of activity intolerance are similar to signs of rejection and infection. In addition, it can be difficult to distinguish clinically between rejection and infection. It is important for the physical therapist to monitor for signs and symptoms of both and to communicate these to the transplant team.

Renal Transplantation

Renal or kidney transplant is the most common organ transplant procedure.[3] In 2012, there were 16,487 recorded kidney transplants in the United States.[1] The goal of renal transplantation is to restore normal renal function to patients with irreversible end-stage renal failure.

The most frequent causes of end-stage renal disease requiring transplantation include the following[9,17]:

- Primary uncontrolled hypertension
- Glomerulonephritis
- Chronic pyelonephritis
- Diabetic nephropathy
- Polycystic kidney disease

Contraindications to renal transplantation include the following[17]:

- Advanced cardiopulmonary disease
- Active vasculitis
- Morbid obesity

Cadaveric versus Living Donor Renal Transplantation

Kidney transplants may be cadaveric or living donor. Cadaveric kidneys may be maintained for as long as 72 hours before transplantation and, as a result, are the last organs to be harvested. Although less commonly performed, living donor kidney transplants are preferred to cadaveric transplantation. Most living donor nephrectomies are performed laparoscopically with a 2- to 3-inch incision in the lower quadrant, minimizing pain and allowing donors to mobilize quickly after surgery.[1,10,32] Because the body can function well with one kidney, the kidney donor can lead a normal, active life after recovering from the surgery. There is no increased risk of kidney disease, hypertension, or diabetes, and life expectancy does not change for the donor.[18]

The benefits of a living donor transplant for the recipient include longer allograft and patient survival rates. According to UNOS data as of April 2013, the 5-year kidney graft survival rate is 79.8% for living donors compared to 66.6% for cadaveric donors, and patient 5-year survival rates are 90.1% and 81.8%, respectively.[1] The higher success rate of the recipients of living

donor transplants can be attributed to the following: potentially healthier recipients since undergoing procedure electively, more thorough pretransplant evaluation resulting in closer genetic matches, lower incidence of acute tubular necrosis (ATN) postoperatively, and lower requirement for immunosuppressive medications resulting in a lower risk for infection/malignancy.[18,33]

Unfortunately, a shortage of donor kidneys continues, with more than 5000 individuals removed from the waiting list due to death in 2009.[1] Strategies to expand the donor pool are evolving and include the following[32]:

- Use of more ECD kidneys.
- Desensitization protocols—use of intravenous immunoglobulin and plasmapheresis before transplant to modulate antibodies and reduce the recipient's potential immune response. This may allow the use of organs that are traditionally deemed incompatible based on blood type and/or a positive cross-match.
- Kidney Paired Donation (KPD)—a potential recipient with a willing but incompatible donor is matched to another incompatible donor recipient pair with reciprocal incompatibility. Donor chains that incorporate this concept are developing.

Renal Transplant Procedure

The renal allograft is not placed in the same location as the native kidney. It is placed extraperitoneally in the iliac fossa through an oblique lower abdominal incision.[3,10,34] The renal artery and vein of the donated kidney are attached to the recipient's internal iliac artery and iliac vein, respectively. The ureter of the donated kidney is sutured to the bladder and a urinary catheter is placed for approximately 5 days to allow for healing.[10] The recipient's native kidney is not removed unless it is a source of infection or uncontrolled hypertension. The residual function may be helpful if the transplant fails and the recipient requires hemodialysis.[34,35]

The advantages of renal allograft placement in the iliac fossa include the following[36]:

- A decrease in postoperative pain because the peritoneal cavity is not entered
- Easier access to the graft postoperatively for biopsy or any reoperative procedure
- Ease of palpation and auscultation of the superficial kidney to help diagnose postoperative complications
- The facilitation of vascular and ureteral anastomoses, because it is close to blood vessels and the bladder

Indication of Renal Function Posttransplant

Restoration of renal function is characterized by:
- Immediate production of urine and massive diuresis (excellent renal function is characterized by a urine output of 800 to 1000 ml per hour)[25]
- Declining levels of BUN and serum creatinine

However, there is a 20% to 30% chance of delayed graft function, and dialysis may be required for a few days to several weeks.[1,34] Dialysis is discontinued once urine output increases and serum creatinine and BUN begin to normalize. With time, normal kidney function is restored, and the dependence on dialysis is eliminated.[34]

Postoperative Care and Complications

Volume status is strictly assessed, and intake and output records are precisely recorded. Daily weights should be measured at the same time using the same scale. When urine volumes are extremely high, intravenous fluids may be titrated. Other volume assessment parameters include inspection of neck veins for distention, skin turgor and mucous membranes for dehydration, and extremities for edema. Auscultation of the chest is performed to determine the presence of adventitious breath sounds, such as crackles, which indicate the presence of excess volume.[17]

The most common signs of rejection specific to the kidney are an increase in BUN and serum creatinine, decrease in urine output, increase in blood pressure, weight gain greater than 1 kg in a 24-hour period, and ankle edema.[17,18,34] A percutaneous renal biopsy under ultrasound guidance is the most definitive test for acute rejection.[34] ATN may occur posttransplantation because of ischemic damage from prolonged preservation, and dialysis may be required until the kidney starts to function.[18]

Ureteral obstruction may occur owing to compression of the ureter by a fluid collection or by blockage from a blood clot in the ureter, and may be visible on ultrasound. The placement of a nephrostomy tube or surgery may be required to repair the obstruction and prevent irreversible damage to the allograft.[34]

Urine leaks may occur at the level of the bladder, ureter, or renal calyx. They usually occur within the first few days of transplantation.[34] Renal ultrasounds are performed to assess for fluid collections, and radionucleotide scans view the perfusion of the kidney. Other potential complications include posttransplant diabetes mellitus (PTDM); renal artery thrombosis or leakage at the anastomosis; hypertension; hyperkalemia; renal abscess or decreased renal function; and pulmonary edema.[3,19,34] Thrombosis most often occurs within the first 2 to 3 days after transplantation.[34] The most common cause of decreased urine output in the immediate postoperative period is occlusion of the urinary catheter due to clot retention, in which case aseptic irrigation is required.[17]

✎ CLINICAL TIP

Individuals who have undergone a kidney transplant tend to have impaired exercise capacity for a number of reasons, including renal osteodystrophy, anemia, and muscle dysfunction/wasting.[37] Although kidney transplant recipients will benefit from rehabilitation, it is often underused in this population. Physical therapists should advocate for physical therapy services at discharge for appropriate individuals.

Physical Therapy for Renal Transplant Recipients

- Daily fluid intake of 2 to 3 liters is generally recommended for kidney transplant recipients.[22,38] Therapists should assist patients in adhering to fluid recommendations from the medical team during therapy sessions.

- In the immediate postoperative period, blood pressure (BP) needs to be maintained to ensure adequate perfusion to the newly grafted kidney. Therapists should check with the physician for specific parameters, but generally the systolic BP should be kept above 110 mmHg. Kidney transplant recipients may be normotensive at rest; however, they respond to exercise with a higher-than-normal blood pressure.[39]

- Consistent BP monitoring for the life span of the transplant is necessary because many transplant recipients develop hypertension over time, and cardiovascular disease is the leading cause of death in kidney transplant recipients.[40]

Liver Transplantation

The liver is the second most commonly recorded organ transplanted in the United States, with 6256 patients undergoing liver transplant surgery in 2012.[1] Indications for liver or hepatic transplantation include the following[7,41,42]:

- End-stage hepatic disease
- Primary biliary cirrhosis
- Chronic hepatitis B or C
- Fulminant hepatic failure (FHF) resulting from an acute viral, toxic, anesthetic-induced, or medication-induced liver injury
- Congenital biliary abnormalities
- Sclerosing cholangitis
- Wilson's disease
- Budd-Chiari syndrome
- Biliary atresia
- Confined hepatic malignancy (hepatocellular carcinoma)
- Hereditary metabolic diseases (such as familial amyloid polyneuropathy)

Contraindications to hepatic transplantation include the following[3,30,41]:

- Advanced cardiac disease
- Myocardial infarction within the previous 6 months
- Severe chronic obstructive pulmonary disease
- Active alcohol use/other substance abuse (required time to be substance-free is determined by center, but is usually greater than 6 months)

Pretransplantation Care

Patients awaiting liver transplant are often deconditioned and malnourished with resulting weakness and muscle loss due to breakdown of muscle protein and fat, which are used as alternative energy sources.[43] Additionally, anasarca and/or ascites often lead to overall weight gain with associated balance impairments. The goals of preoperative physical therapy include aerobic conditioning, strength training, postural education, and maximizing functional mobility with a focus on education regarding postoperative follow-up, fall prevention, home exercise program, and lifestyle modification.

TABLE 14-1 Medical Characteristics of Liver Failure, Their Related Clinical Effects, and Physical Therapy Implications

Medical Characteristics of Liver Failure	Clinical Effects	Physical Therapy Implications
↑ Bilirubin level	Jaundice Dark, tea-colored urine May induce nausea and anorexia	None
↓ Albumin synthesis	Accumulation of ascites fluid in the peritoneal cavity causes abdominal swelling and increased abdominal girth May promote protein loss and a negative nitrogen balance May lead to anasarca (total body edema)	May cause pressure on the diaphragm, leading to respiratory and nutritional difficulties Monitor for dyspnea with activity Patient may have an altered center of gravity and decreased balance May lead to muscle atrophy and skin fragility
Altered clotting ability	Increased prothrombin time and partial thromboplastin time	Prolonged bleeding time Patient bruises easily Monitor patient safety and prevention of falls
Impaired glucose production	Low blood sugar	Patient may have decreased energy
Portal hypertension	Presence of esophageal varices May lead to hepatic encephalopathy	Bleeding may occur spontaneously Patient may have altered mental status and decreased safety awareness
Diminished phagocytic activity	Spontaneous bacterial peritonitis or cholangitis	None
Failure to absorb vitamin D	Osteoporosis may result	May develop compression or pathologic fractures
Impaired cerebral function	Lack of awareness, decreased attention span, lethargy, personality changes, disorientation, coma	Patient may be confused with treatment Maintain safety and monitor for changes to communicate with medical team

↑, Elevated; ↓, decreased.

Data from Sigardson-Poor KM, Haggerty LM: Nursing care of the transplant recipient, Philadelphia, 1990, Saunders, p 149-151; Braddom RL, editor: Physical medicine and rehabilitation, ed 2, Philadelphia, 2000 and 2007, Saunders, pp 139 and 1145; Findlay JY et al: Critical care of the end-stage liver disease patient awaiting liver transplantation, Liver Transplantation 17:496-510, 2011.

Table 14-1 provides some characteristics of liver failure, their clinical effects, and their implications for physical therapy.

Types of Liver Transplants

Orthotopic Cadaveric Liver Transplantation

Orthotopic liver transplantation involves removal of the diseased liver and insertion of a cadaveric liver into the normal anatomic position via a midline sternotomy and continuous laparotomy.

Cadaveric Split Liver Transplant

Split liver transplants are sometimes used to expand the donor pool. Surgeons divide an adult cadaveric liver in situ into two functioning allografts.[1] Usually, the smaller left lobe is donated to a child, and the larger right lobe is given to an adult.[44]

Living Adult Donor Liver Transplant

A single lobe of the liver from a living adult is transplanted into the recipient. Because of the unique ability of the liver to regenerate, the donor's and recipient's livers will grow back to normal size within several months.[18] At 1 year follow-up, there was no significant difference in bilirubin, albumin, and international normalized ratio (INR) of the donors compared to pretransplant. In spite of this, the use of living donors in liver transplant has declined steadily since its peak in 2001, likely due to concerns about higher donor morbidity and mortality relative to what is seen with kidneys.[1]

Domino Liver Transplant

Domino liver transplant (DLT) is a technique used in the treatment of several hereditary metabolic diseases including familial amyloid polyneuropathy (FAP). Patients with these diseases have aberrant or deficient protein production in the liver; however, it is structurally and functionally normal. In a domino liver transplant, these individuals receive a donated cadaveric liver and in turn donate their explanted liver to the domino recipient, another patient on the waiting list. Because of the natural history of these disease processes, it can take years for any symptomatic disease to develop in domino recipients, if at all. Individuals who are chosen to receive these domino livers are usually older and more marginal transplant candidates, and it is thought that they might not otherwise be offered a transplant.[42]

Indication of Liver Function Posttransplant

- Once the graft is vascularized in the operating room, the functioning liver starts to produce bile.[17] Thus, prompt outflow of bile through the biliary T tube, which is inserted at the time of surgery, is an early indicator of proper function of the transplanted liver.[12] Thick, dark-green bile drainage indicates good liver function. A sudden drop in amount of bile or change to a light yellow color indicates an alteration in liver function.[12]

- The most sensitive laboratory indices of liver function are the coagulation factors, prothrombin time (PT), partial thromboplastin time (PTT), and INR. Alteration in liver function is reflected very early by prolonged coagulation times. A steady downward trend to normalization of the PT and PTT should occur postoperatively.[17]

- The LFTs should reveal a progressive decline after transplantation. The exact values can vary from patient to patient and with volume status; more accurate levels are determined 6 to 12 hours after surgery.[17]

- In the immediate postoperative period, hypokalemia is another sign that the liver is functional. Once the graft is vascularized, hepatocytes extract potassium from the blood. On the other hand, hyperkalemia often signifies cell death and that the hepatocytes are nonfunctional.[17]

- Normal to slightly elevated blood glucose levels indicate that the liver is able to store glycogen and convert it to glucose.[3]

> ### ✎ CLINICAL TIP
>
> Patients may have prolonged clotting time reflected in the lab results (PT/PTT/INR). An INR of greater than 4.0 increases the risk of uncontrolled bleeding with injury. Check the guidelines at your facility for physical therapy intervention for the patient with an elevated INR, and communicate with the team.

Postoperative Care and Complications

Postoperatively, liver transplant recipients may emerge with several Jackson-Pratt (JP) suction drains and a biliary T tube. The JP drains lie over the superior surface of the liver and drain blood-tinged fluid. The JP drains are gradually removed after surgery as the drainage decreases, but often one is left in place for up to a week after surgery.[18,25] The T tube, which is placed in the bile duct, allows for monitoring the amount, color, and consistency of the bile. It remains in place for up to 12 weeks postoperatively and is removed once the bilirubin level falls.[18,30]

Primary graft failure (PGF) is a sign of acute hepatic failure that may be seen immediately postoperatively. It is characterized by a markedly abnormal liver function; prolonged PT, PTT, or both; oliguria; metabolic acidosis; hyperkalemia; hypoglycemia; and coma. In the event of primary graft failure, retransplantation is immediately required.

Acute kidney injury (AKI) is relatively common following liver transplant. Several factors influence the development of AKI after liver transplant, including intraoperative hypotension, severity of liver disease, preoperative renal function, and drug-induced toxicity. Calcineurin inhibitors are frequently used after liver transplant but may lead to renal injury, and they are now used in reduced doses and at a later time postsurgery.[31] Other potential medical complications include PTDM, abscess, atelectasis, and pneumonia secondary to ascites or peritonitis.[7]

Acute rejection specific to a transplanted liver includes elevated LFTs (especially an increase in bilirubin) and prolonged PT, PTT, or both; jaundice; right upper-quadrant pain; clay-colored stools; tea-colored urine; decreased quantity of bile; thin, watery, light-colored bile through the T tube; and increased ascitic drainage. A liver biopsy is the definitive diagnostic test for rejection and is able to distinguish between early rejection and ischemic injury.[30]

Surgical complications include hepatic artery thrombosis, biliary leak, or stricture. These complications present with a rising bilirubin level and are identical in appearance to an acute rejection episode.[3] Consequently, recipients undergo routine Doppler ultrasound of the abdomen to check for fluid collections and patency of the hepatic artery and portal vein.[30] A cholangiogram, which examines the patency of the biliary tree drainage system, may be performed to rule out bile duct obstruction. Surgical intervention is indicated if the biliary obstruction cannot be corrected by a percutaneous transhepatic cholangiogram. Portal vein thrombosis is evident if ascites persist or variceal hemorrhage develops.[19]

Long-term evidence shows cardiovascular complications related to obesity, diabetes, and hyperlipidemia in post–liver transplant patients. Corticosteroids used to treat rejection are the primary risk factor for development of these postoperative complications; however, studies indicate a significant decrease in these complications when steroids are withdrawn by 3 to 4 months posttransplant.[45] Exercise and diet modification can play a role in preventing these complications.[46] Survival rates for liver transplant recipients are improving with 86% to 90% 1-year survival and 72% to 78% 5-year survival (higher in living vs. cadaveric).[1] Fatigue has also been found to be a significant chronic problem following liver transplant.[2]

> ### ✎ CLINICAL TIP
>
> Typical length of stay in the hospital after liver transplant ranges from 1 to 3 weeks.[10] An individualized home exercise program with follow-up home or outpatient physical therapy is recommended because of the high incidence of obesity and diabetes in post–liver transplant patients. In addition, energy conservation techniques may help to reduce activity limitations in recipients during periods of increased fatigue.

Physical Therapy for Liver Transplant Recipients

- Deep breathing and physical activity are beneficial during the early postoperative course. Liver transplant recipients are susceptible to atelectasis and pneumonia because of the long operative procedure and large incision that hinders full chest expansion and cough effectiveness. Postoperatively, many recipients still have ascites from weeping of sodium-rich and albumin-rich fluid from the liver's surface.[12]

- Along with ascites and postsurgical fluid retention, liver transplant recipients have an increased abdominal girth and lower extremity edema that lead to a shift in the patient's center of gravity and impaired balance. Often, patients have an increase in lumbar lordosis and complain of low back pain.

Combined Liver-Kidney Transplantation

It has been estimated that approximately one quarter of all liver transplant candidates have impaired renal function; consequently renal transplant may also be indicated. Consensus statements have been developed to describe indications for combined liver-kidney transplants. Factors used in this determination include the degree and duration of renal injury, length of time undergoing renal replacement therapy, the degree of proteinuria, and findings from renal biopsy.[47]

Pancreas Transplantation

Indication for Pancreas Transplant

Pancreas transplant candidates have insulin-dependent, type 1 diabetes mellitus and are preuremic (without urea in the blood). These patients have severe brittle diabetes and metabolic imbalances, such as hypoglycemic unawareness and subcutaneous insulin resistance.[48,49] Pancreas transplantation attempts to stabilize or prevent the devastating target organ complications of type 1 diabetes by returning the patient to normoglycemia and improving the patient's quality of life.[3] Ideally, pancreas transplantation should be performed before secondary complications of diabetes (such as retinopathy, peripheral neuropathy, vasculopathy, and end-stage renal disease) develop. Because pancreas transplantation alone is not a lifesaving procedure and has a high incidence of rejection and surgical complications, the patient's condition is evaluated carefully to determine whether the benefits outweigh the risks of transplantation.[50]

Contraindications to pancreas transplantation include the following[49,50]:

- Age greater than 50 years (relative)
- Morbid obesity
- Active smoking
- Severe cardiovascular disease

Living donor pancreas transplantation, in which the segment of the body and tail of the pancreas are used from a living donor, may be performed; however, whole-organ cadaveric pancreas transplantation is preferred. The donor pancreas is placed intraperitoneally in the right iliac fossa through either an oblique lower-abdominal or a midline incision.[19,51] The recipient's native pancreas is left intact. The new pancreas vasculature is anastomosed to the iliac vessels, and insulin is delivered to the systemic circulation.[50]

Enteric Drainage versus Bladder Drainage

Pancreatic exocrine secretions can be drained through two different techniques. For both approaches the pancreas is transplanted with a segment of the donor duodenum. In an enteric approach, the duodenum is anastomosed to a loop of the recipient's small bowel. With this technique, concerns have included the risk of contaminating the field with the bowel and associated leaks and infections. Bladder drainage is obtained by anastomosing the donor duodenum with the recipient's urinary bladder.[49,50,52] This permits exocrine secretions to be expelled with the urine and allows monitoring of urine amylase as a marker for rejection.[49,52] The disadvantage of bladder drainage is that urologic and metabolic complications are common, including metabolic acidosis, volume depletion, dehydration, pancreatitis from reflux of urine, urinary tract infections, and urethral stricture formation.[53] Enteric conversion may be required if there are persistent metabolic issues.[49,52] Because of the significant complications noted with bladder drainage, enteric drainage has become the preferred technique at most transplant centers, with more than 80% of transplants using this since 2003.[50] Ultimately, the decision of which technique to use is the choice of the transplant surgeon.[49]

Indication of Pancreatic Function Posttransplant

Within 24 hours, the transplanted pancreas should be producing insulin. Analysis of blood glucose response and C-peptide levels (a protein produced by the pancreas) is used to determine a successful pancreatic transplant. Immediately after transplantation, blood sugar levels are monitored every hour, because glucose levels typically drop 50 mg/dl each hour, and dextrose infusion may be necessary.[52] The blood glucose level should range between 80 and 150 mg/dl within a few hours after the transplantation.[19] C-peptide levels are elevated, and blood sugar level returns to normal within 2 to 3 days postoperatively.[7] After a diet is started, serum glucose is monitored four times a day. Recipients should return to normal or near-normal fasting plasma glucose levels, glycosylated hemoglobin levels (which represent the average blood glucose level over the previous several weeks), and glucose tolerance tests.[48,54] Generally within a week to 10 days, the recipient weans from insulin and becomes insulin independent with normal carbohydrate metabolism for an indefinite period.[19,54] The need for strict adherence to a diet and constant blood sugar monitoring should diminish.[7] Long-term follow-up studies indicate that the insulin independence can be sustained for at least 5 years.[54]

Postoperative Care and Complications

The recipient may be placed on strict bed rest for a few days postoperatively to prevent kinking of the vascular allografts that may result from a position shift of the pancreas.[19] A Foley catheter is left in place for at least the first week to prevent distention of the bladder and leakage from a bladder anastomosis.[19] During the first postoperative day, a baseline radionuclide blood flow study of the pancreas and a Doppler ultrasonography of the allograft vasculature are performed. Repetition of these studies and operative intervention are performed urgently with any sign of pancreatic dysfunction.[19]

Acute rejection after pancreas transplantation is difficult to diagnose. Nonspecific clinical criteria, such as fever, allograft tenderness, weight gain, ileus, abdominal pain, hematuria, leukocytosis, and hyperglycemia, can be used in combination to detect acute pancreas rejection.[49,53] Hyperglycemia does not occur until 80% to 90% of the graft has been destroyed.[25] A decrease in bicarbonate, urine pH, or urine amylase levels of more than 25% from baseline, an elevation of serum amylase, or a combination of these factors also indicates acute pancreas rejection in a bladder-drained pancreas transplant recipient.[17,19,20,53] Percutaneous ultrasound-guided or cystoscopic biopsy of the transplanted pancreas is used as a sensitive histologic method to confirm acute graft rejection.[20,49]

> ✎ **CLINICAL TIP**
>
> Remind pancreas transplant recipients to drink enough fluids to rehydrate themselves during and after exercise. Hydration is critical in patients with a bladder-drained pancreas. Recipients must take in 3 to 4 liters of fluid per day.[52]

Pancreatic Islet Cell Transplantation

Pancreatic islet β cells are responsible for the production of insulin. In this experimental procedure for type 1 diabetes being performed at some U.S. centers, islet cells are first isolated and removed from the pancreas of a deceased donor. Radiographic (x-ray or ultrasound) guidance is used to place a catheter through the recipient's abdomen and into the portal vein. Following purification, the cells are injected through the catheter, and once implanted, they begin to produce and release insulin in the recipient. The clear advantage of this technique is its minimally invasive nature, typically requiring only local anesthesia. However, there is still a potential for hemorrhage and thrombosis, and the immunosuppression requirements have significant side effects. Preliminary results show that insulin independence is achieved in the majority of recipients; however, it has been difficult to maintain over time.[55]

Pancreas-Kidney Transplantation

Types of Pancreas-Kidney Transplants

Simultaneous Pancreas-Kidney Transplants

Typically, simultaneous pancreas-kidney (SPK) transplants are offered to patients who have type 1 diabetes mellitus with diabetic nephropathy and renal insufficiency. SPK transplants are more common than a non-lifesaving pancreas transplantation alone, accounting for approximately 80% of pancreas transplants, as physicians are reluctant to use potent immunosuppressive drugs in patients with diabetes before they need a concomitant renal transplant.[50,54] The benefits of a successful SPK transplant include normoglycemia, elimination of dialysis, prevention of reoccurring diabetic nephropathy in the kidney graft, higher quality of life compared to individuals on dialysis, and higher 10-year survival compared to individuals receiving a kidney transplant alone.[1,48,54]

SPK transplants may be cadaveric or from living donors, in which case a segmental pancreas transplant is performed. Using an abdominal midline incision, the pancreatic graft is implanted first on the right side of the pelvis, after which the kidney graft is implanted on the left.[20,51]

Pancreas-after-Kidney Transplants

A pancreas-after-kidney (PAK) transplant is performed on a patient with type 1 diabetes who has already received a functioning kidney transplant, or individuals following an SPK with a failing pancreas graft.

Postoperative Care and Complications

In SPK transplants, pancreas rejection episodes frequently occur concurrently with renal allograft rejection. Rejection of the donor pancreas is more difficult to diagnose; therefore acute rejection of both allografts is recognized by deterioration in kidney function.[52,54] When rejection is clinically suspected, kidney biopsy specimens are obtained.

The SPK transplant involves a more complex surgical procedure, with more complications, longer hospitalizations, more frequent rehospitalizations, greater morbidity, and a higher incidence of rejection and immunosuppression required than renal transplant alone.[50,52] The advantages noted earlier, including near-perfect glucose metabolism and the prevention of further secondary diabetic complications, help to justify the increased risk.[52]

Cardiac Transplantation

Candidates for heart transplantation have irreversible end-stage cardiac disease, no other surgical or medical options, and a poor prognosis for survival longer than 6 to 12 months.[2,3,12] Patients typically present with low exercise tolerance, cachexia, generalized weakness, decreased muscle mass, marginal blood pressure, dyspnea, and poor peripheral perfusion.[56]

Common indications for heart transplants include the following[2,3,6,12,29]:

- Severe left ventricular disease (ejection fraction less than 20% to 25%)
- Cardiomyopathy
- Ischemic heart disease
- Congenital heart disease
- Valvular disease
- Inoperable coronary artery disease, with angina refractory to medical management
- Malignant cardiac dysrhythmias unresponsive to medical or surgical therapy, or both
- Primary cardiac tumors with no evidence of spread to other systems

Contraindications to cardiac transplantation include the following[3,6,17,29,57]:

- Autoimmune disorders
- Irreversible kidney, liver, or lung disease
- Fixed pulmonary hypertension
- Unresolved pulmonary infarction
- Relative: active peptic ulcer disease, type 1 diabetes mellitus with secondary complications, chronic obstructive

pulmonary disease (COPD) with a forced expiratory volume in 1 second (FEV_1) of less than 50%, age greater than 65

Pretransplantation Care

Although heart failure continues to be a significant problem, the number of cardiac transplants (approximately 2300 annually) has remained relatively unchanged.[1] With demand for hearts much higher than the supply, ventricular assist devices (VAD) and the total artificial heart (TAH) are being used as bridges to cardiac transplant.[58] Physical therapists often treat patients with these devices awaiting cardiac transplant. A thorough understanding of not only the precautions and contraindications, but the evidence related to physical therapy intervention and outcomes is essential. Please refer to Chapter 18 for information on pertinent physical therapy implications when working with patients who have these devices. The management of individuals with end-stage heart failure requiring transplant is often very intensive and requires ongoing hospitalization compared to other solid organ transplants. The physical therapist may be involved with helping to condition transplant candidates before transplant and helping to maximize quality of life in the hospital.

Orthotopic and Heterotopic Heart Transplantation

Orthotopic and heterotopic transplantation are the two types of heart transplant procedures. The more common orthotopic procedure involves a median sternotomy with removal of the recipient's heart and the insertion of the donor heart in the normal anatomic position.[6,13,59,60] There are two variations on the orthotopic technique. In the standard biatrial technique, the recipient's native atria are left in place and a large atrial anastomosis is used to connect the donor with the recipient. In the bicaval technique, the recipient's native atria are totally excised. The newer bicaval technique maintains the normal anatomy of the atria and evidence suggests it may result in fewer surgical and postoperative complications, including reduced sinoatrial node dysfunction.[61,62]

Heterotopic or "piggy-back" transplants, which retain the diseased heart, are rare and are used for patients with pulmonary hypertension. Whether orthotopic or heterotopic heart transplantation is performed, temporary epicardial pacing wires and mediastinal and pleural chest tubes are inserted before closure of the chest wall (see Chapter 18).[16]

Indication of Cardiac Function Posttransplant

Following the initial separation of the heart from bypass, the allograft requires active hemodynamic support and management. The exact type of support (pharmacological, epicardial pacing, and/or mechanical) and how long it will be required varies tremendously between recipients. Important indicators of function include arterial pressure, right atrial pressure or central venous pressure, left atrial or pulmonary artery wedge pressure, cardiac output, and ejection fraction. Hemodynamic monitoring devices typically include a pulmonary artery catheter and an arterial line (see Chapter 18). In addition, transesophageal echocardiography (TEE) and transthoracic echocardiography (TTE) can be used to assess heart function both intraoperatively and postoperatively. After surgery, continuous pulse oximetry and electrocardiography (ECG) is used, and the patient's complete blood count, arterial blood gas, serum electrolyte, metabolic functions, and immunosuppressant levels are monitored closely.[6,62]

With reperfusion in the operating room, most recipients display a normal sinus rhythm. Sinus node dysfunction may occur following surgical trauma or ischemia and result in bradycardia or a slow junctional rhythm. Although this is much less with the bicaval technique, it is treated with atrial or atrioventricular pacing or chronotropic drugs when it occurs. It may take the new heart a few days to achieve a stable intrinsic rhythm, and the heart may vary from bradycardia to tachycardia. The target is to maintain the heart rate between 90 and 100 bpm to optimize cardiac output.[6,62]

It is typical for the transplanted heart to demonstrate a functional decline over the first 12 hours due to the effects of ischemia, reperfusion, and myocardial edema. During this period of myocardial depression, the transplanted heart may be affected temporarily by decreased diastolic compliance, diminished systolic function, and impaired contractility.[6,19] Support for heart dysfunction typically begins with pharmacotherapy, including inotropes, and advances to an intraaortic balloon pump (IABP) and mechanical support such as VADs only when initial measures have failed. Cardiac rate and function usually return to normal within 3 to 4 days, at which time intravenous medications, mechanical support, and pacing mechanisms are weaned.[6]

Postoperative Care and Complications

Immediate postoperative care for cardiac transplant recipients is similar to that of patients who have undergone cardiothoracic surgery. In the initial postoperative period, mediastinal drainage is promoted by elevating the head of the bed to a 30-degree angle and turning the patient every 1 to 2 hours.[6] Chest tubes are typically removed 2 days postoperatively once chest drainage is less than 25 ml per hour, and pacing wires are removed 7 days after transplantation if there were no events of bradycardia.[6]

Early postoperative management is focused on maintaining hemodynamic stability as described previously. Aside from sinus node dysfunction and myocardial depression, other potential complications after heart transplant include mediastinal bleeding, thrombosis or leakage of anastomosis, PGF, right heart failure, biventricular heart failure, pulmonary hypertension, pericardial effusion, renal dysfunction, immunosuppressant-induced hypertension, and PTDM.[6,13,21,57,62]

Heart transplant recipients have an increased risk of excessive postoperative bleeding and cardiac tamponade.[19] Owing to chronic congestive heart failure, patients usually have passive liver congestion, which increases the risk of bleeding.[57] Many patients also receive anticoagulation therapy preoperatively to prevent thrombus formation. However, inadequate heparin reversal may occur and, depending on the severity of anticoagulation, treatment includes transfusion of platelets or fresh-frozen plasma.[57]

PGF occurs within 24 hours after transplant when there is severe mechanical dysfunction without obvious anatomical or immunological cause (such as hyperacute rejection) that requires two or more inotropes or mechanical support. This can result in left ventricular, right ventricular, or biventricular failure.[62] Right heart failure is the most common cause of cardiac dysfunction postoperatively.[57] It may be caused by a preexisting elevated pulmonary vascular resistance (PVR), donor size mismatch in which the donor heart is too small for the recipient, long ischemic time, and acute rejection.[57] Clinical evidence of right ventricular heart failure includes hypotension, low cardiac output, an elevated central venous pressure, and low urinary output.[19] Right atrial pressures, pulmonary artery pressure, PVR, cardiac output, and signs of right-sided heart failure are monitored closely.[6]

Many cardiac transplant recipients have preexisting renal insufficiency due to their low cardiac output, congestive heart failure, and long-term diuretic use.[6,57] After transplantation, cardiopulmonary bypass and use of nephrotoxic immunosuppressants can cause renal failure in the transplant recipient.[6]

Objective characteristics of acute rejection specific to cardiac transplant recipients include new cardiac arrhythmias, hypotension, pericardial friction rub, ventricular S_3 gallop, decreased cardiac output, peripheral edema, pulmonary crackles, and jugular vein distention.[13,16,17] Subjectively, recipients may report vague symptoms of decreased exercise tolerance, fatigue, lethargy, or dyspnea. However, the most reliable technique to diagnose rejection is by performing periodic endomyocardial biopsy. The initial biopsy is performed 5 to 10 days after transplantation under fluoroscopy and local anesthesia using a catheter inserted through the right internal jugular vein into the right ventricle.[16,57] The frequency of surveillance biopsies varies between transplant institutions and tends to decrease over time.[16,19] If the cardiac transplant recipient has frequent arrhythmias (which often indicate ischemia), periodic coronary angiography is performed to detect allograft coronary disease.[13,17]

Physical Therapy for Cardiac Transplant Recipients

Phase I cardiac rehabilitation usually begins 2 to 3 days postoperatively, once the patient is hemodynamically stable. It is important to recognize that the transplanted heart is physiologically different due to several factors (Table 14-2):

1. Ischemia: Procurement of the organ subjects the heart to ischemia and reperfusion, which may reduce myocardial contractility and impair function.[63]
2. Denervation: The extrinsic nervous supply to the donor heart is severed during the procurement surgery so the heart receives no efferent input from the autonomic nervous system and provides no direct afferent input to the central nervous system. The heart is unaffected by the recipient's sympathetic and parasympathetic nervous system, which normally controls the rate and contractility. In the absence of this neural regulation, the denervated heart depends on circulating catecholamines and the Frank-Starling mechanism to regulate cardiac output.[6,12,16,63]
3. Diastolic dysfunction: Impaired filling is fairly common due to myocardial scarring and fibrosis.[63]

TABLE 14-2 Physiologic Changes Following Cardiac Transplantation

	Resting	Submaximal Exercise	Maximal Exercise	Post-activity	Physical Therapy Implications
Heart rate (HR)	Higher than normal (~90-115 bpm; rate of sinoatrial node)	Delayed increase (~3-5 min) from circulating catecholamines	Reduced peak (~150 bpm) HR reserve less than normal	Max HR achieved in first few minutes of recovery Delayed return to baseline	Use Borg RPE scale with target 11-13 in postoperative phase[16] Extend warm-up and cool-down by 5-10 minutes
Blood pressure (BP)	Higher than normal systolic and diastolic Orthostatic hypotension common (absence of reflex tachycardia)[6]	Higher than normal systolic Appropriate response with exercise Diastolic may fall with reduced peripheral resistance	Slightly reduced peak	Delayed return to baseline	Monitor BP before, during, and after activity Target resting BP: systolic BP 80-150 mm Hg; diastolic BP <90 mm Hg[60] Allow time to adapt to position changes[76]
Cardiac output (CO)	Normal to slightly less than normal	Delayed increase Initial increase due to increase of stroke volume via Frank-Starling law Later due to increased HR from circulating catecholamines	Below normal	Delayed return to baseline	Extend warm-up and cool-down by 5-10 minutes Watch for signs/symptoms of activity intolerance

Data from Squires RW: Exercise therapy for cardiac transplant recipients, Prog Cardiovasc Dis 53(6):429-436, 2011.

4. Skeletal muscle structural and biochemical abnormalities: Heart transplant recipients have been found to have impaired aerobic metabolic enzyme activity, lower capillary density, endothelial dysfunction with impaired peripheral and coronary vasodilation during exercise, and an increased proportion of type II fibers.[63]

Additional considerations for physical therapy include:

- Patients may be asked to follow sternal precautions, which may limit shoulder range of motion, pushing, pulling, and lifting for up to 6 to 8 weeks.[63] However, the exact definition of these precautions varies by institution and also often by surgeon. Emerging evidence suggests that traditional sternal precautions may be overly restrictive and impede healing and restoration of functional mobility.[64] In transplant recipients though, immunosuppressants may contribute to delayed healing. It is recommended that therapists consider talking to the medical team to assess the patient's risk for sternal complications and determine restrictions on an individualized basis.

- Exercise prescription should be progressive and based on the patient's activity tolerance, typically beginning with active supine exercises without resistance to ambulation and stationary biking. Extended warm-up and cool-down periods are essential, and the RPE scale should be used to monitor and prescribe exercise. Vital signs are monitored before, during, and immediately after exercise. For most, oxygen saturation will be normal at rest and with exercise.[63]

- Most recipients will not experience typical anginal symptoms due to denervation, although there is some evidence for limited regeneration in the first few months to years posttransplant.[63] The physical therapist should monitor the ECG for arrhythmias and stay alert for other sign/symptoms of activity intolerance, including fatigue, dyspnea, lightheadedness, and increased RPE.[13,16,17,60,65]

- When monitoring the ECG, there may be two P-waves if both donor and recipient sinoatrial nodes are present. The recipient-generated P-wave does not cross the surgical suture line, however, so there should only be one QRS wave from the donor heart.[57,66]

- Overall, adult heart transplant recipients have an approximately 30% to 40% lower exercise capacity (oxygen consumption) than do healthy age-/sex-matched controls.[67] The cause of this is likely multifactorial, with potential factors including the physiological differences outlined above, tissue damage from rejection episodes, general pretransplant deconditioning, and long-term immunosuppressant use.[67] Because early cardiac rehabilitation has been found to improve exercise capacity and quality of life posttransplant, physical therapists should be sure to discuss potential

participation in outpatient cardiac rehabilitation with the medical team and recipient before hospital discharge.[68]

Lung Transplantation

Lung transplantation is indicated for end-stage pulmonary disease due to a variety of medical conditions. Major indications include the following[4,5,24]:

- COPD (with FEV_1 of less than 20% of predicted value)
- Cystic fibrosis (with FEV_1 of less than 30% of predicted value)
- Emphysema
- Bronchiectasis
- Primary pulmonary hypertension
- Pulmonary fibrosis
- Eisenmenger's syndrome (a congenital heart disease)
- Alpha$_1$-antitrypsin deficiency
  Less-frequent indications include the following:
- Sarcoidosis (see Appendix 13-A)
- Eosinophilic granuloma
- Scleroderma
  Contraindications to lung transplantation include the following[3,24]:
- Poor left ventricular cardiac function
- Significant coronary artery disease
- Significant dysfunction of other vital organs (e.g., liver, kidney, central nervous system)
- Active cigarette smoking
- Autoimmune disorders
- Poor nutritional status (malnutrition or obesity)

Types of Lung Transplants

There are three types of surgical procedures for lung transplantation:

Single-Lung Transplantation

This is the most common surgical technique and is indicated for all types of end-stage lung disease, except cystic fibrosis and bronchiectasis.[4] It involves a single anterolateral or posterolateral thoracotomy in which the right or left cadaveric lung is transplanted into the recipient.[24]

Double-Lung or Bilateral Lung Transplantation

With double-lung transplantation, the left and right lungs are transplanted sequentially into one recipient, with the least functional lung resected and replaced first.[24] The incision used is a bilateral anterior thoracotomy in the fourth or fifth intercostal space, or the surgeon may choose a transverse sternotomy to create a "clamshell" incision.[24] This may be used for individuals with cystic fibrosis, bronchiectasis, or pulmonary hypertension.[4,25]

Living Donor Lobar Transplantation

Transplantation of lobes involves bilateral implantation of lower lobes from two blood-group–compatible living donors.[4] The donor's lungs are larger than the recipient's for the donor lobes

---

✎ CLINICAL TIP

Complaints of chest pain from the recipient may be due to the sternal incision and musculoskeletal manipulation during surgery but are likely noncardiac because of denervation.[69]

to fill each hemithorax.[4] This procedure is rare and is performed primarily for patients with cystic fibrosis.[1,19]

Preoperative Care

Patients awaiting lung transplant often present with decreased work capacity in both respiratory and skeletal muscles, and daily physical activity that is significantly lower than what has been found for individuals with chronic disease.[70] Preoperative physical therapy should focus on improving functional mobility and exercise capacity with the goal of increasing quality of life and activity tolerance postoperatively. The preoperative program should include resistive training with focus on proximal muscles of the upper and lower extremities, core, and respiratory muscles, as well as aerobic training. Interval training may allow potential recipients to better tolerate exercise. Caution should be used with upper-extremity exercise because it may lead to dyssynchronous thoracoabdominal breathing and dyspnea in individuals with severe respiratory disease.[2] The literature supports using tools, such as the 6-minute walk distance (6MWD) (see Chapter 23), muscle endurance test (using timed stair climbing), and shuttle test, to assist in objectively demonstrating training effects. The 6MWD has been has been found to be a strong predictor of mortality both before and after lung transplant; however, further research is needed to determine if rehabilitation focused on improving this before transplant will increase survival.[71] Physical therapists also play a role in using airway clearance techniques (see Chapter 4), as patients are often admitted with pulmonary decompensation while waiting for transplantation.[72]

Indication of Lung Function Posttransplant

For patients with pulmonary vascular disease, single-lung and double-lung transplantation results in an immediate and sustained normalization of pulmonary vascular resistance and pulmonary arterial pressures.[4] This is accompanied by an immediate increase in cardiac output. Arterial oxygenation generally returns to normal, and supplemental oxygen is no longer required, usually by the time of hospital discharge.[4]

The maximum improvement in lung function and exercise capacity is achieved within 3 to 6 months after transplantation, once the limiting effects of postoperative pain, altered chest wall mechanics, respiratory muscle dysfunction, and acute lung injury have subsided.[4,5] After double-lung transplantation, normal pulmonary function is usually achieved. However, in single-lung transplantation, lung function improves but does not normalize fully, owing to the disease and residual impairment of the remaining nontransplanted lung. Lung volumes and flow rates improve to two thirds of normal in single-lung transplantation.[5] Most lung transplant recipients are therefore able to resume an active lifestyle, free of supplemental oxygen, with less dyspnea and improved exercise tolerance.

Postoperative Care and Complications

Ineffective postoperative airway clearance occurs after lung transplantation. Recipients present with an impaired cough reflex, incisional pain, altered chest wall musculoskeletal function, and diminished mucociliary clearance.[72]

Bronchopulmonary hygiene is a crucial part of the postoperative care, as it helps mobilize secretions and prevent atelectasis and mucous plugging. It may also help to improve activity tolerance if performed before exercise, as airflow obstruction has been found to limit daily physical activity levels in transplant recipients.[70]

Postoperative complications that may develop in the denervated transplanted lung include pulmonary edema or effusion, acute respiratory distress syndrome, dehiscence of the bronchial anastomosis, and anastomotic stenosis.[4] Single-lung transplant recipients may experience complications of ventilation-perfusion mismatch and hyperinflation owing to the markedly different respiratory mechanics in each hemithorax.[19] The rate of infection in lung transplant recipients is higher than that of other organ transplant recipients, because the graft is exposed to the external environment through the recipient's native airway. The patient's white blood cell (WBC) and absolute neutrophil count are monitored closely.[7] Bacterial pneumonia and bronchial infections are very common complications that usually occur in the first 30 days.[4,19] Bronchoalveolar lavage is used to diagnose opportunistic infections.[2]

Clinical manifestations of acute pulmonary rejection in lung transplant recipients include dyspnea, nonproductive cough, leukocytosis, hypoxemia, pulmonary infiltrates as seen on chest x-ray, sudden deterioration of pulmonary function tests (PFTs), elevated WBC count, need for ventilatory support, fever, and fatigue.[7,17,24] The rejection typically presents with a sudden deterioration of clinical status over 6 to 12 hours.[25] Daily documentation of the oxygen saturation and the FEV_1 is used to monitor and detect early rejection, especially in bilateral lung transplant recipients, because a decline in oxygen saturation or spirometry values in excess of 10% commonly accompany episodes of rejection or infection.[4,5,69] Bronchoscopic lung biopsy, bronchiolar lavages, and cytoimmunologic monitoring of the peripheral blood may be used to diagnose acute rejection.[4,25,69]

Bronchoscopy is performed routinely and whenever rejection is suspected to assess airway secretions, healing of the anastomosis, and the condition of the bronchial mucous membrane.[17] The first bronchoscopy is performed in the operating room to inspect the bronchial anastomosis.[25] To prevent infection and atelectasis, routine fiberoptic bronchoscopy with saline lavage and suctioning are used to reduce accumulation of secretions that the recipient is unable to clear.[19]

Physical Therapy for Lung Transplant Recipients

Following extubation, aggressive bronchopulmonary hygiene should be performed every 2 to 4 hours, while the patient is awake.[17] An effective bronchopulmonary hygiene program should include the following[17]:

1. Reeducation in coughing techniques following denervation (splinted cough with a pillow may assist with pain control)
2. Education in breathing techniques including diaphragmatic breathing
3. Suctioning to remove secretions and help maintain adequate oxygenation (when intubated, a premeasured catheter can be used to prevent damage to the anastomosis)
4. Vibration and gentle percussion (see Chapter 4)

5. Incentive spirometry and use of a flutter device to maximize lung expansion and prevent atelectasis and pneumonia
6. Chest and upper extremity mobilization exercises can be used to help improve thoracic mobility with caution to protect the incision.[2]
7. Postural drainage and positioning (see Chapter 22)
   • As long as they are hemodynamically stable, recipients should sleep in a reverse Trendelenburg position to aid in postural drainage.
   • During the first 24 hours after surgery, patients with double-lung transplants should be turned side to side. Turning is initiated gradually, beginning with 20- to 30-degree turns and assessing vital signs, and then increasing gradually to 90 degrees each way, every 1 to 2 hours. Prolonged periods in supine position are avoided to minimize secretion retention.[17]
   • Patients with single-lung transplants should lie on their nonoperative side to reduce postsurgical edema, assist with gravitational drainage of the airway, and promote optimal inflation of the new lung.[17]

> **✎ CLINICAL TIP**
>
> Initially, most lung transplant recipients are asked to follow thoracotomy precautions including no lifting greater than 10 lb. They are generally restricted to partial weight bearing of their upper extremities, which may limit the use of an assistive device at least temporarily. It is important to check with the medical team for specific precautions and to determine when it is safe to incorporate assistive devices and upper extremity resistance exercises (generally after 6 to 8 weeks).

In spite of improved lung function posttransplant, exercise capacity continues to be impaired (40% to 60% of predicted).[73] Studies indicate that lower extremity skeletal muscle dysfunction, rather than dyspnea, is the primary limiting factor impairing exercise tolerance in patients after lung transplant.[74] This muscle dysfunction includes: decreased muscle mass and strength, reduced proportion of type I fibers, decreased mitochondrial enzyme activity, impaired calcium uptake and release, and an impaired capacity for oxidative metabolism.[73-75] Several factors may contribute to this, such as pretransplant skeletal muscle changes as a result of the disease process and side effects of immunosuppressive drugs given pretransplant and posttransplant, as well as inactivity.[74]

Evidence suggests that structured exercise training programs, including aerobic conditioning and upper and especially lower limb strengthening, may improve functional exercise capacity, skeletal muscle strength, and lumbar bone mineral density in lung transplant recipients.[75] However, further research is still needed to determine optimal exercise guidelines for this population. Multiple rest periods may be required during activity at the beginning of the postoperative period to limit the amount of dyspnea and muscle fatigue. Rest periods can be gradually decreased so that the patient advances toward periods of continuous exercise as endurance improves.

> **✎ CLINICAL TIP**
>
> Always monitor the recipient's oxygen saturation before, during, and after exercise. If the patient is on room air at rest, supplemental oxygen may be beneficial during exercise to reduce dyspnea and improve activity tolerance. The lung transplant recipient should maintain an arterial oxyhemoglobin saturation greater than 90% with activity.[76]

Heart-Lung Transplantation

Heart-lung transplantation (HLT) is performed on patients who have a coexistence of end-stage pulmonary disease and advanced cardiac disease that produces right-sided heart failure.[17]

Indications for heart-lung transplantation include the following[4,9,66]:
• Primary pulmonary hypertension
• COPD
• Cystic fibrosis
• Pulmonary fibrosis
• Eisenmenger's syndrome
• Irreparable cardiac defects or congenital heart disease
• Advanced lung disease and coexisting left ventricular dysfunction or extensive coronary artery disease

The heart and lung of the donor are removed en bloc and placed in the recipient's chest. The anastomosis to join the donor organs is at the trachea, right atrium, and aorta.[9,19] Postoperative HLT care is similar to the heart and lung posttransplant care previously discussed. Rejection of the heart and lung allografts occurs independently of each other.[66] Bacterial pneumonia from contamination in the donor tracheobronchial tree is the most common cause of morbidity and mortality after HLT.[9]

Stem Cell Transplantation

Stem cells are primitive cells found in bone marrow or circulating blood that have the capacity to evolve into specialized cells, including mature blood cells (white cells, red cells, and platelets). Stem cell transplantation (SCT) is performed for a variety of conditions in order to replace defective blood cells and restore hematologic and immunologic functions. However, this approach is only used after conventional methods of treatment have failed. Indications for SCT include the following[12,65,77,78]:
• Malignant disorders (including myelodysplastic syndromes, acute lymphocytic or myelogenous leukemia, chronic myelogenous leukemia, lymphoma, multiple myeloma, neuroblastoma, and selected solid tumors including breast, ovarian, and testicular cancers)
• Nonmalignant hematologic disorders (such as aplastic anemia, sickle cell anemia, and thalassemia)
• Immunodeficiency disorders (severe combined immunodeficiency disease)

Contraindications to SCT include the following[78]:

- Inadequate cardiac function (left ventricular ejection fraction less than 45%)
- Inadequate pulmonary function (forced expiratory capacity and forced vital capacity less than 50%)
- Inadequate renal function (creatinine greater than 2 mg/dl)
- Inadequate hepatic function (bilirubin greater than 2 mg/dl)

When the stem cells are harvested from the bone marrow, the procedure is referred to as a bone marrow transplant (BMT), and when the cells are taken from the blood itself, it is referred to as a peripheral blood stem cell transplant (PBSCT).

The three types of SCT are *allogeneic, syngeneic,* and *autologous* transplants[79]:

1. An *allogeneic transplant* is one in which cells are harvested from an HLA-matched donor who may be related or unrelated. Umbilical cord blood can also be used. A move has been made from standard serological tissue typing toward DNA-based procedures to improve HLA matching. Improved matching has been shown to decrease time to engraftment, decrease incidence of graft versus host disease (GVHD), and improve overall transplant survival.[80]
2. A *syngeneic transplant* is one in which cells are harvested from an identical twin.
3. An *autologous transplant* is one in which the donor and recipient are the same. Cells are harvested from the patient when he or she is healthy or in complete remission, and they are frozen and stored for future reinfusion.

Patient Preparation

Before the SCT, the recipient's body is deliberately immunosuppressed to gain the greatest acceptance of the graft. The recipient undergoes a 2- to 4-day cytoreduction protocol, consisting of ablative chemotherapy, radiation, or both, designed to destroy malignant cells and create space in the bone marrow for the engraftment of new marrow.[7,12,77] New protocols for non-myeloablative transplants are evolving that use lower, less toxic doses during the cytoreduction phase. It is believed that donor graft cells may actually help to attack remaining malignant cells when they react immunologically.[79]

Harvesting

In BMT, the bone marrow is harvested by multiple needle aspirations, most commonly from the posterior and anterior iliac crests of the donor or, less commonly, from the sternum. Five hundred to 2500 ml of aspirated marrow is filtered, heparinized, mixed with peripheral blood, frozen, and stored.[12] The donor may experience some soreness and stiffness at the graft site; however, the body replaces the lost marrow, and most donors are fully recovered within a couple of weeks.[79]

For a PBSCT, the cells are harvested by apheresis. During apheresis, the patient's blood is removed via a central venous catheter or from a large vein in the arm. It is then circulated through a high-speed cell separator in which the peripheral stem cells are removed, frozen, and stored. The plasma cells and erythrocytes are reinfused into the patient. Donors may be given a hematopoietic growth factor before apheresis to increase the number of cells available. Apheresis may cause some temporary constitutional symptoms such as minor bone and muscle aches, lightheadedness, and nausea and vomiting.[7,79]

Reinfusion and Indication of Postprocedure Function

One to 3 days after the last dose of chemotherapy or radiation, the cells are then infused into the patient, much like a blood transfusion, through a central venous access device or Hickman right atrial catheter. The most common side effects of reinfusion are fever, chills, nausea, headache, and flushing.[7,81]

The stem cells that were infused migrate to the recipient's marrow cavities and begin to produce new blood cells, a process known as engraftment. A successful engraftment, which is indicated by an increase in the platelet, RBC, and WBC counts, is decided 10 to 20 days after transplantation.[9,66,81] The hematologic recovery for PBSCT is approximately a week earlier than with BMT because the stem cells procured from the peripheral blood are more mature than those in the bone marrow.[65] Because of this faster hematologic recovery and also a quickened immunologic recovery after allogenic PBSCT, it is becoming more common. Some disadvantages include a longer process for donors and increased fluid to recipients during transplantation with possible fluid overload to the lungs.[82]

Postprocedure Care and Complications

Major complications of SCT include marrow failure, infection, hemorrhage, pneumonia, interstitial pneumonitis, veno-occlusive disease of the liver, and GVHD.[7,12,25,59]

All recipients undergoing SCT experience a period of bone marrow failure, which generally begins within 10 days after the start of chemotherapy or radiation and can last up to 3 to 4 weeks after transplantation. Recipients will likely present with pancytopenia, a marked reduction in red blood cells, white blood cells, and platelets.[12,77,81] During this time, recipients may receive daily transfusions of platelets, lymphocytes, and granulocytes (preferably from the donor) and antimicrobial therapy to counteract the side effects of hemorrhage and infection.[9,77] Daily bone marrow aspirations and complete blood counts (CBCs) are performed to monitor the progress of the grafts and to check for recurrence of malignancy. SCT recipients are at risk for fatal infection because normal immune function may not be regained for 12 to 18 months when the transplanted immune system has fully matured.[12,81] Hemorrhage is also a significant threat due to impaired clotting from the loss of platelets.

Veno-occlusive disease is characterized by obstruction of the hepatic venules by deposits of collagen and fibrin formed from endothelial cell damage with chemotherapy and radiation. Clinical manifestations of veno-occlusive disease include sudden weight gain, increased LFTs, hepatomegaly, right upper quadrant pain, ascites, and jaundice.[77] Veno-occlusive disease may occur 1 to 3 weeks after transplantation and spontaneously resolves within 2 to 3 weeks in approximately half of those affected.[12]

Graft versus host disease is a complication that occurs in approximately 20% to 70% of allogeneic transplant recipients and may be either acute or chronic.[83] It is caused by the donor marrow's production of T lymphocytes that react immunologically to the host recipient and attack the host cells. Acute

GVHD occurs typically between 3 and 30 days after transplantation.[7,77,84] Major organs affected by GVHD are the skin, liver, gastrointestinal tract, and lymphoid system.[7,77] Skin involvement manifests as an erythematous rash that can progress to blistering and desquamation. Liver manifestations include increased liver enzymes and bilirubin, right upper quadrant pain, hepatomegaly, and jaundice. Gastrointestinal tract manifestations include nausea, vomiting, diarrhea, malabsorption, ileus, sloughing of intestinal mucosa, abdominal pain, cramping, and bloody stools.[7,77] GVHD is treated with immunosuppressive medications.[81] GVHD does, however, appear to have a protective effect with some leukemias, as the donor cells may also attack the host malignancy and prevent relapse.[79,83]

Physical Therapy for Stem Cell Transplantation Recipients

Physical therapy is beneficial to stem cell transplantation recipients during their prolonged hospital stay, with an average duration of 5 weeks.[84] Prolonged bouts of malaise, fever, diarrhea, nausea, and pain from inflammation of mucous membranes of the mouth and digestive tract that usually accompany stem cell transplantation can be debilitating to patients. Initially, physical therapists provide a gentle exercise program to prevent deconditioning and muscle atrophy from disuse and improve functional mobility as patients slowly regain their strength. When patients are confined to their rooms because of protective isolation, they often use a stationary bicycle, treadmill, or restorator (a portable device that a patient can pedal seated at the bedside or in a chair) as part of their exercise prescription. Evidence demonstrates the benefits of a posttransplant exercise program, including decreased fatigue and time in the hospital, as well as minimized WBC and platelet drops frequently seen following transplantation.[85] Stem cell transplantation recipients typically require 6 months to a year before they recover full strength and return to a normal lifestyle.[81]

It is important that physical therapists routinely monitor CBCs and consider the implications of abnormal values when designing treatment plans. Values especially important in this population include hemoglobin/hematocrit, white blood cell count (especially the absolute neutrophil count), and platelets (Table 14-3). Caution should also be used with patients who present with temperature above 99.5° F.[85]

General Physical Therapy Guidelines for Transplant Recipients

Physical therapists play an integral role in the rehabilitation of transplant recipients. With the exception of stem cell transplantation recipients, the length of stay (LOS) in an acute care hospital, depending on the type of organ transplantation and barring any complications, ranges from 3 to 16 days. The shortest LOS is generally for kidney recipients and the longest for SPK recipients. Some factors that may prolong hospitalization

TABLE 14-3 Important Lab Values in Transplant

Lab Value	Reference Value	Abnormal Value	Physical Therapy Implications
Absolute neutrophil count (ANC)	2500-6000/mm^3	<1500	Neutropenic precautions (high risk for infection; level implemented depends on facility) Thorough hand washing Physical therapist must glove, gown, mask Reverse isolation Private, sterile, laminar airflow room or possibly HEPA filtered Items entering room must be sterile (exercise equipment) No live plants or flowers (may harbor bacteria) Limited visitors
Platelets (PLT)	150,000-350,000/μl	<50,000 >20,000 10,000-20,000 <10,000 and/or temperature >100.5° F	Thrombocytopenic precautions (risk for spontaneous bleeding; no passive range of motion/stretching) Therapeutic exercise/bike with or without resistance Therapeutic exercise/bike without resistance Hold therapy; no therapeutic exercise
Hemoglobin (Hgb)	12-17 gm/dl	>8 <8-10 <8	Ambulation and self-care as tolerated; resistance exercises allowed* Activities of daily living with assistance for safety; light aerobics and weights (1-2 lb)* Light range-of-motion exercise and isometrics; avoid aerobic or progressive programs*
Hematocrit (Hct)	36%-51%	>25 <25-35 <25	Same as implications for corresponding hemoglobin ranges above

*Should be interpreted along with patient's comorbidities, cause of blood loss, and possibility of transfusion.
   Information from Acute Care Section: Lab values interpretation resources, American Physical Therapy Association. http://www.acutept.org/associations/11622/files/LabValuesResourceUpdate2012.pdf. Accessed March 2012.

include the following: advanced recipient age and comorbidities, use of ECD organs, those donated following cardiac death, or those with increased cold ischemic time.[8,11,18-20,60] Given the short LOS for many transplant recipients, physical therapists are consulted in the early postoperative period to provide treatment and assist the transplant team with a safe discharge plan. If patients are medically stable but need assistance for activities of daily living and ambulation, they will require transfer to a rehabilitation facility for further physical and occupational therapy before discharge home.

Goals

In the acute care setting, the primary physical therapy goals are similar to those of postoperative abdominal or cardiothoracic surgical patients. They include maximizing functional mobility and endurance; improving range of motion, strength, balance, and coordination; and progressing the recipient to his or her maximum independent functional level safely.

Many transplant recipients have experienced end-stage organ disease for years before receiving their transplant and may present with other medical comorbidities. As a result, they are usually physically deconditioned and present with a marked reduction in exercise capacity and skeletal muscle strength owing to long-standing pretransplant physical inactivity. For example, extreme fatigue and weakness are exhibited in patients with chronic liver disease, reduced muscle endurance is seen in patients with chronic heart failure, and decreased oxygen uptake capacity is exhibited in heart and lung disease.[1] Generalized weakness results from the disease process, fluid and electrolyte imbalance, and poor nutrition. After their transplant, recipients generally require a longer time frame to regain their strength and endurance and to achieve their goals.

General Physical Therapy Management for Transplant Recipients

- Coordinate the best time for physical therapy with the patient's nurse each day. The patient may be fatigued after other interventions or medically inappropriate for exercise owing to a decline in medical status, especially in the intensive care unit (ICU) or early in the postoperative course. Visits should also ideally be scheduled after patients have received their pain medications and any breathing treatments. Incisional pain can limit activity progression, deep breathing exercises, and coughing.
- During the ICU stay, it is recommended to keep mean arterial pressure (MAP) above 60 to 70 mm Hg to maintain safe organ perfusion.[86]
- Analyze laboratory values daily, as they may change dramatically from day to day (see Table 14-3):
  - Many recipients have very low platelet counts immediately posttransplantation. Patients with low platelet counts or increased PT/INR, PTT, or both are at risk for bleeding. It is usually contraindicated to perform percussion on patients with a platelet count less than 50,000/mm^3, and caution should be used with suctioning. Other aspects of bronchopulmonary hygiene as described under lung transplantation may still be performed.
  - Anemia is also common posttransplant, and recipients may present with reduced activity tolerance.
  - White blood cells, especially neutrophils, are also commonly affected after transplant and should be monitored carefully in light of the high risk of infection.
  - Each type of solid organ transplant has other specific values that help to indicate graft function and should be followed (e.g., creatinine for kidneys, blood glucose and C-peptide levels for pancreas).
- Infection control is vitally important after transplant. Depending on the type of transplant and the medical status, patients may be placed in a protective isolation room and positive-pressure flow rooms may be used to limit the transfer of airborne pathogens. Strict hand washing and standard precautions are essential, and the use of a face mask is often required of the health care worker entering the room and/or for the patient when they are leaving their room.[60]
- Supine therapeutic exercise in the acute care setting is implemented only if necessitated by the recipient's condition, such as high fever, chills, bed rest restriction secondary to ventilator use, or low platelet count. A high temperature will result in elevated respiratory and heart rates; therefore it is important to avoid strenuous cardiovascular and resisted exercise during this time.
- Timeline to mobilization out of bed after transplant is variable and depends on several factors, including preoperative status, type of transplant, and complications. In less complicated cases such as a standard kidney transplant, mobilization generally begins 1 to 2 days postsurgery.[38] Early ambulation helps to decrease the risk of cardiovascular and pulmonary infection, increase blood circulation, stimulate gastrointestinal function, relieve gas pains, and maintain muscle tone.[18,87]
- Many posttransplant patients retain fluid, especially in the lower extremities. Weight bearing may be painful; however, ambulation for short periods of time should still be encouraged. The recipient's balance may be altered secondary to increased fluid retention, and he or she may require the use of an assistive device. The physical therapist will be required to provide assistance or appropriate guarding to maintain maximum safety.
- Always monitor and document vital signs, oxygen saturation, and RPE (for cardiac transplant recipients) before, during, and after physical therapy intervention. Report any abnormal change in the patient's response to activity to the patient's nurse. An activity log or flow sheet may be used to document daily progress or decline and vital sign responses.
- Many patients experience some form of organ rejection. If approved by the transplant team, exercise generally continues if their rejection episode is mild to moderate.[16,73]
- The adverse effects of immunosuppressants may produce delayed wound healing and can contribute to osteoporosis. Upper-extremity resistive training is important; however, it should be delayed for cardiac and lung transplant recipients until cleared by the medical team (generally around 6 to 8 weeks posttransplant), when wound and tissue healing is complete.[76] All recipients should be instructed in postural

awareness, alignment, exercise, and optimal body mechanics to combat the effects of osteoporosis.[56]

- Consider the implementation of standardized outcomes measures to objectively assess and document patient status and improvement. For example, the 6MWD has been frequently used in patients following heart and lung transplantation and also with patients after liver transplant in the immediate postoperative period.[63,88] Other tests such as the sit-to-stand (STS)-10 and the STS-60 have been studied in patients undergoing dialysis and may be appropriate for patients after kidney transplant.[89]

Activity Progression

Activity posttransplant is progressed gradually by the physical therapist according to foundational exercise principles while monitoring for signs and symptoms of activity intolerance and making appropriate adjustments. Physical therapists should refer to the individual transplant sections for special considerations when designing and implementing programs. Initially most transplant recipients will fatigue easily and require frequent rest periods. Thus shorter and more frequent treatment sessions may be beneficial.

Patient Education

- Physical therapists assist in the education of transplant recipients. Recipients must assume an active role in health care after transplantation. Patients are educated preoperatively about what to expect after transplantation. Initially, the recipient is very weak and may have difficulty learning during the early posttransplant rehabilitation phase. The physical therapist reinforces the activity protocol with the patient. The transplant team usually provides the recipient with a comprehensive guide that includes information on medications, proper diet, exercise, and psychosocial changes. The patient must adhere to the medication protocol posttransplant and be able to monitor for signs and symptoms of infection, rejection, and toxicity to the medications. Patients are instructed to monitor their temperature and weight daily, inspect mouth and gums, maintain proper oral hygiene, and report fever or infectious symptoms.

- On discharge home, transplant recipients should participate in a daily home exercise routine. The physical therapy department or the organ transplant team may have preprinted exercise protocols. Otherwise, the physical therapist should customize an individual exercise program that consists of stretching and strengthening exercises and a walking or aerobic program that includes a warm-up and cool-down period. A gradual increase in ambulation to at least 30 minutes a day is recommended. An activity log may be used to document the patient's progress.

- Strenuous exercise and activities that stretch or put pressure on the incision should be avoided until approximately 2 months after discharge from the hospital with clearance from the attending physician. Contact sports should be avoided for life after transplantation to prevent trauma to the transplanted organ.[18]

Organ transplantation provides a patient with end-stage organ disease an opportunity to improve his or her quality of life by receiving a donated organ, "the gift of life." With ongoing commitment and hard work, transplant recipients can regain an independent, healthy, and active lifestyle.

References

1. Organ Procurement and Transplantation Network: http://optn.transplant.hrsa.gov. Accessed April 13, 2013.*
   *"This work was supported in part by Health Resources and Services Administration contract 234-2005-37011C. The content is the responsibility of the authors alone and does not necessarily reflect the views or policies of the Department of Health and Human Services, nor does mention of trade names, commercial products, or organizations imply endorsement by the U.S. Government."

2. Young MA, Stiens SA: Organ transplantation and rehabilitation. In Braddom RL, editor: Physical medicine and rehabilitation, ed 3, Philadelphia, 2009, Saunders, pp 1433-1451.

3. Black JM, Hokanson-Hawks J, editors: Medical-surgical nursing: clinical management for positive outcomes, ed 8, St Louis, 2009, Saunders, pp 834-835, 1629, 2137-2153.

4. Arcasoy SE, Kotloff RM: Lung transplantation, N Engl J Med 340(14):1081-1091, 1999.

5. Kesten S: Advances in lung transplantation, Dis Mon 45(3):101-114, 1999.

6. Becker C, Petlin A: Heart transplantation: minimizing mortality with proper management, Am J Nurs (Suppl 5):8-14, 1999.

7. Black JM, Matassarin-Jacobs E, editors: Medical-surgical nursing: clinical management for continuity of care, ed 5, Philadelphia, 1997, Saunders, pp 584-585, 641-651, 1148, 1352-1353, 1898-1901, 1931.

8. Olaverri JG et al: Utilization of advanced-age donors in renal transplantation, Transplant Proc 43:3340-3343, 2011.

9. Atkinson LJ, Howard Fortunato N, editors: Operating room technique, ed 8, Boston, 1996, Mosby, pp 897-912.

10. Daniels R, Nicoll L, editors: Contemporary medical surgical nursing, ed 2, Clifton Park, NY, 2012, Delmar Cengage Learning.

11. Manara AR, Murphy PG, O'Callaghan G: Donation after circulatory death, Br J Anaesth 108(s1):i108-i121, 2012.

12. Monahan FD, Neighbors M: Medical-surgical nursing, ed 2, Philadelphia, 1998, Saunders, pp 227-229, 480-483, 1196-1198, 1408-1411, 1448-1455, 1488-1491.

13. Winkel E, DiSesa VJ, Costanzo MR: Advances in heart transplantation, Dis Mon 45(3):62-87, 1999.

14. Ambrosio F et al: The emerging relationship between regenerative medicine and physical therapeutics, Phys Ther 90:1807-1814, 2010.

15. National Institutes of Health: Stem cell information: stem cell basics. http://stemcells.nih.gov/info/basics/basics6.asp. Accessed March 2012.

16. Sadowsky HS: Cardiac transplantation: a review, Phys Ther 76(5):498-515, 1996.

17. Smith SL: Tissue and organ transplantation, St Louis, 1990, Mosby, pp 27-28, 179, 183, 202-203, 218, 220, 245, 257, 267, 287, 309.

18. Jenkins RL, editor: A guide for transplant recipients, Burlington, MA, 2000, Lahey Clinic.

19. Grenvik A, Ayres SM et al, editors: Textbook of critical care, ed 4, Philadelphia, 2000, Saunders, pp 1938-1985.

20. Gruessner RWG, Kendall DM, Drangstveit MB et al: Simultaneous pancreas-kidney transplantation from live donors, Ann Surg 226(4):471-482, 1997.

21. O'Connell JB, Bourge RC, Costanzo-Nordin MR et al: Cardiac transplantation: recipient selection, donor procurement, and medical follow-up, Circulation 86(3):1061-1075, 1992.

22. Murphy F: Managing post-transplant patients in primary care, Pract Nurs 22(6):292-297, 2011.

23. Biancofiore G, Bindi ML, Romanelli AM et al: Fast track in liver transplantation: 5 years' experience, Eur J Anaesthesiol 22:584-590, 2005.

24. Meyers BF, Patterson GA: Lung transplantation: current status and future prospects, World J Surg 23:1156-1162, 1999.

25. Hall JB, Schmidt GA, Wood LDH, editors: Principles of critical care, ed 2, New York,1998, McGraw-Hill, pp 1093-1094, 1325-1339.

26. United Network for Organ Sharing: Transplant living: medications—protecting your transplant. http://www.transplantliving.org/afterthetransplant/medications/typesofsuppressants.aspx. Accessed March 15, 2012.

27. Duncan MD, Wilkes DS: Transplant-related immunosuppression, Proc Am Thorac Soc 2005(2):449-455, 2005.

28. Sheiner PA, Magliocca JF, Bodian CA et al: Long-term medical complications in patients surviving ≥5 years after liver transplant, Transplantation 69(5):781-789, 2000.

29. Zavotsky KE, Sapienza J, Wood D: Nursing implications for ED care of patients who have received heart transplants, J Emerg Nurs 27(1):33-39, 2001.

30. Jenkins RL, editor: Liver transplantation protocol manual, Burlington, MA, 1999, Lahey Clinic, pp 7, 8, 33, 37-41.

31. Razonable RR, Findlay JY, O'Riordan A, et al: Critical care issues in patients after liver transplantation. Liver Transplant 17(5):511-527, 2011.

32. Warren DS, Montgomery RA: Incompatible kidney transplantation: lessons from a decade of desensitization and paired kidney exchange, Immunol Res 47:257-264, 2010.

33. Manske CL: Risks and benefits of kidney and pancreas transplantation for diabetic patients, Diabetes Care 22(Suppl 2):B114-B119, 1999.

34. Bartucci MR: Kidney transplantation: state of the art. AACN Clin Issues 10(2):153-163, 1999.

35. Pizer HF, editor: Organ transplants: a patient's guide, Cambridge, MA, 1991, Harvard University Press, p 155.

36. Nolan MT, Augustine SM, editors: Transplantation nursing: acute and long-term management, Stamford, CT, 1995, Appleton & Lange, pp 201, 213-226.

37. Romano G, Simonella R, Falleti E et al: Physical training effects in renal transplant recipients, Clin Transplant 24(4):510-514, 2010.

38. Gordon EJ, Prohaska TR, Gallant MP et al: Longitudinal analysis of physical activity, fluid intake, and graft function among kidney transplant recipients, Transplant Int 22(10):990-998, 2009.

39. Kjaer M, Beyer N, Secher NH: Exercise and organ transplantation, Scand J Med Sci Sports 9:1-14, 1999.

40. Sanchez ZV, Cashion AK, Cowan PA, et al: Perceived barriers and facilitators to physical activity in kidney transplant recipients, Prog Transplant 17(4):324-331, 2007.

41. Schluger LK, Klion FM: The indications for and timing of liver transplantation, J Intensive Care Med 14(3):109-116, 1999.

42. Kitchens WH: Domino liver transplantation: indications, techniques, and outcomes, Transplant Rev 25:167-177, 2011.

43. Cortazzo MH, Helkowski W, Pippin B et al: Acute inpatient rehabilitation of 55 patients after liver transplantation, Am J Phys Med Rehabil 84:880-884, 2005.

44. Neuberger J: Liver transplantation, QJM 92:547-550, 1999.

45. Wiesner RH, Rakela J, Ishitani MB: Recent advances in liver transplantation, Mayo Clin Proc 78(2):197-210, 2003.

46. Correia TD, Isabel M: Post-liver transplant obesity and diabetes, Curr Opin Clin Nutr Metab Care 6(4):457-460, 2003.

47. Findlay JY, Fix OK, Paugam-Burtz C et al: Critical care of the end-stage liver disease patient awaiting liver transplantation, Liver Transplant 17:496-510, 2011.

48. Shapira Z, Yussim A, Mor E: Pancreas transplantation, J Pediatr Endocrinol Metab 12(1):3-15, 1999.

49. Cicalese L, Giacomoni A, Rastellini C et al: Pancreatic transplantation: a review, Int Surg 84:305-312, 1999.

50. Lam VWT, Pleass HCC, Hawthorne W et al: Evolution of pancreas transplant surgery, Aust N Z J Surg 80(6):411-418, 2010.

51. Hampson FA, Freeman SJ, Ertner J et al: Pancreatic transplantation: surgical technique, normal radiological appearances and complications, Insights Imaging 1(5-6):339-347, 2010.

52. Freise CE, Narumi S, Stock PG et al: Simultaneous pancreas-kidney transplantation: an overview of indications, complications, and outcomes, West J Med 170(1):11-18, 1999.

53. McChesney LP: Advances in pancreas transplantation for the treatment of diabetes, Dis Mon 45(3):88-100, 1999.

54. Hricik DE: Combined kidney-pancreas transplantation, Kidney Int 53:1091-1097, 1998.

55. U.S. Department of Health and Human Services: Pancreatic islet cell transplantation. http://diabetes.niddk.nih.gov/dm/pubs/pancreaticislet/. Accessed March 2012.

56. Arthur EK: Rehabilitation of potential and cardiac transplant recipients, Cardiopulmonary Rec APTA Section 1, 11-13, 1986.

57. Lynn-McHale D, Dorozinsky C: Cardiac surgery and heart transplantation. In L Bucher, S Melander, editors: Critical care nursing, Philadelphia, 1999, Saunders, pp 330-348.

58. Fitzsimmons CL: Sensitivity, ventricular assist devices, and the waiting game in heart transplantation: what's new? Crit Care Nurs Q 27(1):65-77, 2004.

59. Hillegass EA, Sadowsky HS, editors: Essentials of cardiopulmonary physical therapy, Philadelphia, 1994, Saunders, pp 165-166, 314-315.

60. Edinger KE, McKeen S, Bemis-Dougherty A et al: Physical therapy following heart transplant, Phys Ther Pract 1(4):25-33, 1992.

61. Czer LSC, Cohen MH, Gallagher SP et al: Exercise performance comparison of bicaval and biatrial orthotopic heart transplant recipients, Transplant Proc 43(10):3857-3862, 2011.

62. Costanzo MR, Dipchand A, Starling R et al: The International Society for Heart and Lung Transplantation guidelines for the care of heart transplant recipients, J Heart Lung Transplant 29:914-956, 2010.

63. Squires RW: Exercise therapy for cardiac transplant recipients, Prog Cardiovasc Dis 53(6):429-436, 2011.

64. Cahalin LP, LaPier TK, Shaw DK: Sternal precautions: is it time for change? Precautions versus restrictions: a review of literature and recommendations for revision, Cardiopulm Phys Ther J 22(1):5-15, 2011.

65. Goodman CC, Boissonnault WG, editors: Pathology: implications for the physical therapist, Philadelphia, 1998, Saunders, pp 120, 340-344, 363-366, 381, 437-438.

66. Sigardson-Poor KM, Haggerty LM, editors: Nursing care of the transplant recipient, Philadelphia, 1990, Saunders, pp 124, 149-151,187, 208, 210-211, 287.

67. Abdul-Waheed M, Yousuf M, Kelly SJ et al: Does left atrial volume affect exercise capacity of heart transplant recipients? J Cardiothorac Surg 5:113, 2010.

68. Hsu C, Chen S, Su S et al: The effect of early cardiac rehabilitation on health-related quality of life among heart transplant recipients and patients with coronary artery bypass graft surgery, Transplant Proc 43(7):2714-2717, 2011.

69. Reichenspurner H, Dienemann H, Rihl M et al: Pulmonary rejection diagnosis after lung and heart-lung transplantation, Transplant Proc 25(6):3299-3300, 1993.

70. Bossenbroek L, ten Hacken NHT, van der Bij W et al: Cross-sectional assessment of daily physical activity in chronic obstructive pulmonary disease lung transplant patients, J Heart Lung Transplant 28(2):149-155, 2009.

71. Martinu T, Babyak MA, O'Connell CF et al: Baseline 6-min walk distance predicts survival in lung transplant candidates, Am J Transplant 8(7):1498-1505, 2008.

72. Wells CL: Lung transplantation, Acute Care Perspect Spring:14-23, 2007.

73. Mathur S, Levy RD, Reid WD: Skeletal muscle strength and endurance in recipients of lung transplants, Cardiopulm Phys Ther J 19(3):84-93, 2008.

74. Mathur S, Reid WD, Levy RD: Exercise limitation in recipients of lung transplants, Phys Ther 84(12):1178-1187, 2004.

75. Wickerson L, Mathur S, Brooks D: Exercise training after lung transplantation: a systematic review, J Heart Lung Transplant 29(5):497-503, 2010.

76. Frownfelter D, Dean E, editors: Principles and practice of cardiopulmonary physical therapy, ed 3, St Louis, 1996, Mosby, pp 703-719.

77. James MC: Physical therapy for patients after bone marrow transplantation, Phys Ther 67(6):946-952, 1987.

78. Nettina SM, editor: The Lippincott manual of nursing practice, ed 6, Philadelphia, 1996, Lippincott-Raven, pp 791-797.

79. National Cancer Institute: Bone marrow transplantation and peripheral blood stem cell transplantation. http:// www.cancer.gov/cancertopics/factsheet/Therapy/bone-marrow-transplant. Accessed March 2012.

80. Hurley CK, Baxter Lowe LA, Logan B et al: National Marrow Donor Program HLA-matching guidelines for unrelated marrow transplants, Biol Blood Marrow Transplant 9(10):610-615, 2003.

81. McGlave P: Hematopoietic stem-cell transplantation from an unrelated donor, Hosp Pract (Off Ed) 35(8):46, 49, 50, 2000.

82. Barrett L, Ruth L: Bone marrow transplantation. Health. http:// www.healthline.com/galecontent/bone-marrow-transplantation. Accessed June 2008.

83. Hymes SR, Alousi AM, Cowen EW: Graft-versus-host disease. Part I: pathogenesis and clinical manifestations of graft-versus-host-disease, J Am Acad Dermatol 66(4):515.e1-515.e18, 2012.

84. Leger CS, Nevill TJ: Hematopoietic stem cell transplantation: a primer for the primary care physician, CAMJ 170(10):1569-1577, 2004.

85. Scalzitti DA, Sternisha C: Does exercise during hospitalization after stem cell transplantation decrease reports of fatigue and reduce the duration of the hospital stay? Phys Ther 82(7):716-721, 2002.

86. Saner FH et al: Intensive care unit management of liver transplant patients: a formidable challenge for the intensivist, Transplant Proc 40:3206-3208, 2008.

87. Luckmann J, editor: Medical-surgical nursing, Philadelphia, 1980, Saunders, pp 167, 1011.

88. Foroncewicz B, Mucha K, Szparaga B et al: Rehabilitation and 6-minute walk test after liver transplantation, Transplant Proc 43(8):3021-3024, 2011.

89. Segura-Orti E, Martinez-Olmos FJ: Test-retest reliability and minimal detectable change scores for sit-to-stand-to-sit tests, the six-minute walk test, the one-leg heel-rise test, and handgrip strength in people undergoing hemodialysis, Phys Ther 91:1244-1252, 2011.

CHAPTER 15

Fluid and Electrolyte Imbalances

Jaime C. Paz

CHAPTER OBJECTIVES

Provide a description of fluid and electrolyte imbalance including:

1. Clinical manifestations and diagnostic studies
2. Contributing health conditions
3. Medical management
4. Guidelines for physical therapy management

PREFERRED PRACTICE PATTERNS

Regulation of fluid and electrolyte imbalance is multifactorial and applies to many body systems. For this reason, specific practice patterns are not delineated in this chapter.

Please refer to Appendix A for a complete list of the preferred practice patterns in order to best delineate the most applicable practice pattern for a given patient with fluid and electrolyte imbalance.

Maintaining homeostasis among intracellular fluid, extracellular fluid, and electrolytes is necessary to allow proper cell function. Proper homeostasis depends on the following factors:

- Concentration of intracellular and extracellular fluids
- Type and concentration of electrolytes
- Permeability of cell membranes
- Kidney function

Many variables can alter a patient's fluid and electrolyte balance. These imbalances can further result in numerous clinical manifestations, which can subsequently affect a patient's functional mobility and activity tolerance. Recognizing the signs and symptoms of electrolyte imbalance is therefore an important aspect of physical therapy management. In addition, the physical therapist must be aware of which patients are at risk for these imbalances, as well as the concurrent health conditions and medical management of these imbalances.

Fluid Imbalance

The total amount of fluid in the body is distributed between the intracellular and extracellular compartments. Intracellular fluid contains approximately two-thirds of the body's fluid. Extracellular fluid is further made up of interstitial fluid and intravascular fluid, which is the blood and plasma.[1-3] Fluid imbalance occurs when there is a deficit or an excess primarily in extracellular fluid.[1-6] Table 15-1 provides an overview of fluid imbalances.

Loss of Body Fluid

Loss of bodily fluid can occur from inadequate fluid intake, loss of blood (hemorrhage), loss of plasma (burns), or loss of body water (vomiting, diarrhea). A fluid deficit can also result from a fluid shift into the interstitial spaces, such as ascites caused by liver failure or pleural effusion from heart failure. Any of these situations can result in dehydration, hypovolemia (loss of circulating blood), or shock in extreme cases.[1-8]

TABLE 15-1 Fluid Imbalances

Imbalance	Definition	Contributing Factors	Clinical Manifestations	Diagnostic Test Findings
Hypovolemia Fluid volume deficit	Decreased blood volume Decreased extracellular fluid volume	Vomiting, diarrhea, fever, blood loss, uncontrolled diabetes mellitus	Weak, rapid pulse; decreased BP; dizziness; thirst; cool, pale skin over extremities; confusion; muscle cramps	Decreased hemoglobin and hematocrit with whole blood loss; increased hematocrit with plasma fluid shift from intravascular to interstitial spaces; increased BUN, serum sodium levels
Hypervolemia Fluid volume excess	Increased blood volume Decreased extracellular fluid volume	Renal failure, congestive heart failure, blood transfusion, prolonged corticosteroid therapy	Shortness of breath; increased BP; bounding pulse; presence of an S3 heart sound and cough if heart is failing; dependent edema	Decreased hematocrit, BUN; normal serum sodium levels with decreased potassium levels
Hyponatremia	Sodium deficiency (serum sodium level <135 mEq/L)	SIADH (see Chapter 10); diuretic therapy; renal disease; excessive sweating; hyperglycemia; NPO status; congestive heart failure; side effects from anticonvulsants, glycemic agents, antineoplastics, antipsychotics, and sedatives	Lethargy, nausea, apathy, muscle cramps, muscular twitching, confusion (in severe states)	Decreased urine and serum sodium levels; elevated hematocrit and plasma protein levels
Hypernatremia	Sodium excess (serum sodium level >145 mEq/L)	Water deficit; diabetes insipidus (see Chapter 10); diarrhea; hyperventilation; excessive administration of corticosteroid, sodium bicarbonate, or sodium chloride	Elevated body temperature; lethargy or restlessness; thirst; dry, flushed skin; weakness; irritability; hyperreflexia; ataxia; tremors; tachycardia; hypertension or hypotension; oliguria; pulmonary edema	Increased serum sodium and decreased urine sodium levels
Hypokalemia	Potassium deficiency (serum potassium level <3.5 mEq/L)	Inadequate potassium intake, diarrhea, vomiting, chronic renal disease, gastric suction, polyuria, corticosteroid therapy, digoxin therapy	Fatigue; muscle weakness; slow, weak pulse; ventricular fibrillation; paresthesias; leg cramps; constipation; decreased BP	ST depression or prolonged PR interval on ECG, increased arterial pH and bicarbonate levels, slightly elevated glucose levels
Hyperkalemia	Potassium excess (serum potassium level >5 mEq/L)	Excessive potassium intake, renal failure, Addison's disease, burns, use of potassium-conserving diuretics, ACE inhibitors, NSAIDs, chronic heparin therapy	Vague muscle weakness, nausea, initial tachycardia followed by bradycardia, dysrhythmia, flaccid paralysis, paresthesia, irritability, anxiety	ST depression; tall, tented T waves; or absent P waves on ECG; decreased arterial pH level
Hypocalcemia	Calcium deficiency (serum calcium level <8.5 mg/dl)	Inadequate intake or absorption, bone or soft-tissue deposition, blood transfusions, decreased PTH and vitamin D	Confusion, paresthesias, muscle spasms, hyperreflexia	Prolonged QT segment on ECG, hyperactive bowel sounds
Hypercalcemia	Calcium excess (serum calcium >12 mg/dl)	Hyperparathyroidism, bone metastases, sarcoidosis, excess vitamin D	Fatigue, weakness, lethargy, anorexia, nausea, constipation	Shortened QT segment or depressed and widened T waves on ECG

TABLE 15-1 Fluid Imbalances—cont'd

Imbalance	Definition	Contributing Factors	Clinical Manifestations	Diagnostic Test Findings
Hypophosphatemia	Phosphate deficiency (serum phosphate level <2 mg/dl)	Intestinal malabsorption, increased renal excretion	Thrombocytopenia, muscle weakness, irritability, confusion, numbness	Decreased heart rate, hypoxia
Hyperphosphatemia	Phosphate excess (serum phosphate >4.5 mg/dl)	Chemotherapy, laxatives, hypoparathyroidism	Confusion, paresthesias, muscle spasms, hyperreflexia	Prolonged QT segment on ECG, hyperactive bowel sounds
Hypomagnesemia	Magnesium deficiency (serum magnesium <1.5 mEq/L)	Malnutrition, intestinal malabsorption, alcoholism, renal dysfunction, use of loop and thiazide diuretic agents	Depression, confusion, irritability, hyperreflexia, muscle weakness, ataxia, nystagmus, tetanus, convulsions	Tachyarrhythmias
Hypermagnesemia	Magnesium excess (serum magnesium >2.5 mEq/L)	Renal failure, excessive antacid intake	Nausea, vomiting, muscle weakness	Bradycardia, decreased BP

Data from Huether SE: The cellular environment: fluids and electrolytes, acids and bases. In McCance KL, Huether SE, Brashers VL et al, editors: Pathophysiology, the biologic basis for disease in adults and children, ed 6, St Louis, 2010, Mosby, pp 96-125; The body fluid compartments: extracellular and intracellular fluids; edema. In Hall JE, editor: Guyton and Hall textbook of medical physiology, ed 12, Philadelphia, 2011, Saunders, pp 285-301; Porth CM: Alterations in fluids and electrolytes. In Porth CM, editor: Pathophysiology, concepts of altered health states, ed 6, Philadelphia, 2002, Lippincott, pp 693-734; Gorelick MH, Shaw KN, Murphy KO: Validity and reliability of clinical signs in the diagnosis of dehydration in children, Pediatrics 99(5):E6, 1997; Mulvey M: Fluid and electrolytes: balance and disorders. In Smeltzer SC, Bare BG, editors: Brunner and Suddarth's textbook of medical-surgical nursing, ed 8, Philadelphia, 1996, Lippincott; Goodman CC, Kelly Snyder TE: Problems affecting multiple systems. In Goodman CC, Boissonnault WG, editors: Pathology: implications for the physical therapist, Philadelphia, 1998, Saunders; Fall PJ: Hyponatremia and hypernatremia: a systematic approach to causes and their correction, Postgrad Med 107(5):75-82, 2000; Marieb EN editor: Human anatomy and physiology, ed 2, Redwood City, CA, 1992, Benjamin Cummings, p 911.

ACE, Angiotensin-converting enzyme; *BP,* blood pressure; *BUN,* blood urea nitrogen; *ECG,* electrocardiogram; *NPO,* nothing by mouth; *SIADH,* syndrome of inappropriate antidiuretic hormone secretion; *ACE,* angiotensin-converting enzyme; *NSAIDs,* nonsteroidal antiinflammatory drugs; *PTH,* parathyroid hormone.

Clinical manifestations may include decreased blood pressure, increased heart rate, changes in mental status, thirst, dizziness, hypernatremia, increased core body temperature, weakness, poor skin turgor, altered respirations, and orthostatic hypotension.[1-8] Clinical manifestations in children also include poor capillary refill, absent tears, and dry mucous membranes.[8]

> ✎ **CLINICAL TIP**
>
> During casual conversation among physicians and nurses, patients who are hypovolemic are often referred to as being *dry,* whereas patients who are hypervolemic are referred to as being *wet.*

Excessive Body Fluid

Excessive bodily fluid can occur when there is excessive sodium or fluid intake, or sodium or fluid retention. Acute or chronic kidney failure can also result in a fluid volume excess. A shift of water from the intravascular space to the intracellular compartments can also occur as a result of excessive pressure in the vasculature (ventricular failure), loss of serum albumin (liver failure), or fluid overload (excessive rehydration during surgery).[1-6,8]

Clinical manifestations of fluid overload include weight gain, pulmonary edema, peripheral edema, and bounding pulse. Clinical manifestations of this fluid shift may also resemble those of dehydration (e.g., tachycardia and hypotension), as there is a resultant decrease in the intravascular fluid volume.[1-6,8]

> ✎ **CLINICAL TIP**
>
> Patients with interstitial edema may often be referred to as *third-spacing,* which refers to the shift of fluid volume from intravascular to extravascular spaces.

Electrolyte Imbalance

Fluid imbalances are often accompanied by changes in electrolytes. Loss or gain of body water is usually accompanied by a loss or gain of electrolytes. Similarly, a change in electrolyte balance often affects fluid balance. Cellular functions that are reliant on proper electrolyte balance include neuromuscular excitability, secretory activity, and membrane permeability.[9] Clinical manifestations will vary depending on the severity of the imbalance and can include those noted in the Fluid Imbalance section. In extreme cases, muscle tetany and coma can also occur. Common electrolyte imbalances are further summarized in Table 15-1. Alterations in arterial blood gas (ABG) levels are also considered electrolyte imbalances.[10]

Electrolyte levels are generally represented schematically in the medical record in a sawhorse figure, as shown in Figure 15-1. Electrolytes that are out of reference range are either highlighted with a circle or annotated with an arrow (↑ or ↓) to denote their relationship to the reference value.

Medical management includes identification of causative factors and ongoing monitoring of electrolyte imbalances with laboratory testing of blood and urine. These tests include

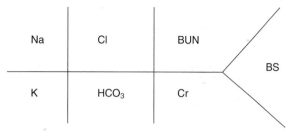

FIGURE 15-1
Schematic representation of electrolyte levels. *BUN,* Blood urea nitrogen; *BS,* blood sugar; *Cl,* chloride; *Cr,* creatinine; *HCO₃,* bicarbonate; *K,* potassium; *Na,* sodium.

measuring levels of sodium, potassium, chloride, and calcium in blood and urine; arterial blood gases; and serum and urine osmolality. Treatment involves managing the primary cause of the imbalance(s), along with providing supportive care with intravenous or oral fluids, electrolyte supplementation, and diet modifications.

Physical Therapy Considerations

- Review the medical record closely for any fluid restrictions that may be ordered for a patient with fluid volume excess. These restrictions may also be posted at the patient's bedside.
- Conversely, ensure proper fluid intake before, during, and after physical therapy intervention with patients who have a fluid volume deficiency.

- Patients who have a fluid volume deficit are at risk for orthostatic hypotension; therefore monitor vital signs carefully and proceed with upright activities very gradually.
- Furthermore, patients who have a sodium deficit may also have fluid restrictions to minimize risk of hyponatremia.
- Slight potassium imbalances can have significant effects on cardiac rhythms; therefore carefully monitor the patient's cardiac rhythm before, during, and after physical therapy intervention. If the patient is not on a cardiac monitor, then consult with the nurse or physician regarding the appropriateness of physical therapy intervention with a patient who has potassium imbalance.
- Patients who are taking antihypertensive medications are at risk for electrolyte imbalances. These medications include thiazide, loop, and potassium-sparing diuretics; β-blockers; angiotensin-converting enzyme (ACE) inhibitors; and angiotensin receptor blockers (ARBs).[11]
- Refer to Chapter 3 for more information on cardiac arrhythmias.
- Refer to Chapter 4 for more information on ABGs.
- Refer to Chapter 9 for more information on fluid and electrolyte imbalances caused by renal dysfunction.
- Refer to Chapter 10 for more information on fluid and electrolyte imbalances caused by endocrine dysfunction.
- Refer to Chapter 19 for more information on antihypertensive medications.

References

1. Huether SE: The cellular environment: fluids and electrolytes, acids and bases. In McCance KL, Huether SE, Brashers VL et al, editors: Pathophysiology, the biologic basis for disease in adults and children, ed 6, St Louis, 2010, Mosby, pp 96-125.
2. The body fluid compartments: extracellular and intracellular fluids; edema. In Hall JE, editor: Guyton and Hall textbook of medical physiology, ed 12, Philadelphia, 2011, Saunders, pp 285-301.
3. Porth CM: Alterations in fluids and electrolytes. In Porth CM, editor: Pathophysiology, concepts of altered health states, ed 6, Philadelphia, 2002, Lippincott, pp 693-734.
4. Rose BD, editor: Clinical physiology of acid-base and electrolyte disorders, ed 2, New York, 1984, McGraw-Hill.
5. Cotran RS, Kumar V, Robbins S et al, editors: Robbins pathologic basis of disease, Philadelphia, 1994, Saunders.
6. Kokko J, Tannen R, editors: Fluids and electrolytes, ed 2, Philadelphia, 1990, Saunders.
7. McGee S, Abernethy WB 3rd, Simel DL: Is this patient hypovolemic? JAMA 281(11):1022-1029, 1999.
8. Springhouse: Portable fluids & electrolytes, Philadelphia, 2008, Lippincott William & Wilkins.
9. Marieb EN, editor: Human anatomy and physiology, ed 2, Redwood City, CA, 1992, Benjamin Cummings, p 911.
10. Fukagawa M, Kurokawa K, Papadakis MA: Fluid & electrolyte disorders. In Tierney LM, McPhee SJ, Papadakis MA, editors: Current medical diagnosis & treatment, New York, 2007, McGraw-Hill.
11. Liamis G, Milionis H, Elisaf M: Blood pressure drug therapy and electrolyte disturbances, Int J Clin Pract 62(10):1572-1580, 2008.

CHAPTER 16

Amputation

Jaime C. Paz

CHAPTER OBJECTIVES

The objectives of this chapter are the following:

1. Provide an overview of the causes and types of lower-extremity amputation
2. Provide an overview of the causes and types of upper-extremity amputation
3. Describe physical therapy management, pertinent to the acute care setting, for patients with either upper or lower-extremity amputation
4. Provide an overview of applicable standardized outcome measures for this patient population

PREFERRED PRACTICE PATTERNS

The most relevant practice patterns for the diagnoses discussed in this chapter, based on the American Physical Therapy Association's *Guide to Physical Therapist Practice*, second edition, are as follows:

- Impaired Motor Function, Muscle Performance, Range of Motion, Gait, Locomotion, and Balance Associated with Amputation: 4J
- Impaired Integumentary Integrity Associated with Skin Involvement Extending into Fascia, Muscle, or Bone and Scar Formation: 7E

Please refer to Appendix A for a complete list of the preferred practice patterns, as individual patient conditions are highly variable and other practice patterns may be applicable.

This chapter provides a brief overview of the most common types of lower-extremity and upper-extremity amputations with subsequent physical therapy management pertinent to the acute care setting. Although the incidence of upper-extremity amputation (UEA) is quite low compared to lower-extremity amputation (LEA), it is important that the acute care physical therapist have an understanding of all types of amputations to properly plan for the management of this patient population.

Lower-Extremity Amputation

Vascular disease and trauma are the primary causes of LEA. In the United States there are approximately 1.6 million persons living with the loss of a limb. Within this population, 38% had an amputation as a result of dysvascular disease along with a concurrent diagnosis of diabetes mellitus (refer to Chapter 10 for more information about diabetes). The number of people living with the loss of a limb is projected to increase to 3.6 million by the year 2050 if the current health status of individuals goes unchanged.[1] Traumatic injury from motorcycle accidents and vehicular collisions with pedestrians accounted for approximately 59% of LEA in the years between 2000 and 2004.[2]

The various locations of LE amputation are shown in Figure 16-1 and are described in Table 16-1.

Upper-Extremity Amputation

UEA is most often the result of trauma, such as automobile collisions, industrial accidents, or penetrating trauma.[2-4] Disease and congenital limb deficiency are also major causes of UEA.[5]

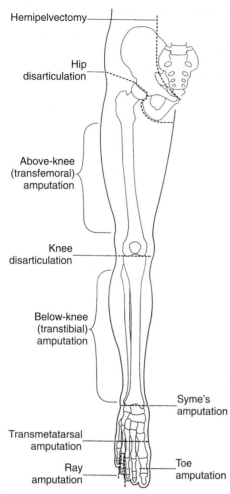

FIGURE 16-1
Levels of amputation. Lower extremity. (From Cameron MH, Monroe LG: Physical rehabilitation: evidence-based examination, evaluation, and intervention, St Louis, 2007, Saunders.)

Despite peripheral vascular disease being a major cause of LE amputation, it often does not create the need for UEA.[3]

The various locations of UEA are shown in Figure 16-2 and are described in Table 16-2.

Physical Therapy Management

The focus of physical therapy in the acute care setting for patients with a new limb amputation is pre-prosthetic management. Prosthetic training, if appropriate, most often occurs in the subacute, outpatient, or home setting and is not discussed specifically in this chapter. The type of amputation may dictate discharge disposition. Patients with UEA are more likely to be discharged home than are patients with LEA, who are more likely to require further care at a skilled nursing facility.[2]

The primary components of physical therapy management for a patient in the acute care setting who has undergone a limb amputation are as follows[6]:

* Wound healing
* Edema control

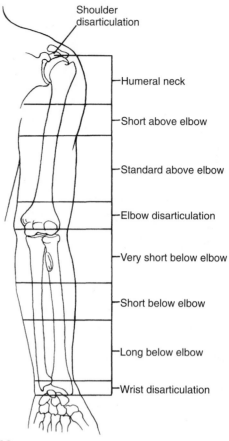

FIGURE 16-2
Upper-extremity amputation. (From Burke SL, Higgins JP, McClinton MA, et al, editors: Hand and upper extremity rehabilitation: a practical guide, ed 3, St Louis, 2006, Churchill Livingstone, p 716.)

* Pain management
* Joint mobility
* Strengthening
* Functional mobility
* Holistic care (including psychosocial needs and comorbidities)

Wound Healing

In order to facilitate prosthetic fitting, the integumentary condition of the residual limb needs to be thoroughly examined for signs of wound healing.[6,7] A poorly healing surgical incision can lead to both infection and delay in prosthetic fitting.[6] In addition, failure of wound healing has been related to a decreased success in ambulation with a prosthetic.[8] Refer to Chapter 12 for more information on wound care management.

> ✎ **CLINICAL TIP**
>
> Patients with peripheral arterial disease and diabetes are at risk for skin breakdown in their sound (nonamputated) lower extremity because this limb will be required to support more weight during the pre-prosthetic time period.[6]

TABLE 16-1 Types of Lower-Extremity Amputations*

Type	Description
Ray	Single or multiple rays can be amputated depending on the patient's diagnosis. If the first ray is amputated, balance is often affected, as weight is transferred to the lateral border of the foot, which may also cause ulceration and skin breakdown. Postoperative weight-bearing status will range from non–weight-bearing to partial weight-bearing status according to the physician's orders.
Transmetatarsal	The metatarsal bones are transected with this procedure as compared to other types of partial foot amputations, which may disarticulate the metatarsals from the cuboid and cuneiform bones. Balance is maintained with a transmetatarsal amputation, because the residual limb is symmetric in shape and major muscles remain intact. An adaptive shoe with a rocker bottom is used to help facilitate push-off in gait.
Syme's amputation (ankle disarticulation)	Often performed with traumatic and infectious cases, this type of amputation is preferred to more distal, partial foot amputations (ray and transmetatarsal) because of the ease of prosthetic management at this level. Patients may ambulate with or without a prosthesis.
Below the knee (transtibial)	Ideal site for amputation for patients with a variety of diagnoses. Increased success rate with prosthetic use. In cases with vascular compromise, the residual limb may be slow to heal. Residual limb length ranges from 12.5 cm to 17.5 cm from the knee joint.
Through-the-knee (disarticulation)	Often performed on elderly and young patients. Maximum prosthetic control can be achieved with this procedure because of the ability to fully bear weight on the residual limb. Also, a long muscular lever arm and intact hip musculature contribute to great prosthetic mobility. The intact femoral condyles, however, leave a cosmetically poor residual limb.
Above the knee (transfemoral)	Traditional transfemoral amputation preserves 50% to 66% of femoral length. Prosthetic ambulation with an artificial knee joint requires increased metabolic demand.
Hip disarticulation (femoral head from acetabulum)	Often performed in cases of trauma or malignancy. The pelvis remains intact; however, patients may experience slow wound healing and may require secondary grafting to fully close the amputation site.
Hemipelvectomy (half of the pelvis is removed along with the entire lower limb)	Also indicated in cases of malignancy. A muscle flap covers the internal organs.

Data from Thompson A, Skinner A, Piercy J, editors: Tidy's physiotherapy, ed 12, Oxford, UK, 1992, Butterworth-Heinemann, p 260; Engstrom B, Van de Ven C, editors: Therapy for amputees, ed 3, Edinburgh, Scotland, 1999, Churchill Livingstone, pp 149-150, 187-188, 208; May B, editor: Amputations and prosthetics: a case study approach, Philadelphia, 1996, FA Davis, pp 62-63; Sanders G, editor: Lower limb amputations: a guide to rehabilitation, Philadelphia, 1986, FA Davis, pp 101-102; Lusardi M, Nielsen C, editors: Orthotics and prosthetics in rehabilitation, Boston, 2000, Butterworth-Heinemann, pp 370-373; Edelstein JE: Prosthetic assessment and management. In O'Sullivan SB, Schmitz TJ, editors: Physical rehabilitation: assessment and treatment, ed 4, Philadelphia, 2001, FA Davis, pp 645-673.

*Unless otherwise stated, the etiology of these amputations is from peripheral vascular disease.

Edema Control

Managing edema in the early postoperative stages has many benefits including pain reduction, facilitating wound healing, and prosthetic fitting. The residual limb may have volume changes for up to 3 months after surgery, and therefore edema control techniques should be maintained until the residual limb is no longer painful, the wound is well healed, and/or the patient is wearing a prosthetic for most of the day.

Several approaches to managing edema include soft dressings (elastic bandages and elastic shrinker socks), semirigid dressings (air splints and *Unna bandage*), and rigid dressings (plastic or plaster). Elastic bandages should be applied in a figure-of-eight pattern to minimize a tourniquet effect.[6] Semirigid dressings such as the *Unna dressing* have been shown to foster wound healing as well to possibly better prepare the residual limb for prosthetic fitting[9]; however, no specific type of dressing has been shown to be the most effective.[6]

> **✎ CLINICAL TIP**
>
> Coordinate with nursing staff during dressing changes in order to visualize the skin and incision without unnecessary disruption to dressings. Monitor dressings for drainage, particularly after therapeutic activities with the limb in a dependent position.

Pain Management

Pain after limb amputation can occur in many areas of the body besides the amputated limb; however, the majority of pain complaints do occur in the residual limb. Several descriptions of pain following amputation exist but are generally categorized into these three types: phantom limb pain, phantom limb sensation, and stump pain. *Phantom limb pain* has been considered a type of neuropathic pain and is defined as a painful sensation

TABLE 16-2 Types of Upper-Extremity Amputations*

Type	Description
Wrist disarticulation	Distal radial ulnar joint function is often retained to maintain rotation of the radius.
Below elbow (transradial) Long below Short below Very short below	Optimum residual limb length for eventual prosthetic fitting is 8 cm above the ulnar styloid. Active prosthetic devices are operated by elbow extension and shoulder flexion, shoulder girdle protraction, or both. Length of residual limb will vary depending on amount of viable tissue below the elbow. Refer to Figure 16-2 for approximate length of these amputations.
Elbow disarticulation	Not a choice location for amputation because of the poor cosmetic look created and decreased postsurgical function of the prosthesis.
Above elbow (transhumeral) Standard above Short above	Often performed as a result of primary malignancy or metastatic disease. Optimum residual limb length for eventual prosthetic fitting is 10 cm above the elbow joint. Length of residual limb will vary depending on amount of viable tissue below the elbow. Refer to Figure 16-2 for approximate length of these amputations.
Humeral neck	Occurs between the glenohumeral joint and deltoid tuberosity. Allows for some attachment of prosthesis.
Shoulder disarticulation	Often performed as a result of primary malignancy or metastatic disease. The head of the humerus is maintained, or the acromion process and clavicle are trimmed to create a rounded appearance.
Forequarter	Often performed as a result of primary malignancy or metastatic disease. Consists of removal of the patient's clavicle, scapula, and arm.

Data from Engstrom B, Van de Ven C, editors: Therapy for amputees, ed 3, Edinburgh, Scotland, 1999, Churchill Livingstone, pp 243-257; Lusardi M, Nielsen C, editors: Orthotics and prosthetics in rehabilitation, Boston, 2000, Butterworth-Heinemann, p 573; Banerjee SN, editor: Rehabilitation management of amputees, Baltimore, 1982, Williams & Wilkins, pp 30-33; Ham R, Cotton L, editors: Limb amputation: from aetiology to rehabilitation, London, 1991, Chapman & Hall, pp 136-143; Theisen L: Management of upper extremity amputations. In Burke SL, Higgins JP, McClinton MA, et al, editors: Hand and upper extremity rehabilitation: a practical guide, ed 3, St Louis, 2006, Churchill Livingstone, p 716.

*Unless otherwise stated, the etiology of these amputations is from trauma.

perceived in the missing limb. *Phantom limb sensation* is any sensation, except for pain, in the missing limb. Examples of phantom limb sensation include tingling, prickling, or pins and needles. *Stump pain* is pain in the residual portion of the amputated limb and may be caused by neuromas, bony spurs, or infection.[10] Factors that affect the prevalence of phantom limb pain include gender (women experience this more than men), upper versus lower limb amputation, and time elapsed since amputation—patients experience less pain as more time passes postoperatively.[11]

Managing pain after amputation includes both medical and rehabilitation components. Preoperative analgesia with nonsteroidal antiinflammatory drugs (NSAIDs) has demonstrated equivocal results in reducing postoperative pain. Postoperative pain management may include the use of opioids, patient-controlled analgesia, local anesthetics such as epidural infusions, NSAIDs, antidepressants, and anticonvulsants.[10] Nonpharmacologic pain interventions include compression bandages, massage, relaxation, ultrasound, transcutaneous electrical stimulation (TENS), and biofeedback.[6]

Joint Mobility, Strengthening, and Functional Mobility

Joint mobility, strengthening, and functional mobility are interrelated aspects that may allow the therapist to achieve different goals with a single therapeutic activity. For example, in order to prevent joint contracture for patients with both UEA and LEA, active movements of all of the joints above the level of the amputation should be performed. Patients who use upper-extremity slings to fixate the arm in elbow flexion and shoulder

internal rotation should be examined regularly for contractures, particularly scapular motion. Active range-of-motion exercises and passive stretching or positioning should be incorporated, as indicated.[3,5,12-15]

For patients with LEA, the physical therapist should provide the patient and members of the nursing staff with education on residual limb positioning, proper pillow placement, and the use of splint boards. Patients with a transtibial amputation will be most susceptible to knee flexion contraction. A pillow should be placed under the tibia rather than under the knee to promote extension. Patients with above-the-knee amputations or disarticulations will be most susceptible to hip flexor and abductor contractures.[3,5,12-15]

During ambulation, patients with UEA tend to flex the trunk toward the side of the amputation and maintain a stiff gait pattern that lacks normal arm swing. Patients often need gait training, balance exercises, posture retraining, or a combination of these to facilitate an efficient gait pattern.[3,5,12-15]

Upper-extremity movements that are required for powering an upper-extremity prosthetic include[3,5,12-15]:
- Below-elbow body-powered prosthesis: elbow extension, shoulder flexion, shoulder girdle protraction, or a combination of these.
- Above-elbow body-powered prosthesis: elbow flexion, shoulder extension, internal rotation, abduction, and shoulder girdle protraction and depression.

Functional mobility training for patients with LEA includes:
- Bed mobility and transfer training, as well as gait training or wheelchair mobility.
- Patients with bilateral above-knee amputations will need a custom wheelchair that places the rear axle in a more

posterior position to compensate for the alteration in the patient's center of gravity when sitting.

> ### ✎ CLINICAL TIP
>
> Be mindful of hand placement for range-of-motion exercises to prevent excessive stresses on new incisions, particularly with transtibial amputations. During functional training for patients with LEA, patients should wear good footwear on the sound limb. This is helpful for both facilitating mobility and potentially preventing falls.

Holistic Care

Patients who undergo limb amputation experience various psychological challenges,[16] including depression, anxiety, body-image anxiety, concern over social functioning, and discomfort, as well as adaptations to a new self-identity. A high rate of depression appears to occur immediately after amputation and between 1 and 2 years postamputation. After this time period, rates of depression appear to decrease to a level found in the general population. Anxiety is also likely to be increased up to 1 year postamputation. A more specific form of anxiety pertaining to body image that includes perceptions of body-image distortion in patients after amputation has been associated with depression, poorer perceived quality of life, higher levels of anxiety, and lower levels of self-esteem. Social discomfort and perceived stigma may also affect physical and social activities. Literature concerning adaptations to a new self-identity is currently limited.[16] As a result of these various psychological challenges, physical therapists must be mindful of these aspects during patient care and refer the patient to appropriate practitioners should these issues arise and possibly affect rehabilitation progression.

Outcome Measures

Numerous tools are available to measure function and outcomes in patients with limb amputation (Table 16-3). The Amputee Mobility Predictor (AMP) has been reported to determine functional level as well as predict functional ability for amputees[17] and can be used for patients both before and after prosthetic fitting and rehabilitation.[18,19] Reliability and validity have also been established for the AMP.[19] More recently the modified Prosthetic Evaluation Questionnaire (PEQ), the version of the SF-36 for veterans (SF-36V), the Orthotics and Prosthetics User's Survey (OPUS), the Patient-Specific Functional Scale

TABLE 16-3 Outcome Measures for Patients with Limb Amputation

Type	Measurement Tool
Self-report	Amputee Activity Survey
	Sickness Impact Profile
	Reintegration to Normal Living
	Prosthetic Profile of the Amputee
	SF-36 Health Status Profile
	Prosthetic Evaluation Questionnaire
	Orthotic Prosthetic User's Survey
	Patient Specific Functional Scale
Professional report	Barthel Index
	Functional Independence Measure
Physical performance instruments	Six-Minute Walk Test
	Two-Minute Walk Test
	Functional Ambulation Profile
	Tinnetti Performance-Oriented Assessment of Mobility
	Timed Get-Up and Go
	Berg Balance Measurement
	Duke Mobility Skills Profile Test
	Functional Reach Test
	Amputee Mobility Predictor

Data from Gailey RS: Predictive outcome measures versus functional outcome measures in the lower limb amputee, J Prosthet Orthot 18(1S):51-60, 2006; Resnik L, Borgia M: Reliability of outcome measures for people with lower-limb amputations: distinguishing true change from statistical error, Phys Ther 91:555-565, 2011.

(PSFS), the Two-Minute Walk Test, the Six-Minute Walk Test, the Timed "Up & Go" (TUG) Test, and the AMP have been studied to examine test-retest reliability as well as to calculate minimal detectable change (MDC) of each measure.[20] All of these aforementioned tools demonstrated good reliability (Interclass coefficient [ICC] > 0.8) when used with patients with one lower-limb amputation.

With regard to MDC, the following should be used as a guide to measure true change (from previous to current measurements) in function for patients who have single-limb LEA[20]:

- Two-Minute Walk Test: 34.3 m
- Six-Minute Walk Test: 45 m
- TUG test: 3.6 seconds
- AMP: 3.4 points

The Medicare Functional Classification Level (MFCL) descriptions are used as a guideline by health care practitioners to determine prosthetic candidacy (Table 16-4). The MFCL is also used by third-party payers to guide their reimbursement for certain types and components of prosthetics.

TABLE 16-4 Medicare Functional Classification Level (MFCL) Descriptions

MFCL	Description	HCFA Modifier
0	Does not have the ability or potential to ambulate or transfer safely with or without assistance, and prosthesis does not enhance quality of life or mobility.	K0
1	Has the ability or potential to use prosthesis for transfers or ambulation on level surfaces at fixed cadence. Typical of the limited and unlimited household ambulator.	K1
2	Has the ability or potential for ambulation with the ability to traverse low-level environmental barriers such as curbs, stairs, or uneven surfaces. Typical of the limited community ambulator.	K2
3	Has the ability or potential for ambulation with variable cadence. Typical of the community ambulator who has the ability to traverse most environmental barriers and may have vocational, therapeutic, or exercise activity that demands prosthetic use beyond simple locomotion.	K3
4	Has the ability or potential for prosthetic ambulation that exceeds the basic ambulation skills, exhibiting high-impact, stress, or energy levels typical of the prosthetic demands of the child, active adult, or athlete.	K4

Adapted from Hafner B, Smith D: Differences in function and safety between Medicare Functional Classification Level-2 and -3 transfemoral amputees and influence of prosthetic knee joint control, J Rehabil Res Dev 46(3):417-433, 2009.
HCFA, Health Care Financing Administration.

References

1. Ziegler-Graham K, MacKenzie E, Ephraim P et al: Estimating the prevalence of limb loss in the United States: 2005 to 2050, Arch Phys Med Rehabil 89(3):422-429, 2008.
2. Barmparas G, Inaba K, Teixeira PGR et al: Epidemiology of post-traumatic limb amputation: a National Trauma Databank analysis, Am Surg 76(11):1214-1222, 2010.
3. Engstrom B, Van de Ven C, editors: Therapy for amputees, ed 3, Edinburgh, Scotland, 1992, Churchill Livingstone.
4. Pomeranz B, Adler U, Shenoy N et al: Prosthetics and orthotics for the older adult with a physical disability, Clin Geriatr Med 22(2):377-394, 2006.
5. Karacoloff LA, Schneider FJ, editors: Lower extremity amputation: a guide to functional outcomes in physical therapy management, Rockville, MD, 1985, Aspen.
6. Edelstein JE: Amputations and prostheses. In Cameron MH, Monroe LG, editors: Physical rehabilitation: evidence-based examination, evaluation, and intervention, St Louis, 2007, Saunders, pp 267-299.
7. Esquenazi A: Amputation rehabilitation and prosthetic restoration. From surgery to community reintegration, Disabil Rehabil 26(14/15):831-836, 2004.
8. Munin MC, Espejo-De Guzman MC, Boninger ML et al: Predictive factors for successful early prosthetic ambulation among lower-limb amputees, J Rehabil Res Dev 38(4):379-384, 2001.
9. Wong CK, Edelstein JE: Unna and elastic postoperative dressings: comparison of their effects on function of adults with amputation and vascular disease, Arch Phys Med Rehabil 81(9):1191-1198, 2000.
10. Chapman S: Pain management in patients following limb amputation, Nurs Stand 25(19):35-40, 2011.
11. Bosmans JC, Geertzen JHB, Post WJ et al: Factors associated with phantom limb pain: a 3½-year prospective study, Clin Rehabil 24(5):444-453, 2010.
12. May B, editor: Amputations and prosthetics: a case study approach, Philadelphia, 1996, FA Davis, pp 86-88.
13. Banerjee SN, editor: Rehabilitation management of amputees, Baltimore, 1982, Williams & Wilkins, pp 30-33, 255-258.
14. Ham R, Cotton L, editors: Limb amputation: from aetiology to rehabilitation, London, 1991, Chapman & Hall, pp 136-143.
15. Theisen L: Management of upper extremity amputations. In Burke SL, Higgins JP, McClinton MA et al, editors: Hand and upper extremity rehabilitation: a practical guide, ed 3, St Louis, 2006, Churchill Livingstone, p 716.
16. Horgan O, MacLachlan M: Psychosocial adjustment to lower-limb amputation: a review, Disabil Rehabil 26(14/15):837-850, 2004.
17. Helm P, Engel T, Holm A, et al: Function after lower limb amputation, Acta Orthop Scand 57:154-157, 1986.
18. Gailey RS: Predictive outcome measures versus functional outcome measures in the lower limb amputee, J Prosthet Orthot 18(1S):51-60, 2006.
19. May BJ, Lockhard MA: Prosthetics & orthotics in clinical practice: a case study approach, Philadelphia, 2011, FA Davis, p 107.
20. Resnik L, Borgia M: Reliability of outcome measures for people with lower-limb amputations: distinguishing true change from statistical error, Phys Ther 91:555-565, 2011.

CHAPTER 17

Physical Therapy Considerations for Patients Who Complain of Chest Pain

Michele P. West

CHAPTER OBJECTIVES

The objectives of this chapter are the following:

1. To describe the physiology and incidence of chest pain
2. To discuss the difference in symptomology of cardiogenic versus noncardiogenic chest pain, as well as "atypical" chest pain patterns in certain patient populations
3. To briefly discuss stable versus unstable angina
4. To provide the physical therapist with a clinical framework for how to proceed if a patient complains of chest pain

PREFERRED PRACTICE PATTERNS

Please refer to Appendix A for a complete list of the preferred practice patterns, as individual patient conditions are highly variable and other practice patterns may be applicable.

Chest pain, a common complaint for which many patients seek medical attention, accounts for approximately 5.5 million emergency department visits per year in the United States. Of these patients, 13% are diagnosed with acute coronary syndrome (ACS).[1] Thus the physical therapist in the acute care setting should be familiar with the various etiologies of cardiogenic and noncardiogenic chest pain and should be competent in taking an efficient history when a patient complains of chest pain.

Physiology of Chest Pain

Cardiogenic chest pain may be ischemic or nonischemic. *Ischemic* chest pain may be caused by atherosclerosis, coronary spasm, systemic or pulmonary hypertension, aortic stenosis, aortic or mitral regurgitation, hypertrophic cardiomyopathy, endocarditis, tachycardia (due to dysrhythmia such as atrial fibrillation), or severe anemia.[2] *Nonischemic* chest pain may be caused by aortic dissection or aneurysm, mitral valve prolapse, or pericarditis.[2] (Refer to the Acute Coronary Syndrome section in Chapter 3 for a description of stable, unstable, and variant [Prinzmetal's] angina and to Figure 3-10 for the possible clinical courses of patients admitted with cardiogenic chest pain.)

Incidence of Chest Pain

The probability of having chest pain caused by coronary artery disease (CAD) is increased if patients present to a primary care setting with four to five of the following variables[3]:

*   Age 55 years or older in men; 65 years or older in women
*   Known CAD or cerebrovascular disease
*   Pain not reproducible by palpation

- Pain worse during exercise
- Patient assumes pain is cardiogenic in origin

Presentation of Chest Pain

Certain patient populations may present with "atypical" anginal patterns. Female patients may not necessarily have mid-chest pain, but rather may have mid-back pain, left-sided chest pain, heaviness or squeezing, or pain in the abdomen.[4] In addition, females often present with indigestion, cold sweats, sleep disturbance, or vague symptoms such as fatigue and anxiety.[5] Elders over the age of 85 often present with anginal equivalents, especially dyspnea or syncope.[5] Patients with diabetes often present with fatigue, dyspnea, nausea and vomiting, or confusion.[5]

Noncardiogenic chest pain can arise from a wide range of diseases and disorders, which makes the differential diagnosis of chest pain challenging. Afferent fibers from the heart, lungs, great vessels, and esophagus enter the same thoracic dorsal ganglia and produce an indistinct quality and location of pain.[6] With overlapping of the dorsal segments, disease that is thoracic in origin may produce pain anywhere between the jaw and epigastrium.[6] Table 17-1 describes the most common differential diagnoses of noncardiogenic chest pain, each with its own distinctive associated signs and symptoms. Refer to Table 8-1 for gastrointestinal pain referral patterns.

Guidelines from the American College of Cardiology (ACC) and American Heart Association (AHA) provide the following as pain descriptions that are less characteristic of myocardial ischemia[7]:

- Pleuritic pain (i.e., sharp or knifelike pain brought on by respiratory movements or cough)
- Primary or sole location of discomfort in the middle or lower abdominal region
- Pain that may be localized at the tip of one finger, particularly over the left ventricular apex
- Pain reproduced with movement or palpation of the chest wall or arms
- Constant pain that persists for many hours
- Very brief episodes of pain that last a few seconds or less
- Pain that radiates into the lower extremities

Physical Therapy Considerations

As this information is ascertained, the physical therapist should discontinue activity (if the patient is not resting) and determine the need for continued seated or supine rest, observe the patient for signs of altered cardiac output (decreased blood pressure), take vital signs, apply supplemental oxygen, and monitor telemetry as necessary based on medical stability.

If the chest pain appears cardiogenic, the physical therapist must determine whether it is stable or unstable. *Stable angina*

TABLE 17-1 Possible Etiologies, Pain Patterns, and Associated Signs of Noncardiogenic Chest Pain

Origin	Possible Etiology	Pain Pattern and Associated Signs and Symptoms
Pulmonary/pleural	Pneumonia, pulmonary embolus, tuberculosis, pleuritis, pneumothorax, mediastinitis, chronic obstructive pulmonary disease	Pain with respiration, of sudden onset, usually well localized (lateral to midline) and prolonged. Pain is associated with abnormal breath sounds, increased respiratory rate, cough, hemoptysis, or pleural rub.
Gastrointestinal	Hiatal hernia, esophagitis, esophageal spasm, gastroesophageal reflux or motility disorder, acute pancreatitis, peptic ulcer, cholecystitis	Pain is epigastric, visceral or burning in nature, of moderate duration or prolonged, and usually related to food/alcohol intake. Pain is relieved by antacids, milk, or warm liquids. Nausea, vomiting, burping, or abdominal pain may be present.
Musculoskeletal	Muscle strain, rib fracture, costochondritis, cervical disk disease, shoulder bursitis or tendonitis, thoracic outlet syndrome	Pain is achy, increased with movement of the head/neck/trunk or upper extremity, or reproducible with palpation. Signs of inflammation may be present, or there may be a history of overuse/trauma.
Psychological	Panic disorder, anxiety, depression, or self-gain	Pain is often precordial with report of pain moving from place to place, moderate duration or situational, and unrelated to movement or exertion. Pain is associated with sighing respirations and accompanied by other evidence of emotional distress/disorder.
Infectious	Herpes zoster (shingles)	Burning, itching pain that is prolonged and in a dermatomal pattern. Pain is localized with a vesicular rash in the area of discomfort.

Data from Cannon CP, Lee TH: Approach to the patient with chest pain. In Libby P, Bonow RO, Mann DL et al, editors: Braunwald's heart disease: a textbook of cardiovascular medicine, ed 8, Philadelphia, 2008, Saunders; Goldman L: Approach to the patient with possible cardiovascular disease. In Goldman L, Ausiello D, editors: Cecil medicine, ed 23, Philadelphia, 2008, Saunders; Runge MS, Ohman EM, Stouffer GA: The history and physical examination. In Runge MS, Patterson C, Stouffer GA, editors: Netter's cardiology, ed 2, Philadelphia, 2010, Saunders.

is considered to be predictable, episodic, reproducible, triggered by physical or psychological stressors, occurring with a constant frequency over time, and relieved by rest or nitroglycerin.[5] *Unstable angina* is considered to be of new onset, occurring at rest or with minimal exertion, progressive in nature with increased frequency and duration of episodes, and refractory to previously effective medication.[5] During an episode of unstable angina, an electrocardiogram may reveal ST segment elevation or depression with or without T-wave inversion that reverses when anginal pain decreases.[4] These electrocardiographic changes are depicted in Figure 17-1. Vital sign findings include:

- Hypotension or hypertension
- Bradycardia or tachycardia
- Irregular pulse

If the patient presents with one or more of these unstable anginal findings, the therapist should stop or defer treatment and immediately notify the nurse and/or physician.

Regardless of the etiology of the patient's complaint of chest pain, the physical therapist must be prepared to gather a reliable chest pain description and respond and/or refer accordingly for prompt medical attention.

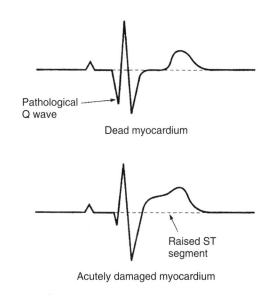

Pathological Q wave

Dead myocardium

Raised ST segment

Acutely damaged myocardium

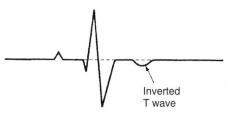

Inverted T wave

Myocardial ischemia
Note: There are a range of other causes for T wave inversion

FIGURE 17-1
Ischemic electrocardiographic changes.

References

1. Bhuiya FA, Pitts SR, McCaig LF: Emergency department visits for chest pain and abdominal pain: United States, 1999-2008. U.S. Department of Health and Human Services. National Center for Health Statistics. http://www.cdc.gov. Accessed July 3, 2012.
2. Runge MS, Ohman EM, Stouffer GA: The history and physical examination. In Runge MS, Patterson C, Stouffer GA, editors: Netter's cardiology, ed 2, Philadelphia, 2010, Saunders, pp 3-14.
3. Bösner S, Haasenritter J, Becker A et al: Ruling out coronary artery disease in primary care: development and validation of a simple prediction rule, CMAJ 182(12):1295-1300, 2010.
4. Goodman CC, Kelly Snyder TE: Screening for cardiovascular disease. In Goodman CC, Kelly Snyder TE, editors: Differential diagnosis for physical therapists: screening for referral, ed 5, Philadelphia, 2012, Saunders, p 253.
5. Brady WJ, Harrigan RA, Chan TC: Acute coronary syndrome. In Marx JA et al, editors: Rosen's emergency medicine, ed 7, St Louis, 2009, Mosby, pp 947-983.
6. Brown JE, Hamilton GC: Chest pain. In JA Marx, editor: Rosen's emergency medicine: concepts and clinical practice, ed 6, Philadelphia, 2006, Mosby.
7. Anderson JL, Adams CD, Antman EM et al: ACC/AHA 2007 guidelines for the management of patients with unstable angina/non ST-elevation myocardial infarction: A report of the American College of Cardiology/American Heart Association Task Force on Practice Guidelines (Writing Committee to Revise the 2002 Guidelines for the Management of Patients with Unstable Angina/Non ST-Elevation Myocardial Infarction): Developed in collaboration with the American College of Emergency Physicians, the Society for Cardiovascular Angiography and Interventions, and the Society of Thoracic Surgeons: Endorsed by the American Association of Cardiovascular and Pulmonary Rehabilitation and the Society for Academic Emergency Medicine, Circulation 116:e148, 2007.

CHAPTER 18

Medical-Surgical Equipment in the Acute Care Setting

Michele P. West

CHAPTER OBJECTIVES

The objectives of this chapter are to provide the following:

1. Describe the various types of medical-surgical equipment commonly used in the acute care setting, including oxygen (O_2) therapy and noninvasive and invasive monitoring and management devices
2. Provide a framework for the safe use of such equipment during physical therapy intervention

PREFERRED PRACTICE PATTERNS

The acute care setting is multifactorial in nature and applies to many body systems. For this reason, specific practice patterns are not delineated in this chapter. Please refer to Appendix A for a complete list of the preferred practice patterns in order to best delineate the most applicable practice pattern for a given diagnosis.

Medical-surgical equipment is used in all areas of the hospital. Some types of equipment are used only in specialty areas, such as the intensive care unit (ICU). The ICU, otherwise known as the critical care unit, is a highly specialized care unit for patients with life-threatening illness or injury. The equipment needed to provide life-sustaining care is numerous. The presence of certain types of equipment in a patient's room can provide the physical therapist with a preliminary idea of the patient's general medical condition and the appropriateness of therapeutic or prophylactic physical therapy intervention, or both. The physical therapist may initially be intimidated by the abundance of medical-surgical equipment (especially in the ICU); however, a proper orientation to such equipment allows the physical therapist to appropriately intervene with safety and confidence.

Oxygen Therapy

The general indication for O_2 therapy is hypoxemia. Hypoxemia is considered to be present when the arterial oxyhemoglobin saturation (SaO_2) is less than 90%, corresponding to an arterial blood O_2 partial pressure (PaO_2) of less than 60 mm Hg.[1] Refer to Table 4-6 for the relation between O_2 saturation as measured by pulse oximetry (SpO_2) and PaO_2 and to Figure 4-7 for the oxyhemoglobin dissociation curve. Other indications for O_2 therapy are severe trauma, shock, acute myocardial infarction, surgery, or carbon monoxide or cyanide poisoning.[1,2] The goal of O_2 therapy is to prevent or reverse hypoxemia by increasing the PaO_2, thereby improving tissue oxygenation, decreasing work of breathing, and decreasing myocardial work.[3]

O_2 moves across the alveolar-capillary membrane by diffusion, the physiologic mechanism by which gas moves across a membrane from a region of higher to lower pressure, and is driven by the partial pressure gradient of O_2 between alveolar air (PaO_2) and pulmonary capillary blood. To improve diffusion, a rise in PaO_2 can be attained by increasing the fraction of inspired O_2 (FiO_2) with supplemental O_2.[4]

Supplemental O_2 is delivered by variable-performance (Table 18-1) or fixed-performance (Table 18-2) systems. Each cannula or mask is designed to provide a range of FiO_2. Variable-performance systems are not intended to meet the total inspiratory requirements of the patient and should not be used if a specific FiO_2 is required. The actual FiO_2 for a given flow rate in a variable system is dependent on a patient's tidal volume and respiratory rate and the type, fit, and placement of the cannula or mask. If a specific FiO_2 is required, then a fixed-performance system is indicated. Fixed-performance systems deliver a specific FiO_2 despite the patient's respiratory rate and pattern.[2]

O_2 delivery devices with masks or reservoirs allow O_2 to collect about the nose and mouth during exhalation, which increases the availability of O_2 during inhalation. As the storage capacity of the mask or reservoir is increased, the FiO_2 for a given flow rate is also increased.[2]

The supplemental O_2 requirements of a patient may fluctuate with activity. Monitoring SaO_2 with pulse oximetry

TABLE 18-1 Variable-Performance Oxygen Delivery for Spontaneously Breathing Adults*

Device/FiO$_2$	Description
Nasal cannula RA $\approx$ 21% FiO_2 1 lpm $\approx$ 24% FiO_2 2 lpm $\approx$ 28% FiO_2 3 lpm $\approx$ 32% FiO_2 4 lpm $\approx$ 36% FiO_2 5 lpm $\approx$ 40% FiO_2 6 lpm $\approx$ 44% FiO_2	**Purpose:** Delivers supplemental O_2 mixed with RA, usually 1-6 lpm. **Consists of:** Prongs, which are attached to an O_2 source via small-bore plastic tubing and are positioned in the patient's nose. The tubing is secured by placing it behind the patient's ears, then under the patient's chin (Figure 18-1, *A*). Otherwise known as nasal prongs. **Clinical implications:** The rule of thumb for the cannula system is that FiO_2 is increased by 3%-4% for each lpm of O_2. Mouth breathing does not necessarily indicate that a patient is not receiving supplemental O_2. If nasal passages are obstructed, O_2 is able to collect in the oral and nasal cavities and is drawn in on inspiration. Flow rates of greater than 6 lpm are unlikely to increase delivered O_2 further and may prove uncomfortable and lead to mucosa irritation. Provide mobile patients with adequate lengths of extension tubing or a portable O_2 tank to enable functional mobility. Patients should be instructed to avoid tripping over or becoming tangled in the tubing. Ensure that the cannula tubing is in place without kinks or external compression during and after a physical therapy session.
Open face tent $FiO_2 \approx$ 30%-55%	**Purpose:** Provides humidified, supplemental O_2 mixed with RA. **Consists of:** A mask that rests under the chin, contacts the cheeks, and is open over the patient's nose. It is secured with an elastic strap around the patient's head. It connects to a humidified O_2 source with large-bore tubing (see Figure 18-1, *B*). **Clinical implications:** A significant amount of mixing with RA occurs, although the capacity of the mask allows O_2 to collect about the nose and mouth. May be more comfortable than a closed face mask for claustrophobic patients or for patients with facial trauma. Moisture may collect in the tubing and should be drained before moving the patient. The mask can easily shift; reposition it under the chin if necessary. The aerosol system is more cumbersome and may make mobilization of the patient more difficult than with nasal prongs. Collaborate with nursing to determine whether nasal prongs or a closed face mask can be used when mobilizing the patient.
Closed face mask 5-6 lpm $\approx$ 40% FiO_2 6-7 lpm $\approx$ 50% FiO_2 7-8 lpm $\approx$ 60% FiO_2	**Purpose:** Delivers supplemental O_2 mixed with RA. The mask has a small capacity but does allow for the collection of O_2 about the nose and mouth. **Consists of:** A dome-shaped mask covering the nose and mouth with ventilation holes on either side. An elastic strap around the patient's head secures it in place. It is connected to an O_2 source via small-bore tubing (see Figure 18-1, *C*). Otherwise known as a simple face mask. **Clinical implications:** The closed face mask interferes with coughing, talking, eating, and drinking and may be very drying and uncomfortable. Patients often remove the mask for these reasons. Educate the patient on the importance of keeping the mask in place.

TABLE 18-1 Variable-Performance Oxygen Delivery for Spontaneously Breathing Adults*—cont'd

Device/FiO$_2$	Description
Transtracheal catheter 1 lpm ≈ 28% FiO$_2$ 2 lpm ≈ 36% FiO$_2$ 3 lpm ≈ 44% FiO$_2$ 4 lpm ≈ 52% FiO$_2$ 5 lpm ≈ 60% FiO$_2$ 6 lpm ≈ 68% FiO$_2$	**Purpose:** Used for long-term O$_2$ therapy. Indicated when there are complications of or suboptimal nasal cannula use, nocturnal hypoxemia despite nasal cannula use, in situations when a patient needs more freedom to mobilize, or for patient preference. Provides continuous supplemental O$_2$ mixed with RA. **Consists of:** A small-bore catheter, which is surgically inserted percutaneously between the second and third tracheal interspaces to provide O$_2$. It is held in place by a narrow strap or chain around the patient's neck. A low flow rate (approximately one half with rest and two thirds with exercise) is used instead of a nasal cannula system owing to the continuous enrichment of the anatomic dead space with O$_2$. **Clinical implications:** Patients with severe bronchospasm, uncompensated respiratory acidosis (pH < 7.3), or steroid use higher than 30 mg per day are excluded from the use of this device. Depending on the surgical technique, the use of this device for O$_2$ delivery is delayed from 1 day to 1 week postoperatively to ensure that a permanent tract is formed between the trachea and skin. This device requires care and attention to hygienic maintenance. The most serious complication is tracheal obstruction resulting from the accumulation of mucus on the outside of the catheter, which can be avoided by routine secretion clearance multiple times per day. There is also a risk of infection around the catheter site and a risk of catheter dislodgement.
Tracheostomy mask or collar FiO$_2$ ≈ 28%-100%	**Purpose:** Provides supplemental, humidified O$_2$ or air at a tracheostomy site. **Consists of:** A mask placed over a stoma or tracheostomy. It is held in place by an elastic strap around the patient's neck. Humidified O$_2$ is delivered by large-bore tubing (see Figure 18-1, D). **Clinical implications:** Significant mixing with RA occurs. Humidification is particularly important for a patient with a tracheostomy, as the tracheostomy bypasses the natural humidification system. Moisture or pulmonary secretions may collect in the mask or tubing and should be drained before moving the patient or lowering the head of the bed. The mask can easily shift; reposition it over the site if necessary. Gently pull the mask away from the patient to access the tracheostomy site for bronchopulmonary secretion clearance.
Partial non-rebreather mask FiO$_2$ ≈ 40%-60%	**Purpose:** Provides a high FiO$_2$ to the patient while conserving the O$_2$ supply. **Consists of:** A closed face mask covering the nose and mouth with ventilation holes on either side, held in place with an elastic strap around the patient's head. A reservoir bag is attached at the base of the mask. The flow of O$_2$ is regulated to permit the initial one third of the expired tidal volume (O$_2$-rich anatomic dead space) to distend the reservoir maximally, therefore allowing some rebreathing of air. The balance of expired air does not enter the reservoir and is vented out the sides of the mask. **Clinical implications:** The partial non-rebreather mask is able to provide a similar FiO$_2$ to the non-rebreather mask at lower flow rates. The closed face mask may interfere with talking, eating, and drinking. High O$_2$ concentration may be drying and uncomfortable; however, humidification is not used with this method, because it interferes with O$_2$ delivery. The reservoir bag should remain at least ⅓ to ½ full on inspiration.
Non-rebreather mask FiO$_2$ ≈ 60%-80%	**Purpose:** Provides the patient with the highest concentration of supplemental O$_2$ available via a face mask in a variable-performance system. **Consists of:** A closed face mask covering the nose and mouth. It is attached to a reservoir bag, which collects 100% O$_2$. A one-way valve between the mask and bag allows O$_2$ to be inspired from the bag through the mask. Additional one-way valves on the side of the mask allow expired gases to exit the mask, thus preventing rebreathing of expired air (see Figure 18-1, E). **Clinical implications:** See Partial non-rebreather mask, above. Physical therapy intervention is usually deferred if a patient requires this type of device to maintain oxygenation. However, bronchopulmonary hygiene may still be indicated.

Data from Cairo JM: Administering medical gases: regulators, flowmeters, and controlling devices. In Cairo JM, Pilbeam SP, editors: Mosby's respiratory care equipment, ed 8, St Louis, 2004, Mosby, pp 60-88; Arata L, Farris L: Oxygen delivery devices. In George-Gay B, Chernicky CC, editors: Clinical medical surgical nursing, Philadelphia, 2002, Saunders, pp 126-127; Christopher KL, Schwartz MD: Transtracheal oxygen therapy, Chest 139(2):435-440, 2011.

FiO$_2$, Fraction of inspired oxygen; lpm, liters per minute; O$_2$, oxygen; RA, room air.
*Listed from least to most oxygen support.

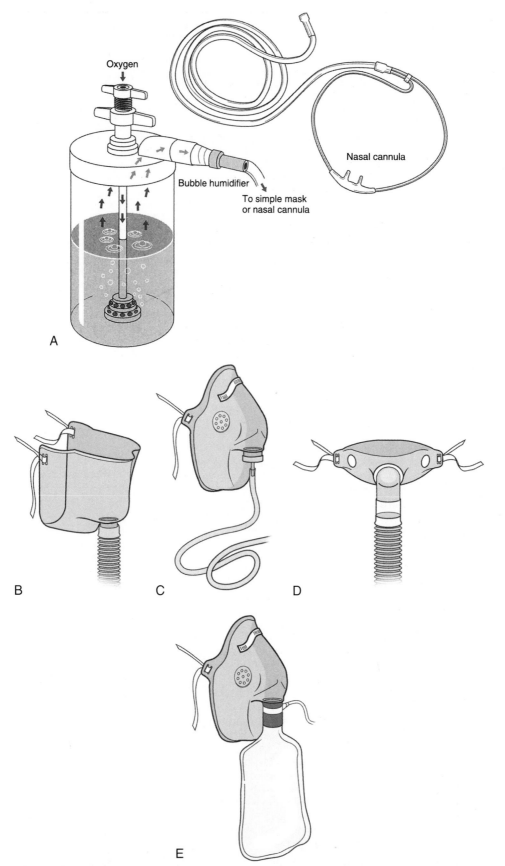

FIGURE 18-1

A, Nasal cannula with humidification. **B,** Open face mask or tent. **C,** Closed face mask. **D,** Tracheostomy mask or collar. **E,** Non-rebreather mask. (**A,** Redrawn from Kersten LD, editor: Comprehensive respiratory nursing: a decision-making approach, Philadelphia, 1989, Saunders. In Hillegass E, Sadowsky HS: Essentials of cardiopulmonary physical therapy, ed 2, Philadelphia, 2002, Saunders. **B** to **E,** From Dewit SC: Fundamental concepts and skills for nursing, ed 4, St Louis, 2014, Saunders.)

TABLE 18-2 Fixed-Performance Oxygen Delivery

Device/FiO_2	Description
Air entrainment mask (Venti mask, Venturi mask) $FiO_2 \approx$ 24%-50%	**Purpose:** Provides a specific concentration of supplemental O_2. **Consists of:** A high-flow system with a closed face mask over the nose and mouth and a jet mixing device located at the base of the mask, which forces 100% O_2 past an entrainment valve. The valve can be adjusted to entrain a specific percentage of RA to mix with the O_2, allowing precise control of FiO_2 (Figure 18-2). **Clinical implications:** The closed face mask interferes with coughing, talking, eating, and drinking and may be very drying and uncomfortable. Patients often remove the mask for these reasons. Educate the patient on the importance of keeping the mask snug in place. Humidification is not used when oxygen flow is < 4 lpm because humidification will interfere with O_2 delivery. Useful for patients with COPD who require a fixed precise FiO_2.
BiPAP (Bilevel positive airway pressure) $FiO_2 \approx$ 21%-100%	**Purpose:** Provides positive inspiratory and positive end expiratory pressure to decrease the work of breathing by reducing the airway pressure necessary to generate inspiration throughout the respiratory cycle. May be used to avoid intubation and mechanical ventilation in cases of acute respiratory failure. Often used in the hospital or home setting for the management of obstructive sleep apnea. **Consists of:** A closed mask with a clear soft gasket around its border, placed over the nose to fit tightly against the patient's face. It is held firmly in place with straps around the top and back of the head. **Clinical implications:** BiPAP may deliver supplemental O_2 at a specific concentration, or it may deliver RA. Patients may feel claustrophobic owing to the tight fit of the mask. The equipment may be noisy; thus the therapist may need to speak loudly to communicate with the patient. Air leaks can occur around the mask. Abrasions on the bridge of the nose can occur and may be prevented with a dressing that provides padding to the area without interfering with the tight fit of the mask. May also cause nasal congestion, nasal dryness, or rhinorrhea. Depending on the patient's oxygen requirements, BiPAP may be turned off, and alternate methods of O_2 delivery may be used to allow the patient to participate in functional activities or an exercise program. The unit may also be placed on a portable intravenous pole or cart for this purpose.
T tube/piece $FiO_2 \approx$ 50%-80%	**Purpose:** Provides a specific concentration of supplemental O_2 to an intubated, spontaneously breathing patient while weaning from a ventilator. **Consists of:** A T-shaped large-bore plastic tube attached directly to an endotracheal or tracheostomy tube. Humidified O_2 is delivered through one end of the T, and expired gas exits the other end. The tubing acts as a reservoir for O_2, allowing a specific concentration of O_2 to be delivered. **Clinical implications:** Tests the patient's true ability to spontaneously breathe and allows for ventilatory muscle training. Patients who are weaning from a ventilator can tire easily. Consult with the medical-surgical team to determine whether the patient will tolerate ventilator weaning (i.e., the use of a T piece) and physical therapy intervention simultaneously, or whether the patient would benefit from bronchopulmonary hygiene to facilitate weaning.

Data from Cairo JM: Administering medical gases: regulators, flowmeters, and controlling devices. In Cairo JM, Pilbeam SP, editors: Mosby's respiratory care equipment, ed 8, St Louis, 2004, Mosby, pp 60-88; Heuer AJ, Scanlon CL: Medical gas therapy. In Wilkins RL, Stoller JK, Scanlon CL, editors: Egan's fundamentals of respiratory care, ed 8, St Louis, 2003, Mosby.

BiPAP, Bilevel positive airway pressure; *FiO_2*, fraction of inspired oxygen; *lpm*, liters per minute; *O_2*, oxygen; *RA*, room air.

(identified as SpO_2) and subsequent titration of O_2 may be indicated during exercise. The physician may order parameters for resting and exercise SpO_2 if a patient has a low activity tolerance or an abnormally low SpO_2 at baseline.

A patient with chronic obstructive pulmonary disease (COPD) who has chronic carbon dioxide retention may become desensitized to the respiratory stimulant effects of carbon dioxide. In these patients, ventilation is driven by means of a reflex ventilatory response to a decrease in PaO_2 and in theory,

providing supplemental O_2 may lead to a reduction in the hypoxic peripheral chemoreceptor ventilatory drive. The hypoxic drive is not usually suppressed until the PaO_2 increases to greater than or equal to 60 mm Hg.[5] Potential respiratory depression or hypercapnia should never contraindicate oxygen therapy in the case of hypoxemia, however.[6] If acute respiratory failure occurs in the patient with COPD, other support measures such as noninvasive positive-pressure ventilation or invasive mechanical ventilation can be used.[7]

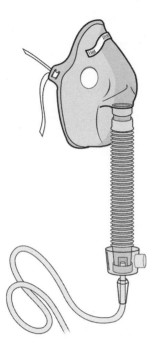

FIGURE 18-2

Air entrainment mask or Venturi mask. (From Dewit SC: Fundamental concepts and skills for nursing, ed 4, St Louis, 2014, Saunders.)

Physical Therapy Considerations

- Note that a green label designates the O_2 supply on hospital walls. A similar gauge supplies pressurized air that is designated by a yellow label.
- The FiO_2 for a given system is dependent on its proper fit and application. Ensure that all connections are intact, that the O_2 is flowing as indicated, and that the cannula or mask is properly positioned.
- Provide extra lengths of O_2 extension tubing if functional mobility will occur farther than 5 or 6 feet from the bedside (i.e., the wall O_2 source). Ensure that the plastic adaptor between two lengths of oxygen supply tubing is secure.
- Ensure that portable O_2 tanks are turned on and have sufficient levels of O_2 before use. Have backup tanks available.
- Observe masks for the accumulation of mucus or clogging. Clear or change the cannula or mask if needed.
- Monitor the patient's skin for potential breakdown due to pressure from the cannula or mask. Provide appropriate padding (such as foam ear protectors) without interfering with the fit of the cannula or mask.
- Significant supplemental O_2 requirements usually indicate a respiratory compromise, which in turn may indicate the need to modify or defer physical therapy intervention.
- Observe the patient for clinical signs of hypoxemia: shortness of breath, use of accessory muscles of breathing, confusion, pallor, or cyanosis.
- Document the type and amount of supplemental O_2 used during physical therapy intervention. This includes different amounts of FiO_2 for rest and exertion or for a recovery period after exercise.

- Oxygen is typically titrated (increased or decreased) according to physician prescription or according to a hospital protocol. The physical therapist should only titrate oxygen if an order to do so exists or if the situation is clinically appropriate. Communicate any changes in FiO_2 to the nurse or respiratory therapist.
- There may be specific guidelines set forth by third-party payers for the qualification of home oxygen. For example, Medicare requires documentation of oxygen saturation levels within 48 hours of durable equipment delivery with a requirement of a resting room air SaO_2 less than or equal to 88%, a room air SaO_2 less than or equal to 88% with exercise, *and* documented improvement of hypoxemia during ambulation with oxygen.[8]

Hemodynamic Monitoring

Monitoring hemodynamic events provides information about the adequacy of a patient's circulation, perfusion, and oxygenation of the tissues and organ systems. The objective of hemodynamic monitoring is to ensure optimal tissue perfusion and oxygen delivery while maintaining adequate mean arterial blood pressure.[9] Many measurements of cardiac and intravascular pressures and volumes are interpreted to direct a therapeutic plan of care. Ideally, hemodynamic monitoring is accurate and reproducible, is as uninvasive as possible, and minimizes harm to the patient.[9] Hemodynamic monitoring can be accomplished using noninvasive (Table 18-3) or invasive (Table 18-4) methods.

Noninvasive, or indirect, hemodynamic monitoring provides physiologic information without the risks of invasive monitoring and can be used in many settings. Invasive, or direct, measurements are obtained by penetrating the skin and inserting a cannula or catheter into a blood vessel, chamber of the heart, or both. The cannula or catheter is attached to a monitoring system, which consists of a transducer, amplifier, and oscilloscope for the display of the vascular waveforms and pressure measurements.[10] Direct monitoring can provide continuous, accurate data; however, thrombosis, infections, air embolisms, and trauma are potential complications.[11]

During invasive hemodynamic monitoring, the level of the right atrium is the standard zero reference point and is identified by the phlebostatic axis—the intersection of the midaxillary line and the fourth intercostal space (Figure 18-3).[10] The nurse will "level" the system using a carpenter's level or laserlight level to align the patient's phlebostatic axis with the transducer. Repositioning the patient may artificially alter waveforms by applying pressure to the catheter, shifting the catheter or stopcock, or shifting the phlebostatic axis relative to the transducer.[10] The transducer is releveled when clinically indicated. Raising the level of the phlebostatic axis relative to the transducer gives false high readings; lowering the phlebostatic axis gives false low readings.[10]

Patients with critical illness will have an alarm set on the hemodynamic monitoring system that sounds when a vital sign(s) is out of the desired parameter.

TABLE 18-3 Noninvasive Medical Monitoring

Device	Description
BP cuff (sphygmomanometer) Normal adult values: Systolic ≈ 100-140 mm Hg Diastolic ≈ 60-90 mm Hg	**Purpose:** Indirectly measures arterial blood pressure. **Consists of:** An inflatable bladder enclosed in a nondistensible cuff, attached to a pressure monitoring device. The device may be a manual aneroid manometer or an automatic oscillometric device. The cuff is typically placed 2.5 cm proximal to the antecubital space. If using a manual cuff, auscultate for Korotkoff sounds (refer to Table 3-7) with a stethoscope over an artery, usually the brachial artery. If using an automatic cuff, follow the manufacturer's directions for operation. **Clinical implications:** Do not use a BP cuff on an extremity with an arterial line, lymphedema, AV fistula or graft, or blood clot, or in an extremity ipsilateral to a mastectomy. Try to avoid measuring BP in an extremity with a peripheral or central intravenous line. Look for signs posted at the patient's bedside stating whether the use of a BP cuff on a particular extremity is contraindicated. Use an appropriately sized cuff. The cuff bladder should be no less than 80% of limb circumference. A cuff that is too small gives a falsely high reading, and a cuff that is too big gives a falsely low reading. The cuff may be placed on the upper extremity distal to the elbow with auscultation of the radial artery. Alternative sites for measurement in the lower extremity are proximal to the popliteal space with auscultation of the popliteal artery or proximal to the ankle with auscultation of the posterior tibial artery. These measurements are best taken with an automatic blood pressure cuff. Avoid contact between stethoscope tubing and the cuff tubing to minimize extraneous sounds. An automatic BP monitor may be used to take a blood pressure measurement if it is too difficult to hear Korotkoff sounds such as in the situation of hypotension. Automatic cuffs may also be helpful when a mean arterial pressure or serial blood pressures are needed, or when the therapist needs both hands (simultaneously) to guard a patient. While an automatic BP cuff is inflating/deflating, be sure to keep the patient's arm and hand still, and free from movement. Be sure to document the location where a blood pressure measurement is taken in your note.
Telemetry (ECG)	**Purpose:** Continuous monitoring of heart rate and rhythm and respiratory rate (see Table 3-9). **Consists of:** Five color-coded electrodes placed on the chest connected to a transmitter that converts the electrical currents from the heart into radio signals. Radio signals are picked up by antennae and transmitted to a central monitor at the nursing station and monitored at a distant site (telemetry). Twelve electrodes are used for a formal ECG. **Clinical implications:** Notify the nurse before physical therapy intervention, as many activities may alter the rate or rhythm or cause artifact (e.g., chest percussion). If an electrode(s) becomes dislodged, reconnect it. One way to remember electrode placement is "white is right" (white electrode is placed on the right side of the chest superior and lateral to the right nipple), "snow over grass" (green electrode is placed below the white electrode on the anterolateral lower-right abdomen), and "smoke over fire" (black electrode is placed on the upper-left rib cage superior and lateral to the left nipple, and the red electrode is placed below the black one on the anterolateral left abdomen). The brown electrode is usually placed centrally in the fourth intercostal space. Do not place electrodes over a pacemaker or defibrillator. Artifact, or poor signal quality, can appear on telemetry because the strength and consistency of the electrical current are interrupted. Causes of artifact include patient movement, poor electrode contact with the skin, or manual techniques for bronchopulmonary hygiene. Patients on telemetry should be instructed to stay in the area monitored by telemetry antennas. Watch the telemetry monitor to get a baseline heart rate and rhythm before physical therapy intervention and to ensure that the telemetry unit is actively connected. Telemetry may be put on hold temporarily for patient travel off the floor, or the batteries in an individual patient box may need replacement. The telemetry box may fit in the pocket of a hospital gown or in a small pocket carrier that is placed around the patient's neck or shoulder for exercise. Telemetry boxes are usually equipped with a "record" button that when pressed will print a rhythm strip of the ECG at the time of an "event" (i.e., when the patient is symptomatic). At some institutions, a designated nurse is stationed at the nursing desk to watch the main telemetry monitor for all patients. If indicated, check in with this nurse and request that the patient's telemetry be carefully watched during physical therapy intervention.

Continued

TABLE 18-3 Noninvasive Medical Monitoring—cont'd

Device	Description
Pulse oximeter Normal SpO_2 (at sea level) ≥ 93%-94%	**Purpose:** A noninvasive method of measuring the percentage of hemoglobin saturated with O_2 in arterial blood. **Consists of:** A probe (hard plastic clip or flexible strip) with an electro-optical sensor placed on a finger, toe, earlobe, forehead, or nose. The pulse oximeter emits two wavelengths of light to differentiate oxygenated from deoxygenated hemoglobin. **Clinical implications:** SpO_2 ≤ 88% indicates the need for supplemental oxygen. The waveform or pulse rate reading should match the ECG or palpated pulse. Monitor changes in pulse oximetry during exercise and position changes. Peripheral vascular disease, arrhythmia (such as atrial fibrillation) sunshine or excessive ambient light, motion artifact, or nail polish may lead to a false reading. In low-perfusion states, such as hypothermia, hypotension (<80 mm Hg in adults), or vasoconstriction, pulse oximetry may understate oxygen saturation. Small changes in the percentage of hemoglobin sites chemically combined (saturated) with oxygen (SaO_2) can correspond to large changes in the partial pressure of oxygen. Refer to Table 4-6 and Figure 4-7.

Data from Albertson B: Vital signs. In Craven R, Hirnle C, Jensen S, editors: Fundamentals of nursing: human health and function, ed 7, Philadelphia, 2013, Wolters Kluwer/Lippincott Williams & Wilkins Health, pp 331-335; Callahan JM: Pulse oximetry in emergency medicine, Emerg Med Clin North Am 26(4):869-879, 2008; Wheaton Franciscan Healthcare: Self-learning telemetry monitoring: applying and maintaining electrodes. http://www.wfhealthcare.org. Accessed July 3, 2012.

AV, Arteriovenous; *BP*, blood pressure; *ECG*, electrocardiography; *SaO₂*, arterial oxyhemoglobin saturation; *SpO₂*, measurement of SaO₂ with pulse oximetry.

TABLE 18-4 Invasive Medical Monitoring

Device/Normal Values	Description
Arterial line (A-line) Normal values: Systolic: 100-140 mm Hg Diastolic: 60-90 mm Hg MAP: 70-105 mm Hg	**Purpose:** To directly and continuously record systolic, diastolic, and MAP; to obtain repeated arterial blood samples; or to deliver medications. **Consists of:** A nontapered Teflon catheter. It is placed in the brachial, radial, or femoral artery. The catheter is usually connected to a transducer that converts a physiologic pressure into an electrical signal that is visible on a monitor. **Clinical implications:** If the A-line is displaced, the patient can lose a significant amount of blood at the insertion site. If bleeding occurs from the line, immediately apply direct pressure to the site while calling for assistance. The normal A-line waveform is a biphasic sinusoidal curve with a sharp rise and a gradual decline (Figure 18-4, *A*). A dampened (flattened) waveform may indicate hypotension, or it may be due to pressure on the line. If a waveform changes during treatment, in the absence of other clinical signs, reposition the patient or limb (if an arterial line is in place) and reassess. If the waveform does not return to baseline, notify the nurse. A patient with a femoral A-line is usually seen bedside. Hip flexion past 60-80 degrees is avoided. After femoral A-line removal, the patient is usually on strict bed rest for 60-90 minutes, with a sandbag placed over the site. Upper-extremity insertion sites are usually splinted with an arm board to stabilize the catheter. The patient with a radial or brachial A-line can usually be mobilized out of bed, although the length of the line limits mobility to a few feet. The transducer may be taped to the patient's hospital gown at the level of the phlebostatic axis (see Figure 18-3) during mobilization.
Central venous catheter Normal value: CVP 2-5 mm Hg or 3-8 cm H_2O	**Purpose:** Indicated for a patient with significant fluid volume deficit and is used as a guide to overall fluid balance. The measurement of CVP as a direct reflection of right heart function. (See the Pulmonary artery catheterization section below.) Also provides vascular access for short-term or long-term use (days to months) for parenteral nutrition, repeated blood sampling, administration of vasoactive or caustic drugs or large fluid volumes, or the initiation of transvenous cardiac pacing. **Consists of:** A single-lumen or multiple-lumen intravenous line placed in the subclavian, basilic, jugular, or femoral vein, terminating in the superior vena cava. **Clinical implications:** Do not use a blood pressure cuff on an extremity with a central line. Greatly reduces the need for repeated venipuncture and reduces risk of vein irritation. A chest x-ray is taken to confirm placement and to rule out iatrogenic pneumothorax. In the ICU setting, the CVP is connected to a transducer leveled to the phlebostatic line and is measured in mm Hg. In the medical-surgical unit, CVP is measured with a water manometer in cm H_2O.

TABLE 18-4 Invasive Medical Monitoring—cont'd

Device/Normal Values	Description
Pacemaker (temporary)	**Purpose:** To provide temporary supportive or prophylactic cardiac pacing postoperatively, for bradydysrhythmias (such as heart block), tachydysrhythmias (such as supraventricular tachycardia), for patients post myocardial infarction, for EPS diagnostic studies, or for permanent pacemaker failure. Refer to the Management section in Chapter 3 for more information on pacemakers. **Consists of:** An external pulse generator connected to an insulated electrical lead and 1 to 3 electrodes. The pacer emits an electrical current that directly causes myocardial depolarization. Pacer is set to deliver a certain number of impulses to the heart per minute. There are four basic types. *Epicardial:* The wires are placed after heart surgery on the epicardium and exit through a mediastinal incision. *Transvenous:* The wires are placed in the right atrium or ventricle via a subclavian or internal jugular central line. *Transcutaneous:* Large electrodes are placed (emergently) on the skin over the anterior and posterior chest. *Transthoracic:* Wire is placed (emergently) in the right ventricle through a transthoracic needle. **Clinical implications:** The presence of a temporary pacemaker does not, in and of itself, limit functional mobility. However, the underlying indication for the pacemaker may limit the patient's activity level. Check for mobility restrictions. Temporary pacing wires and electrodes should be kept dry. Be aware of the location of the generator and wires at all times, especially during mobility activities. If a temporary pacemaker is placed after a coronary artery bypass graft, the wires are usually removed 1 to 3 days after surgery. The patient is usually placed on bed rest for 1 hour after pacing wire removal, with vital sign monitoring every 15 minutes. Patients with temporary pacemakers require continuous ECG monitoring to evaluate pacemaker function. Temporary pacemaker malfunctions can occur and include failure to pace due to a mechanical problem with the pacer, "loss of capture" when the pacing stimulus fails to initiate myocardial depolarization, "rate drift" when pacing occurs at inappropriate times, "undersensing" when the pacer does not detect spontaneous myocardial depolarizations, and "oversensing" when the pacer detects extraneous electrical input, then inappropriately triggers or inhibits output.
Pulmonary artery catheterization (PA line, Swan-Ganz) Normal values: PAS: 20-30 mm Hg PAD: 5-10 mm Hg PAP (mean): 10-15 mm Hg PAOP (mean): 5-12 mm Hg LAP: 5-12 mm Hg RAP: 2-8 mm Hg CVP: 2-5 mm Hg Core temperature: 98.2°-100.2°F (36.8°-37.9°C) CO: 4-6 lpm (at rest) CI: 2.2 lpm/m²	**Purpose:** To directly or indirectly measure PAS, PAD, PAP, PAOP*, LAP, RAP, CVP, core body temperature, CI, and CO in cases of hemodynamic instability, ARDS, acute myocardial infarction, heart failure, or shock states. **Consists of:** A radiopaque, multilumen balloon-tipped catheter inserted through an introducing sheath into a large vein, usually the subclavian, or the brachial, femoral, or internal jugular vein (see Figure 18-4, *B*). The catheter is directed by blood flow into various locations of the heart and terminating in the pulmonary artery, with proper placement confirmed by x-ray. The catheter is connected to a transducer to allow for continuous monitoring. The proximal lumen opens into the right atrium to measure CVP and CO, and for the delivery of fluids or medications. The distal lumen opens into the pulmonary artery to measure PAP and to provide access to mixed venous blood samples. To obtain a PAOP measurement, a balloon at the end of the distal lumen is temporarily inflated. It follows the blood flow from the right ventricle into the pulmonary artery to a distal branch of the pulmonary artery, where it is "wedged" for a short time (up to 15 seconds). **Clinical implications:** The patient with a PA line is usually on bed rest. Avoid head and neck (for subclavian access) or extremity movements that could disrupt the PA line at the insertion site, including the line dressing. PAOP is an indirect measure of LAP. PAP is equal to right ventricle pressure. RAP is equal to CVP. CO equals stroke volume (SV) × heart rate (HR).

Data from Lough ME: Cardiovascular diagnostic procedures. In Urden LD, Stacy KM, Lough ME, editors: Critical care nursing: diagnosis and management, ed 6, St Louis, 2010, Mosby; Dirks JL: Cardiovascular therapeutic management. In Urden LD, Stacy KM, Lough ME, editors: Critical care nursing: diagnosis and management, ed 6, St Louis, 2010, Mosby.

A-line, Arterial line; *ARDS,* acute respiratory distress syndrome; *CI,* cardiac index; *CO,* cardiac output; *CVP,* central venous pressure; *EPS,* electrophysiology study; *ICU,* intensive care unit; *LAP,* left atrial pressure; *MAP,* mean arterial pressure; *PAP,* pulmonary artery pressure; *PAOP,* pulmonary artery occlusion pressure; *PAD,* pulmonary artery diastolic pressure; *PAS,* pulmonary artery systolic pressure; *RAP,* right atrial pressure.

*PAOP (formerly called pulmonary capillary wedge pressure or PAWP).

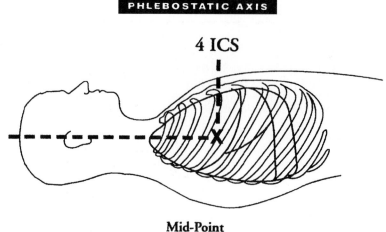

FIGURE 18-3
The phlebostatic axis at the intersection of the fourth intercostal space (*ICS*) and the midpoint of the anterior
(*A*) and posterior (*P*) chest wall. (Courtesy Edwards Lifesciences LLC.)

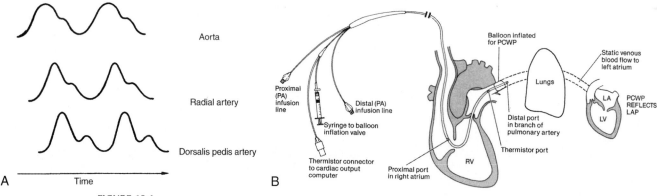

FIGURE 18-4
A, Arterial line tracing from different sites. **B,** Pulmonary artery (*PA*) catheter (four-lumen model) in a branch
of a PA with the balloon inflated; the pulmonary capillary wedge pressure (*PCWP*) reflects left atrial pressure
(*LAP*). *LA,* Left atrium; *LV,* left ventricle; *RV,* right ventricle. (**A,** From Yentis SM, Hirsh NP, Smith GB,
editors: Anaesthesia and intensive care A-Z. An encyclopedia of principles and practice, ed 2, Oxford, UK,
2000, Butterworth-Heinemann, p 45. **B,** From Kersten LD, editor: Comprehensive respiratory nursing: a
decision-making approach, Philadelphia, 1989, Saunders, p 758.)

Intracranial Pressure Monitoring

Intracranial pressure (ICP) and cerebral perfusion pressure
(CPP) may be measured in a variety of ways, depending on how
urgently ICP values are needed and the patient's neurologic or
hemodynamic stability. The purpose of ICP monitoring is the
maintenance of normal CPP and the early identification of
increased ICP before the occurrence of secondary cerebral
damage.[12] Refer to Intracranial and Cerebral Perfusion Pressure
in Chapter 6 for a description of these terms, Table 6-28 for a
description of the early and late signs of increased ICP, and Table
6-29 for a list of treatment options to decrease ICP.

Table 18-5 describes the different types of ICP monitors. For
some ICP monitors, such as the intraventricular catheter, the
sensor and the transducer must be level. Often, the zero point
for the transducer is at the tragus, or the top of the ear. A normal
ICP waveform has a triphasic sinusoidal waveform and should
correspond to heart rate.

Physical Therapy Considerations

- As with hemodynamic monitoring, be aware of the ICP
  value and the corresponding waveform on the monitor. The
  waveform may change shape (plateau wave) if cerebral
  hypoxia or ischemia occurs.[13]
- Momentary elevations in ICP will normally occur. A sustained elevation in ICP longer than 5 minutes is of concern[13]
  and should be reported to the nurse.
- Patients with elevated ICP are often positioned with the
  head of the bed at 30 degrees, which maximizes venous blood
  flow from the brain to help decrease ICP.[13] Therefore be
  aware that lowering the head of the bed may increase ICP.
  Other positions that increase ICP are the Trendelenburg
  position, lateral neck flexion, and extreme hip flexion.

TABLE 18-5 Intracranial Pressure (ICP) Monitors

Device	Description
Epidural sensor	**Purpose:** To monitor ICP. **Consists of:** A fiberoptic pneumatic flow sensor. It is placed in the epidural space (i.e., superficial to the dura) and connects to a transducer and monitor. **Clinical implications:** The transducer does not need to be adjusted (releveled) with position changes. Fair to good reliability. Reliability may decrease if the sensor drifts. A valuable option for patients with severe coagulopathy because it is least invasive.
Subarachnoid bolt	**Purpose:** To directly monitor ICP. **Consists of:** A hollow bolt or screw placed in the subarachnoid space through a burr hole. **Clinical implications:** The physician will determine the level at which the transducer should be positioned. This is documented in the chart and posted at the bedside. The transducer must be repositioned to the appropriate level with position changes. Poor reliability and decreased accuracy at high ICP readings. Complications include infection and blockage of the bolt by clot or brain tissue.
Intraventricular catheter (ventriculostomy)	**Purpose:** To directly monitor ICP and provide access for the sampling and drainage of cerebrospinal fluid (CSF). Occasionally used to administer medications or to instill air or contrast agent for ventriculography. **Consists of:** A small catheter that is placed in the anterior horn of the lateral ventricle through a burr hole. The catheter connects to a transducer and to a drainage bag, where CSF collects. **Clinical implications:** The nondominant hemisphere is the preferable insertion site. There are two different types of drainage systems: intermittent and continuous. The intermittent system allows the nurse to drain CSF for 30-120 seconds by momentarily opening a stopcock when the ICP exceeds the parameters set by the physician. A continuous system allows the drainage of CSF to occur against a pressure gradient when the collection bag is positioned (leveled) above the foramen of Monro. This is usually 15 cm above the external auditory meatus. The transducer must be repositioned to the appropriate level with position changes. Very reliable. The gold standard due to a high level of precision. Complications can include infection, meningitis, ventricular collapse, or catheter occlusion by blood or brain tissue.
Fiberoptic transducer-tipped catheter	**Purpose:** To monitor ICP. Can also be used in conjunction with a CSF drainage device (if the catheter is placed in the parenchyma). **Consists of:** A fiberoptic transducer-tipped catheter. It is placed in the ventricle, within the parenchyma, in the subarachnoid or subdural space, or under a bone flap. **Clinical implications:** The transducer does not need to be adjusted (releveled) with position changes. Very reliable.

Data from Smeltzer SC, Bare BG, Hinkle JL, et al: Management of patients with neurologic dysfunction. In Smeltzer, SC, Bare, BG, Hinkle, JL, et al, editors: Brunner & Suddarth's textbook of medical-surgical nursing, ed 11, Philadelphia, 2007, Lippincott Williams & Wilkins; Baumann JJ: Neurologic clinical assessment and diagnostic procedures. In Urden LD, Stacy KM, Lough ME, editors: Critical care nursing: diagnosis and management, ed 6, St Louis, 2010, Mosby, pp 718-719.

- Additional conditions that increase ICP are the Valsalva maneuver, noxious stimuli, coughing, pain, stress, and frequent arousal from sleep.[13]

Multimodal Neuromonitoring

Multimodal neuromonitoring, or the simultaneous use of multiple types of invasive and noninvasive modalities, are used to care for patients with traumatic brain injury (TBI).[14] This concept of brain monitoring includes common tests and measures combined with newer technologies. The goal is to prevent secondary ischemic and hypoxic injury from changes in brain metabolism after TBI.[14] An overview of these monitoring technologies, which are typically used in larger hospitals that treat a significant population of patients with neurotrauma or after neurosurgery, are listed in Table 18-6.

TABLE 18-6   Multimodal Brain Monitoring Technologies

Technology	Description
Cerebral microdialysis	**Purpose:** To measure glucose, lactate, pyruvate, and glycerol levels in the brain of a patient with severe head trauma. **Consists of:** A catheter with a semipermeable distal-end membrane is placed in the brain parenchyma through a burr hole, open craniotomy, or bolt. Ideally placed in the area of injury. Isotonic fluid is pumped in the catheter so that the catheter acts as an artificial blood capillary. Via diffusion, molecules related to the production of ATP are collected and analyzed on an hourly basis or less, depending on patient status. **Clinical implications:** The recovered metabolites represent 70% of the true interstitial fluid concentrations and are compared to normal values. A result toward a threshold value requires intervention such as permissive hyperglycemia, hypoglycemia prevention, vasopressor use, or positioning. A second catheter may be placed in an uninjured area of the brain for comparison.
Cerebral blood flow (CBF)	**Purpose:** Bedside monitoring of cerebral blood flow and circulation. Perfusion is measured by the ability of brain tissue to carry heat via thermal conduction. **Consists of:** A minimally invasive probe inserted via burr hole is placed in the white matter 2-2.5 cm below the dura in the tissue surrounding the injury. The probe is secured in place with a fixation disc or a bolt. The probe, which has a distal and proximal thermistor and is connected to a cable and monitor, provides a K value that calibrates to body temperature. **Clinical implications:** Reflects real-time perfusion of the brain. The patient may need to be cooled if brain temperature is >38.5° C. A second catheter may be placed in an uninjured area of the brain for comparison. The probe can be seen on computed tomography and radiography, yet is not compatible with magnetic resonance imaging.
Brain tissue oxygenation (P_{BTO_2})	**Purpose:** Directly measures brain oxygen and temperature as a marker of cerebral ischemia and secondary brain injury in the mechanically ventilated patient. **Consists of:** A triple-lumen introducer kit with an oxygen sensor at the distal tip (and other sensors for temperature and ICP) is placed 25 to 35 mm into the brain near the injured area via a double- or triple-lumen bolt. A baseline measurement is taken and compared to an oxygen challenge test whereby the patient receives 100% FiO_2 for 2-5 minutes. The P_{BTO_2} should increase and is ideally 30 mm Hg. **Clinical implications:** Lower P_{BTO_2} values may represent impending hypoxia. Elevated P_{BTO_2} values may represent hyperemia or excessive cerebral blood flow, which could increase ICP. P_{BTO_2} results can be improved during ischemic conditions by decreasing ICP with barbiturates, CSF drainage, or craniotomy. Cerebral oxygen delivery can be increased with isotonic fluid administration, vasopressors, or blood transfusion. Conditions such as pain, shivering, or agitation that decrease brain oxygenation can be managed with sedatives, antiinflammatory agents, or cooling devices.

Data from Cecil S et al: Traumatic brain injury advanced multimodal neuromonitoring from theory to clinical practice, Crit Care Nurse 31(2):25-36, 2011.
ATP, Adenosine triphosphate; *CSF,* cerebrospinal fluid; *FiO₂,* fraction of inspired oxygen; *ICP,* intracranial pressure.

Medical-Surgical Management Devices

Various lines, tubes, catheters, and access devices make up the wide variety of medical-surgical equipment used in the acute care setting. In general, these devices may be peripheral or central, for short-term or long-term use, and inserted or applied at the bedside in a special procedure (e.g., under fluoroscopic guidance) or in the operating room. Table 18-7[15-23] describes

the medical-surgical management devices most commonly encountered in the acute care setting.

Physical Therapy Considerations

The following information applies to medical-surgical equipment, as well as to the O₂ therapy and noninvasive, invasive, and ICP monitoring equipment previously discussed.

Text continued on p. 388

TABLE 18-7 Medical-Surgical Management Devices*

Device	Description
Arteriovenous (AV) fistula or graft	**Purpose:** Provides access for long-term hemodialysis. **Consists of:** The fistula is the surgical joining of a peripheral artery and vein, allowing arterial blood to flow directly to a vein. Usually located in the forearm. The graft is an artificial blood vessel, usually made of Gore-Tex, used to join an artery and vein when a patient's own vessels are not viable for an AV fistula. A minimum of 2 weeks is required before the fistula may be cannulated for dialysis use. **Clinical implications:** Elevate and avoid weight bearing on the involved extremity for 24 hours after surgical procedure. The involved extremity should not be used for phlebotomy, IV infusions, or blood pressure measurements. Avoid pressure or constriction over the site (as in sleeping on or bending the accessed limb for prolonged periods of time). Palpable turbulence is normal in the graft or fistula, which will have a raised, ropelike appearance. Complications can include thrombosis, infection, and vascular steal syndrome.
Central venous catheter	Refer to Table 18-4 for information on central venous catheter.
Chest tube	**Purpose:** Removes and prevents the reentry of air or fluid from the pleural space or mediastinal space and provides negative intrapleural pressure. Used to treat pneumothorax, hemothorax, pleural effusion, empyema, or chylothorax. May also be used for chemical pleurodesis to treat recurrent pleural effusion or pneumothorax. **Consists of:** Tube(s) placed in the pleural or mediastinal space that exits the chest and is usually connected to a drainage system (Figure 18-5). The placement of the tube is determined by indication. Mediastinal chest tubes, placed to drain the pericardium after surgery, exit the chest directly below the sternum. Apical chest tubes drain air, which typically collects in the apices of the pleural spaces. Fluid tends to collect near the bases; in these cases, tubes are placed more inferiorly near the fluid collection. Postoperatively, tubes often exit the chest through the surgical incision. If chest tubes are placed in a nonsurgical situation, they are often placed along the midaxillary line at the appropriate level. Tubes usually connect to a drainage system with three compartments: the drainage collection chamber, the water seal chamber with a one-way valve that prevents air or fluid from reentering the drainage collection chamber, and the suction chamber, which decreases excess pressure in the pleural space. Tubes may be connected to a small one-way valve (Heimlich valve) that allows air or fluid to escape from the pleural space while preventing reentry. **Clinical implications:** Chest tubes may cause discomfort, which may inhibit a cough, deep breath, mobility, or lying on the involved side. The patient may benefit from premedication for pain before treatment. Chest tube is often abbreviated "CT." If the chest tube has been removed from suction, it is often referred to as "chest tube to water seal." The drainage system should be below the level of chest tube insertion. Avoid tipping the collection reservoir. The reservoir may be hung from the side of the bed or taped to the floor to prevent tipping. If the reservoir is overturned, return the drainage container to the upright position and notify the nurse. If the chest tube itself becomes dislodged, stop activity and notify the nurse immediately. If possible, place the patient in an upright sitting position, and monitor the patient's breath sounds, vital signs, and respiratory rate and pattern for possible signs of tension pneumothorax. The occlusive dressing, usually a petrolatum gauze dressing to prevent the influx of air, should remain intact. Do not apply pressure over the insertion site. Prevent kinks in the tubing. The presence of a chest tube should not, in and of itself, limit activity. Position changes and mobility can facilitate drainage. Ask the nurse or doctor whether the chest tube may be temporarily disconnected from suction during mobility activities. If the suction must remain connected, additional lengths of tubing may be added, or a portable suction device may be used during mobility activities. Serial chest x-rays are often performed to determine chest tube placement and effectiveness, and to assist the medical-surgical team in determining the chest tube weaning process.

Continued

TABLE 18-7   Medical-Surgical Management Devices*—cont'd

Device	Description
Lumbar drain (lumbar drainage device, LDD)	**Purpose:** Drainage of CSF from the subarachnoid space in the lumbar spine. For the treatment of CSF leaks/dural tears, shunt infections, or traumatic dural fistulae or to reduce intracranial pressure. **Consists of:** A spinal catheter inserted in L4-5 subarachnoid space, advanced to an appropriate level, and connected to a sterile closed CSF collection system. A clear dressing is typically placed over the insertion site. **Clinical implications:** The position of the patient, the position of the transducer (if any), and the position of the collection bag are determined by the physician and the rationale for the LDD intervention. Changes in the patient's position, in the level of the collection bag, or in the intrathecal pressure affect the amount and rate of drainage. Avoid extremes of hip flexion, extension, or rotation as these positions can impede outflow. CSF is drained to a specific level of the drainage bag, to a specific volume per hour, or to a specific pressure. Patients are usually on bed rest while the drain is in place. Note any mobility and positioning restrictions in the medical record or posted in the patient's room. Patients are often instructed to avoid coughing, sneezing, straining, or the Valsalva maneuver. Complications of LDD by relative presence or overdrainage/underdrainage include infection, lower extremity nerve root irritation, tension pneumocephalus, central herniation of the brain, compression of the brain stem, and subdural hematoma. Monitor the patient for any changes in neurologic status. Notify nursing immediately if any changes are noted. The LDD is typically in place for 3-7 days depending on the rationale for its use.
Midline catheter	**Purpose:** Delivers IV medications or fluids for up to 4-6 weeks. Cannot be used to draw blood. **Consists of:** A 4- to 6-inch peripheral catheter placed via the veins near the antecubital fossa (basilic, cephalic, or brachial veins) and terminating in the axillary vein. **Clinical implications:** Do not use blood pressure cuff on the involved extremity.
Nasoenteric feeding tube (Dobbhoff tube)	**Purpose:** Placed for enteral feedings when patients are unable to take in adequate nutrition by mouth. **Consists of:** A radiopaque, small-diameter tube inserted via the nostril through the esophagus and into the stomach or duodenum, and held in place with tape across the nose. Can be inserted at the bedside, by an interventional radiologist, or surgically. Tube position is confirmed by x-ray before use. **Clinical implications:** The position of the tube in the nostril and the back of the throat can be irritating to the patient and may inhibit a cough. The tube often hangs in front of the patient's mouth and may also hinder airway clearance. The patient may be more comfortable if the tube is positioned away from his or her mouth and taped to the forehead or cheek. The tube can be dislodged easily. Check that the tape is secure. The tube may be safety-pinned to the patient's hospital gown for reinforcement. Notify the nurse if the tube becomes dislodged. Patient may be on aspiration precautions. Patient is typically positioned with the head of the bed ≥30 degrees during feedings. Place feedings on hold when the head of the bed is flat to minimize the risk of regurgitation or aspiration. This small-diameter tube can clog easily; some facilities require that feeding tubes be flushed with water when placed on hold for >15 minutes to minimize the risk of clogging.
Nasogastric tube (NGT)	**Purpose:** Keeps the stomach empty after surgery and rests the bowel by preventing gastric contents from passing through the bowels. Also used for gastric decompression (to relieve pressure and prevent vomiting), for gastric lavage, and to provide access to gastric specimens for laboratory analysis. Some NGTs allow access to the stomach for medications or tube feedings (see Nasoenteric feeding tube section). **Consists of:** A large-bore tube inserted via the nostril, through the esophagus, and into the stomach. Often attached to low-level suction pressure. Held in place with tape across the nose. **Clinical implications:** See Nasoenteric feeding tube section for positioning tips. Review the orders to determine if the patient's NGT may be temporarily disconnected from suction. Ask the nurse to disconnect or "clamp" the NGT from suction for mobilization of the patient. If/when disconnected, monitor the patient for nausea or abdominal distention. When disconnected from suction, the open end should be capped. Monitor the NGT to make sure it remains capped to prevent leaking.

TABLE 18-7 Medical-Surgical Management Devices*—cont'd

Device	Description
Nebulizer	**Purpose:** Delivers inhaled medications, usually bronchodilators and mucolytics. **Consists of:** A handheld chamber with a mouthpiece or a mask through which pressurized air aerosolizes medications that are then inhaled. May deliver medications through ventilator or tracheostomy tubing. **Clinical implications:** Treatment time is usually 10 minutes; however, the medications are usually effective for 3-6 hours. Patients may be better prepared for mobility activities or airway clearance after nebulizer treatments. These treatments are often referred to as "nebs."
Percutaneous endoscopically inserted gastrostomy/ jejunostomy tube (PEG/PEJ tube)	**Purpose:** Provides long-term access for nourishment to patients who are unable to tolerate food by mouth or have a nasoenteral obstruction, or for a patient with confusion/agitation at risk for nasoenteral tube dislodgement. May be used to supplement nutrition taken by mouth. **Consists of:** A feeding tube placed by endoscopy into the stomach (PEG) or jejunum (PEJ) through the abdominal wall. Tube is anchored with a balloon or disc inside the stomach. May also be placed by a surgeon during an operative procedure. **Clinical implications:** Place tube feedings on hold when the head of the bed is flat to minimize the risk of regurgitation/ aspiration. PEJ tube is considered postpyloric; therefore the risk of aspiration from regurgitation is minimized. This small-diameter tube can clog easily; some facilities require that feeding tubes be flushed with water when placed on hold for >15 minutes to minimize the risk of clogging.
Peripheral intravenous (IV) line	**Purpose:** Provides temporary access for delivery of medications, fluids, electrolytes, nutrients, or blood product transfusions. Cannot be used to draw blood. **Consists of:** A short plastic catheter, 1-1¼ inches long and of various diameters, inserted into a small peripheral vein. Ideally used in the cephalic or basilic veins on a noninvolved or nondominant upper extremity. Covered with a transparent dressing and secured in place with tape. May be secured further with a stretch net or arm board. **Clinical implications:** Avoid using blood pressure cuff on the involved extremity if possible. Watch IV tubing for kinks or occlusions. Position the patient to avoid occluding flow. Observe the patient for signs of infiltrated IV or phlebitis: localized pain, edema, erythema, or tenderness. Notify the nurse if signs are present. Notify the nurse if the IV dressing is not intact or appears infiltrated, or if the IV has become dislodged. If the IV is accidentally removed, safely apply direct pressure to the site with gloved hands. The patient may experience pain at an IV site in the thumb or wrist area when weight bearing or using an assistive device.
Peripherally inserted central catheter (PICC line)	**Purpose:** Provides IV access for long-term administration of TPN, medications, fluid, blood products, or chemotherapy. Useful for the patient having head/neck surgery. **Consists of:** A single- or double-lumen catheter placed via the basilic (most common), cephalic, or median cubital vein, terminating in the superior vena cava. Exterior tubing is taped to the arm and covered with a transparent dressing. **Clinical implications:** Wait for x-ray results before mobilizing the patient to confirm proper placement of the line, as improper placement can break the line; cause a hematoma; pierce the lung, causing a pneumothorax; or terminate in a vessel other than the vena cava. Do not use a blood pressure cuff on the involved extremity. Encourage range of motion of the involved extremity. Use of axillary crutches may be contraindicated, especially if the PICC is inserted in the basilic vein.

Continued

TABLE 18-7 Medical-Surgical Management Devices*—cont'd

Device	Description
Rectal pouch/tube	**Purpose:** Temporarily collects and contains bowel drainage (typically large amounts of liquid stool) and protects fragile skin from contact with feces. Also used for infection-control purposes. **Consists of:** An ostomy-type pouch placed externally and secured with an adhesive or a tube placed internally in the rectum, connected to a drainage bag. **Clinical implications:** Both are easily dislodged. Use a draw sheet when moving the patient in bed. Keep the collection bag below the level of insertion.
Sequential compression device (SCD) (pneumatic compression boots)	**Purpose:** Provides intermittent pressure to the lower extremities to promote venous return and prevent deep vein thrombosis (DVT) and venous thromboembolism (VTE) secondary to prolonged or postoperative bed rest or inactivity. **Consists of:** Inflatable sleeves, applied to the lower legs, which intermittently inflate and deflate. In some cases, the sleeve is applied to the leg from the ankle to mid-thigh. **Clinical implications:** Usually worn when the patient is in bed, but can be worn when sitting in a chair. Reapply when patient returns to bed. Best fit occurs when sleeves are applied without air in them. Discontinued when the patient is ambulating on a regular basis. Contraindicated in an extremity in which there is a known DVT. Not used directly over the lower extremity with a fracture, open wound, or acute cellulitis.
Suprapubic catheter	**Purpose:** Drains the bladder temporarily after some bladder or gynecologic surgeries, or permanently in cases of blocked urethra due to a tumor, stricture, periurethral abscess, or a severe voiding dysfunction. **Consists of:** A catheter placed in the bladder through a surgical incision in the lower abdominal wall (above the pubis) that is connected to a closed drainage system. Secured to the abdominal wall with sutures or a body retention seal and covered with a sterile dressing. **Clinical implications:** Keep the collection bag below the level of the bladder. The collection tubing may be taped to the patient's thigh. Avoid pressure over the insertion site. May be removed after a successful voiding trial with the tube clamped. Often more comfortable and allows greater mobility than a urethral catheter.
Surgical drain	**Purpose:** To remove excess air, blood or fluid (serum, lymph, bile, pus, or intestinal secretions) from a surgical site that would otherwise collect internally; to control ecchymosis; and to prevent deep wound infection. **Consists of:** Latex, polyvinyl chloride, or silicone catheters and collection vessels inserted at the time of surgery. Surgical drains are of two basic types: passive (open) or active (closed). Passive drainage is accomplished by gravity or capillary action. Drainage is further facilitated by transient increases in intraabdominal pressure, as with coughing. Passive surgical drains include Penrose, Foley, and Malecot catheters. Active drainage is accomplished by suction from a simple bulb device or with negative pressure from a suction pump. These systems may be closed, like the Hemovac and Jackson-Pratt (JP) drains. **Clinical implications:** Be aware of the location of the drain when moving the patient. The drain or tubing may be taped or pinned to the patient's skin or clothing to prevent tugging. Ask the nurse to temporarily disconnect a drain from suction, if necessary/appropriate. Before mobilization, visually inspect the drain for output. If the drain is three-quarters full to full, ask the nurse to empty the drain so that it works properly. Position changes can cause increased output. Monitor any drains for leakage during a PT session and report this to the nurse.

TABLE 18-7 Medical-Surgical Management Devices*—cont'd

Device	Description
Texas catheter (condom catheter)	**Purpose:** Noninvasively drains and collects urine from the penis. **Consists of:** A condom-like flexible sheath that fits over the penis to drain urine into a collection bag. This noninvasive method of collecting urine has a much lower risk of infection and irritation than does an indwelling catheter and is often the preferred method of managing male urinary incontinence. **Clinical implications:** It is easily dislodged. It may be held in place with a Velcro strap. The drainage bag should always be below the level of the bladder to allow drainage by gravity. Keep the collection bag off the floor. Secure the collection bag or catheter tubing to patient's leg, clothing, or assistive device to prevent the patient from tripping or becoming tangled in the tubing during mobility activities.
Vascular access port (VAP) (Port-A-Cath, MediPort, Pass-port, Infuse-A-Port, BardPort)	**Purpose:** For long-term (>6 months) chemotherapy, TPN, or other intermittent infusion therapy. **Consists of:** A completely indwelling surgically implanted catheter, usually placed in the subclavian or jugular vein, terminating in the superior vena cava. Access to the catheter is obtained through a tunneled portion attached to a port that is implanted in a subcutaneous pocket in the chest wall, usually below the clavicle. May also be placed in the arm, abdomen, flank, or thigh. The subcutaneous titanium or plastic port has a reservoir with a self-sealing silicone septum that is accessed by a special noncoring needle through intact skin. The tunneled portion is anchored to a muscle or subcutaneous tissue with sutures. **Clinical implications:** Once healed and cleared by MD, physical activity is not limited. Patients can usually swim or bathe and exercise without limitation. Appears as a slight protrusion under the skin. Report signs/symptoms of infection or infiltration to the nurse. Complications can include skin breakdown, site infection, extravasation, or thrombosis.
Tunneled central venous catheter (Hickman, Broviac, and Groshong, catheters)	**Purpose:** Used for long-term chemotherapy, TPN, or other infusion therapy. May be used for months to years for continuous or intermittent therapy. **Consists of:** Single-lumen or multilumen silicone catheter surgically implanted into a large vein (such as the subclavian or jugular) with the tip advanced to the superior vena cava. Very similar to a vascular access port; however, access is obtained through a "tailed" portion, which exits the skin from the anterior chest wall superior to the nipple. A Dacron cuff surrounds the tunneled portion just inside the exit site. The cuff causes a subcutaneous inflammatory reaction to occur after insertion, which, when healed, provides fixation and a barrier to venous infection within 7-10 days of implantation. **Clinical implications:** The tailed portion should be taped down to prevent dislodging. Do not perform manual techniques directly over the tail. Patients are allowed to shower once the insertion site is healed; however, tub bathing and swimming are usually limited.
Urinary catheter (Foley catheter)	**Purpose:** Temporarily drains and collects urine from the bladder. Used for urinary incontinence and retention, to assist with postoperative bladder drainage, when accurate measurement of urine output is necessary, or to prevent leakage in patients with stage III to IV pressure ulcers on the buttocks/perineum. **Consists of:** A tube inserted through the urethra into the bladder that drains into a collection bag. It is held in place internally by an inflated cuff. **Clinical implications:** Be aware of the position of the catheter. The collection bag should always be below the level of the bladder to allow drainage by gravity. Secure the collection bag or tubing to the patient's leg, clothing, or assistive device to prevent the patient from tripping or becoming tangled in the tubing during mobility activities. The collection bag should be kept off the floor.

Continued

TABLE 18-7 Medical-Surgical Management Devices*—cont'd

Device	Description
Ventriculoperitoneal shunt (VP); ventriculoatrial shunt (VA)	**Purpose:** Drains excess CSF from the brain into the abdominal cavity/peritoneum (VP) or right atrium of the heart (VA). **Consists of:** A shunt, tunneled under the skin, from the lateral ventricle of the brain to the collection cavity. **Clinical implications:** The patient may be on bed rest for 24 hours after placement. The shunt can often be palpated under the skin. Avoid excess pressure over the shunt. Monitor for signs of increased ICP.
Yankauer suction	**Purpose:** Clears secretions from the oral cavity or the oropharynx. **Consists of:** A handheld clear rigid tube attached to wall suction via tubing. The suction pressure is usually 100 to 120 mm Hg. **Clinical implications:** Some patients use this independently; if so, place within the patient's reach. To keep the Yankauer as clean as possible, it is often stored in the original packaging and rinsed with saline if pulmonary secretions collect on the inside or outside. Patients with a decreased cough reflex or dysphagia or on ventilator support may collect secretions in the mouth or in the back of the throat. Gentle Yankauer suctioning before rolling or other mobility may prevent aspiration of the collected secretions. Yankauer suctioning may stimulate a cough and help clear secretions in patients who are unable to clear secretions independently. If a patient bites down on the Yankauer, do not attempt to pull on the device. Wait for the patient to relax, and then gently slide the Yankauer from the patient's mouth.

Data from Urden LD, Stacy KM, Lough ME, editors: Critical care nursing: diagnosis and management, ed 6, St Louis, 2010, Mosby; Burchell PL, Powers KA: Focus on central venous pressure monitoring in an acute care setting, Nursing (Dec):39-43, 2011; Domke MN: Get a positive outcome from negative pressure, Nursing Made Incredibly Easy! (Jan/Feb):20-29, 2010; American Association of Neuroscience Nurses: Reference series for clinical practice. Care of the patient with a lumbar drain, ed 2, pp 1-15. http://www.aann.org. Accessed July 5, 2012; Craven R, Hirnle C, Jensen S, editors: Fundamentals of nursing: human health and function, ed 7, Philadelphia, 2013, Wolters Kluwer/Lippincott Williams & Wilkins Health; Fink J: Aerosol drug therapy. In Wilkins RL, Stoller JK, Scanlon CL, editors: Egan's fundamentals of respiratory care, ed 8, St Louis, 2003, Mosby, pp 775-780; Minkler MA: What are those tubes for? What you need to know about central venous access devices, EMS Mag 37(5):46, 48, 50 passim, 2008; McEwen DR: Wound healing, dressings and drains. In Rothcock JC, editor: Alexander's care of the patient in surgery, ed 14, St Louis, 2011, Mosby, pp 265-266; Ferrar-Hoffman DL, Krizman SJ: Neurosurgery. In Rothcock JC, editor: Alexander's care of the patient in surgery, ed 14, St Louis, 2011, Mosby, pp 866-867; Simmons KF, Scanlon CL: Airway management. In Wilkins RL, Stoller JK, Scanlon CL, editors: Egan's fundamentals of respiratory care, ed 8, St Louis, 2003, Mosby, p 654.

AV, Arteriovenous; *CSF,* cerebrospinal fluid; *CVP,* central venous pressure; *TPN,* total parenteral nutrition.

*Listed in alphabetical order.

- Before entering a patient's room, review the medical record, particularly new orders, recent progress notes, and test results. Review graphic sheets for vital signs, noting trends or variations from the norms.
- Note whether any particular precautions protecting the patient or the caregiver from specific pathogens are in place (e.g., contact precautions). Refer to Table 13-3 for a summary of infection prevention precautions.
- Practice standard precautions. The likelihood of encountering bodily fluids is increased in the acute care setting, especially in the ICU.
- Discuss your planned intervention with the nurse. Scheduled procedures may take precedence over this intervention, or it may coordinate well with another planned procedure.
- On entering the patient's room, take inventory. Observe the patient's appearance and position. Systematically observe the patient, and verify the presence of all documented lines. Develop a consistent method of surveying the room: left to right, or top of bed to bottom of bed, to ensure that all lines and equipment are observed and considered in your treatment plan. Take note of all readings on the monitors before intervention.
- Anticipate how your intervention may change the patient's vital signs and how this will likely appear on the monitors. Be aware of which readings may change artificially owing to relative position change.
- Using appropriate precautions, gently trace each line from the patient to its source. Ask for assistance, if needed, to untangle any lines or to free any lines that might be under the patient.
- Ensure that there is no tension on each line before attempting to move the patient.
- Never attempt to free a line that cannot be completely visualized!
- Discuss with the nurse whether any lines can be removed or temporarily disconnected from the patient before your treatment.
- Ask for appropriate assistance when mobilizing the patient.

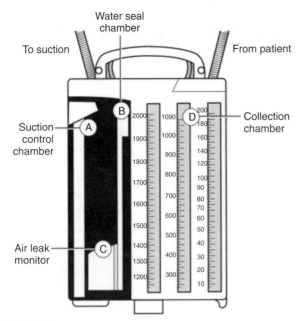

To suction

Water seal
chamber

From patient

Suction
control
chamber

A

B

D

Collection
chamber

2000
1900
1800
1700
1600
1500
1400
1300
1200

1090
1000
900
800
700
600
500
400
300

200
180
160
140
120
100
90
80
70
60
50
40
30
20
10

Air leak
monitor

C

FIGURE 18-5
Tubing attachment to three-chamber collection unit. (From Phillips N:
Berry and Kohn's operating room technique, ed 12, St Louis, 2013, Mosby.)

- Most invasive monitoring systems have two alarm controls: one to silence or discontinue the alarm for a few minutes, and another to disable or turn off the alarm. Do not silence an alarm without permission from the nurse! It is not recommended that the physical therapist disable an alarm.
- If available and appropriate, use a portable telemetry monitor to maintain the continuity of the ECG when mobilizing a patient who has continuous ECG monitoring away from the bedside.
- On completion of your treatment, ensure that all appropriate alarms are turned on and that the patient is positioned with the appropriate safety and communication measures in place. Notify the nurse of any change in the patient's status.

References

1. AARC clinical practice guideline: oxygen therapy for adults in the acute care facility-2002 revision and update. http://www.aarc.org. Accessed June 9, 2012.
2. Heuer AJ, Scanlon CL: Medical gas therapy. In Wilkins RL, Stoller JK, Scanlon CL, editors: Egan's fundamentals of respiratory care, ed 8, St Louis, 2003, Mosby, pp 827-861.
3. Cray L: Respiratory Function. In Craven R, Hirnle C, Jensen S, editors: Fundamentals of nursing human health and function, ed 7, Philadelphia, 2013, Wolters Kluwer, p 756.
4. Cairo, JM: Administering Medical Gases: Regulators, flowmeters, and controlling devices. In Cairo JM, Pilbeam SP, editors: Mosby's respiratory care equipment, ed 8, St Louis, 2004, Mosby, pp 60-88.
5. Shapiro, SD, Reilly JJ, Rennard SI: Chronic bronchitis and emphysema. In Murray & Nadel's textbook of respiratory medicine, ed 5, Philadelphia, 2010, Saunders, p 955.
6. American Thoracic Society/European Respiratory Society Task Force: Standards for the diagnosis and management of patients with COPD, version 1.2. New York, 2004, American Thoracic Society [updated September 8, 2005]. http://www.thoracic.org/go/copd. Accessed June 24, 2012.
7. Global Initiative for Chronic Obstructive Lung Disease (GOLD): Global strategy for the diagnosis, management and prevention of COPD 2011. http://www.goldcopd.org. Accessed June 24, 2012.
8. Department of Health and Human Services, Centers for Medicare and Medicaid Services: Oxygen therapy supplies: complying with documentation & coverage requirements. ICN 904883, December 2011. http://www.cms.org. Accessed June 24, 2012.
9. Rhodes A, Grounds RM, Bennett ED: Hemodynamic monitoring. In Textbook of critical care, ed 6, Philadelphia, 2011, Saunders, p 533.
10. Lough ME: Cardiovascular diagnostic procedures. In Urden LD, Stacy KM, Lough ME, editors: Critical care nursing: diagnosis and management, ed 6, St Louis, 2010, Mosby, pp 323-326.
11. Sturgess DJ, Morgan TJ: Haemodynamic monitoring. In Bersley AD, Soni N, editors: Oh's intensive care manual, ed 6, Boston, 2008, Butterworth-Heinemann, p 107.
12. Rabinstein AA: Principles of neurointensive care. In Bradley's neurology in clinical practice, ed 6, Philadelphia, 2012, Saunders, pp 802-818.
13. Smeltzer SC, Bare BG, Hinkle JL, et al: Management of patients with neurologic dysfunction. In Smeltzer SC, Bare BG, Hinkle JL, et al, editors: Brunner & Suddarth's textbook of medical-surgical nursing, ed 11, Philadelphia, 2007, Lippincott Williams & Wilkins, pp 2171-2180.
14. Cecil S et al: Traumatic brain injury: advanced multimodal neuromonitoring from theory to clinical practice, Crit Care Nurse 31(2):25-37, 2011.
15. Urden LD, Stacy KM, Lough ME, editors: Critical care nursing: diagnosis and management, ed 6, St Louis, 2010, Mosby.
16. Burchell PL, Powers KA: Focus on central venous pressure monitoring in an acute care setting, Nursing (Dec):39-43, 2011.
17. Domke MN: Get a positive outcome from negative pressure, Nursing Made Incredibly Easy! (Jan/Feb):20-29, 2010.
18. American Association of Neuroscience Nurses: Reference series for clinical practice. Care of the patient with a lumbar drain, ed 2, pp 1-15. http://www.aann.org. Accessed July 5, 2012.
19. Craven R, Hirnle C, Jensen S, editors: Fundamentals of nursing: human health and function, ed 7, Philadelphia, 2013, Wolters Kluwer/Lippincott Williams & Wilkins Health.
20. Fink J: Aerosol drug therapy. In Wilkins RL, Stoller JK, Scanlon CL, editors: Egan's fundamentals of respiratory care, ed 8, St Louis, 2003, Mosby, pp 775-780.
21. Minkler MA: What are those tubes for? What you need to know about central venous access devices, EMS Mag 37(5):46, 48, 50 passim, 2008.
22. McEwen DR: Wound healing, dressings and drains. In Rothcock JC, editor: Alexander's care of the patient in surgery, ed 14, St Louis, 2011, Mosby, pp 265-266.
23. Ferrar-Hoffman DL, Krizman SJ: Neurosurgery. In Rothcock JC, editor: Alexander's care of the patient in surgery, ed 14, St Louis, 2011, Mosby, pp 866-867.

APPENDIX 18A: MECHANICAL VENTILATION

Sean M. Collins
Jaime C. Paz

OBJECTIVES OF MECHANICAL VENTILATION

Mechanical ventilatory support provides positive pressure to inflate the lungs. Patients with acute illness, serious trauma, exacerbation of chronic illness, or progression of chronic illness may require mechanical ventilation.[1]

PHYSIOLOGIC OBJECTIVES OF MECHANICAL VENTILATION[2,3]

- Support or manipulate pulmonary gas exchange
- Increase lung volume
- Reduce or manipulate the work of breathing

CLINICAL OBJECTIVES OF MECHANICAL VENTILATION[2,3]

- Reverse hypoxemia and acute respiratory acidosis
- Relieve respiratory distress
- Reverse ventilatory muscle fatigue
- Permit sedation, neuromuscular blockade, or both
- Decrease systemic or myocardial oxygen consumption and intracranial pressure
- Stabilize the chest wall
- Provide access to tracheal-bronchial tree for pulmonary hygiene
- Provide access for delivery of an anesthetic, analgesic, or sedative medication

The following are indications for mechanical ventilation[2,4]:

- Apnea
- Acute hypercapnia that is not quickly reversible with standard treatment
- Partial pressure of arterial oxygen of less than 50 mm Hg with supplemental oxygen
- Respiratory rate of more than 30 breaths per minute
- Vital capacity less than 10 liters per minute
- Negative inspiratory force of less than 25 cm H_2O
- Protection of airway from aspiration of gastric contents
- Reversal of respiratory muscle fatigue[5]

Types of Mechanical Ventilatory Support

There are two primary methods to deliver mechanical ventilatory support, noninvasive and invasive. Noninvasive mechanical ventilation is used mainly for patients with exacerbations of chronic obstructive pulmonary disease (COPD) and cardiogenic pulmonary edema who are able to protect their airways.[6] Invasive mechanical ventilation involves the use of an artificial airway and is described further in the following sections. Non-invasive mechanical ventilation consists of an interface to connect the patient to the ventilator tubing. Six types of interfaces are currently available: full-face (or oronasal) mask, total face mask, mouthpieces, nasal mask, nasal pillows or plugs, and a helmet.[6] Noninvasive systems are further described in Table 18A-2. The use of either method to deliver mechanical ventilator support is dependent on several variables based on available evidence.[6]

Process of Invasive Mechanical Ventilation

Intubation

Intubation is the passage of an artificial airway (tube) into the patient's trachea (Figure 18A-1), generally through the mouth (endotracheal tube intubation) or occasionally through the nose (nasotracheal intubation). Intubation is considered for the following reasons[4,7]:

- The presence of upper airway obstruction
- Inability to protect the lower airways from aspiration

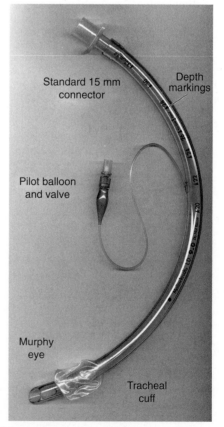

FIGURE 18A-1

A typical endotracheal tube. (From Durbin CG: Airway management. In Cairo JM, Pilbeam SP, editors: Mosby's respiratory care equipment, ed 7, St Louis, 2004, Mosby.)

- Inability to clear pulmonary secretions
- Hypoxemia despite supplemental oxygen
- Respiratory acidosis
- Progressive general fatigue including mental status deterioration
- The need for positive pressure ventilation

The process of removing the artificial airway is called *extubation*.

When patients require ventilatory support for a prolonged time period, a tracheostomy is considered. According to one author, it is best to allow 1 week of endotracheal intubation; then, if extubation seems unlikely during the next week, tracheostomy should be considered.[1] Recent recommendations also state that, depending on the patient's condition, transfer out of the intensive care unit (ICU) can generally be considered at the same time tracheostomy is being considered.[8] However, a patient can also be intubated for many weeks without tracheostomy, depending on the clinical situation.

A tracheostomy tube is inserted directly into the anterior trachea below the vocal cords, generally performed in the operating room. Benefits of tracheostomy include:

- Reduced laryngeal injury
- Improved oral comfort
- Decreased airflow resistance
- Increased effectiveness of airway care
- Feasibility of oral feeding and vocalization[7]

If the patient is able be weaned from ventilatory support, humidified oxygen can be delivered through a tracheostomy mask (see Chapter 18, Table 18-1).

Cuff

Approximately 0.5 inches from the end of an endotracheal or tracheal tube is a cuff (balloon). The cuff is inflated to (1) ensure that all of the supplemental oxygen being delivered by the ventilator via the artificial airway enters the lungs and (2) help hold the artificial airway in place. Cuff inflation pressure should be adequate to ensure that no air is leaking around the tube; however, cuff pressures should not exceed 20 mm Hg. High cuff pressures have been linked to tracheal damage and scarring, which can cause tracheal stenosis.

> ✎ **CLINICAL TIP**
>
> A cuff leak should be suspected if the patient is able to phonate or audible sounds come from his or her mouth. Cuff leaks can occur if the endotracheal tube is shifted (positional leak) or if the pressure decreases in the cuff. If a cuff leak is suspected, then the respiratory therapist or nurse should be notified. (Physical therapists who specialize in critical or cardiopulmonary care may be able to add air to the cuff according to the facility's guidelines.)

Positive Pressure Ventilators

Positive pressure ventilators are classified based on the method used to stop the inspiratory phase and allow expiration (cycling method) to occur.[7]

There are three basic cycling methods:

1. Pressure cycled
2. Volume cycled
3. Time cycled[9]

Ventilators can also be classified by control mode, the three modes being:

1. Volume controlled
2. Pressure controlled
3. Dual targeted[10]

For our purposes these two classification approaches are interchangeable. Pressure-cycled (or controlled) ventilators stop inspiration at a preset pressure, volume-cycled (or controlled) ventilators stop inspiration at a preset volume, and time-cycled ventilators stop inspiration at a preset time interval. Dual-targeted ventilators combine features from both pressure and volume control systems. These methods allow for increased control of certain variables during inspiration. However, holding only one variable constant for the termination of positive pressure inhalation allows other factors to affect inspiration and potentially cause barotrauma or reduced inspiratory volumes. These factors include position changes and manual techniques.

For example, with a volume-cycled ventilator, a preset volume will be delivered regardless of the patient's position, and reductions in chest wall expansion owing to a patient's position (e.g., side lying) may increase the pressure placed on the dependent lung tissue and result in barotrauma. Conversely, in the same scenario, if a patient is on a pressure-cycled ventilator, then pressure will be delivered to the predetermined level, but because the patient's position may hinder chest expansion, a resultant lower volume of inspired air may be delivered, because the preset pressure limit was reached. Dual-targeted ventilators provide the clinician with more than one cycling option, and certain modes of ventilation allow for more than one parameter to determine the inspiratory phase (as discussed throughout this appendix).

Wide-bore plastic tubing is used to create the mechanical ventilator's circuit. The terminal end of this circuit directly connects to an endotracheal or tracheal tube or, less commonly, to a face mask.[7] Some ventilator circuits have an extra port at their terminal end for an "in-line" suction catheter, which allows for suctioning without the removal of the ventilator circuit from the patient.[7]

> ✎ **CLINICAL TIP**
>
> Being aware of the cycling (control) method, the therapist can pay attention to changes in the pressure or tidal volume (V_T) associated with interventions.

Modes of Ventilation

Modes of ventilation can range from providing total support (no work performed by the patient) to minimal support (near-total work performed by the patient). Modes of ventilation are geared toward allowing the patient to do as much of the work of breathing as is physiologically possible, while meeting the intended objectives of ventilatory support. Even short periods (11 days) of complete dependence on positive pressure ventilation can lead to respiratory muscle atrophy and concomitant reductions in diaphragm strength (25%) and endurance (36%).[11] Figure 18A-2 provides a schematic of the conventional modes of ventilation based on the amount of support they provide. Characteristics of conventional and alternative modes of ventilation are presented in Tables 18A-1 and 18A-2, respectively.

Ventilatory Settings

Ventilatory settings are parameters established to provide the necessary support to meet the patient's individual ventilatory and oxygenation needs.[5,12] Establishment of the ventilatory settings is dependent on the patient's (1) arterial blood gas levels, (2) vital signs, (3) airway pressures, (4) lung volumes, and (5) pathophysiologic condition, including the patient's ability to spontaneously breathe.[5,12] Ventilator settings, subdivided into those that influence oxygenation and those that influence ventilation, are presented in Table 18A-3.

Complications of Mechanical Ventilation

Auto Positive End-Expiratory Pressure

Auto positive end-expiratory pressure (PEEP) occurs when lung volumes fail to return to functional residual capacity before the onset of the next inspiration. The process leading to auto PEEP is referred to as *dynamic hyperinflation*.[2,5] The primary consequence of dynamic hyperinflation is increased air trapping, which results in physiologic dead space due to pulmonary

shunting (perfusion is delivered to alveolar units that are not receiving fresh ventilation), which decreases gas exchange. Ultimately, this leads to an increased work of breathing owing to higher respiratory demand, as well as altered length-tension relationships of the inspiratory muscles. Auto PEEP and concomitant air trapping can occur when the minute ventilation or respiratory rate is too high; the inspiratory-expiratory ratios are not large enough, or the endotracheal tube is too narrow or kinked; there is excess water condensation in the tubing; or in patients with obstructive lung disease. A combination of the aforementioned factors can increase the likelihood of auto PEEP. In patients with chronic obstructive pulmonary disease who are on ventilator modes that allow them to initiate ventilator-assisted breaths (assisted ventilation, assist/control ventilation, synchronous intermittent mandatory ventilation [SIMV], pressure-supported ventilation [PSV]), the therapist should realize that activity could increase the patient-generated respiratory rate. Some modes will then, given the initiation of a breath, provide a set volume of air (assisted ventilation, assist/control ventilation, SIMV) that could increase the likelihood of hyperinflation owing to auto PEEP. This can also happen in modes that do not deliver a set volume of air (PSV), because inspiration is assisted with positive pressure.

Barotrauma

Barotrauma refers to damage to the lungs caused by excessive airway pressure. Many of the alternative modes of ventilation are geared toward reducing this complication (see Table 18A-2). In the normal lung, spontaneous inhalation without ventilatory support takes place because of negative pressure. The volume of inhaled air is limited by the return of intrapulmonary pressure back to atmospheric pressure in the lungs during inhalation. Because mechanical ventilation is predominantly delivered with

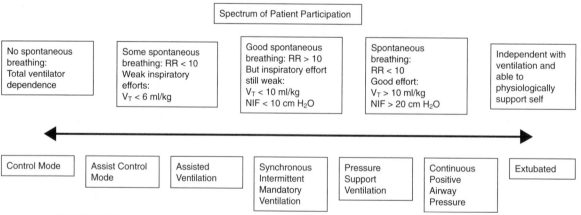

FIGURE 18A-2

Schematic of mechanical ventilator modes: the ability of patients to participate in the process of ventilation and oxygenation in part determines the mode of ventilation. Parameters used to determine the patient's ventilatory effort include the presence of spontaneous breaths, the number of breaths per minute he or she initiates (respiratory rate [RR]), the volume of those breaths per breath (tidal volume [V_T]), and the negative inspiratory force (NIF) generated with those breaths. The values indicated above are examples of patient characteristics along the spectrum from complete ventilatory dependence to independence. The effectiveness of the patient's efforts needs to be assessed based not only on the above parameters, but on "outcome" variables, such as oxygenation (PaO_2, oxygen saturation as measured by pulse oximetry), ventilation ($PaCO_2$), and overall status (hemodynamic stability, symptoms).

TABLE 18A-1 Conventional Modes of Ventilation

Modes	Characteristics
Control ventilation (CV)	Total control of the patient's ventilation: preset rate; FiO_2; V_T; flow rate; I:E ratio. Patients may be sedated or pharmacologically paralyzed. No active respiratory muscle activity is necessary.
Assist ventilation (AV)	Patient controls respiratory pattern and rate; breath initiated by patient creates negative airway pressure in circuit; once initiated, the volume is delivered with either a preset volume or pressure and flow rate; respiratory muscles are still working. Patient can trigger RRs that are too high, leading to respiratory alkalosis or auto PEEP (refer to Complications of Mechanical Ventilation).
Assist control (AC)	Combination of CV and AV; delivers breath of predetermined tidal volume with the patient's inspiratory effort.[1] If the patient does not initiate a breath within a specified time period, the ventilator will deliver a breath to maintain preset RR.
Synchronized intermittent mandatory ventilation (SIMV)	Delivers breaths intermittently at preset time intervals with a preset RR, V_T, and flow rate. Patient is allowed to breathe spontaneously through a separate circuit between machine-delivered breaths. However, like AV, it will assist a patient-initiated breath. Mandatory breaths are only delivered when the patient is not initiating enough breaths to allow a preset minute ventilation.
Pressure-supported ventilation (PSV)	Patient-initiated breaths are augmented with a preset flow of gas from the ventilator to maintain constant inspiratory pressure; when the inspiratory flow drops to a preset value, the flow of gas terminates. Patient controls RR, inspiratory time, and flow; patient and ventilator determine V_T and minute ventilation. The V_T received from the machine is related not only to the patient's effort but also to the amount of pressure provided by the ventilator.
Continuous positive airway pressure (CPAP)	Intended to decrease work of breathing by reducing the airway pressure necessary to generate inspiration throughout the respiratory cycle while the patient is spontaneously breathing. Positive pressure is constantly maintained above atmospheric pressure. Most commonly used during weaning from the mechanical ventilator or in an attempt to postpone intubation (can be delivered via an endotracheal tube or a specially designed face mask, respectively). Commonly used at night for the treatment of sleep apnea.

Data from Marino P: The ICU book, ed 3, Philadelphia, 2006, Lippincott Williams & Wilkins; Slutsky AS: Mechanical ventilation. American College of Chest Physicians' Consensus Conference, Chest 104:1833, 1993; Chestnutt MS, Murray JA, Prendergast TJ: Pulmonary disorders. In Tierney LM, McPhee SJ, Papadakis MA, editors: Current medical diagnosis & treatment, New York, 2008, McGraw-Hill; Chandrashekar R, Perme C: Monitoring and life support equipment. In Hillegass EA, editor: Essentials of cardiopulmonary physical therapy, ed 3, St Louis, 2011, Saunders.

FiO_2, Fraction of inspired oxygen; *I:E ratio,* inspiratory time to expiratory time ratio; *PEEP,* positive end-expiratory pressure; *RR,* respiratory rate; *V_T,* tidal volume.

positive inspiratory pressure, these normal physiologic mechanisms for preventing such trauma are bypassed, and pressures in the lung exceed normal pressures. Another consideration is that many of the lung conditions requiring mechanical ventilation do not uniformly affect the lungs (adult respiratory distress syndrome, pneumonia). Inhalation volumes are delivered to those areas that are still normal, which can overdistend (causing high pressure) as a result. This can produce stress fractures in the walls of the alveoli, thus exacerbating the acute lung condition.[13,14] Infants who are mechanically ventilated are five times more likely to develop bronchopulmonary dysplasia than are infants who are not mechanically ventilated.[15] It is thought that barotrauma exacerbates the acute lung injury associated with adult respiratory distress syndrome.[1] Other complications associated with barotrauma include pneumothorax and subcutaneous emphysema.[5]

Other possible complications of mechanical ventilation are as follows[2,5,12]:

- Improper intubation can result in esophageal or tracheal tears. If the artificial airway is mistakenly placed in the esophagus and is not detected, gastric distention can occur with the initiation of positive pressure.

- Ventilator-associated pneumonia (VAP)—a form of health care–associated infection that occurs in patients who are mechanically ventilated longer than 48 hours. VAP is highly problematic as it results in increased length of stay for patients both in the ICU and in the hospital. Mortality is also increased 27% to 43% if a patient has VAP. Risk factors include immunosuppression, underlying lung conditions, body position, level of consciousness, endotracheal tubing, ventilator circuits, and hospital personnel not following standard precautions. Prevention consists of good oral hygiene to the patient before intubation, avoiding saline lavage during suctioning, changing positions frequently, and preventing aspiration by keeping the head of the bed up 30 degrees.[16]

- Oxygen toxicity: Oxygen levels that are too high and maintained for a prolonged time can result in the following:
  - Substernal chest pain that is exacerbated by deep breathing
  - Dry cough
  - Tracheal irritation
  - Pleuritic pain with inspiration
  - Dyspnea

TABLE 18A-2 Alternative Modes of Ventilation

Mode	Characteristics
Pressure control ventilation	Delivers a preset airway pressure for a predetermined inspiratory time interval. Inspiratory time is usually prolonged, and patients are generally sedated because of discomfort due to the prolonged mechanical inspiration. V_T is determined by lung compliance; useful in cases in which barotrauma is thought to exacerbate the acute lung injury (ARDS); now also available in ACV or SIMV modes.
High-frequency oscillation ventilation	A technique of ventilation that is administered with frequencies of 100-3000 breaths per minute and consequently small tidal volumes of 1-4 ml/kg. Primary advantage is dramatic reduction of airway pressure and has shown beneficial results in neonates and adults with ARDS, particularly those adults who do not respond positively to conventional mechanical ventilatory modes.
Inverse ratio ventilation	A rarely used technique involving the use of an inspiratory to expiratory ratio of more than 1 to 1; can be delivered as a pressure-controlled or volume-cycled mode. The proposed benefit is the recruitment of a greater number of lung units during the respiratory pause and longer inspiration. Potential risk of generating auto PEEP and dynamic hyperinflation (refer to Complications of Mechanical Ventilation).
Mandatory minute ventilation (minimum minute ventilation or augmented minute ventilation)	Only set parameter is the minute ventilation; if spontaneous, unassisted breaths do not meet that minute ventilation, the ventilator makes up the difference by supplying mechanical breaths. Used primarily in weaning patients from a ventilator.
Noninvasive positive-pressure ventilators (NPPV)	Delivery of ACV, SIMV, and PSV modes of ventilation via a nose mask or face mask to reduce the need for intubation. Bilevel positive airway pressure (BiPAP), also called *bilevel pressure assist,* is a form of NPPV that employs PSV and PEEP. Shown to be useful in reducing in-hospital mortality in COPD patients and long-term use in patients with neuromuscular diseases.
Proportional assist ventilation (PAV)	Offers patient autonomy because every breath is initiated and stopped by the patient; pressure assistance by the machine is proportional to a combination of the inspired volume and the inspiratory flow rate.
Negative-pressure ventilators	Exposes the chest wall to subatmospheric pressure during inspiration to reduce intrapleural pressure, thereby allowing air to enter the lungs. Efficacy has not been demonstrated in patients with COPD and is unproven for acute respiratory failure.
Airway pressure release ventilation (APRV)	Lungs are kept inflated with a preset airway pressure, and exhalation occurs during cyclic reductions in pressure. Advocated for protecting the lung from high peak airway pressures, although no benefit has been demonstrated over conventional methods.
Adaptive support ventilation	A mode of ventilation that accommodates a patient's breathing pattern by changing the number of mandatory breaths and pressure support level until a calculated tidal volume is reached.
Pressure-regulated volume control	Provides volume support to a patient while keeping peak inspiratory pressures (PIP) at the lowest level by altering inspiratory time and peak flow. Useful in patients with changing airway compliance or characteristics.
High-frequency jet ventilation	Uses a nozzle and injector to deliver jets of gas directly into the lung at high rates. Indicated for the neonatal population who has pulmonary hypoplasia, restrictive lung disease, and persistent pulmonary hypertension. Typically used in tandem with a conventional ventilator.
Partial liquid ventilation	Uses perfluorocarbon liquids (does not mix with surfactant and has a high solubility for O_2 and CO_2). Lungs are filled with the liquid to approximately functional residual capacity, and then standard mechanical ventilation is attempted. Has not demonstrated benefits above conventional ventilator modes, and still requires much research before being used routinely.

Data from Marino P: The ICU book, ed 3, Philadelphia, 2006, Lippincott Williams & Wilkins; Slutsky AS: Mechanical ventilation. American College of Chest Physicians' Consensus Conference, Chest 104:1833, 1993; Chestnutt MS, Murray JA, Prendergast TJ: Pulmonary disorders. In Tierney LM, McPhee SJ, Papadakis MA, editors: Current medical diagnosis & treatment, New York, 2008, McGraw-Hill; Fan E, Stewart TE: New modalities of mechanical ventilation: high-frequency oscillatory ventilation and airway pressure release ventilation, Clin Chest Med 27(4):615-625, 2006; Chang DW. In Clinical application of mechanical ventilation, ed 3, New York, 2006, Thomson Delmar Learning; Chandrashekar R, Perme C: Monitoring and life support equipment. In Hillegass EA editor: Essentials of cardiopulmonary physical therapy, ed 3, St Louis, 2011, Saunders; Pilbeam SP, Cairo JM: Mechanical ventilation: physiological and clinical applications, ed 4, St Louis, 2006, Mosby; DeTurk WE, Cahalin LP: Cardiovascular & pulmonary physical therapy: an evidence-based approach, ed 2, New York, 2011, McGraw-Hill.

ACV, Assist/control ventilation; *ARDS,* adult respiratory distress syndrome; *COPD,* chronic obstructive pulmonary disease; *I:E ratio,* inspiratory time to expiratory time ratio; *PEEP,* positive end-expiratory pressure; *PSV,* pressure-supported ventilation; *SIMV,* synchronous intermittent mandatory ventilation; V_T, tidal volume.

TABLE 18A-3 Ventilator Settings

Purpose	Setting	Characteristic
Oxygenation	Fraction of inspired oxygen (FiO$_2$)	The percentage of inspired air that is oxygen; at normal respiratory rate (RR), tidal volume (V$_T$), and flow rates, an FiO$_2$ of 21% (ambient air) yields a normal oxygen partial pressure of 95-100 mm Hg; an increase in the percentage of oxygen delivered to the alveoli results in a greater PaO$_2$ and therefore a greater driving force for the diffusion of oxygen into the blood. FiO$_2$ of 60% has been set as the threshold value to avoid toxicity with prolonged use.
	Positive end-expiratory pressure (PEEP)	The pressure maintained by the mechanical ventilator in the airways at the end of expiration; normal physiologic PEEP (maintained by sufficient surfactant levels) is considered to be 5 cm H$_2$O. Settings are adjusted as needed to maintain functional residual capacity above closing capacity to avoid closure of alveoli. Closure of alveoli can result in shunting of blood past the alveoli without gas exchange, which results in decreased oxygenation.
Ventilation	RR	Set according to the amount of spontaneous ventilatory efforts by the patient; different ventilatory modes, described in Tables 18A-1 and 18A-2, are prescribed according to the patient's needs; patients who are unable to generate any spontaneous breaths are fully ventilated at respiratory rates of 12-20 breaths per minute. This rate is decreased accordingly for those who are able to generate spontaneous breaths. The amount of volume delivered with each breath is adjusted with respiratory rate to control partial pressure of arterial carbon dioxide (PaCO$_2$).
	V$_T$	Excessive volume leads to increased airway pressures, and therefore pressures are routinely monitored to prevent barotrauma. At times, hypercapnia is allowed to prevent high lung pressures due to the delivered volume and noncompliance of lung tissue, termed *permissive hypercapnia*.
	Inspiratory flow rate	Set to match the patient's peak inspiratory demands; if this match is not correct, it can cause the patient discomfort while breathing with the ventilator. High flow rates deliver greater volume in less time and therefore allow longer expiratory times (prevents hyperinflation); however, this also leads to greater peak airway pressure and the possibility of barotrauma. If the rate is too slow, the patient may attempt to continue to inhale against a closed circuit, resulting in respiratory muscle fatigue.
	Inspiratory-to-expiratory ratio	The inspiratory-to-expiratory ratio is set with the goal of allowing the ventilator to be as synchronous as possible with the patient's respiratory ratio. For patients who are not spontaneously breathing, this ratio is set according to what is required to maintain adequate ventilation and oxygenation.
	Sensitivity	Pressure change is required in the airway to trigger an ACV or PSV breath; typically −1 to −3 cm H$_2$O. If mechanical sensors respond poorly, then respiratory muscle fatigue can occur. If the sensors are too sensitive, then hyperventilation can develop.

Data from Marino P: The ICU book, ed 3, Philadelphia, 2006, Lippincott Williams & Wilkins; Slutsky AS: Mechanical ventilation. American College of Chest Physicians' Consensus Conference, Chest 104:1833, 1993; Howman SF: Mechanical ventilation: a review and update for clinicians, Hosp Physician December:26-36, 1999. *ACV*, Assist/control ventilation; *PaO$_2$*, oxygen saturation as measured by pulse oximetry; *PSV*, pressure-supported ventilation.

- Nasal stiffness and congestion
- Sore throat
- Eye and ear discomfort
- Cardiovascular: High positive pressures can result in decreased cardiac output from compression of great vessels by overinflated lungs.

Weaning from Mechanical Ventilation

The process of decreasing or discontinuing mechanical ventilation in a patient is referred to as *the weaning process*.[12] A contributing factor to a successful wean from ventilatory support is the resolution or stability of the condition that led to the need for ventilatory support.[17] A spontaneous breathing trial (SBT) is typically performed to evaluate a patient's readiness to begin the weaning process. The trial consists of the patient breathing spontaneously for 15 to 30 minutes while being closely monitored.[9]

The patient criteria for an attempt at weaning from mechanical ventilation are as follows:
- Spontaneous breathing
- Fraction of inspired oxygen less than 50% and PEEP less than 5 cm H$_2$O with oxygen saturation as measured by pulse oximetry greater than 90%
- Maximal inspiratory pressure greater than −30 cm H$_2$O: Pressures greater than −30 have been associated with successful extubation, while pressures greater than −15 are associated with an inability to maintain spontaneous breathing[18]
- Respiratory rate less than 35 breaths per minute
- Tidal volume greater than 325 ml[18]
- Respiratory rate/V$_T$ ratio less than 105. (A respiratory rate/V$_T$ ratio greater than 105 indicates shallow and rapid

breathing and is a powerful predictor of an unsuccessful wean[18,19])

Examples of weaning methods are as follows:

- SIMV: Decreasing the number of breaths per minute that the ventilator provides requires the patient to increase his or her spontaneous breaths. This is commonly used after surgery, while patients are waking up from anesthesia. These patients typically have not been on support for an extended period of time and do not usually have a lung condition that required them to be intubated in the first place. As soon as respiratory drive and spontaneous breathing return, it is expected that the patient can be removed from ventilatory support.

- T-piece: Breathing off of the ventilator, while still intubated, for increasing periods of time. This technique is something of an all-or-none method. Patients need to have the respiratory drive to breathe spontaneously and the capability to generate adequate V_T to attempt this weaning process. The process aims to improve respiratory muscle strength and endurance with prolonged time periods of independent ventilation.

- PSV: The patient spends periods of time with decreased pressure support to increase his or her spontaneous ventilation. Two factors can be manipulated with PSV: (1) to increase strength load on the respiratory muscles and reduce the PSV, and (2) to increase endurance requirement on the respiratory muscles and increase the length of time that PSV is reduced.

Currently it is the consensus that the T-piece and PSV methods of weaning are superior to the SIMV method.[17,20]

In addition, two techniques have been developed to possibly enhance the patient's ability to wean off the ventilator: automatic tube compensation (ATC) and proportional-assist ventilation (PAV). Both of these techniques are designed to lessen the resistive load of the artificial airways and associated ventilator tubing, thus decreasing the patient's work of breathing and possibly increasing tolerance of the weaning process.[17]

Five major factors to consider during a patient's wean are as follows[12]:

1. Respiratory demand (the need for oxygen for metabolic processes and the need to remove carbon dioxide produced during metabolic processes) and the ability of the neuromuscular system to cope with the demand
2. Oxygenation
3. Cardiovascular performance
4. Psychological factors
5. Adequate rest and nutrition

Signs of increased distress during a ventilator wean are as follows[5,12]:

- Increased tachypnea (more than 30 breaths per minute)
- Drop in pH to less than 7.25 to 7.30 associated with an increasing $PaCO_2$
- Paradoxical breathing pattern (refers to a discoordination in movements of the abdomen and thorax during inhalation; see Chapter 4)
- Oxygen saturation as measured by pulse oximetry less than 90%

- Change in heart rate of more than 20 beats per minute
- Change in blood pressure of more than 20 mm Hg
- Agitation, panic, diaphoresis, cyanosis, angina, or arrhythmias

Physical Therapy Considerations

A patient who is mechanically ventilated may require ventilatory support for a prolonged period of time. Patients who require prolonged ventilatory support are at risk for developing pulmonary complications, skin breakdown, joint contractures, and deconditioning from bed rest. Physical therapy intervention, including bronchopulmonary hygiene and functional mobility training, can help prevent or reverse these complications despite mechanical ventilation. Reports in the literature indicate that patients who were on mechanical ventilation for longer than 4 days were able to safely participate in activities such as sitting at the edge of the bed, sitting in a chair, and ambulating distances up to 100 feet at time of discharge from the ICU setting. These patients were determined to be physiologically ready for activity if (1) they were responsive to verbal stimulation, (2) their FiO_2 was 0.6 or less, (3) their positive end-expiratory pressure was 10 cm H_2O or less, and (4) they had an absence of orthostatic hypotension and catecholamine drips.[21] Furthermore, early activity provided by a multidisciplinary team, including physical therapy, has been shown to decrease length of hospital stay,[22] with a recent review of early mobilization of critically ill patients concluding that available evidence supports physical therapy as safe and effective with a significant effect on outcomes.[23]

Bronchopulmonary Hygiene

Patients on ventilatory support are frequently suctioned as part of their routine care. Physical therapists working with patients on their bronchopulmonary hygiene and airway clearance should use suctioning as the last attempt to remove secretions. Encouraging the process of huffing and coughing during treatment will improve or maintain cough effectiveness (huffing is performed without glottis closure, which cannot be achieved when intubated), owing to activation of the expiratory muscles. If patients have difficulty with a deep inspiration for an effective huff or cough, then manual techniques, postural changes, or assistive devices such as an adult manual breathing unit (AMBU bag) can be used to facilitate depth of inspiration.

Weaning from Ventilatory Support

During the weaning process, the physical therapist can play a vital role on an interdisciplinary team responsible for coordinating the wean. Physical therapists offer a combined understanding of the respiratory difficulties faced by the patient, the biomechanics of ventilation, the principles of exercise (weaning is a form of exercise), and the general energy requirements of functional activities. Physical therapists can work with the multidisciplinary team to optimize the conditions under which the patient attempts each wean (time of day, activities before and after the wean, position during the wean) and parameters to be manipulated during the wean (frequency, intensity, duration). Patients should be placed in a position that facilitates the biomechanics of their ventilation.[24] For many patients, this is seated and may also include the ability to sit forward with the arms supported.

Biofeedback to increase V_T and relaxation has been shown to improve the effectiveness of weaning and reduce time on the ventilator.[25] Inspiratory muscle-resistive training has also been shown to increase respiratory muscle strength and endurance to facilitate weaning success,[26] particularly in patients who have previously demonstrated a failure to wean.[27]

References

1. Marino P: The ICU book, ed 3, Philadelphia, 2006, Lippincott Williams & Wilkins.
2. Slutsky AS: Mechanical ventilation. American College of Chest Physicians' Consensus Conference, Chest 104:1833, 1993.
3. Huang YT, Singh J: Basic modes of mechanical ventilation. In Papadakos PJ, Lachman B, editors: Mechanical ventilation, Philadelphia, 2007, Saunders Elsevier, pp 247-256.
4. Chestnutt MS, Murray JA, Prendergast TJ: Pulmonary disorders. In Tierney LM, McPhee SJ, Papadakis MA, editors: Current medical diagnosis & treatment, New York, 2008, McGraw-Hill.
5. Tol G, Palmer J: Principles of mechanical ventilation, Anaesth Intensive Care Med 11(4):125-128, 2010.
6. Nava S, Hill N: Non-invasive ventilation in acute respiratory failure, Lancet 374:250-259, 2009.
7. Chandrashekar R, Perme C: Monitoring and life support equipment. In Hillegass EA editor: Essentials of cardiopulmonary physical therapy, ed 3, St Louis, 2011, Saunders, pp 451-460.
8. Huntziner A: NAMDRC recommendations for prolonged mechanical ventilation, Am Fam Physician 73(7):1277-1284, 2006.
9. Pilbeam SP, Cairo JM: Mechanical ventilation: physiological and clinical applications, ed 4, St Louis, 2006, Mosby.
10. DeTurk WE, Cahalin LP: Cardiovascular & pulmonary physical therapy: an evidence-based approach, ed 2, New York, 2011, McGraw-Hill, pp 588-642.
11. Anzueto A, Peters JI, Tobin MJ et al: Effects of prolonged mechanical ventilation on diaphragmatic function in healthy adult baboons, Crit Care Med 25:1187-1190, 1997.
12. Gerold KB: Physical therapists' guide to the principles of mechanical ventilation, Cardiopulm Phys Ther 3:8, 1992.
13. Costello ML, Mathieu-Costello O, West JB: Stress fracture of alveolar epithelial cells studied by scanning electron microscopy, Am Rev Respir Dis 145:1446-1455, 1992.
14. Mathieu-Costello O, West JB: Are pulmonary capillaries susceptible to mechanical stress? Chest 105(Suppl):102S-107S, 1994.
15. Heimler R, Huffman RG, Starshak RJ: Chronic lung disease in premature infants: a retrospective evaluation of underlying factors, Crit Care Med 16:1213-1217, 1988.
16. Augustyn B: Ventilator-associated pneumonia: risk factors and prevention, Crit Care Nurse 27(4):32-36, 38-39; quiz 40, 2007.
17. Eskandar N, Apostolakos MJ: Weaning from mechanical ventilation, Crit Care Clin 23(2):263-274, 2007.
18. Eskandar, Siner JM: Liberation from mechanical ventilation: what monitoring matters? Crit Care Clin 23(3):613-638, 2007.
19. Yang KL, Tobin MJ: A prospective study of indexes predicting the outcome of trials of weaning from mechanical ventilation, N Engl J Med 324:1446-1495, 1991.
20. Dries DJ: Weaning from mechanical ventilation, J Trauma 43:72-384, 1997.
21. Baily P et al: Early activity is feasible and safe in respiratory failure patients, Crit Care Med 35(1):139-145, 2007.
22. Morris PE, Holbrook A, Thompson C et al: A mobility protocol for acute respiratory failure patients delivered by an ICU mobility team shortens hospital stay, Crit Care Med 34(A20), 2006.
23. Adler J, Malone D: Early mobilization in the intensive care unit: a systematic review, Cardiopulm Phys Ther J 23(1):5-13, 2012.
24. Shekleton ME: Respiratory muscle condition and the work of breathing—a critical balance in the weaning patient, AACN Clin Issues Crit Care 2:405-414, 1991.
25. Holliday JE, Hyers TM: The reduction of wean time from mechanical ventilation using tidal volume and relaxation biofeedback, Am Rev Respir Dis 141:1214-1220, 1990.
26. Aldrich TK, Karpel JP, Uhrlass RM et al: Weaning from mechanical ventilation: adjunctive use of inspiratory muscle resistive training, Crit Care Med 17, 1989, 143-147, 1989.
27. Martin AD, Smith BK, Davenport PD et al: Inspiratory muscle strength training improves weaning outcomes in failure to wean patients: a randomized trial, Crit Care 15: R84, 2011.

APPENDIX 18B: MECHANICAL CIRCULATORY ASSIST DEVICES

Jaime C. Paz

Circulatory assist devices are designed to support patients in hemodynamic collapse, cardiogenic shock, or cardiopulmonary arrest, or prophylactically during invasive procedures. Circulatory assist devices are either percutaneous or surgically implanted. The purpose of this appendix is to describe each of these types of circulatory assist devices and to describe the implications to physical therapy evaluation or treatment.

There are four types of percutaneous devices:
1. Intraaortic balloon pump (IABP)
2. Percutaneous cardiopulmonary support (PCPS)
3. Left ventricular assist devices: TandemHeart, Impella
4. Extracorporeal membrane oxygenation (ECMO)

Surgical devices include ventricular assist devices (VAD) and total artificial hearts (TAH). Ventricular assist devices are manufactured by companies such as Thoratec and MicroMed. Total artificial hearts are manufactured by companies such as SynCardia and AbioMed.

Percutaneous Devices

Intraaortic Balloon Pump

The main function of the IABP is to lessen the work (decreased myocardial oxygen demand) of the heart by decreasing afterload in the proximal aorta through a vacuum effect created by rapid balloon deflation. The IABP also improves coronary artery perfusion (increased myocardial oxygen supply) by increasing diastolic pressure in the aorta and thereby displacing blood proximally into the coronary arteries.[1] The IABP consists of a catheter with a sausage-shaped balloon at the end of it, all of which is connected to an external pump-controlling device. The catheter is inserted percutaneously into the femoral artery and is threaded antegrade until it reaches the proximal descending thoracic aorta.

Figure 18B-1 illustrates the balloon inflating during ventricular filling (diastole) and deflating during ventricular contraction (systole). The deflation of the balloon just before the aortic valve opening decreases afterload and therefore reduces resistance to the ejection of blood during systole. The blood in the aorta is then propelled forward into the systemic circulation. The inflation of the balloon during diastole assists with the perfusion of the coronary and cerebral vessels. This process is referred to as *counterpulsation,* because the inflation and deflation of the balloon occur opposite to the contraction and relaxation of the heart.[1]

Indications for IABP include the following[1-7]:
- Acute left ventricular failure, refractory to other management
- Unstable angina, refractory to other management
- Recent acute myocardial infarction
- Cardiogenic shock
- Acute mitral valve regurgitation
- Weaning patients from cardiopulmonary bypass
- Ventricular septal defect
- Refractory ventricular dysrhythmias
- Adjunctive therapy in high-risk or complicated catheterization and angioplasty
- Preoperative management for high-risk cardiac surgery patients

The ratio of heartbeats to counterpulsations of the IABP indicates the amount of circulatory support an individual requires (e.g., 1 to 1 is one counterpulsation to one heartbeat; 1 to 4 is one counterpulsation to every fourth heartbeat; a ratio of 1 to 1 provides maximum circulatory support). Weaning from an IABP involves gradually decreasing the number of counterpulsations to heartbeats, with the goal being 1 counterpulsation for every fourth heartbeat, as tolerated, before discontinuing the IABP. Although weaning the IABP is generally performed by decreasing the number of counterpulsations, weaning also can be performed by gradually decreasing the amount of inflation pressure of the balloon in the aorta.[1]

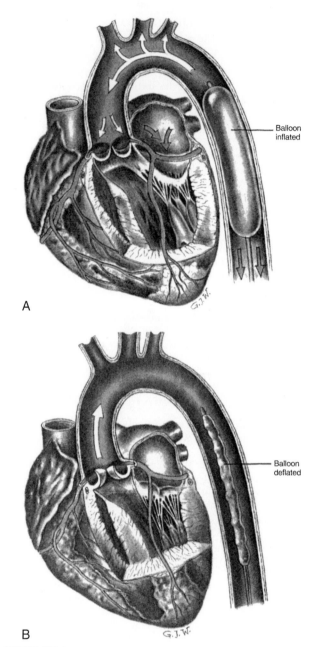

A

B

FIGURE 18B-1
Mechanisms of action in intraaortic balloon pump. **A,** Diastolic balloon inflation augments coronary blood flow. **B,** Systolic balloon deflation decreases afterload. (From Urden LD: Thelan's critical care nursing: diagnosis and management, ed 5, St Louis, 2006, Mosby.)

Potential complications of IABP include the following[1,8-11]:
- Transient loss of peripheral pulse
- Limb ischemia
- Thromboembolism
- Compartment syndrome
- Aortic dissection
- Local vascular injury—hematoma, pseudoaneurysm (false aneurysm)
- Thrombocytopenia, hemolysis
- Cerebrovascular accident
- Infection

- Balloon rupture
- Balloon entrapment

Physical Therapy Considerations

- Length of time on IABP as well as poor ejection fraction and a history of vascular disease increases the risk of limb ischemia and vascular complications.[12,13]
- During IABP, the lower extremity in which femoral access is obtained cannot be flexed at the hip, and the patient's head cannot be raised higher than 30 degrees in bed in order to prevent the intraaortic balloon catheter from migrating.[14]
- If the IABP becomes dislodged, allow 1 to 2 seconds of bleeding to allow any clots to be removed before applying firm pressure, and then call for the nurse or doctor.[14]
- Once the IABP is removed, the patient should be on bed rest for a minimum of 8 hours and should avoid exercising the extremity to prevent bleeding.[14]
- Patients may require range of motion or strengthening exercises for the hip and knee after the IABP is removed. The ankle can be ranged while the patient is on the IABP.[14]
- The patient is at risk for skin breakdown due to limited mobility and decreased perfusion to the affected extremity. Therefore patients benefit from pressure-reducing or pressure-relieving mattresses; frequent repositioning; and assessment of vascular, motor, and sensory function.[14]
- To prevent pulmonary complications while on bed rest, patients benefit from frequent repositioning and deep breathing and coughing exercises.

Enhanced External Counterpulsation

Enhanced external counterpulsation (EECP) is a noninvasive technique that reduces angina and extends time to exercise-induced myocardial ischemia in patients with symptomatic coronary disease. This type of treatment is primarily performed in outpatient clinics by EECP technicians under the supervision of a cardiologist. Information provided here is brief because EECP is not used by the acute care physical therapist.

EECP uses the sequential inflation of three sets of pneumatic cuffs wrapped around the lower extremities. The cuffs are inflated sequentially from calf to thigh to buttock at the onset of diastole, producing aortic counterpulsation, diastolic augmentation, and increased venous return (Figure 18B-2).

At the onset of systole, the external pressure in the cuffs is released rapidly, producing a decrease in systolic pressure.[13] In contrast to IABP, EECP provides long-lasting increase in coronary blood flow (12 months).[14] A treatment procedure involves 1 to 2 hours per day for a total of 35 hours of therapy. The patient lies supine for the treatment. On completion of the 35 sessions, studies have shown that the time to exercise-induced ischemia is delayed significantly and the frequency of angina is reduced significantly compared with patients who did not receive EECP.[14,15]

Percutaneous Cardiopulmonary Support

Percutaneous cardiopulmonary support (PCPS) provides full hemodynamic support and oxygenation of venous blood. It is similar to the support provided during coronary artery bypass

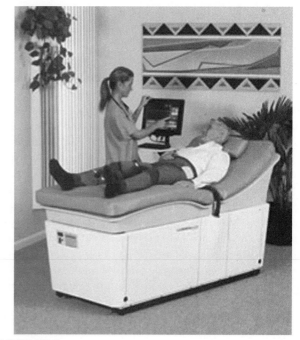

FIGURE 18B-2
Enhanced external counterpulsation (EECP). (Courtesy Vasomedical, Westbury, NY.)

graft surgery and valve replacement surgery. PCPS involves placing large-bore catheters in the central arterial and venous circulation. Blood from the venous catheter is removed from the patient and pumped through an external heat exchanger and oxygenator; it is then returned under pressure to the systemic arterial circulation via the arterial cannula. The femoral artery and the femoral vein are commonly a source of entry into the body for PCPS.[15,16] PCPS requires continuous, highly technical support and is inserted in a catheterization laboratory. PCPS is in general not suitable for long-term applications because of the large-bore cannulas, resulting in significant pressure gradients and eventually hemolysis.[17] The mean duration for PCPS is 62 hours.[18]

Indications for PCPS include the following[16,17]:

- Cardiogenic shock and cardiopulmonary arrest
- High-risk percutaneous transluminal coronary angioplasty (PTCA)
- Pulmonary embolism
- Intractable ventricular arrhythmias
- Hypothermia
- Beating heart donor preservation for transplantation

> ✎ **CLINICAL TIP**
>
> Because of the large cannulations required during this procedure, assess the patient for local vascular or neurologic changes after the cannulae are removed.

Left Ventricular Assist Devices

Percutaneous left ventricular assist devices (pLVAD) provide short-term circulatory assist without the need for cardiac surgery. Currently there are two types of percutaneous LVAD available: TandemHeart and Impella.

TandemHeart

The TandemHeart is an extracorporeal (external) continuous flow centrifugal assist device (Figure 18B-3). Cannulas are inserted percutaneously through the femoral vein and are advanced across the interatrial septum into the atrium. The pump withdraws oxygenated blood from the left atrium back to the pump via the cannula in the femoral vein before it is ejected into the left ventricle. The blood returns via the cannula in the femoral vein to the pump resting extracorporeally on the upper thigh. The pump propels the blood by means of a magnetically driven impeller through the outflow port, and returns it to one or both femoral arteries via arterial cannulas.[19] Some of the blood in the femoral arteries continues in a forward flow through the arterial system to perfuse the lower extremities, and some returns in a reverse flow back up to the aorta to provide perfusion to the coronary arteries, the upper extremities, and the head. The reverse flow is possible because there is no forward flow from the left ventricle to the aorta. Through this pumping action, the TandemHeart can provide a cardiac output of up to 4 L/min.[20,21]

By unloading the left ventricle, decreasing myocardial oxygen consumption, and decreasing left atrial filling pressures, this percutaneous LVAD can provide short-term support from a few hours to 14 days in the intensive care unit. This gives time for the native heart to recover.[19]

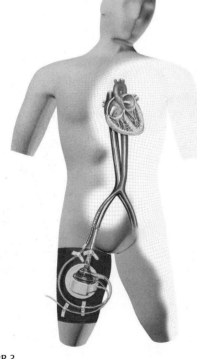

FIGURE 18B-3
TandemHeart percutaneous VAD. (Courtesy Cardiac Assist, Pittsburgh, PA.)

Indications for the TandemHeart include the following[19-22]:
- High-risk percutaneous coronary interventions
- Cardiogenic shock
- Bridge to cardiac transplantation
- Bridge to long-term mechanical circulatory support, such as a surgically implanted left ventricular assist device

Potential complications of the TandemHeart include the following[21-23]:
- Bleeding
- Thromboembolism
- Transseptal cannula dislocation
- Arterial cannula dislocation
- Lower extremity ischemia
- Infection

Physical Therapy Considerations
- Avoid hip flexion greater than 20 degrees to prevent the cannula from kinking or displacing.
- Use a knee immobilizer to prevent flexion of the hip.
- Keep the head of the bed elevated less than 20 degrees.
- Use the reverse Trendelenburg position less than 30 degrees.
- When the cannulae are removed, do not allow hip flexion for at least 4 to 6 hours.

Impella Recover System

The Impella Recover System is a minimally invasive percutaneous ventricular unloading catheter that allows the heart to rest and recover by actively unloading the ventricle and reducing myocardial workload and oxygen consumption, while increasing cardiac output, coronary perfusion, and end organ perfusion. There are two types of percutaneous catheters available in this system: the Impella LP2.5 and the Impella LP5.0. The Impella LP2.5 can provide up to 2.5 liter/min of cardiac output and can provide support for up to 5 days, whereas the Impella LP5.0 can provide up to 5 liter/min of cardiac output and can provide support for up to 10 days. Figure 18B-4 illustrates an Impella LP 2.5.

Either catheter is inserted percutaneously in the cardiac catheterization laboratory into the femoral artery; however, the Impella LP5.0 requires a small cut-down of the femoral artery. The inflow cannula miniaturized pump is inserted through the aortic valve under guidance into the left ventricle to pump blood from the left ventricle into the ascending aorta. An advantage of the Impella over the TandemHeart is that there is no need for a transseptal puncture and no extracorporeal blood.[21,22]

Indications for the Impella include the following[19,21]:
- Impella LP2.5
  - High-risk percutaneous coronary interventions
  - Post percutaneous coronary intervention support
  - Acute myocardial infarction with low cardiac output
- Impella LP5.0
  - Postcardiotomy low cardiac output syndrome
  - Post percutaneous coronary intervention support
  - Myocarditis
  - Cardiogenic shock
  - Acute heart failure
  - Bridge to next decision

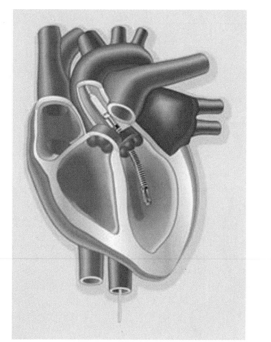

FIGURE 18B-4
Illustration of the Impella LP 2.5. (Courtesy AbioMed, Danvers, MA.)

Potential complications of the Impella include the following[21,22]:
- Bleeding
- Thromboembolism
- Critical limb ischemia
- Pump displacement
- Infection

✎ CLINICAL TIP

There are currently no specific guidelines that relate to hip range of motion (ROM) or mobility of the patient. Typically these patients are critically ill, so if you are consulted to evaluate a patient with an Impella, follow your hospital's guidelines related to ROM and mobility guidelines. Consider the risk of kinking or displacing the femoral cannula in your clinical decision making.

Extracorporeal Membrane Oxygenation

Extracorporeal membrane oxygenation involves the use of a device external to the body for direct oxygenation of blood, assistance with the removal of carbon dioxide, or both. The primary indication for ECMO is cardiac or respiratory failure that is not responding to maximal medical therapy and conventional mechanical ventilation. The pediatric population with respiratory failure seems to benefit from this therapy the most; however, the successful use of ECMO in the adult population has improved as a result of technological advances.[24,25]

Patient situations that may require ECMO include the following:
- Neonatal respiratory distress syndrome
- Congenital heart diseases
- Postcardiotomy cardiac or pulmonary support
- Cardiac arrest
- Cardiogenic shock
- Primary respiratory failure
- Post lung or heart transplantation or VAD placement
- "Bridge to bridge" therapy for patients have the potential to receive an implantable device[26]

As illustrated in Figure 18B-5, the ECMO system consists of a venous drainage cannula, a reservoir for blood, a pumping device that uses a centrifugal or a roller system, an oxygenator, and an arterial or a second venous return cannula.[24,27]

The pumping device is used to help a failing ventricle circulate blood, whereas the oxygenator device assists the failing respiratory system to fully oxygenate the patient. Patients who have respiratory failure require concurrent mechanical ventilation to prevent atelectasis while on ECMO. However, less positive pressure is required to oxygenate blood when on ECMO, resulting in a decreased incidence of barotrauma.[24]

The system that uses the venous drainage to arterial return cannula (V-A mode) is primarily performed on patients who require cardiac or cardiorespiratory. The V-A mode can be achieved in the following three ways[24]:
1. Femoral vein to the ECMO system and back to the femoral artery
2. Right atrium to the ECMO system and back to the ascending aorta
3. Femoral vein to the ECMO system and back to the ascending aorta

The system that uses the venous drainage to venous return cannula (V-V mode) is primarily used for patients who only have respiratory failure. The V-V mode is the preferred mode and can be achieved in the following two ways[24]:
1. Internal jugular vein to the ECMO system and back to the common femoral vein
2. Common femoral vein drainage to the ECMO system and back to the contralateral common femoral vein

Patients who are on V-A mode ECMO are typically anticoagulated with heparin and may require the use of IABP to further assist the ventricle. Patients on the V-V mode may require sedation and/or medical paralysis to help improve oxygenation to organs and tissues by minimizing the metabolic demands of an awake person.[24]

The following are potential complications of ECMO[27,28]:
- Bleeding
- Lower limb ischemia
- Thrombocytopenia
- Thromboembolism
- Failure of the oxygenator device

Physical Therapy Considerations
- The physical therapist generally does not start direct handling of a patient on ECMO until the ECMO apparatus is disconnected because of the risk of dislodgment in patients with severe medical conditions.[27]
- However, if working with a patient with ECMO is indicated, reducing the patient's stress level decreases the amount of energy expenditure while on ECMO.[27]

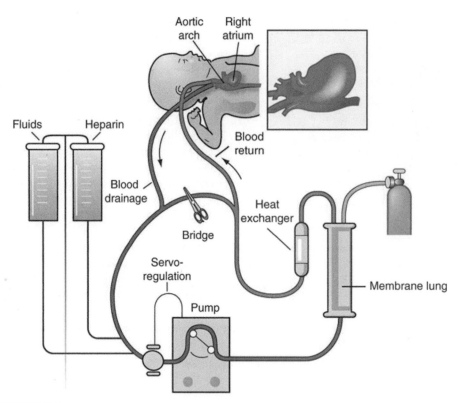

FIGURE 18B-5

Illustration of extracorporeal membrane oxygenation. (From Shanley CJ, Bartlett RH: Extracorporeal life support: techniques, indications, and results. In Cameron JL, editor: Current surgical therapy, ed 4, St Louis, 1992, Mosby-Year Book, pp 1062-1066.)

- Rolling or turning the patient is not recommended because of risk of dislodging the cannula.
- ROM should only be performed if the benefits heavily outweigh the risks. If ROM is performed, avoid ROM near the cannula insertion site.
- Many neonates require physical therapy once the ECMO is removed to assess the patients for neurological impairments such as cognitive changes, developmental dysfunction, and hypotonia.[29]

Surgical Devices

Ventricular Assist Devices

A ventricular assist device is a mechanical pump that provides prolonged circulatory assistance in patients who have acute or chronic ventricular failure. First used over 30 years ago, multiple devices have been designed and clinically tested, with ongoing clinical trials developing the future generation of pumps.[30] Patients are appropriate for VAD implantation if they are categorized as New York Heart Association (NYHA) Class III or IV and Stage D from the American College of Cardiology/ American Heart Association Stages.[31] The pumps are either temporary or permanent. If the pump is temporary, it is referred to as a *bridge to heart transplantation (BTT)*. If the pump is permanent, it is referred to as *destination therapy (DT)*. Reports in the literature indicate that VAD therapy is highly beneficial in alleviating symptoms and improving outcomes, including survival rates and quality of life in patients with Class IV heart failure.[32] The life expectancy of patients who receive VAD implantation for DT is approximately 1 to 2 years.[33,34]

Additional indications for VAD implantation in patients with advanced heart failure include optimal maximal medical therapy, a cardiac index less than 1.8 liters per minute, a pulmonary capillary wedge pressure greater than 25 mm Hg, and a systolic blood pressure below 90 mm Hg. The VAD restores cardiac output and blood pressure, as well as providing a reduction in left ventricular pressure and volume. A reduction in left ventricular workload further produces a decrease in pulmonary venous and arterial pressures along with reducing pulmonary vascular resistance. The VAD also improves perfusion to all body organs, which results in improved autonomic function and normalization of the neurohormonal and cytokine milieu that is present in heart failure.[35]

Generally, the left ventricle is most commonly assisted with an LVAD, but occasionally, the right ventricle also needs assistance from a right ventricular assist device (RVAD). In more severe situations, both ventricles need to be assisted (BiVAD). Pharmacologic support with angiotensin-converting enzyme inhibitors, angiotensin receptor blockers, and beta blockers such as carvedilol is provided to patients with LVADs in order to minimize systemic hypertension and help preserve right heart function.[36] In 20% to 30% of cases where the LVAD provides pressure and volume unloading of the left ventricle, the increase in venous return to the right ventricle results in right ventricle volume overload. This can be treated with inotropes or pulmonary vasodilators, but in some instances an RVAD is necessary.[35]

Ventricular assist devices consist of a pump, a driveline providing electric or pneumatic energy, a system controller, and a console. The pumps generally fall into two main categories: pulsatile pumps and axial (continuous) flow pumps. Pulsatile pumps tend to be larger than axial flow pumps because of the number of components necessary to engineer the pump. They are capable of producing a stroke volume of 65 to 95 ml, generating a cardiac output of 10 liters of blood flow per minute. Continuous-flow pumps have fewer moving parts and require less power to operate. Axial-flow pumps are capable of rotating at speeds of 7,000 to 12,500 revolutions per minute to produce a cardiac output up to 10 liters per minute.[37]

The mechanical pump can be intracorporeal (internal) or extracorporeal (external) to the patient. An intracorporeal VAD is designed to support the left ventricle and consists of a pump that is surgically placed in a preperitoneal or intraabdominal position with the inflow conduit draining the left ventricle through the apex of the heart and an outflow conduit ejecting blood into the ascending aorta (Figure 18B-6, *A*). The power source line exits the abdomen and leads to an external device. An extracorporeal VAD can be univentricular or biventricular and consists of a pump(s) that is completely external to the patient, but with inflow and outflow conduits entering the abdomen, shunting blood from the heart to the great vessels (see Figure 18B-6, *B*). This type of VAD may be placed paracorporeally (lying on top of the abdomen) and may be referred to as a "paracorporeal VAD."[38] Extracorporeal pumps will need to be adequately supported during functional mobility.

> ### ✎ CLINICAL TIP
>
> An axial-flow pump provides continuous flow, so there are no distinct systolic and diastolic phases. For this reason a traditional blood pressure cannot be measured. An average blood pressure or mean arterial pressure (MAP) can be measured instead using a Doppler ultrasound.[39]

The various types and general characteristics of intracorporeal and extracorporeal VADs are described briefly in Table 18B-1. The VADs described in this table are either FDA approved or in investigational stages. It is beyond the scope of this appendix to describe in detail all aspects of each type of VAD; however, physical therapists working with patients who have a VAD need to be familiar with the type of device that the patient is using, as well as the safety features of the VAD.

Complications from VAD implantation can either be machine or patient related. Device-related complications may include

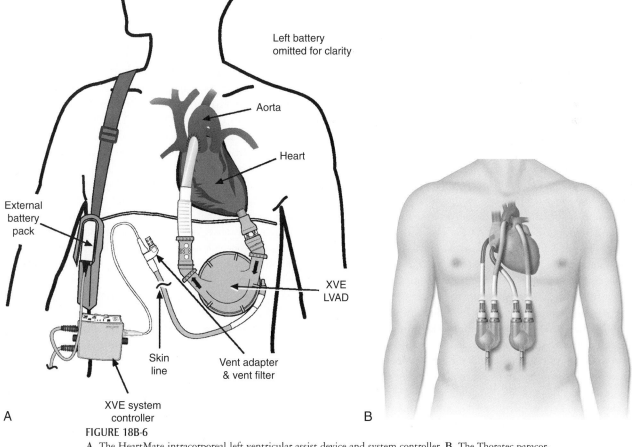

FIGURE 18B-6

A, The HeartMate intracorporeal left ventricular assist device and system controller. **B,** The Thoratec paracorporeal ventricular assist device. (**A,** Courtesy Thoratec Corporation, Pleasanton, CA. **B,** Courtesy Thoratec Corporation, Pleasanton, CA.)

TABLE 18B-1 Ventricular Assist Devices

Device	Pump Mechanism	Position	Purpose
AbioMed AB 5000*	Pulsatile	Extracorporeal	BTR
Thoratec Centrimag*	Continuous	Extracorporeal	RVAD, TCS
Thoratec IVAD*	Pulsatile	Intracorporeal	BTT
Thoratec PVAD*	Pulsatile	Extracorporeal	BTT
Thoratec HeartMate II*	Continuous	Intracorporeal	BTT, DT
HeartAssist5 Pediatric Ventricular Assist System*	Continuous		BTT (children age 5-16 yr)
Berlin Heart INCOR I†	Continuous	Intracorporeal	BTR, BTT, DT
Berlin Heart EXCOR*	Pulsatile	Extracorporeal	BTR pediatric population
Jarvik 2000†	Continuous	Intracorporeal	BTT, DT
DuraHeart LVAD†	Continuous	Intracorporeal	BTT, DT
HeartWare HVAD	Continuous	Intracorporeal	BTT

Data from Thoratec Corporation. http://www.thoratec.com/medical-professionals/vad-product-information/index.aspx. Accessed February 5, 2013; Timms D: A review of clinical ventricular assist devices, Med Eng Phys 33:1041-1047, 2011; U.S. Food and Drug Administration: http://www.fda.gov/MedicalDevices/ProductsandMedicalProcedures/DeviceApprovalsandClearances/Recently-ApprovedDevices/ucm302715.htm. Accessed February 5, 2013; AbioMed: http://www.abiomed.com/products. Accessed February 5, 2013; MicroMed Cardiovascular: HeartAssist 5. http://www.micromedcv.com/united_states/medical-professionals/certs-approvals.html. Accessed February 5, 2013.

BTR, Bridge to recovery; *BTT,* bridge to transplant; *DT,* destination therapy; *TCS,* temporary circulatory support.

*FDA approved.

†Investigational.

any of the following: disconnection of the lead and drivelines, valve dysfunction, and/or deterioration in the pump mechanism requiring either repair or replacement with another VAD.[33,40] Each VAD has an educational manual outlining the relevant details of the components, operation, and safety features. For example, the physical therapist must know how to respond emergently in the event of a pump failure. Pulsatile pumps can be hand pumped if the pump fails. Physical therapists should be competent in hand pumping should an emergency situation arise.[41] Axial (continuous) flow pumps cannot be hand pumped, so in the presence of axial flow pump failure, follow your hospital's emergency code procedure.

Patient-related complications may include any of the following: infection, arrhythmias, gastrointestinal distress, thromboembolic events including stroke, respiratory failure, and death.[33,40] Patients with pulsatile pumps who require defibrillation can be defibrillated after the pump is disconnected from power and hand pumping is started. Patients with an axial flow pump can be defibrillated per Advanced Cardiac Life Support (ACLS) guidelines without disconnecting the pump from power.

The combination of technological improvements and a lack of donor organs has increased the use of VADs in patients with advanced heart failure. Reports in the literature indicate that patients with a VAD can be mobilized safely in the hospital and that their exercise tolerance (as demonstrated by 6-minute walk test distance, peak VO$_2$, and subjective reports) can be improved while awaiting transplantation or while continuing with destination therapy.[39,41-44] Patients with LVAD implantation also demonstrate quality-of-life improvements as measured by the Kansas City Cardiomyopathy questionnaire and Minnesota Living with Heart Failure questionnaire, which correlate to an improved functional capacity denoted by NYHA classification.[33,40]

Physical Therapy Intervention

The following are general goals and guidelines for the physical therapist when working with a patient who has a VAD.

Whether a patient is awaiting heart transplantation (BTT) or not (DT), the primary goals of physical therapy for the patient with an implanted VAD are to optimize mobility and functional capacity. The patient's length of stay and achievement of goals is likely dependent on their medical status along with the primary purpose of VAD implantation (BTT or DT). Patients with VADs can benefit from outpatient cardiac rehabilitation once discharged from the hospital. Physical therapy can be initiated on postoperative day 1, depending on hemodynamic stability.[39,41] In some cases, physical therapy may already be working with patients preoperatively.

Open-heart surgery via a sternotomy is required in order to implant the VAD and its components. Therefore your facility's guidelines for sternal precautions will need to be observed for approximately 8 weeks postimplantation. Also, as these patients have undergone sternotomy, it is essential to prevent postoperative pulmonary complications by auscultating lung sounds, establishing cough effectiveness, and performing airway clearance techniques.[41,45] Sternal precautions that have been reported in the literature include[46]:

- Not lifting more than 10 lb of weight bilaterally
- Abstaining from bilateral or unilateral upper-extremity sports
- No driving or hand-over-head activities
- Limiting active shoulder elevation greater than 90 degrees
- Lifting of 1- to 3 lb (0.45 to 1.36 kg) is allowed in the absence of sternal instability (i.e., no detectable pain, movement, or cracking in the sternum)
- Limit range of motion if mild pain or "pulling" sensations occurs in the incisional area[47]

Postoperatively, patients may have symptoms of pain at the exit site of the access lines in the abdomen and may need appropriate premedication with analgesics before therapy.[42] Pain at exit sites can promote a kyphotic or scoliotic posture that could lead to an obstruction in the LVAD driveline, resulting in a possible reduction in flow rates to meet activity demands.[41] Patients may also have symptoms of nausea due to the position of the internal pump within the peritoneal region of the trunk and may need antiemetic medication before therapy. An abdominal binder for all activity should be worn to protect the exit site of the driveline and allow scar tissue to form and reduce shearing forces at the exit site, thereby decreasing the risk of infection at the drive site. Abdominal binders may need to be customized to fit the patient appropriately and modified to provide an attachment for the system controller.

Hemodynamic monitoring is affected by both patient and mechanical factors. The patient's native heart is still contracting; therefore the patient's electrocardiogram will reflect the native heart's electrical activity. The native heart rate response at rest and with activity will likely be blunted as a result of taking beta blockers. A peripheral pulse can typically be palpated in a patient with a pulsatile pump, and a traditional blood pressure can be measured. Furthermore, because the VAD is performing a majority of the patient's cardiac output, the patient's peripheral pulse is indicative of the parameters set on the VAD.[41] A flow rate of 3 to 4 liters per minute is considered adequate in most devices to achieve a sufficient cardiac output, which is displayed on the screen of the power base monitor of the VAD.[39,41] To help maintain an adequate flow rate, fluids are often not restricted in these patients,[39] but it is helpful to ascertain any precautions before working with them.

The rate or speed of a VAD can be fixed or automatic/adaptive. VADs that have automatic rates or speeds are able to adjust their rate or speed according to the demands of the patient. However, keeping the pump at a fixed rate or fixed speed improves the pump's longevity, if the patient can tolerate it.[37,41] Physical therapists can monitor several parameters to gauge the appropriate intensity and response to exercise or activity. These parameters may include the patient's rating of perceived exertion (RPE) with the Borg Scale, BP or MAP, and oxygen saturation. An RPE of 11 to 13 out of 20 has been reported to be an appropriate intensity level to safely exercise and achieve training benefits for this patient population.[41] Based on the type of VAD and settings a MAP between 70 and 95 mm Hg at rest and with activity has been reported as a reference value for most patients.[39] For more detail refer to the review by Scheiderer.[47a]

Patients with VADs still have heart failure; therefore a supervised resistance exercise program is an important part of their exercise prescription.[48] Vigorous upper-extremity resistance training is deferred until sternal precautions are discontinued. Indications to stop exercise in a patient with a VAD are the same as when treating any patient with cardiac disease (refer to Chapter 3 for more guidelines). In addition, if a patient demonstrates a drop in the pump flow or speed or rate, this may indicate pump failure, occlusion of a tube, and/or bleeding.[41] Therefore stop exercise, investigate the cause, and seek assistance as necessary.

During mobility, VADs can be powered by batteries, making the patient independent to move without the electric power source. Physical therapists must be knowledgeable about the battery life. It is important to always carry extra batteries and a system controller when mobilizing the patient away from the patient's room. Most hospitals require the patient and caregivers to be independent in switching batteries before mobilizing away from the unit. Since patients will need to learn how to manage mobilizing with the VAD equipment, physical therapists can prescribe the appropriate training to assist the patient in preparation for this activity. For example, postural exercises can assist the patient in gaining strength to carry the batteries in the battery holster.

Patients should be educated to avoid strong static discharges (e.g., television or computer screens), swimming, and contact sports. Patients can shower provided they use a waterproof shower kit that protects the VAD.[49] Patients with electric pumps can be discharged to home once they reach the appropriate level of independence. This type of pump can be powered by batteries, whereas patients with pneumatic pumps are confined to the hospital.

Total Artificial Heart

A total artificial heart (TAH), which is implantable and sustainable, has been under investigation for over 30 years.[50] Two devices, the SynCardia CardioWest Temporary TAH system and the AbioCor Implantable Replacement Heart, have been approved by the Food and Drug Administration for use in patients with end-stage congestive heart failure. The SynCardia device is approved for use as bridge to transplantation,[51] and the AbioCor device is approved under the Humanitarian Device Exemption program for use in patients without other alternatives.[52,53]

Indications for the CardioWest include cardiogenic shock, biventricular failure, multiple organ failure, unsuccessful medical management, need for mechanical circulatory support such as LVAD, and eligibility for heart transplantation.[54,55] Implantation of the CardioWest involves removal and subsequent replacement of the native atria, ventricles, and valves, thus avoiding the need for medications such as inotropic or antiarrhythmic agents.[54,56] However, a combination of anticoagulants may be applied for these patients, beginning with unfractionated heparin progressing to warfarin and then to aspirin.[55]

The CardioWest consists of an external drive console that sends pneumatic pulses, from compressed air tanks, through 7-foot drivelines into two independent ventricles that have unidirectional inflow and outflow valves. The drive console also has a backup battery, which is activated automatically in cases of power failure and can also serve as a power supply during mobility. Noninvasive monitoring is provided by a laptop computer on the console.[54-56] Figure 18B-7 illustrates the CardioWest TAH.

The AbioCor Implantable Replacement Heart is indicated for patients over the age of 18 who are not likely to live more than 30 days, have failed to improve with maximal medical therapies, and are not eligible for heart transplantation.[53,57,58]

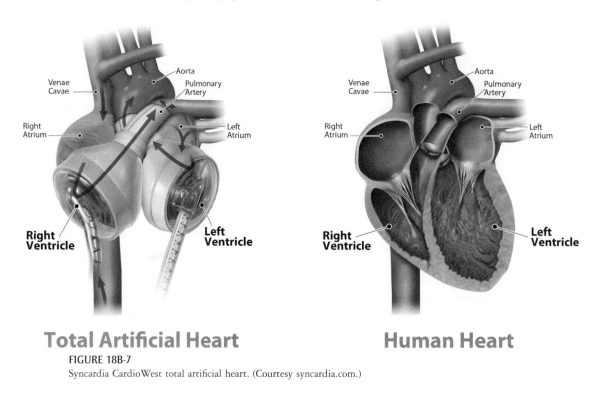

Total Artificial Heart

Human Heart

FIGURE 18B-7
Syncardia CardioWest total artificial heart. (Courtesy syncardia.com.)

The AbioCor system replaces the native heart with a combination of internal and external components.

The internal components consist of a pump with two blood sacs, an internal controller that monitors and controls the pump mechanics, an internal rechargeable battery that functions as an emergency or backup power source, and an internal transcutaneous energy transfer (TET) coil.[58,59] The internal TET coil transmits external power to the internal battery, which can operate for approximately 20 minutes when disconnected from the main power source.[59] The external components include an external TET coil, radiofrequency communication system, portable power sources, and a computer console. The portable power sources are two external battery packs, which can provide power for this system for 2 to 4 hours.[58,59]

Although the native heart is totally replaced with the AbioCor system, medications are still necessary to ensure stability. Vasoactive agents and anticoagulants are provided, respectively, to control blood pressure and minimize thrombotic complications.[59] In addition, the TET coils help to minimize infection risk as these coils are transcutaneous and there is no need to penetrate the skin.[58,59] Replacing the native heart with a mechanical heart also results in no electrocardiogram to examine.[59]

Physical Therapy Considerations

More literature pertinent to physical therapy has been documented for the CardioWest TAH, and thus the considerations provided will apply only to this device. Hemodynamic stability needs to be established by the medical team before out-of-bed mobility can occur. Reports in the literature indicate that rehabilitation has begun approximately 4 to 7 days postimplantation.[54,55,60]

Safe exercise and increased endurance with TAH devices has also been documented.[54,55,60]

- Because these devices are still undergoing clinical trials in the United States, monitoring guidelines and exercise progression are similar to those in patients with cardiac disease and those with implanted VADs.[54,60]
- Specific training needs to be completed by staff working with the CardioWest TAH before initiating care and rehabilitation.[54,60]
- Device rate, flow and volume, blood pressure, symptoms of orthostasis, oxygen saturation, and exercise intolerance (rating of perceived exertion [RPE]) should be monitored throughout each treatment session. The device is typically set at a fixed beat rate of 90 to 130 beats per minute with the cardiac output automatically increasing up to 9.5 liters per minute.[54,60]
- Physical therapy should be modified or terminated when the patient is short of breath (at least 5/10 on modified 10-grade dyspnea scale) or reports exercise intolerance (greater than 13/20 on Borg RPE scale), becomes orthostatic, systolic blood pressure is less than 80 mm Hg or decreases by more than 20 mm Hg, device flow is less than 3 liters per minute, the device alarms, and if the therapist notices neurological changes, such as ataxia, or bleeding. The medical team should also be consulted for assistance during these events.[54,60]
- Patients with TAH have demonstrated a blunted blood pressure response during exercise, and therefore clinicians should be watchful for potential episodes of hypotension.[60]
- For the CardioWest TAH, ensuring pain control and proper posture is helpful to prevent driveline occlusion by splinting and/or altered trunk positions. Patients should

not be positioned on the side of the driveline or their stomach.[54]

- Infection control is also essential for patients with the CardioWest device, particularly in the areas where drivelines exit the body.[54,55]

- Sternal precautions will be necessary if working with the patient for the first 8 to 10 weeks after implantation.[54,60]
- Ensure all equipment is operational before ambulation. Assistance will be needed to move the large console during ambulation.[54,55,60]

References

1. Krishna M, Zacharowski K: Principles of intra-aortic balloon pump counterpulsation, Cont Edu Anaesth Crit Care Pain 9(1):24-28, 2009.
2. Ishihara M, Sato H, Tateishi H et al: Intraaortic balloon pumping as a postangioplasty strategy in acute myocardial infarction, Am Heart J 122:385, 1991.
3. Lincoff AM, Popma SJ, Ellis SG et al: Percutaneous support devices for high risk or complicated coronary angioplasty, J Am Coll Cardiol 17:770, 1991.
4. Ohman EM, Califf RM, George BS et al: Use of intraaortic balloon pumping as adjunct to reperfusion therapy in acute myocardial infarction: the Thrombolysis and Angioplasty in Myocardial Infarction (TAMI) Trial Study Group, Am Heart J 121:895, 1991.
5. Rajai HR, Hartman CW, Innes BJ et al: Prophylactic use of intraaortic balloon pump in aortocoronary bypass for patients with left main coronary artery disease, Ann Surg 187:118, 1978.
6. Tremper RS: Home study program. Intra-aortic balloon pump therapy—a primer for perioperative nurses, AORN J 84(1):33-42, 2006.
7. Dyub AM, Whitlock RP, Abouzahr LL et al: Preoperative intra-aortic balloon pump in patients undergoing coronary bypass surgery: a systematic review and meta-analysis, J Cardiac Surg 23(1):79-86, 2008.
8. Barnett MG, Swartz MT, Peterson GJ et al: Vascular complications from intraaortic balloons: risk analysis, J Vasc Surg 19:81, 1994.
9. Cook L, Pillar B, McCord G et al: Intra-aortic balloon pump complications: a five-year retrospective study of 283 patients, Heart Lung 28(3):195-202, 1999.
10. Funk M, Ford CF, Foell DW et al: Frequency of long-term lower limb ischemia associated with intraaortic balloon pump use, Am J Cardiol 70:1195, 1992.
11. Patel JJ, Kopisyansky C, Boston B et al: Prospective evaluation of complications with percutaneous intraaortic balloon counterpulsation, Am J Cardiol 76:1205, 1995.
12. Dick P, Mlekusch W, Delle-Karth G et al: Decreasing incidence of critical limb ischemia after intra-aortic balloon pump counterpulsation, Angiology 60(2):235-241, 2009.
13. Parissis H, Leotsinidis M, Akbar MT et al: J Cardiothorac Surg 5:20, 2010. doi:10.1186/1749-8090-5-20. http://www.cardiothoracicsurgery.org/content/5/1/20. Accessed September 26, 2011.
14. Reid MB, Cottrell D: Nursing care of patients receiving: intra-aortic balloon counterpulsation, Crit Care Nurse 25:40-49, 2005.
15. Baxley WA, Roubin GS, Knobloch J: Support systems for percutaneous cardiac interventions. In Stack RS, Roubin GS, O'Neill WW, editors: Interventional cardiovascular medicine: principles and practice, ed 2, Philadelphia, 2002, Churchill Livingstone, pp 572-584.
16. Field ML, Al-Alao B, Mediratta N et al: Open and closed chest extrathoracic cannulation for cardiopulmonary bypass and extracorporeal life support: methods, indications, and outcomes, Postgrad Med J 82(967):323-331, 2006.
17. Von Segesser LK: Cardiopulmonary support and extracorporeal membrane oxygenation for cardiac assist, Ann Thorac Surg 68:672-677, 1999.
18. Hannan RL, Ojito JW, Ybarra MA et al: Rapid cardiopulmonary support in children with heart disease: a nine-year experience, Ann Thorac Surg 82:1637-1642, 2006.
19. Francesca S, Palanichamy N, Kar B et al: First use of the TandemHeart percutaneous left ventricular assist device as a short-term bridge to cardiac transplantation, Tex Heart Inst J 33:490-491, 2006.
20. Frank CM, Palanichamy N, Kar B et al: Use of a percutaneous ventricular assist device for treatment of cardiogenic shock due to critical aortic stenosis, Tex Heart Inst J 33:487-489, 2006.
21. Lee MS, Makkar RR: Percutaneous left ventricular support devices, Cardiol Clin 24:265-275, 2006.
22. de Souza CF, De Lima VC: Percutaneous mechanical assistance for the failing heart, J Interv Cardiol 23(2):195-202, 2010.
23. Aragon J, Lee M, Kar S et al: Percutaneous left ventricular assist device: "TandemHeart" for high-risk coronary intervention, Catheter Cardiovasc Interv 65(3):346-352, 2005.
24. Kaplon RJ, Smedira NG: Extracorporeal membrane oxygenation in adults. In Goldstein DJ, Oz MC, editors: Cardiac assist devices, Armonk, NY, 2000, Futura, pp 263-273.
25. Mulroy J: Acute respiratory distress syndrome. In Bucher L, Melander S, editors: Critical care nursing, 1999, Philadelphia, Saunders, pp 457-458.
26. Fitzgerald D, Ging A, Burton N et al: The use of percutaneous ECMO support as a "bridge to bridge" in heart failure patients: a case report, Perfusion 25(5):321, 2010.
27. Lowes LP, Palisano RJ: Review of medical and developmental outcome of neonates who received extracorporeal membrane oxygenation, Pediatr Phys Ther 7:15-22, 1995.
28. Zwischenberger JB, Upp JR: Emergencies during extracorporeal membrane oxygenation and their management. In Zwischenberger JB, Bartlett RH, editors: ECMO: Extracorporeal cardiopulmonary support in critical care, Ann Arbor, MI, 1995, Extracorporeal Life Support Organization, p 221.
29. Hofkosh D, Feldman HM, Thompson AE et al: Ten years of extracorporeal membrane oxygenation: neurodevelopmental outcome, Pediatrics 87:549-555, 1991.
30. Smedira NG: Implantable left ventricular assist devices. In Braunwald E, editor: Harrison's advances in cardiology, New York, 2003, McGraw-Hill, pp 538-542.
31. Russell SD, Miller LW, Pagani FD: Advanced heart failure: a call to action, Congest Heart Fail 14:316-321, 2008.
32. Rose EA, Gelijns AC, Moskowitz AJ et al: Long-term mechanical left ventricular assistance for end-stage heart failure, N Engl J Med 345:1435-1443, 2001.
33. Slaughter MS, Rogers JG, Milano CM et al: Advanced heart failure treated with continuous-flow left ventricular assist device, N Engl J Med 361:2241, 2009.
34. Lietz K, Long JW, Kfoury AG et al: Outcomes of left ventricular assist device implantation as destination therapy in the post-REMATCH era: implications for patient selection, Circulation 116:497-505, 2007.
35. Burkhoff D, Klotz S, Mancini D: LVAD-induced reverse remodeling: basic and clinical implications for myocardial recovery, J Card Fail 12(3):227-239, 2006.
36. Klodell C, Staples E, Beaver T et al: Managing the post-left ventricular assist device patient, Congest Heart Fail (Greenwich, Conn) 12(1):41-45, 2006.

37. Song X, Throckmorton AL, Untaroiu A et al: Axial flow blood pumps, ASAIO J 49:355-364, 2003.
38. Smedira NG, Vargo RL, McCarthy PM: Mechanical support devices for end-stage heart failure. In Brown DL, editor: Cardiac intensive care, Philadelphia, 1998, Saunders, pp 697-703.
39. Nissinoff J, Tian F, Therattil M et al: Acute inpatient rehabilitation after left ventricular assist device implantation for congestive heart failure, PM R 3:586-589, 2011.
40. Allen JG, Weiss ES, Schaffer JM et al: Quality of life and functional status in patients surviving 12 months after left ventricular assist device implantations, J Heart Lung Transplant 29(3):278-285, 2010.
41. Humphrey R, Buck L, Cahalin L et al: Physical therapy assessment and intervention for patients with left ventricular assist devices, Cardiopulm Phys Ther 9(2):3-7, 1998.
42. Buck LA: Physical therapy management of three patients following left ventricular assist device implantation: a case report, Cardiopulm Phys Ther 9(2):8-14, 1998.
43. Morrone TM, Buck LA, Catanese KA et al: Early progressive mobilization of patients with left ventricular assist devices is safe and optimizes recovery before heart transplantation, J Heart Lung Transplant 15:423-429, 1996.
44. Kennedy MD, Haykowsky M, Humphrey R: Function, eligibility, outcomes, and exercise capacity associated with left ventricular assist devices, J Cardiopulm Rehabil 23:208-217, 2003.
45. Sendura M, Mehtap M, Oztekin O: Physical therapy in the intensive care unit in a patient with biventricular assist device, Cardiopulm Phys Ther 22(3):31-34, 2011.
46. Cahalin L, Lapier T, Shaw D: Sternal precautions: is it time for change? Precautions versus restrictions—a review of literature and recommendations for revision, Cardiopulm Phys Ther J 22(1):5-15, 2011.
47. Crabtree TD, Codd JE, Fraser VJ et al: Multivariate analysis of risk factors for deep and superficial sternal infection after coronary artery bypass grafting at a tertiary care medical center, Semin Thorac Cardiovasc Surg 16:53-56, 2004.
47a. Scheiderer R, Belden C, Haney C et al: Exercise guidelines for inpatients status post VAD placement: a systematic review of the literature, Cardiopulmonary Phys Ther 24(2):33-39, 2013.
48. Davies EJ, Moxham T, Rees K et al: Exercise based rehabilitation for heart failure. Cochrane Database Syst Rev 4: CD003331, 2010.
49. Thoratec Corporation: Frequently asked questions. http://www.thoratec.com/patients-caregivers/living-with-vad/faqs.aspx#. Accessed September 28, 2011.
50. Cooley DA: The total artificial heart, Nat Med 9(1):108-111, 2003.
51. U.S. Food and Drug Administration: http://www.fda.gov/MedicalDevices/ProductsandMedicalProcedures/DeviceApprovalsandClearances/Recently-ApprovedDevices/ucm080816.htm
52. U.S. Food and Drug Administration: http://www.fda.gov/MedicalDevices/ProductsandMedicalProcedures/DeviceApprovalsandClearances/Recently-ApprovedDevices/ucm077536.htm
53. Nosé Y: FDA approval of totally implantable permanent total artificial heart for humanitarian use, Artif Org 31(1):1-3, 2007.
54. Nicholson C, Paz J: Total artificial heart and physical therapy management, Cardiopulm Phys Ther 21(2):13-21, 2010.
55. Allen Y, Collins R, Lester C et al: Managing the failing heart: total circulatory assist—a case study, Progress Transplant 19(1):13-17, 2009.
56. Platis A, Larson DF: CardioWest temporary total artificial heart, Perfusion 24(5):341-348, 2009.
57. Texas Heart Institute: http://texasheart.org/Research/Devices/abiocor.cfm. Accessed February 11, 2013.
58. Samuels L: The AbioCor totally implantable replacement heart, Am Heart Hosp J 1(1):91-96, 2003.
59. Frazier OH, Dowling RD, Gray LA Jr et al: The total artificial heart: where we stand, Cardiology 101(1-3):117-121, 2004.
60. Kohli SH, Canada J, Arena R et al: Exercise blood pressure response during assisted circulatory support: comparison of the total artificial heart with a left ventricular assist device during rehabilitation, J Heart Lung Transplant 30:1207-1213, 2011.

Margarita V. DiVall
Kelsea A. Ziegler

CHAPTER OBJECTIVE

The objective of this chapter is to provide:

1. An overview of the pharmacologic agents that are commonly prescribed as an adjunct to the medical-surgical management of a wide variety of diseases and disorders

PREFERRED PRACTICE PATTERNS

Pharmacology is multifactorial in nature and applies to many body systems. For this reason, specific practice patterns are not delineated in this chapter. Please refer to Appendix A for a complete list of the preferred practice patterns in order to best delineate the most applicable practice pattern for a given diagnosis.

The medications in this chapter are organized according to systems (see the following index table). Both generic and common brand name(s) are listed for each agent. Depending on the practice setting, you may see generic names being used all the time (acute, inpatient setting) or brand names used (outpatient setting). Many drugs are available as extended-release formulations. In that case, several letters may be added to the generic/brand name of the drug. Among the common abbreviations are XL, XT, and ER (extended release); SR (sustained release); and CR (controlled release). Pharmacy laws mandate the dispensing of a generic medication if generic is available, even if the physician writes a prescription using a brand name. A physician may indicate "No substitution" on the prescription if he or she desires only the brand name to be dispensed. For each type of medication in this chapter, a description of the indication(s), mechanism of action, and side effects, as well as important physical therapy (PT) considerations, is presented in tables.[1,2] Note that some pharmacologic agents are listed in another chapter or appendix.

The following is a list of tables in this chapter, organized according to body system and drug classes.

Text continued on p. 445

Table	Topic
Cardiovascular System	
Table 19-1	Antiarrhythmic Agents
Table 19-2	Anticoagulants
Table 19-3	Antihypertensive Agents
Table 19-3a	Combination Drugs for Hypertension
Table 19-4	Antiplatelet Agents
Table 19-5	Lipid-Lowering Agents
Table 19-6	Positive Inotropes (Pressors)
Table 19-7	Thrombolytics (Also Known as Fibrinolytics)
Respiratory System	
Table 19-8	Adrenocortical Steroids (Glucocorticoids)
Table 19-9	Antihistamines
Table 19-10	Bronchodilators
Table 19-11	Leukotriene Modifiers and Other Nonsteroidal Antiinflammatory Agents
Table 19-12	Mast Cell Stabilizers
Musculoskeletal System	
Table 19-13	Disease-Modifying Antirheumatic Drugs (DMARDs)
Table 19-14	Muscle Relaxants and Antispasmodic Agents
Central Nervous System	
Table 19-15	Antianxiety Medications
Table 19-16	Anticonvulsants
Table 19-17	Antidepressants
Table 19-18	Antipsychotics
Table 19-19	Mood Stabilizers
Table 19-20	Multiple Sclerosis Medications
Table 19-21	Parkinson's Medications
Oncology	
Table 19-22	Antiemetic Medications
Table 19-23	Chemotherapy
Vascular System and Hematology	
Table 19-24	Colony-Stimulating Factors
Gastrointestinal System	
Table 19-25	Antacids
Table 19-26	Antidiarrheal Medications
Table 19-27	Antispasmodic Medications
Table 19-28	Cytoprotective Medications
Table 19-29	Histamine-2 Receptor Antagonists (H₂RAs)
Table 19-30	Laxatives
Table 19-31	Proton Pump Inhibitors (PPIs)
Genitourinary System	
Table 19-32	Benign Prostatic Hyperplasia (BPH) Therapy
Table 19-33	Oral Contraceptives
Infectious Disease	
Table 19-34	Antibiotics
Table 19-35	Antifungal Agents
Table 19-36	Antitubercular Agents
Table 19-37	Antiretroviral Medications
Table 19-38	Antiviral Medications
Endocrine System	
Table 19-39	Hypoglycemic Agents
Table 19-40	Treatment of Hyperparathyroidism
Table 19-41	Treatment of Osteoporosis
Table 19-42	Treatment of Thyroid Disorders
Organ Transplantation	
Table 19-43	Immunosuppressants

Cardiovascular System

TABLE 19-1 Antiarrhythmic Agents

Indications: Treatment and prevention of arrhythmias.
Precautions: All antiarrhythmic drugs are proarrhythmic. Monitor vital signs, ECG, and side effects.

Class: Mechanism of Action	Generic Name (Common Brand Name[s])	Adverse Effects	PT Considerations
Class I: Sodium channel blockers—slow the fast sodium channels, thereby controlling rate of depolarization		Class common side effects: anticholinergic, nausea, vomiting, dizziness, drowsiness, fatigue	Monitor for orthostasis.
Class Ia	Disopyramide (Norpace) Procainamide (Pronestyl) Quinidine (Biquin, Cardioquin)	CHF Lupus, fever, hematologic toxicity Hypotension, diarrhea, tinnitus	Monitor for orthostasis.
Class Ib	Lidocaine (Xylocaine), tocainide (Tonocard), mexiletine (Mexitil)	Disorientation, slurred speech, tinnitus, seizures, tremor	Monitor for orthostasis.
Class Ic	Flecainide (Tambocor)	Visual disturbances, dyspnea, tachycardia, syncope	Monitor for orthostasis.
	Propafenone (Rythmol)	Angina, CHF, AV block, ECG abnormalities, syncope, constipation	
Class II: Beta blockers	See Table 19-3		
Class III: Agents in this class prolong the action potential and refractory period in myocardial tissue; decrease AV conduction and sinus node function	Amiodarone (Cordarone, Pacerone), dronedarone (Multaq)	Amiodarone: ECG abnormalities, bradycardia, hypotension (IV form), pulmonary fibrosis, hepatotoxicity, thyroid dysfunction, corneal deposits, photosensitivity, constipation, blue-gray skin discoloration Dronedarone: designed to reduce toxicities associated with amiodarone, but possibly less effective; postmarketing case reports of acute liver and renal failure, torsades	This drug concentrates in the tissues and causes toxicities in the heart, eyes, thyroid, and lungs. Any new symptoms should be reported. This agent has numerous drug-drug interactions.
	Dofetilide (Tikosyn)	Arrhythmias, dizziness, insomnia, headache, GI side effects	Requires initiation in inpatient setting with constant telemetry monitoring due to high risk of arrhythmias in the first 3 days.
	Ibutilide (Corvert)	Arrhythmias, hypotension, bradycardia, headaches	
	Sotalol (Betapace, Betapace AF)	Bradycardia, chest pain, fatigue, dizziness, dyspnea, CHF, GI side effects	Has beta-blocking properties and is associated with similar side effects.
Class IV: Nondihydropyridine calcium channel blockers	See Table 19-3		

Miscellaneous

Slows conduction time through the AV node, interrupting the reentry pathways through the AV node	Adenosine (Adenocard, Adenoscan)	Facial flushing, headache, dizziness, chest pressure, dyspnea	
Direct suppression of the AV node conduction to increase effective refractory period and decrease conduction velocity	Digoxin (Lanoxin)	Anorexia, lethargy, confusion, visual disturbances, ECG abnormalities, arrhythmias	

AV, Atrioventricular node; *CHF,* chronic heart failure; *ECG,* electrocardiogram; *GI,* gastrointestinal; *IV,* intravenous.

TABLE 19-2 Anticoagulants

Indications: Prevention and treatment of DVT and PE, prevention of ischemic stroke in patients at high risk (e.g., atrial fibrillation patients), during ACS/MI.

Adverse Effects for all of these agents: Excessive bleeding.

PT Considerations for all of these agents: Do not perform deep-tissue massage; exercise fall precautions; monitor signs and symptoms of bleeding: Hct, Hgb, bleeding from the nose, gums, or GI tract (blood in the stool or vomit); monitor bruising, mental status changes (stroke).

Class: Mechanism of Action	Generic Name (Common Brand Name[s])	Adverse Effects	PT Considerations
Coumarin derivatives: Interfere with synthesis of vitamin K–dependent clotting factors that decrease prothrombin	Warfarin (Coumadin)	Systemic cholesterol microembolism (purple toe syndrome); rare	Monitor INR; goal INR is 2-3 for majority of patients; lower INR values are associated with high risk of thrombotic events; INR > 3 associated with increased bleeding risk. Warfarin has many drug-drug and drug-food interactions.
Direct thrombin inhibitors: Directly inhibits thrombin, can be used to treat heparin-induced thrombocytopenia and as an alternative to heparin in allergic patients	Argatroban (Argatroban), bivalirudin (Angiomax), dabigatran (Pradaxa), lepirudin (Refludan)	Anaphylaxis (with lepirudin)	aPTT monitoring is necessary with goal values 1.5-2.5 times control. Goal range differs by institution (typically 60-80 seconds); high aPTT values are associated with increased bleeding risk; argatroban causes false-positive elevations in INR, and goal INR during concomitant argatroban warfarin therapy is 4-5; dabigatran is the only oral agent in this class.
Factor Xa inhibitor: Selective inhibitor of factor Xa	Fondaparinux (Arixtra), rivaroxaban (Xarelto)	Thrombocytopenia	Monitor neurological impairment if patient is receiving neuraxial anesthesia or is undergoing spinal puncture; rivaroxaban is oral agent, whereas fondaparinux needs to be injected subcutaneously.
Heparin: Prolongs clotting time by inhibiting the conversion of prothrombin to thrombin	Heparin sodium	Heparin-induced thrombocytopenia type 1 (small decline in platelet count, self-resolving, more common) and type 2 (>50% decrease in platelets, an allergic reaction, requires immediate treatment; rare)	aPTT monitoring is necessary with goal values 1.5-2.5 times control. Goal range differs by institution (typically 60-80 seconds); high aPTT values are associated with increased bleeding risk. Low doses administered SC for prophylaxis do not require aPTT monitoring.
Low-molecular-weight heparins	Dalteparin sodium (Fragmin), enoxaparin sodium (Lovenox)	Heparin-induced thrombocytopenia (see Heparin); less common than with heparin	No special lab monitoring required.

ACS, Acute coronary syndrome; *aPTT,* activated partial thromboplastin time; *DVT,* deep venous thrombosis; *Hct,* hematocrit; *Hgb,* hemoglobin; *INR,* international normalized ratio; *MI,* myocardial infarction; *OTC,* over-the-counter; *PE,* pulmonary embolism; *PT,* physical therapy.

TABLE 19-3 Antihypertensive Agents

Indications: Treatment of hypertension, heart failure, arrhythmias, ischemic heart disease.
Precautions: Monitor vital signs and the potential for orthostasis with most antihypertensive agents.

Class: Mechanism of Action	Generic Name (Common Brand Name[s])	Adverse Effects	PT Considerations
Adrenergic agonists: Stimulate alpha2-adrenoceptors in the brain stem, thus activating an inhibitory neuron, resulting in reduced sympathetic outflow from the CNS, producing a decrease in peripheral resistance, renal vascular resistance, heart rate, and blood pressure	Clonidine (Catapres, Catapres TTS—transdermal patch)	Drowsiness, dizziness, dry mouth, orthostasis, headache, lethargy, weakness	Clonidine can also be used as an epidural to control pain. It takes 2-3 days to see full efficacy after the first application of the transdermal patch. Clonidine levels will slowly decline over 2-3 days after patch removal.
Adrenergic antagonists: Competitively inhibit postsynaptic alpha-adrenergic receptors, which results in vasodilation of veins and arterioles and a decrease in total peripheral resistance and blood pressure	Doxazosin (Cardura), prazosin (Minipress), tamsulosin (Flomax), terazosin (Hytrin)	Drowsiness, dizziness, first dose syncope, palpitations, orthostasis, weakness	These agents should not be used for treatment of HTN due to increased cardiovascular mortality (ALLHAT trial) compared to other antihypertensives. These are commonly used to treat BPH. Tamsulosin is the most selective for prostate and causes the least amount of cardiovascular side effects. Tamsulosin can also be used to treat kidney stones (in both men and women).
Angiotensin-converting enzyme (ACE) inhibitors: Inhibit conversion of angiotensin I to angiotensin II and therefore act to decrease excess water and sodium retention while also preventing vasoconstriction	Captopril (Capoten), enalapril (Vasotec), fosinopril (Monopril), lisinopril (Prinivil, Zestril), perindopril (Aceon), quinapril (Accupril), ramipril (Altace), trandolapril (Mavik), moexipril (Univasc)	Common: Cough, hypotension, dizziness, hyperkalemia Serious: renal failure, angioedema, anaphylaxis, neutropenia	Report to other providers changes in urine output, muscle cramps (indicative of hyperkalemia), and swelling or redness in the face and neck area (indicative of angioedema).
Angiotensin II receptor blockers (ARBs): Selectively antagonize angiotensin II and therefore act to decrease excess water and sodium retention while also preventing vasoconstriction	Azilsartan (Edarbi), candesartan (Atacand), eprosartan (Teveten), irbesartan (Avapro), losartan (Cozaar), olmesartan (Benicar), telmisartan (Micardis), valsartan (Diovan)	Common: hypotension, dizziness, hyperkalemia Serious: renal failure, angioedema, anaphylaxis	Refer to ACE inhibitors above.
Beta-blockers: Decrease myocardial oxygen demand by decreasing sympathetic input to myocardium, therefore decreasing heart rate and contractility	Beta-1 selective: Acebutolol (Sectral), atenolol (Tenormin), esmolol (Brevibloc), metoprolol (Lopressor, Toprol XL) Non-selective beta 1 and 2: Nadolol (Corgard), pindolol (Visken), propranolol (Inderal) Alpha and beta blockers: Carvedilol (Coreg), labetalol (Normodyne)	Common: smooth muscle spasm (bronchospasm), exaggeration of therapeutic cardiac actions (bradycardia), fatigue, insomnia, masking of hypoglycemic symptoms in diabetics (except diaphoresis), impaired glucose tolerance, lipid abnormalities, exercise intolerance Serious: AV block	Negative inotropic effects prevent heart rate to increase in response to exercise; use Borg RPE scale to monitor exertion rather than checking the pulse; check blood sugar in diabetics before exercise and administer a carbohydrate snack with blood sugar ≤ 100 mg/dl before exercise

Continued

TABLE 19-3 Antihypertensive Agents—cont'd

Class: Mechanism of Action	Generic Name (Common Brand Name[s])	Adverse Effects	PT Considerations
Calcium-channel blockers: Inhibit calcium ion from entering the "slow channels" or select voltage-sensitive areas of vascular smooth muscle and myocardium during depolarization, producing a relaxation of coronary vascular smooth muscle and coronary vasodilation; increases myocardial oxygen delivery in patients with vasospastic angina; non-DHP CCB also slow automaticity and conduction of AV node	Non-DHP: verapamil (Isoptin, Calan, Verelan, Covera-HS), diltiazem (Cardizem, Tiazac, Cartia XT) DHP: amlodipine (Norvasc), felodipine (Plendil), nifedipine (Procardia XL, Adalat CC), isradipine (DynaCirc), nicardipine (Cardene)	Bradycardia, hypotension, AV block, CHF, constipation and gingival hyperplasia (with verapamil) Hypotension, peripheral edema, flushing, palpitations, headaches, gingival hyperplasia (with nifedipine)	Non-DHP CCB will decrease the heart rate and prevent heart rate increase in response to exercise similarly to beta-blockers. DHP-CCBs have more effects in the peripheral vasculature vs. non-DHP CCBs, which have more central cardiac effects.
Diuretics			
Thiazide diuretics: Inhibit sodium reabsorption in the distal tubules causing increased excretion of sodium and water as well as potassium and hydrogen ions	Chlorthalidone (Hygroton), hydrochlorothiazide (Esidrix, HydroDIURIL), metolazone (Zaroxolyn)	Hypotension, orthostasis, volume depletion, hypokalemia, hyponatremia, photosensitivity, hyperuricemia, hyperglycemia	All diuretics can cause volume depletion. Monitor weight, urine output for changes in renal function, orthostasis, serum electrolytes (will decrease), signs and symptoms of gout (due to increase in uric acid).
Loop diuretics: Inhibit reabsorption of sodium and chloride in the ascending loop of Henle, thus causing increased excretion of water, sodium, chloride, magnesium, phosphate, and calcium	Bumetanide (Bumex), furosemide (Lasix), torsemide (Demadex)	Hyperglycemia, hyperuricemia, hypokalemia, hypocalcemia, hypomagnesemia, hypotension, excessive urination, dehydration, orthostasis	
Potassium-sparing diuretics: Interfere with potassium/sodium exchange (active transport) in the distal tubule, cortical collecting tubule, and collecting duct; spironolactone is an aldosterone antagonist	Amiloride (Midamor), spironolactone, triamterene (Dyrenium)	Hyperkalemia, dizziness, hypotension With spironolactone: Gynecomastia, breast pain, hyperkalemia, hyponatremia, dehydration, hyperchloremic metabolic acidosis in decompensated hepatic cirrhosis, inability to achieve or maintain an erection, irregular menses, amenorrhea, postmenopausal bleeding	

TABLE 19-3 Antihypertensive Agents—cont'd

Class: Mechanism of Action	Generic Name (Common Brand Name[s])	Adverse Effects	PT Considerations
Carbonic anhydrase inhibitors: Inhibit carbonic anhydrase enzyme, resulting in reduction of hydrogen ion secretion at renal tubule and an increased renal excretion of sodium, potassium, bicarbonate, and water	Acetazolamide (Diamox), dichlorphenamide (Daranide), methazolamide (Neptazane)	Flushing, dizziness, drowsiness, fatigue, allergic reactions, hyperglycemia or hypoglycemia, hypokalemia, hyponatremia, metabolic acidosis, kidney stones, hepatic insufficiency, myopia	Due to toxicities, these are not used as diuretics, but can be used to treat glaucoma, acute mountain sickness, or metabolic alkalosis.
Nitrates: Relax vascular smooth muscle; decreased venous ratios and arterial blood pressure; reduce left ventricular work; decrease myocardial O$_2$ consumption. In addition to hypertension indication, often used in patients with ischemic heart disease	Amyl nitrite (Aspirol, Vapor-ole; inhalation), nitroglycerin (NTG) (dosage forms: sublingual, spray, percutaneous ointment, oral, sustained release, IV) (Nitro-Bid, Nitrostat; Nitro-Dur, Transderm-Nitro, Nitrodisc; transdermal patch), isosorbide dinitrate (Isordil, Sorbitrate; sublingual, oral, chewable), isosorbide mononitrate (ISMO)	Hypotension, orthostasis, flushing, tachycardia, headache, dizziness	Patients with ischemic heart disease should always carry rapid-acting NTG (sublingual or spray). In case of angina, administer 1 tab or spray up to 3 times every 5 minutes and call 911. Sublingual NTG tabs have specific storage requirements that should be followed (avoid heat, moisture, light). If tablets no longer have their shape, NTG is likely to be expired and may not be effective. Monitor for orthostasis.
Renin inhibitors: Renin inhibitor, resulting in blockade of the conversion of angiotensinogen to angiotensin I	Aliskiren (Tekturna)	Dizziness, rash, hyperkalemia, increases in serum creatinine, cough, increase in serum CK, diarrhea	New class of antihypertensive agents. Monitor muscle cramps associated with hyperkalemia. Monitor urine output and weight for renal dysfunction.
Vasodilators: Direct vasodilation of arterioles (with little effect on veins) with decreased systemic resistance	Hydralazine (Apresoline), minoxidil (Loniten)	Headache, hypotension, compensatory sympathetic reflex causing increased heart rate, lupus with long-term hydralazine	Monitor blood pressure and heart rate. Patients at risk for orthostasis. *Use caution.*

ACE, Angiotensin-converting enzyme; *ARB,* angiotensin receptor blocker; *BPH,* benign prostatic hypertrophy; *CCB,* calcium channel blockers; *CK,* creatinine kinase; *CNS,* central nervous system; *DHP,* dihydropyridine; *HTN,* hypertension; *IV,* intravenous; *NTG,* nitroglycerin; *RPE,* rating of perceived exertion.

TABLE 19-3A Combination Drugs for Hypertension

Many patients require antihypertensive therapy with multiple agents. General principles of HTN management include combining multiple agents with different mechanisms of action to achieve optimal blood pressure goals. This approach allows for greater efficacy and lower toxicity rather than maximizing the dose of individual agents. To facilitate patient adherence, there are a number of fixed-dose formulations that allow patients to take multiple medications in one pill. In the majority of cases, these combinations are only available by brand name and are considerably more expensive than individual components that may be available generically. The fixed-dose combinations may also be more difficult to titrate at the start of therapy as opposed to individual components. PTs should consider the side effects and monitoring of all individual components of the combination antihypertensives. (See Table 19-3.)

Combination Type	Fixed-Dose Combination, mg*	Trade Name
ACEIs and CCBs	Amlodipine–benazepril hydrochloride (2.5/10, 5/10, 5/20, 10/20) Enalapril-felodipine (5/5) Trandolapril-verapamil (2/180, 1/240, 2/240, 4/240)	Lotrel Lexxel Tarka
ACEIs and diuretics	Benazepril-hydrochlorothiazide (5/6.25, 10/12.5, 20/12.5, 20/25) Captopril-hydrochlorothiazide (25/15, 25/25, 50/15, 50/25) Enalapril-hydrochlorothiazide (5/12.5, 10/25) Fosinopril-hydrochlorothiazide (10/12.5, 20/12.5) Lisinopril-hydrochlorothiazide (10/12.5, 20/12.5, 20/25) Moexipril-hydrochlorothiazide (7.5/12.5, 15/25) Quinapril-hydrochlorothiazide (10/12.5, 20/12.5, 20/25)	Lotensin HCT Capozide Vaseretic Monopril/HCT Prinzide, Zestoretic Uniretic Accuretic
ARBs and diuretics	Azilsartan medoxomil–chlorthalidone (40/12.5, 40/25) Candesartan-hydrochlorothiazide (16/12.5, 32/12.5) Eprosartan-hydrochlorothiazide (600/12.5, 600/25) Irbesartan-hydrochlorothiazide (150/12.5, 300/12.5) Losartan-hydrochlorothiazide (50/12.5, 100/25) Olmesartan medoxomil–hydrochlorothiazide (20/12.5, 40/12.5, 40/25) Telmisartan-hydrochlorothiazide (40/12.5, 80/12.5) Valsartan-hydrochlorothiazide (80/12.5, 160/12.5, 160/25)	Edarbyclor Atacand HCT Teveten-HCT Avalide Hyzaar Benicar HCT Micardis-HCT Diovan-HCT
ARB and rennin inhibitor	Valsartan-aliskiren (160/150), (320/300)	Valturna
ARBs, calcium-channel blocker, and diuretics	Olmesartan medoxomil–amlodipine-hydrochlorothiazide (20/5/12.5), (40/10/25) Valsartan-amlodipine-hydrochlorothiazide (320/10/25)	Tribenzor Exforge HCT
BBs and diuretics	Atenolol-chlorthalidone (50/25, 100/25) Bisoprolol-hydrochlorothiazide (2.5/6.25, 5/6.25, 10/6.25) Metoprolol-hydrochlorothiazide (50/25, 100/25) Nadolol-bendroflumethiazide (40/5, 80/5) Propranolol LA–hydrochlorothiazide (40/25, 80/25) Timolol-hydrochlorothiazide (10/25)	Tenoretic Ziac Lopressor HCT Corzide Inderide LA Timolide
Centrally acting drug and diuretic	Methyldopa-hydrochlorothiazide (250/15, 250/25, 500/30, 500/50) Reserpine-chlorthalidone (0.125/25, 0.25/50) Reserpine-chlorothiazide (0.125/250, 0.25/500) Reserpine-hydrochlorothiazide (0.125/25, 0.125/50)	Aldoril Demi-Regroton, Regroton Diupres Hydropres
Diuretic and diuretic	Amiloride-hydrochlorothiazide (5/50) Spironolactone-hydrochlorothiazide (25/25, 50/50) Triamterene-hydrochlorothiazide (37.5/25, 75/50)	Moduretic Aldactazide Dyazide, Maxzide
HTN and lipid lowering	Amlodipine-atorvastatin (5/10, 5/20, 5/40, 5/80, 10/10, 10/20, 10/40, 10/80)	Caduet
Renin inhibitor and calcium-channel blocker	Aliskiren-amlodipine (150/5), (300/10)	Tekamlo
Renin inhibitor, calcium-channel blocker and diuretic	Aliskiren-amlodipine-hydrochlorothiazide (300/10/25)	Amturnide

ACEIs, Angiotensin-converting enzyme inhibitors; *ARBs*, angiotensin receptor blockers; *BBs*, beta blockers; *CCBs*, calcium channel blockers; *HTN*, hypertension.
*Some drug combinations are available in multiple fixed doses. Each drug dose is reported in milligrams.

TABLE 19-4 Antiplatelet Agents

Indications: Primary and secondary prevention of coronary heart disease, stroke; peripheral arterial disease; adjunct therapy with anticoagulants during acute coronary syndrome; prevention of thrombosis after stent placement.
Precautions: Combination of these agents with other antiplatelet or anticoagulant drugs increases the risk of bleeding.

Class: Mechanism of Action	Generic Name (Common Brand Name[s])	Adverse Effects	PT Considerations
Glycoprotein IIb/IIIa inhibitors: Block the platelet glycoprotein IIb/IIIa receptor, the binding site for fibrinogen, von Willebrand factor, and other ligands. Inhibition of binding at this final common receptor blocks platelet aggregation and prevents thrombosis	Abciximab (ReoPro) Eptifibatide (Integrilin) Tirofiban (Aggrastat)	Produce potent antiplatelet effect with high risk of bleeding	Only used for short-term therapy, typically, in combination with other antiplatelet and anticoagulant agents; high risk of bleeding.
Salicylates: Inhibit cyclooxygenase; block prostaglandin synthetase action, which prevents formation of the platelet-aggregating substance thromboxane A_2	Aspirin (many brand names, available OTC) Aspirin/dipyridamole (Aggrenox)	Well tolerated at 81-325 mg Common: dyspepsia, minor bleeding Serious: anaphylaxis, bronchospasm, severe bleeding	Many NSAIDs may decrease the antiplatelet effects of aspirin; if used concomitantly, patient should take aspirin 2 hours before NSAID.
Thienopyridine: Blocks ADP receptors, which prevent fibrinogen binding at that site and thereby reduce the possibility of platelet adhesion and aggregation	Clopidogrel (Plavix), prasugrel (Effient), ticagrelor (Brilinta)	Common: dyspepsia, gastritis, minor bleeding, dyspnea (ticagrelor)	Serious: bleeding.

ADP, Adenosine diphosphate; *NSAID*, nonsteroidal antiinflammatory drug; *PT*, physical therapy.

TABLE 19-5 Lipid-Lowering Agents

Indications: Treatment of dyslipidemia.

Class: Mechanism of Action	Generic Name (Common Brand Name[s])	Adverse Effects	PT Considerations
Bile acid sequestrants: Bind bile acids including glycocholic acid in the intestine, impeding their reabsorption. Increase the fecal loss of bile salt–bound LDL-C.	Cholestyramine (Questran), colesevelam (WelChol), colestipol (Colestid)	Constipation, dyspepsia, flatulence	These drugs cause significant GI discomfort. Ask the patient when his or her symptoms are less severe to schedule your sessions.
Cholesterol absorption inhibitor: Inhibits absorption of cholesterol at the brush border of the small intestine. This leads to a decreased delivery of cholesterol to the liver, reduction of hepatic cholesterol stores, and an increased clearance of cholesterol from the blood; decreases total C, LDL-cholesterol (LDL-C), ApoB, and triglycerides (TG) while increasing HDL-cholesterol (HDL-C).	Ezetimibe (Zetia)	Dizziness, headache, diarrhea	This medication is well tolerated. Often combined with a statin for additional LDL reduction.

Continued

TABLE 19-5 Lipid-Lowering Agents—cont'd

Class: Mechanism of Action	Generic Name (Common Brand Name[s])	Adverse Effects	PT Considerations
Fibric acid derivatives: Fenofibric acid is believed to increase VLDL catabolism by enhancing the synthesis of lipoprotein lipase; as a result of a decrease in VLDL levels, total plasma triglycerides are reduced by 30% to 60%; modest increase in HDL occurs in some hypertriglyceridemic patients.	Bezafibrate (Bezalip), fenofibrate (Antara, Lipofen, Tricor), gemfibrozil (Lopid)	Constipation, LFT abnormalities	Monitor for hepatotoxicity: yellow skin/sclera, abdominal pain. If combined with a statin, higher potential for hepatotoxicity and muscle toxicity.
Fish oil (omega-3 fatty acids): Mechanism has not been completely defined. Possible mechanisms include inhibition of acetyl CoA:1,2 diacylglycerol acyltransferase, increased hepatic beta-oxidation, or a reduction in the hepatic synthesis of triglycerides.	Fish oil is available in many formulations OTC. Because of concern over impurities of OTC formulations, there is a product available by prescription only. Trade name: Omacor	Dyspepsia, fishy odor, taster perversion	
HMG-CoA reductase inhibitors (statins): Inhibit 3-hydroxy-3-methylglutaryl coenzyme A (HMG-CoA) reductase, the rate-limiting enzyme in cholesterol synthesis (reduces the production of mevalonic acid from HMG-CoA); results in a compensatory increase in the expression of LDL receptors on hepatocyte membranes and a stimulation of LDL catabolism.	Atorvastatin (Lipitor), fluvastatin (Lescol), lovastatin (Mevacor), pitavastatin (Livalo), pravastatin (Pravachol), rosuvastatin (Crestor), simvastatin (Zocor)	Headache, GI toxicity, hepatotoxicity, muscle pain and weakness, rhabdomyolysis (rare)	LFTs must be monitored routinely, monitor for hepatotoxicity. Patients with muscle pain not related to exercise should be referred to their providers to check for muscle breakdown (CK levels are typically checked).
Nicotinic acid: inhibits the synthesis of very low-density lipoproteins.	Niacin (Niacor; Niaspan; Slo-Niacin [OTC]).	Edema, flushing, hypotension, orthostasis, palpitations, tachycardia, hyperglycemia, hyperuricemia, hepatotoxicity	Monitor blood pressure and heart rate and orthostasis, signs and symptoms of hyperglycemia, and gout. Monitor for hepatotoxicity.

Combinations: Advicor (lovastatin + niacin), Caduet (atorvastatin + amlodipine), Pravigard PAC (aspirin + pravastatin), Vytorin (ezetimibe + simvastatin).
CK, Creatinine kinase; *GI,* gastrointestinal; *HDL,* high-density lipoprotein; *HMG-CoA,* hydroxy-3-methylglutaryl coenzyme A; *LDL,* low-density lipoprotein; *LFTs,* liver function tests; *OTC,* over-the-counter; *TG,* triglycerides; *VLDL,* very-low-density lipoprotein.

TABLE 19-6 Positive Inotropes (Pressors)

Indications: Administered intravenously for hemodynamic support in patients with cardiovascular and/or respiratory collapse, severe heart failure, severe sepsis with hemodynamic instability; some agents are used for resuscitation during cardiovascular arrest.

Mechanism of Action	Generic Name (Common Brand Name[s])	Adverse Effects	PT Considerations
Agents in this class increase cardiac output via stimulating alpha, beta, and/or dopaminergic receptors.	Dopamine, dobutamine, epinephrine (Adrenalin, EpiPen), norepinephrine (Levophed), phenylephrine (Neo-Synephrine), vasopressin (Pitressin)	Increase BP and HR, chest pain, ischemia, ACS, arrhythmia	These agents are used acutely, typically in unstable patients in the ICU setting. Outpatient intermittent infusions can be used in severe heart failure. Monitor vitals and avoid exertion.

ACS, Acute coronary syndrome; *BP,* blood pressure; *HR,* heart rate; *ICU,* intensive care unit.

TABLE 19-7 Thrombolytics (Also Known as Fibrinolytics)

Indications: ACS, ischemic stroke, severe PE, clot lysis in IV catheters (very small doses).

Mechanism of Action	Generic Name (Common Brand Name[s])	Adverse Effects	PT Considerations
Initiate fibrinolysis by binding to fibrin and converting plasminogen to plasmin	Alteplase (Activase, Cathflo), reteplase (Retavase), streptokinase (Streptase), tenecteplase (TNKase), urokinase (Abbokinase)	Bleeding at various sites, including intracranial hemorrhage	These agents are used acutely, typically in unstable patients. Risk of bleeding is very high and may outweigh the benefit of clot lysis and restoration of blood flow. PT will probably not be done in patients immediately post thrombolysis.

ACS, Acute coronary syndrome; *IV,* intravenous; *PE,* pulmonary embolism; *PT,* physical therapy.

Respiratory System

TABLE 19-8 Adrenocortical Steroids (Glucocorticoids)

Indications: Stabilize and limit the inflammatory response (bronchoconstriction) in the respiratory tract in patients with asthma and COPD (inhaled and systemic); to decrease cerebral edema or inflammation in neoplastic or inflammatory diseases, or both (systemic); relief of seasonal or perennial rhinitis (intranasal and inhaled).

Mechanism of Action	Generic Name (Common Brand Name[s])	Adverse Effects	PT Considerations
Prevent the accumulation of inflammatory cells at the infection site, inhibit lysosomal enzyme release and chemical mediators of inflammatory response, reduce capillary dilatation and permeability	Systemic: Dexamethasone (Decadron), fludrocortisone (Florinef), hydrocortisone (Cortef, Solu-Cortef), methylprednisolone (Depo-Medrol, Medrol), prednisone (Deltasone, Sterapred, Sterapred DS), prednisolone (Orapred, Pediapred, Prelone), triamcinolone (Aristocort) Inhaled: Beclomethasone (Beclovent, Vanceril), budesonide (Pulmicort), flunisolide (AeroBid), fluticasone propionate (Flovent, Advair [in combination with salmeterol]), triamcinolone acetonide (Azmacort) Intranasal: Beclomethasone dipropionate (Beconase, Vancenase), budesonide (Rhinocort), fluticasone propionate (Flonase), mometasone furoate monohydrate (Nasonex), triamcinolone acetonide (Nasacort)	Common side effects: Headache, vertigo, diaphoresis, nausea, vomiting. In susceptible patients: euphoria, insomnia, seizure, muscle weakness, cushingoid features (chronic use), decreased wound healing (chronic use), ecchymosis, skin atrophy (chronic use), thromboembolism, hypertension, hyperglycemia, hypokalemia Serious reactions: adrenal insufficiency, steroid psychosis, immunosuppression (chronic use), peptic ulcer, congestive heart failure, osteoporosis (chronic use) Inhaled: oral thrush, change of voice quality Intranasal: local mucosal irritation	Systemic steroids: Monitor blood pressure (will increase) and blood glucose (will increase); modalities that increase the risk of bruising or skin tears should be avoided; be aware of the risk of osteoporosis with chronic use—exercise caution when exercising and prescribe weight-bearing exercises that promote bone health; reinforce compliance—abrupt discontinuation leads to adrenal insufficiency crisis Inhaled steroids: emphasize compliance to maintain disease control, patients should rinse mouth after use to prevent thrush; chronic use and high doses increase the risk of systemic side effects, especially osteoporosis

COPD, Chronic obstructive pulmonary disease; *PT,* physical therapy.

TABLE 19-9 Antihistamines

Indications: To decrease inflammation and bronchoconstriction associated with hypersensitivity reactions, such as allergic rhinitis.

Mechanism of Action	Generic Name (Common Brand Name[s])	Adverse Effects	PT Considerations
Reduce or prevent the physiologic effects of histamine by competing for histamine binding sites	Azelastine (Astelin), chlorpheniramine maleate (Chlor-Trimeton), cetirizine (Zyrtec), clemastine (Tavist), desloratadine (Clarinex), diphenhydramine (Benadryl, various), fexofenadine (Allegra), loratadine (Alavert, Claritin)	Drowsiness, dizziness, decreased coordination, orthostatic hypotension, hypotension, hypertension, palpitations, bradycardia, tachycardia, epigastric distress, urinary frequency, thickening of bronchial secretions, dry mouth	If patient experiences drowsiness, avoid scheduling PT session within a few hours of administration with short-acting formulations. Many are available in 12h and 24h formulations, so ask patient when he or she feels the most sedation.

PT, Physical therapy.

TABLE 19-10 Bronchodilators

Indications: To relieve bronchospasm associated with obstructive pulmonary disease, asthma, and exercise-induced bronchospasm.

Mechanism of Action	Generic Name (Common Brand Name[s])	Adverse Effects	PT Considerations
Anticholinergics: Block the action of acetylcholine at parasympathetic sites in bronchial smooth muscle causing bronchodilation. Also decrease mucous secretion and play greater role in the management of COPD	Ipratropium bromide (Atrovent), tiotropium (Spiriva)	Bronchitis, palpitations, dizziness, dry mouth	Short-acting beta-2 agonists are often referred to as "rescue" inhalers. In patients with asthma and COPD, maintenance therapy should minimize the use of short-acting beta-2 agonists. Observe if patients are using their rescue inhalers too often, and refer them to their health care provider to titrate maintenance therapy. Encourage patients who have exertion- or exercise-induced bronchospasm to administer beta-2 agonists 10-15 minutes before therapy sessions. Bronchodilator administration can also facilitate chest PT effectiveness.
Beta-2 agonists: Relax bronchial smooth muscle by action on beta-2-receptors with little effect on heart rate	Short-acting: Albuterol (Proventil, Ventolin), arformoterol (Brovana), epinephrine (various), isoproterenol (Isuprel), levalbuterol (Xopenex), metaproterenol (Alupent), pirbuterol (Maxair) Long-acting: formoterol (Foradil), salmeterol (Serevent) Ultra-long-acting: indacaterol (Arcapta Neohaler)	Common: tachycardia, palpitations Rare: increased blood pressure, angina, hypokalemia	
Theophylline: Causes bronchodilatation, diuresis, CNS and cardiac stimulation, and gastric acid secretion by blocking phosphodiesterase, which increases tissue concentrations of cyclic adenine monophosphate (cAMP)	Theophylline (Elixophyllin, Quibron, Theo-24, TheoCap, Theochron, Uniphyl)	Appropriate therapeutic range is 5-20 mcg/ml At therapeutic concentrations: nervousness, insomnia, tachycardia, nausea and vomiting 15-25 mcg/ml: GI upset, diarrhea, nausea/vomiting, abdominal pain, nervousness, headache, insomnia, agitation, dizziness, muscle cramp, tremor 25-35 mcg/ml: Tachycardia, occasional PVCs >35 mcg/ml: Ventricular tachycardia, frequent PVCs, seizure	Monitor for signs and symptoms of toxicity. Theophylline has many drug interactions, and levels can rapidly change. Caffeine intake will exacerbate side effects.

Combination: Advair (fluticasone + salmeterol); Combivent (albuterol + ipratropium); Dulera (mometasone + formoterol); Symbicort (budesonide + formoterol).
CNS, Central nervous system; *COPD,* chronic obstructive pulmonary disease; *GI,* gastrointestinal; *PT,* physical therapy; *PVC,* premature ventricular contraction.

TABLE 19-11 Leukotriene Modifiers and Other Nonsteroidal Antiinflammatory Agents

Indications: Long-term control of asthma or COPD in adults and children.

Mechanism of Action	Generic Name (Common Brand Name[s])	Adverse Effects	PT Considerations
Leukotriene receptor antagonist—selective competitive inhibitor of LTD_4 and LTE_4 receptors; 5-lipooxygenase inhibitor	Montelukast (Singulair), zafirlukast (Accolate), zileuton (Zyflo)	Montelukast and zafirlukast are well tolerated with infrequent cough, dizziness, fatigue, dyspepsia. Zileuton can cause hepatotoxicity.	Monitor for abdominal pain, yellow skin, and sclera appearance with zileuton.
Phosphodiesterase type 4 inhibitor	Roflumilast (Daliresp)	Nausea, reduced appetite and weight loss, abdominal pain, diarrhea, sleep disturbances, headache, back pain, dizziness.	This medication has a lot of drug interactions, so make sure to educate patients to avoid making medication changes without discussions with providers.

COPD, Chronic obstructive pulmonary disease; LTD_4, leukotriene D_4; LTE_4, leukotriene E_4; PT, physical therapy.

TABLE 19-12 Mast Cell Stabilizers

Indications: Long-term control of asthma in adults and children, allergic rhinitis, exercise-induced asthma.

Mechanism of Action	Generic Name (Common Brand Name[s])	Adverse Effects	PT Considerations
Decrease histamine release from mast cells; block early and late reaction to allergen; inhibit acute response to exercise, cold dry air, and sulfur oxide	Cromolyn (Intal), nedocromil (Tilade)	Well tolerated; unpleasant taste with nedocromil	May take up to 2 weeks to see complete response. Effective to prevent exercise-induced asthma

PT, Physical therapy.

Musculoskeletal System

TABLE 19-13 Disease-Modifying Antirheumatic Drugs (DMARDs)

Indications: Treatment of rheumatoid arthritis (RA). Refer to Chapter Appendix 13A.

Unlike the NSAIDs and acetaminophen, DMARDs can reduce and prevent joint damage and preserve joint integrity and function. The American College of Rheumatology recommends initiation of DMARDs within the first 3 months of diagnosis of rheumatoid arthritis (RA) in patients with ongoing joint pain despite adequate treatment with nonsteroidal antiinflammatory drugs, significant morning stiffness, active synovitis, persistent elevations in erythrocyte sedimentation rate and C-reactive protein levels, and/or radiographic evidence of joint damage. Methotrexate is considered a first-line agent among DMARDs because of its long-term efficacy, low cost, and acceptable toxicity profile. DMARDs lose efficacy over time, and patients are typically placed on combination regimens of different DMARDs; with time, more expensive, toxic agents may need to be tried. Many DMARDs do not begin to work immediately; effect may not be seen for 3 to 6 months. DMARDs are potent antiinflammatory agents that can lead to immunosuppression. PTs should exercise infection-control measures such as good hand hygiene, sanitizing of equipment, and avoiding contact with patients if feeling sick. DMARDs are listed in alphabetical order and not in order of preference in the table below. Corticosteroids are frequently used as part of RA therapy, typically for short courses (see Table 19-8).

Mechanism of Action	Generic Name (Common Brand Name[s])	Adverse Effects	PT Considerations
Selective costimulation modulator; inhibits T-cell (T-lymphocyte) activation. Activated T lymphocytes are found in the synovium of rheumatoid arthritis patients.	Abatacept (Orencia)	Headache, nausea, high risk of infections (54% incidence), COPD exacerbations, hypertension, dizziness, cough, back pain, infusion-related reactions	Monitor blood pressure (may increase). Monitor for and report any new symptoms associated with infections: increase in WBC, fever, cough, skin infections.

Continued

TABLE 19-13 Disease-Modifying Antirheumatic Drugs (DMARDs)—cont'd

Mechanism of Action	Generic Name (Common Brand Name[s])	Adverse Effects	PT Considerations
Blocks biologic activity of interleukin-1.	Anakinra (Kineret)	Injection site reactions are very common. Also, headache, nausea, diarrhea, sinusitis, flulike symptoms, abdominal pain, and infections	Monitor skin appearance for injection site reactions. Exercise infection-control measures.
Bind and inhibit tumor necrosis factor (TNF), which produces potent antiinflammatory effect.	Anti–tumor necrosis factor therapy: Adalimumab (Humira), certolizumab pegol (Cimzia), etanercept (Enbrel), golimumab (Simponi), infliximab (Remicade)	Rash, headache, nausea, cough Serious: associated with infections, including serious mycobacterial, fungal, and opportunistic complications	Patients are at high risk for infection. Monitor for any signs and symptoms including fever, productive cough, and increase in WBC. Exercise infection-control measures.
Antagonizes purine metabolism and may inhibit synthesis of DNA, RNA, and proteins; may also interfere with cellular metabolism and inhibit mitosis.	Azathioprine (Imuran)	Dose-related bone marrow suppression, stomatitis, diarrhea, rash, and liver failure	Monitor WBC (will decrease; patients will be at high risk for infection), hematocrit (will decrease; patient will complain of fatigue), platelets (will decrease; the risk of bleeding will increase).
Mechanism is unknown; appear to suppress the synovitis possibly through stimulation of protective interleukins 6 and 10.	Gold compounds Gold sodium thiomalate (Myochrysine), aurothioglucose (Solganal), auranofin (Ridaura)	With IM injections, patients can experience injection reactions: flushing, weakness, dizziness, sweating, syncope, hypotension Common: rash ranging from simple erythema to exfoliative dermatitis; oral formulation causes nausea, diarrhea, taste disturbances Rare: renal disease, leukopenia, thrombocytopenia	Monitor skin appearance for rash. Avoid scheduling PT sessions immediately and soon after the IM injection (injections are scheduled every 2-3 weeks and then monthly). Ensure that the injection site has no adverse reaction before initiating therapy.
May inhibit interleukin 1 (IL-1) release by monocytes, thereby decreasing macrophage chemotaxis and phagocytosis.	Hydroxychloroquine (Plaquenil)	Rash, abdominal cramping, diarrhea, myopathy, skin pigment changes, peripheral neuropathy Serious: retinal damage that can lead to vision loss	Monitor for muscle pain not associated with exercise. Monitor for tingling and numbness of the extremities. Patients should be evaluated by ophthalmologist every 6-12 months. Report any vision changes.
Inhibits dihydro-orotate dehydrogenase (an enzyme involved in the de novo pyrimidine synthesis) and has antiproliferative and antiinflammatory effect	Leflunomide (Arava)	Diarrhea, alopecia, hypertension, rash, hepatotoxicity	Monitor liver function (abdominal pain, yellow skin and sclera). Risk of hepatotoxicity is higher when used in combination with methotrexate.
Inhibits dihydrofolate reductase and interferes with DNA synthesis, repair, and cellular replication.	Methotrexate (Rheumatrex)	Nausea, vomiting, and stomatitis are common Serious: hepatotoxicity, bone marrow suppression, pulmonary toxicity	Ask patients about GI side effects to optimize scheduling PT session. Monitor WBC (will decrease; use infection-control measures), hematocrit (will decrease; patient will complain of fatigue), and platelets (will decrease; patient will be at a higher risk of bleeding).

TABLE 19-13 Disease-Modifying Antirheumatic Drugs (DMARDs)—cont'd

Mechanism of Action	Generic Name (Common Brand Name[s])	Adverse Effects	PT Considerations
Sulfasalazine is broken down by intestinal flora into 5-aminosalicylic acid and sulfapyridine. Sulfapyridine likely inhibits endothelial cell proliferation, reactive oxygen species, and cytokines.	Sulfasalazine (Azulfidine)	Headache, GI intolerance, taste perception disturbances, rash, leukopenia, thrombocytopenia	Ask patient about GI side effects to optimize scheduling of the session. Use infection-control measures if WBC decreases (wash hands, sanitize equipment, avoid contact with patient if sick). Use caution if platelet count decreases (patient will be at higher risk of bleeding).
Interleukin-6 (IL-6) inhibitor	Tocilizumab (Actemra)	Serious: severe infections	Monitor for signs and symptoms of infection. Monitor liver function in adults and children.

COPD, Chronic obstructive pulmonary disease; *GI,* gastrointestinal; *IM,* intramuscular; *PT,* physical therapy; *WBC,* white blood cells.

TABLE 19-14 Muscle Relaxants and Antispasmodic Agents

Baclofen, tizanidine, dantrolene, and botulinum toxin are best reserved for spasticity, as opposed to acute musculoskeletal conditions. Adverse effects common to all muscle relaxants include drowsiness, dizziness, and GI effects. CNS depression is additive with other CNS depressants (e.g., opioids).

Mechanism of Action	Generic Name (Common Brand Name[s])	Adverse Effects	PT Considerations
Structural analog of GABA; inhibits spinal reflexes	Baclofen (Lioresal) [available for intrathecal administration]	Withdrawal syndrome (e.g., hallucinations, psychosis, seizures)	Useful for spasticity and muscle spasms. Causes only transient drowsiness. Be aware of the withdrawal syndrome and educate patients on avoiding abrupt discontinuation.
Acetylcholine release inhibitor and a neuromuscular blocking agent used to relieve spasm and cervical dystonia	Botulinum toxin A (Botox, Dysport, Myobloc)	Muscular weakness, dysphagia, dry mouth, injection site discomfort, fatigue, headache, neck pain, musculoskeletal pain, dysphonia, injection site pain, and eye disorders	Monitor for side effects and efficacy of injections.
Acts in brain stem and spinal cord to relieve muscle spasm, pain, and tenderness	Cyclobenzaprine (Flexeril, Amrix extended-release capsules)	Sedation, anticholinergic side effects (e.g., dry mouth), can cause cardiovascular side effects at higher doses	Structurally related to a tricyclic antidepressant; has drug interactions—advise your patients to alert health care providers with any medication change; schedule PT sessions when patient is least drowsy.
Interferes with calcium release from the sarcoplasmic reticulum	Dantrolene (Dantrium)	Dose-dependent hepatotoxicity (onset between 3 and 12 months of therapy)—most common in women over 35 and can be severe (fatalities reported); dose-dependent diarrhea	Monitor for signs and symptoms of hepatotoxicity (e.g., abdominal pain, icterus, and jaundice); establish optimum time for PT based on side effects.

Continued

TABLE 19-14 Muscle Relaxants and Antispasmodic Agents—cont'd

Mechanism of Action	Generic Name (Common Brand Name[s])	Adverse Effects	PT Considerations
Muscle relaxation through neuronal inhibition via GABA receptors	Diazepam (Valium), lorazepam (Ativan), and other benzodiazepines	Sedation	Schedule PT sessions when patient is least drowsy.
Inhibits motor neurons by stimulating alpha-2 receptors; structurally related to clonidine	Tizanidine (Zanaflex)	Hypotension, hepatotoxicity (usually reversible, rarely fatal), hallucinations/delusions, withdrawal (hypertension, tachycardia, hypertonia)	Monitor blood pressure; avoid abrupt discontinuation; this agent has many drug interactions (avoid drugs that prolong QT interval)—advise patients to notify providers of any medication changes.
Unknown mechanism; may act as an analgesic	Orphenadrine (Norflex)	Anticholinergic (e.g., dry mouth, urinary retention)	Has long half-life, which may be problematic if side effects are serious.
Unknown mechanism; may act as a sedative	Carisoprodol (Soma), chlorzoxazone (Parafon Forte), metaxalone (Skelaxin), methocarbamol (Robaxin)	Sedation; some will exhibit hypersensitivity with these agents; mild withdrawal syndrome; methocarbamol causes urine discoloration (brown, black, green)	Sedation is common, so time PT sessions during time of least sedation. Metaxalone is least drowsy of these agents.

CNS, Central nervous system; *GABA,* gamma-aminobutyric acid; *PT,* physical therapy.

Central Nervous System

TABLE 19-15 Antianxiety Medications

Indications: Treatment of generalized anxiety disorder, panic disorder, agoraphobia, obsessive-compulsive disorder, social anxiety disorder, various phobias, posttraumatic stress disorder, anxiety, sleep problems.
Precautions: The acronym LOT can be used to remember the three benzodiazepines with short half-lives that are preferred in elderly patients: L (lorazepam), O (oxazepam), and T (temazepam).

Mechanism of Action	Generic Name (Common Brand Name[s])	Adverse Effects	PT Considerations
Benzodiazepines: Potentiate the actions of GABA, an inhibitory neurotransmitter	Alprazolam (Xanax), chlordiazepoxide (Librium), clobazam (Onfi), clonazepam (Klonopin), diazepam (Valium), estazolam (ProSom), flurazepam (Dalmane), halazepam (Paxipam), lorazepam (Ativan), oxazepam (Serax), prazepam (Centrax), quazepam (Doral), temazepam (Restoril), triazolam (Halcion)	Sedation, dizziness, confusion, blurred vision, diplopia, syncope, residual daytime sedation, psychomotor and cognitive impairment	Lorazepam, oxazepam, temazepam have shorter half-lives and no active metabolites and are preferred in elderly. Increased risk of falls in this population. High potential for abuse. Schedule session when the patient is least sedated and provide education about minimizing fall risk. Do not abruptly discontinue BZD to avoid withdrawal and seizures.
Buspirone: Poorly understood; stimulates presynaptic 5-HT1A receptors	Buspirone (BuSpar)	GI upset, headache, nervousness, less sedating	Onset of anxiolytic effect longer than with BZDs (2-3 weeks).
Sedative-hypnotic agents: GABA receptor agonists; ramelteon affects melatonin receptors	Eszopiclone (Lunesta), ramelteon (Rozerem), zaleplon (Sonata), zolpidem (Ambien)	Dizziness, somnolence, confusion	Shorter half-lives allow for less sedation in the morning.

BZD, Benzodiazepine; *GABA,* gamma-aminobutyric acid; *GI,* gastrointestinal; *5-HT,* 5-hydroxytryptamine.

TABLE 19-16 Anticonvulsants

Indications: Treat and prevent seizures; many of the agents in this class can be used for other indications such as treatment of neuropathic pain and migraine prevention.

Mechanism of Action	Generic Name (Common Brand Name[s])	Adverse Effects	PT Considerations
Multiple mechanisms of action: Enhancement of sodium channel inactivation, reducing current through T-type calcium channels, enhancement of GABA activity, antiglutamine activity	Carbamazepine (Tegretol, Carbatrol)	Rash, nausea, vomiting, drowsiness, dizziness, neutropenia, SIADH, osteomalacia, folic acid deficiency, hepatotoxicity, aplastic anemia.	Many drug interactions, complex pharmacokinetics, therapeutic drug level 4-12 mcg/ml. Monitor for hepatotoxicity.
	Ethosuximide (Zarontin)	Aggressiveness, ataxia, disturbance in sleep, dizziness, drowsiness, euphoria, fatigue, headache, hyperactivity, inability to concentrate, irritability, lethargy, mental depression (with cases of overt suicidal intentions), night terrors, paranoid psychosis.	Monitor changes in mood, aggression, suicidal ideations.
	Ezogabine (Potiga)	The most common adverse reactions (incidence ≥4% and approximately twice placebo) are dizziness, somnolence, fatigue, confusional state, vertigo, tremor, abnormal coordination, diplopia, disturbance in attention, memory impairment, asthenia, blurred vision, gait disturbance, aphasia, dysarthria, and balance disorder.	Fatigue and somnolence can impact effective physical therapy; offer balance training.
	Fosphenytoin (Cerebyx), phenytoin (Dilantin)	Nausea, vomiting, drowsiness, dizziness, peripheral neuropathy, acne, hirsutism, gingival hyperplasia, folate deficiency, hepatic failure, Steven-Johnson syndrome.	Many drug interactions; therapeutic drug levels 10-20 mcg/ml.
	Felbamate (Felbatol)	Weight loss, hepatotoxicity, aplastic anemia.	
	Gabapentin (Neurontin), pregabalin (Lyrica)	Well-tolerated, somnolence, ataxia, weight gain.	Popular for treatment of neuropathic pain.
	Lamotrigine (Lamictal)	Rash, Steven-Johnson syndrome.	Refer to the prescriber if rash develops.
	Levetiracetam (Keppra)	Behavioral symptoms (aggression, hyperkinesias, irritability, neurosis), somnolence, fatigue.	
	Oxcarbazepine (Trileptal), tiagabine (Gabitril)	Dizziness, somnolence, headache, ataxia, fatigue, vertigo.	
	Phenobarbital (Barbital, Luminal, Solfoton)	Drowsiness, dizziness, incoordination, decreased cognition, hepatic failure, Steven-Johnson syndrome.	High potential for abuse, very sedating, therapeutic drug levels 15-40 µg/ml.
	Topiramate (Topamax), zonisamide (Zonegran)	Drowsiness, dizziness, difficulty with concentration, loss of appetite, mood changes, metabolic acidosis, kidney stones, weight loss, oligohydrosis (inability to sweat).	Make sure patient stays well hydrated; patients who develop oligohydrosis may overheat easily and need to stay well hydrated.
	Valproic acid (Depakon, Depakene, Depakote)	Nausea and vomiting, significant weight gain, alopecia, tremor, thrombocytopenia, fatal hepatotoxicity, fatal hemorrhagic pancreatitis.	Design an exercise regimen to minimize weight gain; monitor abdominal pain for liver and pancreatic toxicity.

GABA, Gamma-aminobutyric acid; *Steven-Johnson syndrome,* Severe and life-threatening hypersensitivity complex that affects the skin and the mucous membranes; *SIADH,* syndrome of inappropriate antidiuretic hormone secretion.

TABLE 19-17 Antidepressants

Indications: Treatment of depression and other psychological disorders such as panic, obsessive compulsive disorder, etc.; some agents in this class can be used to treat neuropathic pain (TCAs) or to prevent migraines (TCAs, SSRIs). It takes 4-6 weeks before full efficacy of drug therapy can be assessed.

Mechanism of Action	Generic Name (Common Brand Name[s])	Adverse Effects	PT Considerations
Monoamine oxidase (MAO) inhibitors: Increase the synaptic concentrations of NE, 5-HT, and DA by inhibiting monoamine oxidase (breakdown enzyme)	Phenelzine (Nardil), tranylcypromine (Parnate)	Orthostatic hypotension, weight gain, sexual dysfunction, anticholinergic effects, hypertensive crisis	These agents are reserved for those with depression refractory to other treatments due to many drug-drug interactions (contraindicated with other drugs that increase 5-HT and/or NE) and dietary restrictions (avoid tyramine-containing foods).
Norepinephrine-dopamine reuptake inhibitor (NDRI): Inhibits NE and DA reuptake	Bupropion (Wellbutrin, Zyban)	GI upset, insomnia, anxiety, headache, decreases seizure threshold	Used for smoking cessation. Causes less sexual dysfunction, but monitor for seizures
Selective serotonin reuptake inhibitors (SSRIs): Selectively inhibit 5-HT reuptake	Citalopram (Celexa), escitalopram (Lexapro), fluoxetine (Prozac, Sarafem), fluvoxamine (Luvox), paroxetine (Paxil), sertraline (Zoloft)	GI complaints, nervousness, insomnia, headache, fatigue, sexual dysfunction. Safer in overdose. SSRI withdrawal syndrome: flulike symptoms, dizziness, nausea, tremor, anxiety, and palpitations	These are considered first-line treatment due to good tolerability profile. Patients should not abruptly discontinue SSRIs (taper over 2-4 weeks, with the exception of fluoxetine)
Serotonin-norepinephrine reuptake inhibitors (SNRI): Inhibit reuptake of NE and 5-HT	Duloxetine (Cymbalta), venlafaxine (Effexor)	GI upset, anxiety, headache, dose-related hypertension	Duloxetine has an indication for the treatment of diabetic neuropathic pain. Monitor blood pressure.
Serotonergic (dual-acting): Inhibit serotonin reuptake similar to SSRIs and serve as partial agonists at 5-HT$_{1A}$ receptor	Vilazadone (Viibryd)	Diarrhea, nausea, dizziness, dry mouth, insomnia, and decreased libido	This agent appears to be as effective as SSRIs but causes more GI upset; dose titration can minimize GI upset. Schedule PT sessions when patients experience less side effects.
Tricyclic antidepressants (TCAs): Increase synaptic concentration of 5-HT and/or NE in the CNS	Amitriptyline (Elavil), clomipramine (Anafranil), desipramine (Norpramin), doxepin (Sinequan), nortriptyline (Pamelor)	Orthostatic hypotension, tachycardia, sedation, anticholinergic effects, arrhythmias (prolongs QT), weight gain, sexual dysfunction	Establish the time of the day when sedation is minimal to schedule PT sessions. TCAs are deadly in overdose (they block sinoatrial node). Drug serum levels can be obtained to guide therapy.
Mirtazapine: Increases 5-HT and NE in the synapses; antagonizes 5-HT2A and 5-HT3 receptors	Mirtazapine (Remeron)	Fewer GI side effects and less anxiety; sedation, increased appetite, weight gain, constipation, elevation of LFTs and TG	Sedation is more pronounced with this medication. Schedule PT sessions when patient is most alert. Design exercise program to minimize weight gain
Nefazodone: Inhibits 5-HT and NE uptake and blocks 5-HT2A receptors	Nefazodone (Serzone)	GI upset, sedation, dry mouth, constipation, lightheadedness, minimal sexual dysfunction, orthostasis, high incidence of hepatotoxicity	Monitor abdominal pain and yellow appearance for hepatotoxicity
Trazodone: Inhibits 5-HT reuptake and blocks 5-HT2A receptors	Trazodone (Desyrel)	Extremely sedating, orthostatic hypotension, priapism; no anticholinergic and cardiovascular side effects	Commonly used for insomnia due to sedating properties. Schedule sessions later in the afternoon if sedation persists into the morning

CNS, Central nervous system; *GI*, gastrointestinal; *5-HT*, 5-hydroxytryptamine; *LFTs*, liver function tests; *MAO*, monoamine oxidase; *NE*, norepinephrine; *PT*, physical therapy; *SDRI*, serotonin-dopamine reuptake inhibitor; *SNRI*, serotonin-norepinephrine reuptake inhibitor; *SSRI*, selective serotonin reuptake inhibitor; *TCA*, tricyclic antidepressant; *TG*, triglycerides.

TABLE 19-18 Antipsychotics

Indications: Treatment of various schizoaffective disorders, such as schizophrenia. Can be used to treat aggressive behaviors associated with bipolar disorders and dementia.

Mechanism of Action	Generic Name (Common Brand Name[s])	Adverse Effects	PT Considerations
Typical (conventional antipsychotics): Block postsynaptic dopamine-2 receptors. Share anticholinergic, antihistamine, and alpha-blocking properties (often producing undesirable side effects)	Chlorpromazine (Thorazine), fluphenazine (Prolixin), haloperidol (Haldol), thioridazine (Mellaril)	Sedation, orthostasis, weight gain, anticholinergic side effects (dry mouth, urinary retention, constipation, confusion), extrapyramidal side (EPS) effects (dystonia, akathisia, pseudoparkinsonism, tardive dyskinesia [TD])	Monitor for orthostasis and sedation. EPS can interfere with therapy sessions. Tardive dyskinesia is irreversible. Report first signs of TD to health care providers. (Symptom triad characteristic of TD: splayed writhing fingers; grimacing, bruxism, lip smacking; protrusion of tongue.) Design exercise programs to minimize weight gain.
Atypical antipsychotics: Weak dopamine and dopamine-2 receptor blockers that block serotonin and alpha-adrenergic, histamine, and muscarinic receptors in the CNS	Aripiprazole (Abilify), asenapine (Saphris), clozapine (Clozaril), iloperidone (Fanapt), lurasidone (Latuda), olanzapine (Zyprexa), paliperidone (Invega), quetiapine (Seroquel, Seroquel XR), risperidone (Risperdal), ziprasidone (Geodon)	Sedation, orthostasis, weight gain, new-onset diabetes, possible dose-related EPS with some agents (incidence of EPS is significantly less than with conventional agents), QT prolongation; hypersalivation and agranulocytosis with clozapine	Monitor for sedation, orthostasis, QT prolongations, signs and symptoms of hyperglycemia (excessive thirst, urination). Design programs to minimize weight gain. With clozapine, WBC count is monitored every 2 weeks; if patient becomes neutropenic, use precautions to minimize exposure to viral and bacterial illness.

CNS, Central nervous system; *EPS,* extrapyramidal side; *TD,* tardive dyskinesia; *WBC,* white blood cell.

TABLE 19-19 Mood Stabilizers

Indications: Bipolar disorders (acute treatment and prophylaxis of manic episodes).

Mechanism of Action	Generic Name (Common Brand Name[s])	Adverse Effects	PT Considerations
Lithium: Unknown; facilitates GABA and influences reuptake of serotonin and norepinephrine	Lithium (Lithobid, Eskalith CR, Cibalith-S)	Tremor, polydipsia, polyuria, nausea, diarrhea, weight gain, hypothyroidism, mental dulling	Lithium has narrow therapeutic range. Therapeutic levels are 0.6-1.2 mEq/L (acute) and 0.8-1.0 mEq/L (maintenance). Monitor signs and symptoms of lithium toxicity*

Divalproex sodium (Depakote and Carbamazepine (Tegretol) are anticonvulsant medications that can be used as mood stabilizers. See Table 19-16.

*Mild lithium toxicity (1.5-2 mEq/L): GI upset, muscle weakness, fatigue, fine hand tremor, difficulty with concentration and memory; moderate toxicity (2-2.5 mEq/L): ataxia, lethargy, nystagmus, worsening confusion, severe GI upset, coarse tremor, increased deep-tendon reflexes; severe toxicity (> 3 mEq/L): severe impaired consciousness, coma, seizures, respiratory complications, death.

GABA, Gamma-aminobutyric acid.

TABLE 19-20 Multiple Sclerosis Medications

Indications: To prevent relapse and/or maintain remission and/or delay multiple sclerosis progression.

Multiple sclerosis (MS) is a complex disorder. Pharmacological treatment of MS falls into three categories: symptomatic therapy, treatment of acute attacks, and disease-modifying therapies. Acute exacerbations are managed with high doses of systemic corticosteroids (e.g., methylprednisolone), whereas many of the medications described in other tables are used for managing symptoms of MS, such as agents to treat constipation, spasticity, depression, and other symptoms. This table reviews disease-modifying agents used to prevent relapse, maintain remission, and delay disease progression.

Mechanism of Action	Generic Name (Common Brand Name[s])	Adverse Effects	PT Considerations
Fingolimod: First oral disease modifying drug for MS. It is a sphingosine 1-phosphate receptor agonist	Fingolimod (Gilenya)	Pronounced first-dose bradycardia (rarely bradyarrhythmia or first-degree AV block). Can rarely cause infections, macular edema, decrease in FEV_1, elevated LFTs, and increase in blood pressure.	Avoid scheduling therapy after first dose administration. Monitor vision changes, exercise tolerance, and blood pressure.
Glatiramer: Mechanism is not completely understood, but glatiramer appears to mimic the antigenic properties of myelin basic protein and induce antiinflammatory lymphocytes, thereby reducing inflammation, demyelination, and axonal damage	Glatiramer (Copaxone)	Mild pain and itching at the injection site. Approximately 10% experience a one-time transient reaction consisting of chest tightness, flushing, and dyspnea beginning several minutes after injection and lasting up to 20 minutes.	This agent is relatively well tolerated. The one-time transient injection reaction present similarly to angina, so be aware of it if working with patients initiated on glatiramer.
Interferon: Mechanism is not completely understood, but likely effect is caused via immunomodulation. Interferon augments suppressor cell function, reduces INF-gamma secretion by activated lymphocytes, and activates macrophages. It also suppresses T-cell proliferation and increases the production of natural killer cells.	Interferon beta 1a (Avonex, Rebif); interferon beta 1b (Betaseron, Extavia)	Commonly cause injection site redness and swelling, as well as flulike symptoms (fevers, chills, myalgias). Less common: tachycardia, depression, thyroid dysfunction, elevated LFTs, thrombocytopenia.	Flulike symptoms typically occur for up to 24 hours post injection (most patients receive injections once a week), so scheduling therapy sessions at least a day after injection is best. Monitor injection sites for signs and symptoms of possible infection.
Mitoxantrone: Chemotherapeutic agent that works in MS by suppressing T cells, B cells, and macrophages that are thought to lead the attack on the myelin sheath.	Mitoxantrone (Novantrone)	Cardiotoxic with maximum lifetime dose of 140 mg/m². Other side effects include nausea, alopecia, and upper respiratory and urinary tract infections.	Monitor for signs and symptoms of congestive heart failure, such as edema, shortness of breath, and exercise intolerance.

AV, Atrioventricular; *FEV*₁, forced expiratory volume over 1 second; *INF*, interferon; *LFTs*, liver function tests.

TABLE 19-21 Parkinson's Medications

Indications: Treat signs and symptoms associated with Parkinson's disease.

Mechanism of Action	Generic Name (Common Brand Name[s])	Adverse Effects	PT Considerations
Amantadine: Antiparkinsonian activity may be due to its blocking the reuptake of dopamine into presynaptic neurons or by increasing dopamine release from presynaptic fibers.	Amantadine (Symmetrel)	Orthostasis, peripheral edema, anxiety, ataxia, dizziness, hallucinations, insomnia, somnolence, anorexia, GI upset	Rarely used; often combined with other agents.
Anticholinergics: Possess both anticholinergic and antihistaminic effects; may also inhibit the reuptake and storage of dopamine, thereby prolonging the action of dopamine.	Benztropine (Cogentin), biperiden (Akineton) procyclidine (Kemadrin), orphenadrine (Disipal, Norflex), trihexyphenidyl hydrochloride (Artane, Trihexy-5)	Dry mouth, blurred vision, constipation, nausea, urinary retention, tachycardia, somnolence, confusion	First line for tremor-predominant disease; can be used to treat motor complications (dyskinesias) of dopaminergic agents.
COMT inhibitors: Inhibit catechol-O-methyltransferase (COMT). Combined with levodopa resulting in more sustained levodopa serum levels, thereby providing for increased CNS levels of dopamine, the active metabolite of levodopa.	Entacapone (Comtan), tolcapone (Tasmar)	Nausea, dyskinesias, orthostasis, dizziness, hallucinations, diarrhea, brown-orange urine discoloration. Hepatotoxicity with tolcapone	These drugs are added to levodopa in order to optimize motor function and reduce motor complications. Patients should be taking one of these with each dose of levodopa.
Dopamine agonists: Centrally active dopamine agonists exert their therapeutic effect by directly stimulating postsynaptic dopamine receptors in the nigrostriatal system.	Bromocriptine mesylate (Parlodel), pergolide mesylate (Permax), pramipexole (Mirapex), ropinirole hydrochloride (Requip)	Nausea and vomiting, dizziness or fainting; sudden, unpredictable attacks of sleepiness (these can be very dangerous if they occur while a person is driving); orthostatic hypotension; confusion or hallucinations; depression; insomnia; dyskinesias; irregular heart rate and chest pain	These are first line in younger patients. Compared to levodopa, the motor complications are less common; however, sleep attacks are more common. Determine the pattern of side effects before scheduling a session. Pergolide has been withdrawn from the market because of heart valve damage (March 2007).
Levodopa/carbidopa: Levodopa converts into dopamine; carbidopa is a peripheral decarboxylase inhibitor that does not allow for conversion of levodopa into dopamine in the periphery. Carbidopa does not penetrate the blood-brain barrier and allows for levodopa to convert to dopamine in the brain at the site of dopamine deficiency.	Levodopa (Dopar, Larodopa), carbidopa (Lodosyn) Levodopa/carbidopa (Sinemet, Sinemet CR)	Orthostasis, hypertension, arrhythmias, dizziness, confusion, nightmares, hallucinations, psychosis, gait abnormalities, increased libido, GI upset, sialorrhea, discoloration of urine and sweat, hemolytic anemia, pancytopenia, LFT elevations, choreiform and involuntary movements, paresthesia, bone pain, shoulder pain, muscle cramps, weakness, hiccups, dyskinesias	Many side effects occur because of some peripheral conversion to dopamine. Onset of action is 30 minutes for Sinemet and 60 minutes for Sinemet CR. Timing your exercise session during the peak activity of Sinemet is best. Patients will require increased dose and frequency as the disease progresses. Motor abnormalities and dyskinesias are predominant side effects that require management.
Selegiline: Potent irreversible inhibitor of monoamine oxidase with specificity for MAO-B at commonly used doses. MAO-B plays a major role in metabolism of dopamine, so selegiline increases dopamine concentrations in the brain.	Selegiline (Eldepryl, Emsam, Zelapar)	Headache, insomnia, dizziness, nausea, hypotension, orthostasis, diarrhea, weight loss	At doses higher than 20 mg per day (recommended dose is 10 mg per day), MAO-B specificity is lost and patients can experience hypertensive crisis with any other serotonergic, sympathomimetic drugs and foods.

Combination: Stalevo (levodopa + carbidopa + entacapone).
CNS, Central nervous system; *MAO*, monoamine oxidase.

Oncology

TABLE 19-22 Antiemetic Medications

Indications: Prevention and treatment of nausea and vomiting from any causes, including chemotherapy and radiation-induced and postoperative nausea and vomiting.

Mechanism of Action	Generic Name (Common Brand Name[s])	Adverse Effects	PT Considerations
5-HT3 receptor antagonists: Selective 5-HT3-receptor antagonists; block serotonin, both peripherally on vagal nerve terminals and centrally in the chemoreceptor trigger zone	Dolasetron (Anzemet), granisetron (Kytril), ondansetron (Zofran), palonosetron (Aloxi)	Well tolerated; headache, constipation, dizziness	Nausea and vomiting is common for the first 24 hours post chemotherapy, but can occur for up to 5 days. Assess severity and frequency before scheduling therapy.
Benzamides: Block dopamine receptors and (when given in higher doses) also blocks serotonin receptors in chemoreceptor trigger zone of the CNS	Metoclopramide (Reglan)	Drowsiness, fatigue, acute dystonic reactions, akathisia, confusion, neuroleptic malignant syndrome (rare), Parkinsonian-like symptoms, diarrhea	Monitor vitals and extrapyramidal symptoms.
Butyrophenones: Antiemetic effect is a result of blockade of dopamine stimulation of the chemoreceptor trigger zone	Droperidol (Inapsine), haloperidol (Haldol)	QT prolongation, restlessness, anxiety, extrapyramidal symptoms, seizure, altered central temperature regulation, sedation, drowsiness	Monitor for QT prolongation on ECG (high risk for torsades); schedule the session when the patient is least sedated.
Cannabinoids: Unknown, may inhibit endorphins in the brain's emetic center, suppress prostaglandin synthesis, and/or inhibit medullary activity through an unspecified cortical action	Dronabinol (Marinol)	Palpitations, vasodilation/facial flushing, euphoria, dizziness, paranoia, somnolence, amnesia, anxiety, ataxia, hallucinations	Assess adverse side effects before scheduling the session; can also be used as an appetite stimulant in cachexia.

CNS, Central nervous system; *ECG,* electrocardiogram; *5-HT,* 5-hydroxytryptamine.

TABLE 19-23 Chemotherapy

Indications: Treat malignancy; some chemotherapeutic agents are used to treat autoimmune and inflammatory disorders such as Crohn's disease and rheumatoid arthritis.

Chemotherapy has the greatest effect on rapidly dividing cells. Most of the potent agents work through damaging DNA. Therapeutic effects are seen when cancer cells are killed, while adverse effects are seen when human cells that rapidly divide are damaged. These include hair follicles, lining of the stomach and the rest of the GI tract, and bone marrow. Universal side effects: Most chemotherapeutic agents cause nausea and vomiting, mucosal ulceration, myelosuppression (decreased white blood cells, red blood cells, and platelets), and alopecia. As the result of myelosuppression, these patients are often immunocompromised and are at high risk for infection and are at increased risk of bleeding. Most chemotherapeutic agents are also carcinogenic, teratogenic, and mutagenic. Most chemotherapeutic agents cause sterility. These side effects are not discussed with each class of agents. Only the most commonly used agents are listed as examples of each class.

In general, physical therapists should avoid working with patients when their blood counts are at nadir (lowest point) and right after chemotherapy cycle administration (nausea and vomiting is most common in the first 24 hours but can occur for up to 5 days). However, a full evaluation of the patient will ultimately determine if physical therapy intervention, depending on its nature, is appropriate. Always use infection-control measures with cancer patients. Make sure that your hands are cleaned properly and any equipment is cleaned/sterilized. Avoid close contact with cancer patients if you are sick. Special measures may be necessary with patients who are neutropenic (decreased white blood cell count), such as facial masks and isolation from other patients. Although this table attempts to highlight the major side effects of each class of chemotherapeutic agents, adverse events profiles vary from agent to agent within the same class, and careful review of a specific agent's side effects is recommended when working with cancer patients.

TABLE 19-23 Chemotherapy—cont'd

Mechanism of Action	Generic Name (Common Brand Name[s])	Adverse Effects	PT Considerations
Alkylating agents: Form covalent bonds with nucleic acids and proteins resulting in cross-linking of DNA stands and inhibition of DNA replication	Carmustine (BICNU), cyclophosphamide (Cytoxan, Neosar), dacarbazine (DTIC-Dome), ifosfamide (Ifex), melphalan (Alkeran), temozolomide (Temodar), thiotepa (Thioplex)	Pulmonary fibrosis (carmustine) and interstitial pneumonitis, hemorrhagic cystitis (cyclophosphamide and ifosfamide), encephalopathy (ifosfamide)	Monitor for signs of pulmonary toxicity, renal function—urinary output, blood in the urine. Mesna (an adjuvant medication) and hydration are administered with cyclophosphamide and ifosfamide to decrease the risk of hemorrhagic cystitis.
Antimetabolites: Act by falsely inserting themselves in place of a pyrimidine or purine ring, causing interference in nucleic acid synthesis	Capecitabine (Xeloda), cytarabine (Cytosar-U, DepoCyt), fludarabine (Fludara), fluorouracil (5-FU, Adrucil), gemcitabine (Gemzar), mercaptopurine (Purinethol), methotrexate (Rheumatrex)	Hand-foot syndrome (redness, tenderness, and possibly peeling of the palms and soles), severe diarrhea, fatigue, neurotoxicity (cytarabine, fludarabine, methotrexate), rash and fever, flulike symptoms (gemcitabine), renal toxicity, conjunctivitis (cytarabine), hemolytic uremic syndrome (gemcitabine), tumor lysis syndrome, hepatotoxicity (methotrexate, mercaptopurine)	Monitor for tingling and swelling of the palms and soles, bruising, bleeding, diarrhea.
Antitumor antibiotics: Block DNA and/or RNA synthesis through various mechanisms	Anthracyclines: doxorubicin (Adriamycin, Doxil), daunorubicin (Cerubidine, Daunoxome), idarubicin (Idamycin), mitoxantrone (Novantrone) Alkylating-like: mitomycin (Mutamycin) Chromomycin: dactinomycin (Cosmegen) Miscellaneous: bleomycin (Blenoxane), pralatrexate (Folotyn)	Severe nausea and vomiting, stomatitis, and alopecia; acute and chronic heart failure (anthracyclines); secondary acute myelogenous leukemia; pulmonary fibrosis and interstitial pneumonitis with bleomycin; renal toxicity with dactinomycin	All anthracyclines have limits on cumulative lifetime dosing due to cardiotoxicity. Delayed nausea and vomiting is common with anthracyclines. Monitor vitals, shortness of breath, fatigue, and edema for signs of heart failure.
Biologic response modifiers and monoclonal antibodies: Biologic response modifiers activate the body's immune-mediated host defense mechanisms to cancerous cells. Monoclonal antibodies bind to specific antigens on malignant cells and cause apoptosis, an antibody-mediated toxicity, or complement-mediated lysis.	Immunologic therapies: aldesleukin (Proleukin), interferon-alpha 2b (Intron A), levamisole (ergamisol) Monoclonal antibodies: alemtuzumab (Campath), bevacizumab (Avastin), brentuximab vedotin (Adcetris), cetuximab (Erbitux), denileukin diftitox (Ontak), gemtuzumab (Mylotarg), ibritumomab (Zevalin), ipilimumab (Yervoy), ofatumumab (Arzerra), rituximab (Rituxan), sipuleucel-T (Provenge), tositumomab (Bexxar), trastuzumab (Herceptin)	Hypotension and hypersensitivity on infusion; cardiac, pulmonary, and renal impairment; depression, diarrhea (brentuximab), fever, fatigue, chills, nausea, musculoskeletal pain; tumor lysis (rituximab); bleeding, hemorrhage, hypertension, proteinuria, rash (bevacizumab and brentuximab); cutaneous and infusion reactions, interstitial lung disease (cetuximab); hypothyroidism (tositumomab), sensory neuropathy (brentuximab)	Patients are typically premedicated with Tylenol and Benadryl to decrease infusion-related reactions. Monitor for hypertension, fever, and organ toxicity (lung: respiratory problems; heart: blood pressure, pulse, exercise tolerance; kidney: urine output, weight, serum creatinine)
Histone deacetylase inhibitor: Induces cell cycle arrest and apoptosis	Romidepsin (Istodax)	Loss of appetite, nausea, vomiting, fatigue, infections	Monitor blood cells for anemia, leukopenia, neutropenia, and thrombocytopenia

Continued

TABLE 19-23 Chemotherapy—cont'd

Mechanism of Action	Generic Name (Common Brand Name[s])	Adverse Effects	PT Considerations
Hormones and antagonists: Act on hormone-dependent tumors by inhibiting or decreasing the production of disease-causing hormone	Androgens: testosterone (Delatestryl), fluoxymesterone (Halotestin) Antiandrogens: abiraterone (Zytiga), dutasteride/ tamsulosin (Jalyn), flutamide (Eulexin), bicalutamide (Casodex), nilutamide (Nilandron) Antiestrogens: tamoxifen (Nolvadex) Aromatase inhibitors: exemestane (Aromasin), anastrozole (Arimidex), letrozole (Femara) Estrogens: ethinyl estradiol (Estinyl) GNRH agonists: abarelix (Plenaxis) LHRH agonists: goserelin (Zoladex), leuprolide (Lupron, Eligard), triptorelin (Trelstar) Progestins: megestrol (Megace), medroxyprogesterone (Provera)	Edema, menstrual disorders, hot flashes, transient bone and muscle pain, thromboembolic events, gynecomastia, elevated liver enzymes, diarrhea, impotence, decreased libido, endometrial cancer (tamoxifen), bone loss (LHRH and aromatase inhibitors); hypotension and syncope (abarelix)	Note weight changes, abnormal vaginal bleeding, body and bone pain. Monitor for embolic disorders (DVT: pain and swelling in the extremities; PE: shortness of breath, chest pain)
Microtubule inhibitors: Inhibit growth phase of microtubules leading to apoptotic cell death	cabazitaxel (Jevtana), eribulin (Halaven)	Diarrhea, nausea, fatigue, anemia, leukopenia, neutropenia, and thrombocytopenia	Monitor blood cell counts; fatigue caused by anemia may interfere with PT; patients with low platelet count have high risk of bleeding.
Plant alkaloids: Inhibit replication of cancerous cells through various mechanisms	Camtothecins: irinotecan (Camtosar), topotecan (Hycamtin) Epipodophyllotoxins: etoposide (VePesid), Teniposide (Vumon) Taxanes: docetaxel (Taxotere), paclitaxel (Taxol, Abraxane) Vinca alkaloids: vinblastine (Velban), vincristine (Oncovin), vinorelbine (Navelbine)	Edema (docetaxel), hypotension/ hypersensitivity upon administration (paclitaxel), neurotoxicity (vincristine), diarrhea, headache, secondary malignancies (epipodophyllotoxins), syndrome of inappropriate antidiuretic hormone secretion (vinca alkaloids)	Monitor for peripheral neuropathy, blood pressure decrease. Acute and late-onset diarrhea may interfere with therapy sessions.
Platinum compounds: Alkylating-like, cause inhibition of DNA synthesis	Carboplatin (Paraplatin), cisplatin (Platinol-AQ), oxaliplatin (Eloxatin)	Nephrotoxicity, peripheral neurotoxicity, ototoxicity	These agents are associated with severe acute and delayed nausea and vomiting; monitor hearing and urinary output, as well as symptoms of peripheral neuropathy
Kinase inhibitors: Inhibit tyrosine kinase, rapamycin kinase (everolimus), serine-threonine kinase (vemurafenib)	Crizotinib (Xalkori), dasatinib (Sprycel), erlotinib (Tarceva), everolimus (Afinitor), gefitinib (Iressa), imatinib (Gleevec), pazopanib (Votrient), sunitinib (Sutent), vandetanib (Caprelsa), vemurafenib (Zelboraf)	Hepatotoxicity, hypertension, fluid retention, weight gain, neutropenia, GI effects, muscle cramps (imatinib); rash, interstitial lung disease (erlotinib); rash, acne (gefitinib); disorder of vision (crizotinib)	

DNA, Deoxyribonucleic acid; *DVT,* deep venous thrombosis; *GNRH,* gonadotropin-releasing hormone, *LHRH,* luteinizing hormone–releasing hormone; *PE,* pulmonary embolism; *PT,* physical therapy; *RNA,* ribonucleic acid.

Vascular System and Hematology

TABLE 19-24 Colony-Stimulating Factors

Indications: Stimulate formation of white and red blood cells.

Mechanism of Action	Generic Name (Common Brand Name[s])	Adverse Effects	PT Considerations
Erythropoiesis-stimulating: Induces erythropoiesis by stimulating the division and differentiation of committed erythroid progenitor cells; induces the release of reticulocytes from the bone marrow into the bloodstream, where they mature to erythrocytes	Darbepoetin alpha (Aranesp), epoetin alpha (Epogen, Procrit)	Hypertension, thrombotic and vascular events, edema, DVT, fever, dizziness, insomnia, headache, pruritus, GI upset, arthralgias, seizures (rare)	Monitor hemoglobin and hematocrit; higher values are associated with thromboembolic complications; monitor blood pressure
Granulocyte-stimulating: Stimulates the production, maturation, and activation of neutrophils. Sargramostim also stimulates the production, maturation, and activation of eosinophils, monocytes, and macrophages	Filgrastim (Neupogen, G-CSF), pegfilgrastim (Neulasta, G-CSF), sargramostim (Leukine, GM-CSF)	Hypertension, edema, chest pain, fever, headache, chills, rash, pruritus, weakness, bone pain, arthralgias, myalgias, GI upset; increase in serum creatinine, bilirubin, serum glucose, and cholesterol (sargramostim)	Monitor for musculoskeletal pain; vital signs. G-CSF and GM-CSF is often used in severely neutropenic patients (high infection risk)—use infection-control measures.

G-CSF, Granulocyte-colony stimulating factor; *GI,* gastrointestinal; *GM-CSF,* granulocyte-macrophage colony-stimulating factor; *GI,* gastrointestinal; *DVT,* deep venous thrombosis.

Gastrointestinal System

TABLE 19-25 Antacids

Indications: Acid suppression for treatment of mild GERD and heartburn; adjunct therapy with more potent acid suppressive therapy (PPIs and H_2RAs) for breakthrough symptoms; can be used as phosphate binders in patients with renal disease.
There are a variety of antacids on the market. All are available over the counter. Antacids contain cations such as aluminum, calcium, magnesium, or a combination. Sodium bicarbonate can also be used as an antacid. Only the most common antacids are presented below. Antacids that contain calcium or magnesium have more ANC (acid neutralizing capacity) per milliliter of suspension or tablet (i.e., they are more potent). Alginic acid acts as an absorbent and is sometimes added to antacid formulations. Combination products are available with improved GI side-effect profile.

Mechanism of Action	Generic Name (Common Brand Name[s])	Adverse Effects	PT Considerations
Antacids neutralize gastric acid and inhibit conversion of pepsinogen to pepsin, thus raising the pH of gastric contents; alginic acid reacts with sodium bicarbonate in saliva to form sodium alginate viscous solution, which floats on the surface of gastric contents and acts as a protective barrier	Aluminum based: aluminum carbonate (Badaljel), aluminum hydroxide (Amphojel, ALternaGEL)	Constipation, hypophosphatemia and bone demineralization; toxicity in patients with renal disease—bone abnormalities	Constipation can interfere with PT; monitor for aluminum toxicity in patients with reduced renal function.
	Calcium based: calcium carbonate (TUMs)	Constipation	Constipation can interfere with PT.
	Magnesium based: magnesium hydroxide	Diarrhea; toxicity in patients with renal disease—deep tendon reflex reduction, muscle weakness, arrhythmias	Diarrhea can interfere with PT; monitor for signs and symptoms of toxicity in patients with reduced renal function.
	Sodium bicarbonate (Alka-Seltzer)	Water retention, edema, exacerbation of hypertension, and heart failure	Avoid in patients with cardiovascular disease.

Combination therapy: aluminum hydroxide + magnesium hydroxide (Maalox), magaldrate (Riopan), alginic acid + aluminum hydroxide + magnesium hydroxide (Gaviscon), calcium carbonate + magnesium hydroxide (Mylanta).
GI, Gastrointestinal; *PT,* physical therapy.

TABLE 19-26 Antidiarrheal Medications

Indications: Treatment of diarrhea.

Mechanism of Action	Generic Name (Common Brand Name[s])	Adverse Effects	PT Considerations
Inhibit/decrease GI motility	Diphenoxylate/atropine (Lomotil), loperamide (Imodium), opium tincture	Constipation; sedation, drowsiness, dizziness (especially with opium tincture)	Assess for presence of CNS depression and timing of diarrhea to optimize scheduling of the PT session.

CNS, Central nervous system; *GI*, gastrointestinal; *PT*, physical therapy.

TABLE 19-27 Antispasmodic Medications

Indications: Treatment of irritable bowel syndrome.

Mechanism of Action	Generic Name (Common Brand Name[s])	Adverse Effects	PT Considerations
Selectively inhibit gastrointestinal smooth muscle (via anticholinergic properties) and reduce stimulated colonic motor activity	Dicyclomine (Bentyl), hyoscyamine (Hyosin, Levsin, Levbid)	Dizziness, lightheadedness, drowsiness, xerostomia, nausea, constipation, blurred vision	Monitor for dizziness and blurred vision.

TABLE 19-28 Cytoprotective Medications

Indications: Protect GI mucosa from drug-induced or stress-related ulceration.

Mechanism of Action	Generic Name (Common Brand Name[s])	Adverse Effects	PT Considerations
Sucralfate: Forms a complex by binding with positively charged proteins in exudates, forming a viscous pastelike, adhesive substance, which serves as a protective coating that protects the lining against peptic acid, pepsin, and bile salts. Misoprostol: Synthetic prostaglandin E_1 analog that replaces the protective prostaglandins consumed with prostaglandin-inhibiting therapies (e.g., NSAIDs)	Misoprostol (Cytotec), sucralfate (Carafate)	Diarrhea, abdominal pain (misoprostol); constipation (sucralfate)	GI side effects may interfere with PT session. Sucralfate will bind other drugs and reduce their efficacy. Misoprostol is teratogenic and should not be used in women who are pregnant or may become pregnant.

Combination: misoprostol + dicolfenac (Arthrotec).

GI, Gastrointestinal; *NSAIDs*, nonsteroidal antiinflammatory drugs; *PT*, physical therapy.

TABLE 19-29 Histamine-2 Receptor Antagonists (H$_2$RAs)

Indications: Acid suppression for treatment of GERD, heartburn, peptic ulcer disease; treatment and prevention of NSAID-induced ulcers; prevention of stress ulcers and drug-induced ulcers; treatment of *H. pylori*.

Mechanism of Action	Generic Name (Common Brand Name[s])	Adverse Effects	PT Considerations
Suppress gastric acid secretion by reversibly blocking histamine-2 receptors on the surface of the gastric parietal cell	Cimetidine (Tagamet), famotidine (Pepcid), nizatidine (Axid), ranitidine (Zantac)	Very well tolerated; headache, nausea, diarrhea, constipation have been reported; confusion can occur in elderly who take high doses; gynecomastia and impotence (cimetidine)	Drug therapy should not influence PT; however, report any new signs and symptoms of GI upset or bleeding, which can occur in case of therapy failure.

Combination therapy: Ranitidine bismuth citrate (Tritec)—used specifically for the treatment of *Helicobacter pylori;* calcium carbonate + magnesium hydroxide + famotidine (Pepcid Complete OTC).

GERD, Gastroesophageal reflux disease; *GI*, gastrointestinal; *NSAID*, nonsteroidal antiinflammatory drug; *PT*, physical therapy.

TABLE 19-30 Laxatives

Indications: Treatment of constipation.

Mechanism of Action	Generic Name (Common Brand Name[s])	Adverse Effects	PT Considerations
Bulk-forming: Absorb water in the intestine to form a viscous liquid that promotes peristalsis and reduces transit time	Methylcellulose (Citrucel), polycarbophil (Fiber-lax, FiberCon), psyllium (Metamucil)	Impaction above strictures, fluid overload, gas and bloating	Patients should ensure that they drink plenty of water to prevent bowel obstruction.
Emollients: Reduce surface tension of the oil-water interface of the stool resulting in enhanced incorporation of water and fat, allowing for stool softening	Docusate (Colace), mineral oil (Fleet mineral oil enema, various)	Mineral oil decreases absorption of vitamins and many drugs	Ask patients about bowel habits and adverse effects, such as nausea, cramping, or flatulence, in order to identify the best time for PT session.
Osmolar agents: Produce an osmotic effect in the colon with resultant distention promoting peristalsis	Glycerin (Fleet glycerin suppositories), magnesium citrate (Citroma), magnesium sulfate (various), lactulose (Enulose, Generlac), polyethylene glycol (MiraLax)	Nausea, bloating, cramping, rectal irritation; magnesium toxicity in renally impaired patients	
Stimulants: Stimulate peristalsis by directly irritating the smooth muscle of the intestine	Bisacodyl (Dulcolax), senna (Senokot)	Gastric irritation, fluid and electrolyte abnormalities	
Lubiprostone: Bicyclic fatty acid that acts locally at the apical portion of the intestine as a chloride channel activator, increasing intestinal water secretion	Lubiprostone (Amitiza)	Headache, nausea, diarrhea	

Combination: docusate + senna (PeriColace).
PT, Physical therapy.

TABLE 19-31 Proton Pump Inhibitors (PPIs)

Indications: Acid suppression for treatment of GERD, peptic ulcer disease; treatment and prevention of NSAID-induced ulcers; treatment of acute GI bleed; prevention of stress ulcers and drug-induced ulcers; treatment of *Helicobacter pylori*.

Mechanism of Action	Generic Name (Common Brand Name[s])	Adverse Effects	PT Considerations
Suppress gastric acid secretion specifically by inhibiting the H^+-ATPase, K^+-ATPase enzyme system of the secretory surface of the gastric parietal cell	Esomeprazole (Nexium), omeprazole (Prilosec), lansoprazole (Prevacid SoluTab), pantoprazole (Protonix), rabeprazole (Aciphex)	Very well tolerated; headache, nausea, diarrhea, constipation have been reported; increase the incidence of *Clostridium difficile*–associated diarrhea	Drug therapy should not influence PT; however, report any new signs and symptoms of GI upset or bleeding that can occur in case of therapy failure.

Combination therapy: lansoprazole + amoxicillin + clarithromycin (Prevpac)—This combination is in terms of packaging only. Medications are not combined into one pill, but rather packaged together for convenience to improve compliance with this commonly utilized *H. pylori* regimen.

ATP, Adenosine 5′-triphosphate; *GERD,* gastroesophageal reflux disease *GI,* gastrointestinal; *NSAID,* nonsteroidal antiinflammatory drug; *PT,* physical therapy.

Genitourinary System

TABLE 19-32 Benign Prostatic Hyperplasia (BPH) Therapy

Indications: Treatment of symptomatic benign prostatic hyperplasia.

Mechanism of Action	Generic Name (Common Brand Name[s])	Adverse Effects	PT Considerations
Alpha-1 blockers: Competitively inhibit postsynaptic alpha1-adrenergic receptors in prostatic stromal and bladder neck tissues. This reduces the sympathetic tone-induced urethral stricture causing BPH symptoms	Alfuzosin (Uroxatral), doxazosin (Cardura), prazosin (Minipress), tamsulosin (Flomax), terazosin (Hytrin)	Dizziness, palpitations, orthostatic hypotension, syncope, headache, drowsiness, urinary frequency	Monitor blood pressure (hypotension). Patients will be at risk for orthostasis; use caution when exercising.
5-Alpha-reductase inhibitors: Competitive inhibitor of both tissue and hepatic 5-alpha reductase. This results in inhibition of the conversion of testosterone to dihydrotestosterone and markedly suppresses serum dihydrotestosterone levels	Dutasteride (Avodart), finasteride (Proscar)	Impotence, decreased libido, weakness, postural hypotension, edema, gynecomastia	Patients will be at risk for orthostasis; use caution when exercising.

PT, Physical therapy.

TABLE 19-33 Oral Contraceptives

A variety of formulations are used for contraception, including injection, transdermal, and intravaginal options. Oral contraceptives typically combine an estrogen and a progestin. There are some progestin-only contraceptives, including oral pills and injections. For the purposes of this chapter, numerous contraceptive formulations are not listed. PTs are advised to recognize the active ingredients of the particular contraceptive preparation and refer to the table below for drug information.

Mechanism of Action	Generic Name (Common Brand Name[s])	Adverse Effects	PT Considerations
Estrogens: Prevent development of dominant follicle by suppression of FSH; do not block ovulation	Ethinyl estrogen (various), mestranol (various)	Nausea, vomiting, breakthrough bleeding, spotting, breast tenderness, weight gain. Serious: venous thrombosis, pulmonary embolism, other thromboembolic disorders	Most patients tolerate oral contraceptives well. PTs should be monitoring for serious adverse effects. Remember the mnemonic ACHES: abdominal pain, chest pain, headaches, eye problems, swelling and/or aching in the legs and thighs
Progestins: Block ovulation; contributes to production of thick and impermeable cervical mucus; contribute to involution and atrophy of the endometrium	Desogestrel, norgestrel, levonorgestrel, ethynodiol diacetate, norethindrone, norethindrone acetate, norethynodrel, ulipristal (various)	Depression, headache, irritability, acne	

FSH, Follicle-stimulating hormone; *PT,* physical therapy.

Infectious Disease

TABLE 19-34 Antibiotics

Indications: Treatment and prophylaxis of infections.

Mechanism of Action	Generic Name (Common Brand Name[s])	Adverse Effects	PT Considerations
Aminoglycosides: Inhibit bacterial protein synthesis by binding to 30S ribosomal subunit and inhibiting bacterial RNA synthesis	Amikacin (Amikin), gentamicin (Garamycin), neomycin (Kantrex), streptomycin, tobramycin (AKTob, TOBI, Tobrex)	Nephrotoxicity, ototoxicity	Serum levels of aminoglycosides require monitoring. High trough levels (at the end of the dosing interval) are associated with renal toxicity. Trough levels for gentamicin and tobramycin should be < 2 mcg/ml. Monitor urine output, serum creatinine for renal function. Report any changes in patient's hearing.
Carbapenems: Inhibit cell wall synthesis, thereby causing cell lysis and death	Ertapenem (Invanz), imipenem-cilastatin (Primaxin), meropenem (Merrem)	Nausea, vomiting, diarrhea, leukopenia, thrombocytopenia, seizures (imipenem-cilastatin only)	Monitor for GI side effects.
Cephalosporins: Inhibit mucopeptide synthesis in the bacterial cell wall, which leads to cell lysis and death	First generation: cefadroxil (Duricef), cefazolin (Ancef, Kefzol), cephalexin (Keflex), cephapirin (Cefadyl), cephradine (Anspor) Second generation: cefaclor (Ceclor), cefonicid (Monocid), cefotetan (Cefotan), cefoxitin (Mefoxin), cefprozil (Cefzil), cefuroxime (Ceftin), loracarbef (Lorabid) Third generation: cefixime (Suprax), cefdinir (Omnicel), cefoperazone (Cefobid), cefotaxime (Claforan), cefpodoxime (Vantin), ceftazidime (Fortaz), ceftibuten (Cedax), ceftizoxime (Cefizox), ceftriaxone (Rocephin) Fourth generation: cefepime (Maxipime) Fifth generation: ceftaroline (Teflaro)	Allergic/hypersensitivity reactions GI side effects with oral administration: nausea, vomiting, diarrhea Serious: seizure, nephrotoxicity	Monitor for rash, hives, swelling in the face and neck for allergic reactions. Ask patients about GI side effects to optimize the time of therapy session. Monitor for resolution of infection.
Fluoroquinolones: Inhibit bacterial DNA topoisomerase and disrupts DNA replication	Ciprofloxacin (Cipro), gatifloxacin (Tequin), levofloxacin (Levaquin), lomefloxacin (Maxaquin), moxifloxacin (Avelox), ofloxacin (Floxin)	Nausea, dyspepsia, headache, dizziness, insomnia, hypoglycemia or hyperglycemia, QT prolongation, tendonitis, photosensitivity, rash, urticaria	Monitor blood sugar (may increase or decrease), especially in patients with diabetes. ECG should be checked for QT prolongation, which predisposes patients to arrhythmias. Tendon rupture has been reported; avoid any exercise that can increase that risk further. Use caution if utilizing UV light as part of therapy.

Continued

TABLE 19-34 Antibiotics—cont'd

Mechanism of Action	Generic Name (Common Brand Name[s])	Adverse Effects	PT Considerations
Macrolides and ketolides: Bind to 50S RNA subunit, thereby inhibiting RNA synthesis	Macrolides: azithromycin (Zithromax), clarithromycin (Biaxin), erythromycin (Ery-tab, various), fidaxomicin (Dificid) Ketolide: telithromycin (Ketek)	GI upset: erythromycin can stimulate GI motility and result in diarrhea; clarithromycin has the least GI side effects; QT prolongation, ototoxicity; fidaxomicin is used to treat *Clostridium difficile*–associated diarrhea	Ask patients about GI side effects to optimize the time of the therapy session. Predisposes patients to arrhythmias; monitor ECG for QT prolongation.
Lipoglycopeptides: Inhibit bacterial wall synthesis and disrupt bacterial cell membrane function	Telavancin (Vibativ)	Taste disturbance, nausea, vomiting, and foamy urine	Ask patients about GI side effects to optimize the time of the therapy session.
Penicillins: Bind to penicillin-binding proteins and inhibit cell wall synthesis in the bacteria, causing lysis and cell death	Natural penicillins: penicillin G (Pfizerpen), penicillin G procaine (Wycillin), penicillin G benzathine (Bicillin LA), penicillin V (Pen-Vee K) Penicillinase-resistance penicillins: oxacillin (Prostaphilin), Nafcillin (Nafcil, Unipen), Dicloxacillin (Dynapen, Dycill) Aminopenicillins: ampicillin (Omnipen), amoxicillin (Amoxil, Trimox) Carboxypenicillins: carbenicillin (Geopen), ticarcillin (Ticar) Ureidopenicillins: mezlocillin (Mezlin), piperacillin (Pipracil) Extended-spectrum penicillins plus beta-lactamase inhibitors: amoxicillin-clavulanic acid (Augmentin), ampicillin-sulbactam (Unasyn), piperacillin-tazobactam (Zosyn), ticarcillin-clavulanic acid (Timentin)	Allergic/hypersensitivity reactions in 3%-10% of patients GI side effects with oral administration: nausea, vomiting, diarrhea Serious: seizure (rare), hepatotoxicity (oxacillin, nafcillin)	Monitor for rash, hives, swelling in the face and neck for allergic reactions. Ask patients about GI side effects to optimize the time of therapy session. Monitor for resolution of infection
Sulfonamides: Interfere with bacterial folic acid synthesis	Sulfadiazine, sulfamethizole (Urobiotic), sulfamethoxazole/trimethoprim (Septra), sulfisoxazole (Gantrisin)	Hypersensitivity reactions, dermatologic reactions: rash, urticaria, Stevens-Johnson syndrome, photosensitivity	Monitor for changes in skin appearance; utilize caution when using UV light therapy.
Tetracyclines: Inhibit bacterial protein synthesis by binding to 30S ribosomal subunit	Demeclocycline (Declomycin), doxycycline (Vibramycin), minocycline (Minocin), tetracycline (Sumycin)	Photosensitivity reactions, hepatotoxicity, diarrhea, nausea, anorexia. Minocycline use is associated with dizziness, ataxia, vertigo, skin and mucous membrane pigmentation	Use caution if using UV light therapy. Monitor for vestibular side effects of minocycline therapy.

TABLE 19-34 Antibiotics—cont'd

Mechanism of Action	Generic Name (Common Brand Name[s])	Adverse Effects	PT Considerations
Miscellaneous			
Inhibits 50S subunit, thereby inhibiting RNA synthesis	Clindamycin (Cleocin)	Nausea, vomiting, diarrhea, abdominal pain, thrombophlebitis	Monitor for GI side effects. Diarrhea can be especially problematic with this drug; high incidence of *C. difficile* colitis (do not recommend over-the-counter antidiarrhea medications).
Binds to components of the cell membrane of susceptible organisms and causes rapid depolarization, inhibiting intracellular synthesis of DNA, RNA, and protein	Daptomycin (Cubicin)	Diarrhea, nausea, vomiting, constipation, weakness, arthralgias, increase in CPK	CPK should be checked at baseline and monitored periodically.
Binds to 23S ribosomal subunit of the 50S RNA subunit, which inhibits bacterial translation	Linezolid (Zyvox)	Myelosuppression	Monitor WBC (will decrease; use infection-control measures), hematocrit (will decrease; patient will complain of fatigue), and platelets (will decrease; patient will be at a higher risk of bleeding).
After diffusing into the organism, interacts with DNA to cause a loss of helical DNA structure and strand breakage resulting in inhibition of protein synthesis and cell death in susceptible organisms	Metronidazole (Flagyl)	Nausea, vomiting, unusual/metallic taste, dark urine, dizziness, headache	Monitor for GI adverse effects
Quinupristin inhibits late-phase protein synthesis; dalfopristin inhibits early-phase protein synthesis through binding to 50S subunit of bacterial RNA	Quinupristin-dalfopristin (Synercid)	Thrombophlebitis and severe injection site reactions, hyperbilirubinemia, arthralgias and myalgias	Monitor bilirubin (will increase, patient's skin and mucosal membranes will become more yellow, patient will complain of itching). Arthralgias and myalgias are common and can lead to drug discontinuation
Inhibits bacterial cell wall synthesis; may inhibit RNA synthesis	Vancomycin (Vancocin)	Nephrotoxicity, ototoxicity, thrombophlebitis, histamine release during or after infusion (red-man syndrome): swelling and redness in the neck and face	Avoid scheduling sessions immediately after vancomycin infusion due to possibility of "red-man syndrome." Monitor urine output and serum creatinine for renal toxicity. Report any changes in patient's hearing.

CPK, Creatine phosphokinase; *DNA,* deoxyribonucleic acid; *ECG,* electrocardiogram; *GI,* gastrointestinal; *PT,* physical therapy; *RNA,* ribonucleic acid; *WBC,* white blood cells.

TABLE 19-35 Antifungal Agents

Indications: Treatment and prevention of fungal infections.

Mechanism of Action	Generic Name (Common Brand Name[s])	Adverse Effects	PT Considerations
Binds to ergosterol in the fungal cell wall, leading to increased permeability and cell death	Amphotericin B (Fungizone), amphotericin B lipid complex (Abelcet), amphotericin B liposomal (AmBisome), amphotericin B cholesteryl sulfate complex (Amphotec)	Infusion reactions: fevers, chills, hypotension, rigors, pain, thrombophlebitis, anaphylaxis. Nephrotoxicity (common and dose-limiting); electrolyte disturbances: hypokalemia, hypocalcemia, hypomagnesemia; anemia; increase LFTs and bilirubin. The incidence of renal and infusion-related side effects is lower with lipid formulations	Avoid scheduling PT sessions immediately after amphotericin infusion. Monitor urine output and serum creatinine for renal toxicity; LFTs, abdominal pain, yellow skin appearance for hepatic failure; electrolytes (will decrease); hematocrit and hemoglobin (will decrease)
Azoles: Inhibit fungal cytochrome P450 14-alpha-demethylase, thereby decreasing ergosterol concentrations	Fluconazole (Diflucan), itraconazole (Sporanox), ketoconazole (Nizoral), voriconazole (Vfend)	Nausea, vomiting, abdominal pain, diarrhea, increase in LFTs, rash, pruritus, photosensitivity (voriconazole only)	Monitor for GI side effects; abdominal pain, yellow skin appearance for hepatotoxicity
Inhibits synthesis of β-(1,3)-D-glucan, an essential component of the cell wall of susceptible fungi	Caspofungin (Cancidas)	Increased LFTs, histamine-release reactions, such as rash, pruritus, anaphylaxis; infusion reactions: fever, nausea, vomiting, myalgias	Avoid scheduling therapy sessions immediately after caspofungin infusion. Monitor for hypersensitivity reactions

LFTs, Liver function tests; *PT,* physical therapy.

TABLE 19-36 Antitubercular Agents

Indications: Treatment and prevention of mycobacterial infections, including tuberculosis.

Mechanism of Action	Generic Name (Common Brand Name[s])	Adverse Effects	PT Considerations
Inhibits folic acid synthesis	Aminosalicylic acid (Paser)	Nausea, vomiting, abdominal pain, diarrhea, hypersensitivity reactions: fever, joint pain, skin eruptions	Monitor for GI side effects and allergic reactions.
Capreomycin is a cyclic polypeptide antimicrobial. Mechanism of action is unknown.	Capreomycin (Capastat)	Nephrotoxicity and ototoxicity in 30% of patients; elevated LFTs; hypersensitivity reactions	Monitor urine output and serum creatinine. Report any changes in patient's hearing.
Structurally similar to D-alanine and inhibits cell wall synthesis by competing for incorporation into the bacterial cell wall	Cycloserine (Seromycin)	Headache, vertigo, confusion, psychosis, seizures	Assess CNS toxicity before therapy.
Inhibits bacterial cellular metabolism	Ethambutol (Myambutol)	Optic neuritis with decreased visual acuity, loss of red-green color discrimination	Report any changes in vision.
Inhibits peptide synthesis	Ethionamide (Trecator)	Hepatitis (rare)	Monitor for hepatotoxicity (abdominal pain, yellow skin discoloration).
Unknown, but may include the inhibition of mycolic acid synthesis resulting in disruption of the bacterial cell wall	Isoniazid (Nydrazid), commonly abbreviated as INH	Peripheral neuropathy, hepatotoxicity, agranulocytosis, thrombocytopenia	Monitor for tingling and pain in the extremities; hepatotoxicity (abdominal pain, yellow skin discoloration); monitor WBC (will decrease; use infection-control measures), hematocrit (will decrease; patient will complain of fatigue), and platelets (will decrease; patient will be at a higher risk of bleeding).

TABLE 19-36 Antitubercular Agents—cont'd

Mechanism of Action	Generic Name (Common Brand Name[s])	Adverse Effects	PT Considerations
Converted to pyrazinoic acid in susceptible strains of *Mycobacterium*, which lowers the pH of the environment; exact mechanism of action unknown	Pyrazinamide (Tebrazid), commonly abbreviated as PZA	Hepatotoxicity, gout	Monitor for hepatotoxicity (abdominal pain, yellow skin discoloration); monitor for pain in joints (could indicate gout).
Inhibits RNA synthesis	Rifampin (Rifadin)	Nausea, vomiting, diarrhea, abdominal pain, headache, dizziness, mental confusion, hepatotoxicity, thrombocytopenia, leukopenia, renal insufficiency	Monitor for hepatotoxicity (abdominal pain, yellow skin discoloration); monitor WBC (will decrease; use infection-control measures), hematocrit (will decrease; patient will complain of fatigue), and platelets (will decrease; patient will be at a higher risk of bleeding); urine output and serum creatinine for renal insufficiency.

Combinations: rifampin + isoniazid (IsonaRif; Rifamate), rifampin + isoniazid + pyrazinamide (Rifater).

CNS, Central nervous system; *GI,* Gastrointestinal; *LFTs,* liver function tests; *PT,* physical therapy; *RNA,* ribonucleic acid; *WBC,* white blood cells.

TABLE 19-37 Antiretroviral Medications

Indications: Treatment of HIV/AIDS.

Treatment options for HIV/AIDS have expanded dramatically over the past decade. There are currently six classes of antiretroviral drugs. Antiretroviral therapy (ART) typically consists of three to five agents from different drug classes. Newer combination drugs allow patients to decrease the number of pills taken per day. Antiretroviral therapy is associated with much toxicity. Class common toxicities: All nucleoside reverse transcriptase inhibitors (NRTIs) can cause nausea, vomiting, and hepatic steatosis with lactic acidosis. Nonnucleoside reverse transcriptase inhibitors (NNRTIs) are associated with rash and hepatotoxicity (rash to one agent in this class does not predict rash to another agent in this class). Protease inhibitors (PIs) can cause lipodystrophy (syndrome characterized by hyperglycemia, hyperlipidemia, fat redistribution, buffalo hump, and truncal obesity), nausea, vomiting, diarrhea, and hepatotoxicity. Each individual agent within these classes has other side effects that are listed in the table below. Physical therapists should use Universal Precautions (avoid direct contact with infected body fluids). Resistance to antiretrovirals can develop fast in the setting of insufficient viral suppression. It is very important for patients to take all of their medications as prescribed or to hold all of their antiretroviral medications (as opposed to only one or two) in case of intolerable side effects. All members of the health care team should provide support for patients with HIV/AIDS and reinforce the importance of adherence to medication regimens. Antiretroviral drugs have many drug-drug and drug-food interactions. Patients should be referred to a pharmacist/physician if any over-the-counter medications or supplements are recommended. Each antiretroviral drug has a commonly used abbreviation, which may lead to confusion and medical errors.

Mechanism of Action	Generic Name (Common Brand Name[s], Abbreviation[s])	Adverse Effects	PT Considerations
NRTIs: Nucleotide analogs that compete with nucleotides for incorporation into replicating DNA, thereby aborting viral replication process	Abacavir (Ziagen, ABC)	Hypersensitivity reactions (can present as combination of the following symptoms: fever, rash, nausea, vomiting, diarrhea, abdominal pain, dyspnea, cough, pharyngitis, malaise, fatigue. HLA-B*5701 testing is performed before initiation to identify those at risk for hypersensitivity Possible increased risk of cardiovascular disease in patients with risk factors	PTs should monitor for symptoms of hypersensitivity. Patient should be referred to the prescriber at once if hypersensitivity is detected because of the potential for serious anaphylactic reactions if therapy is not discontinued. In patients with multiple cardiovascular risk factors, report any new symptoms.
	Didanosine (Videx EC, ddI)	Peripheral neuropathy, pancreatitis, diarrhea, nausea	This medication must be taken on an empty stomach. Ask patients about diarrhea to optimize scheduling therapy sessions. Monitor abdominal pain for pancreatitis and tingling and numbness in the extremities for peripheral neuropathy.

Continued

TABLE 19-37 Antiretroviral Medications—cont'd

Mechanism of Action	Generic Name (Common Brand Name[s], Abbreviation[s])	Adverse Effects	PT Considerations
	Emtricitabine (Emtriva, FTC), lamivudine (Epivir, 3TC)	Well tolerated; increased pigmentation on palms/soles	These agents are also active against hepatitis B. Acute withdrawal of it can result in hepatitis flare—monitor for new/increased abdominal pain.
	Stavudine (Zerit, D4T)	Peripheral neuropathy, pancreatitis, lipoatrophy, hyperlipidemia, rapidly ascending progressive neuromuscular weakness	Monitor abdominal pain for pancreatitis and tingling and numbness in the extremities for peripheral neuropathy. Report any neuromuscular weakness to the prescriber.
	Tenofovir (Viread, TDF)	Diarrhea, flatulence, renal insufficiency, asthenia, headache	Monitor urine output and serum creatinine for renal failure. This agent is also active against hepatitis B. Acute withdrawal of it can result in hepatitis flare—monitor for new/increased abdominal pain.
	Zidovudine (Retrovir, AZT, ZDV)	Headache, hyperpigmentation of skin and nails, anemia, neutropenia, myopathy	Monitor WBC (will decrease) and hematocrit (will decrease; patient will report fatigue). Report any muscle pain/weakness not associated with exercise.
NNRTIs: Inhibit reverse transcriptase, an enzyme involved in viral replication	Efavirenz (Sustiva, EFV)	Drowsiness, dizziness, insomnia, abnormal dreaming, agitation, hallucinations	Assess CNS side effects when scheduling PT sessions. Afternoon may be a preferred time because patients take this medication at bedtime and may still complain of side effects in the morning.
	Etravirine (Intelence, ETR)	Nausea, hypersensitivity reactions with rash, hepatic failure	Should be taken after a meal; tablets can be dispersed in water if patient has difficulty swallowing. Monitor for rash, nausea, and abdominal pain.
	Nevirapine (Viramune, Viramune XR, NVP)	Severe rash and hepatotoxicity; medication should be titrated up to decrease the incidence of rash; should be avoided in men and women with CD4 counts > 250 and 400 cells/mm^3, respectively, because of higher risk of liver toxicity	Report any indication of rash, abdominal pain, yellow skin appearance.
	Rilpivirine (Edurant, RPV)	Depression, insomnia, headache, rash	Should be taken with food; interacts with acid-reducing agents and can prolong QTc interval—monitor. Monitor mood and sleep.
Protease inhibitors: Inhibit protease, an enzyme involved in viral replication	Atazanavir (Reyataz, ATV)	Hyperbilirubinemia, prolonged PR interval on ECG, asymptomatic first-degree heart block, nephrolithiasis; does not have a negative effect on lipids	Report yellow skin/sclera appearance. Monitor HR and ECG. Encourage patients to drink a lot of noncaffeinated fluids to prevent kidney stones.
	Darunavir (Prezista, DRV)	Rash, abdominal pain, constipation	Incidence of rash is higher in those with sulfa allergy (but not contraindicated).
	Fosamprenavir (Lexiva, FPV)	Rash, nausea, diarrhea	Incidence of rash is higher in those with sulfa allergy (but not contraindicated); interacts with acid-reducing medications.

TABLE 19-37 Antiretroviral Medications—cont'd

Mechanism of Action	Generic Name (Common Brand Name[s], Abbreviation[s])	Adverse Effects	PT Considerations
	Indinavir (Crixivan, IDV)	Nephrolithiasis (kidney stones), hyperbilirubinemia	Remind patients to consume at least 48 ounces of fluid per day to prevent kidney stones.
	Lopinavir/ritonavir (Kaletra, KAL, LPV/r)	GI intolerance, asthenia, prolonged PR, rare cases of second- and third-degree heart block, prolonged QT interval	Tablets should be swallowed whole and can be taken with or without food. Solution should be taken with food to improve absorption. Ask patients about GI side effects to optimize the time of the therapy session. Monitor ECG.
	Nelfinavir (Viracept, NFV)	Diarrhea	Ask patients about GI side effects to optimize the time of the therapy session. Should be taken with food.
	Ritonavir (Norvir)	Severe GI intolerance, taste disturbances, asthenia, paresthesias	Ritonavir is commonly used in small doses to boost pharmacokinetics of another PI and is better tolerated in lower doses.
	Saquinavir (Invirase-HBC or tab, SQV)	GI intolerance, increases QTc—avoid in patients with cardiovascular disease or drugs that cause QT prolongation	Ask patients about GI side effects to optimize the time of the therapy session; monitor ECG.
	Tipranavir (Aptivus, TPV)	Hepatotoxicity, GI intolerance, increased risk of intracranial hemorrhage, rash	Monitor LFTs; ask patients about GI side effects to optimize the time of the therapy session. Rash is more common in those with sulfa allergy (not contraindicated); interacts with antacids.
Fusion inhibitor: Inhibits the fusion of HIV-1 virus with CD4 cells by blocking the conformational change in gp41 required for membrane fusion and entry into CD4 cells	Enfuvirtide (Fuzeon, T-20, ENF)	Injection-site reactions occur in all patients: itching, swelling, redness, pain or tenderness, induration, nodules and cysts; hypersensitivity reactions: rash, fever, nausea, vomiting, chills, rigors, hypotension, elevated LFTs	Monitor injection-site reactions for signs and symptoms of infection (warm, swollen). Report any signs and symptoms associated with hypersensitivity.
CCR5 inhibitor: Binds to CCR5 co-receptor on CD4 cell and prevents HIV entry into the cell in CCR5-tropic infections (note that genetic testing to establish CCR5 tropism is required)	Maraviroc (Selzentry, MVC)	Hepatotoxicity (maybe preceded by systemic hypersensitivity reaction), dizziness/postural hypotension, cough, rash, musculoskeletal symptoms, abdominal pain	Monitor and report pruritic rash, abdominal pain. Be aware of postural hypotension.
Integrase inhibitor: Inhibits the catalytic activity of HIV-1 integrase, an HIV-1 encoded enzyme that is required for viral replication.	Raltegravir (Isentress, RAL)	Diarrhea, nausea, headache, increased LFTs, myopathy, and rhabdomyolysis have been reported	Typically well tolerated; monitor for abdominal pain, gastrointestinal intolerance. Report any new muscle pain not associated with exercise; risk of myopathy is higher in combination with other drugs that can cause myopathy, such as statins.

Combinations: lamivudine + zidovudine (Combivir), lamivudine + abacavir (Epzicom), lamivudine + abacavir + zidovudine (Trizivir), tenofovir + emtricitabine (Truvada), efavirenz + tenofovir + emtricitabine (Atripla), rilpivirine + emtricitabine + tenofovir (Complera).

AIDS, Acquired immunodeficiency syndrome; *ART,* antiretroviral therapy; *CNS,* central nervous system; *DNA,* deoxyribonucleic acid; *EC,* enteric coated; *ECG,* electrocardiogram; *GI,* gastrointestinal; *HIV,* human immunodeficiency virus; *HR,* heart rate; *LFTs,* liver function tests; *NNRTI,* nonnucleoside reverse transcriptase inhibitor; *NRTI,* nucleoside reverse transcriptase inhibitor; *PI,* protease inhibitor; *PT,* physical therapy; *WBC,* white blood cell.

TABLE 19-38 Antiviral Medications

Indications: Treatment and prevention of viral illnesses.

Mechanism of Action	Generic Name (Common Brand Name[s])	Adverse Effects	PT Considerations
Inhibit DNA synthesis and viral replication by competing with deoxyguanosine triphosphate for viral DNA polymerase and being incorporated into viral DNA.	Acyclovir (Zovirax), famciclovir (Famvir), ganciclovir (Cytovene, Vitrasert), penciclovir (Denavir), valganciclovir (Valcyte; rapidly converts into ganciclovir in the body)	Malaise, headache, nausea, vomiting; topical administration can produce local redness and irritation; acyclovir IV can lead to nephrotoxicity; ganciclovir can cause neutropenia, anemia, thrombocytopenia	With IV acyclovir, monitor urine output and serum creatinine for renal function; monitor blood counts (will decrease).
Protease inhibitor indicated for treatment of genotype 1 hepatitis C in combination with peginterferon alpha and ribavirin.	Boceprevir (Victrelis)	Rash (discontinue all treatment components if progressive or severe), fatigue, itching, nausea, anemia	Monitor for rash and report to the prescriber. Fatigue that can be related to anemia may interfere with effective PT.
Cidofovir diphosphate suppresses CMV replication by selective inhibition of viral DNA synthesis. Incorporation of cidofovir into growing viral DNA chain results in reductions in the rate of viral DNA synthesis.	Cidofovir (Vistide)	Chills, fever, pain, nausea, vomiting, diarrhea, anemia, neutropenia, weakness, renal failure	This drug is administered every other week. Ask patients about toxicity to optimally schedule therapy. Monitor urine output and serum creatinine for renal function. Monitor WBC (will decrease) and hematocrit (will decrease, patient will report fatigue).
Noncompetitive inhibitor of many viral RNA and DNA polymerases as well as HIV reverse transcriptase.	Foscarnet (Foscavir)	Fever, headache, hypokalemia, hypocalcemia, hypomagnesemia, hypophosphatemia, nausea, diarrhea, vomiting, anemia, granulocytopenia, renal toxicity	Monitor temperature (will increase), electrolytes (will decrease), blood counts (will decrease).
Exert immunomodulating effect through suppression of cell proliferation, enhancement of the phagocytic activity of macrophages and augmentation of the specific cytotoxicity of lymphocytes for target cells, and inhibition of virus replication in virus-infected cells.	Interferon-alpha2b (Intron A) and peginterferon-alpha2b (Peg-Intron, Sylatron)	Most frequently reported adverse reactions were "flulike" symptoms, particularly fever, headache, chills, myalgia, and fatigue. These agents are poorly tolerated and affect almost every organ system. Serious effects include hypotension, arrhythmia, cardiomyopathy, hemorrhagic stroke, depression and suicidal behavior, bone marrow suppression, thyroid abnormalities, peripheral neuropathy, and hepatotoxicity	If working with patients on interferon therapy, become familiar with the adverse event profile and monitor for new symptoms, which should be reported to the prescriber. Fatigue and flulike symptoms will likely interfere with PT.
Inhibits influenza virus neuraminidase, with the possibility of alteration of virus particle aggregation and release.	Oseltamivir (Tamiflu), zanamivir (Relenza)	Nausea, vomiting, abdominal pain, neuropsychiatric events (self-injury, confusion, delirium)	Monitor for CNS toxicity.
Inhibits replication of RNA and DNA viruses; inhibits influenza virus RNA polymerase activity and inhibits the initiation and elongation of RNA fragments resulting in inhibition of viral protein synthesis	Ribavirin (Copegus; Rebetol)	Fatigue, headache, insomnia, nausea, anorexia, anemia, fever, depression, irritability, dizziness, alopecia, pruritus, neutropenia, anemia, thrombocytopenia, myalgia, arthralgias, muscle pain, cough, dyspnea, flulike syndrome	This medication is very toxic with high incidence of side effects. Careful determination of readiness for physical therapy should be performed.
Protease inhibitor indicated for treatment of genotype 1 hepatitis C in combination with peginterferon alpha and ribavirin	Telaprevir (Incivek)	Fatigue, anemia (over 40% of patients need erythropoiesis-stimulating agent), nausea, headache, dysgeusia (distortion of the sense of taste)	Fatigue and anemia (patient will complain of fatigue and exercise intolerance) are most likely to interfere with PT. Anemia should be corrected to facilitate effective PT.

CMV, Cytomegalovirus; *CNS,* central nervous system; *DNA,* deoxyribonucleic acid; *HIV,* human immunodeficiency virus; *IV,* intravenous; *PT,* physical therapy; *RNA,* ribonucleic acid.

Endocrine System

Diabetes

PTs should be familiar with signs and symptoms of hyperglycemia (polyuria, polydipsia, polyphagia, fatigue), hypoglycemia (shakiness, dizziness, sweating, hunger, headache, pale skin color, sudden moodiness or behavior changes, clumsy or jerky movements, seizure, difficulty paying attention, confusion, tingling sensations around the mouth), and ketoacidosis (shortness of breath, breath that smells fruity, nausea and vomiting, very dry mouth, coma). Because of the effect of exercise on blood glucose, physical therapists must pay special attention to patients with diabetes.

Well-controlled insulin-treated diabetic patients with adequate serum insulin concentrations will usually have an exercise-induced fall in blood glucose concentrations that is much larger than that in normal subjects. Several factors contribute to this response: (1) exogenous insulin cannot be shut off, thereby maintaining muscle glucose uptake and inhibiting hepatic glucose output; and (2) increased temperature and blood flow associated with exercise may speed insulin absorption from subcutaneous depots (storage/collection sites where a drug remains before its release into the bloodstream).

In contrast, exercise can cause a paradoxical elevation in blood glucose concentrations in diabetic patients with poor metabolic control (blood glucose concentration above 250 mg/dl, hypoinsulinemia, and some ketonuria). In these patients, the lack of insulin impairs glucose uptake by muscles and cannot prevent an increase in hepatic glucose output that is mediated by counterregulatory hormones. Blood glucose should be managed before, during, and after exercise. If the blood sugar (BS) is greater than 250 mg/dl, exercise should be delayed until better control is achieved. Alternatively, if the BS is close to or lower than 100 mg/dl, a carbohydrate snack should be consumed before the exercise begins. Make sure that patients are wearing proper footwear to reduce the chance of skin ulcer formation.

TABLE 19-39 Hypoglycemic Agents

Indications: Treatment of hyperglycemia in patients with diabetes mellitus or drug-induced hyperglycemia.

Mechanism of Action	Generic Name (Common Brand Name[s])	Adverse Effects	PT Considerations
Alpha-glucosidase inhibitors: Inhibit pancreatic α-amylase and intestinal brush border alpha-glucosidases, resulting in delayed hydrolysis of ingested complex carbohydrates and disaccharides and absorption of glucose	Acarbose (Precose), miglitol (Glyset)	Abdominal pain, diarrhea, flatulence	GI side effects may interfere with PT session; has an advantage of decreasing postprandial blood sugars; should be taken with each meal (skip a meal, skip a dose). Do not cause hypoglycemia if used as monotherapy (i.e., the only agent used). Use only simple sugars (i.e., glucose tabs) to treat hypoglycemic episodes, because these drugs delay the breakdown of complex carbohydrates.
Amylin analog: Synthetic analog of human amylin co-secreted with insulin by pancreatic beta cells; prolongs gastric emptying time, reduces postprandial glucagon secretion, and reduces caloric intake through centrally mediated appetite suppression	Pramlintide (Symlin)	Nausea (50% of patients), hypoglycemia (in combination with insulin)	Administered subcutaneously with meals; can be used in type 1 and type 2 diabetes as adjunct therapy with insulin. Can cause weight loss.
Biguanides: Decreases hepatic glucose production, decreasing intestinal absorption of glucose, and improves insulin sensitivity (increases peripheral glucose uptake and utilization)	Metformin (Glucophage)	Nausea, vomiting, diarrhea, flatulence, lactic acidosis	No hypoglycemia and possible weight loss are advantages of this agent; GI side effects may interfere with PT session; lactic acidosis is rare, but fatal in 50% of cases; risk factors for lactic acidosis include age > 80, reduced renal function, liver disease, ischemic/acidotic states, use of contrast dye for imaging (hold metformin for at least 48 hours postprocedure).

Continued

TABLE 19-39 Hypoglycemic Agents—cont'd

Mechanism of Action	Generic Name (Common Brand Name[s])	Adverse Effects	PT Considerations
Dopamine receptor agonist: Activates the postsynaptic dopamine receptors to inhibit prolactin secretions and also stimulates the receptors to improve motor function. The mechanism of action of improving glycemic control is poorly understood. It contributes to resetting circadian rhythms in individuals with type 2 diabetes. Central effects may reverse some of the metabolic changes associated with insulin resistance and obesity.	Bromocriptine mesylate (Cycloset)	Constipation, diarrhea, nausea, asthenia, dizziness, headache, rhinitis, fatigue	Oral therapy for type 2 DM; take with food within 2 hours of waking. Should avoid activity until drug effects are realized. This should be taken as an adjunct with other hypoglycemic agents, such as metformin. Although it does not cause hypoglycemia, it can be poorly tolerated and has only modest benefit, so other alternatives should be tried first.
DPP-IV inhibitors: Inhibit dipeptidyl peptidase IV (DPP-IV) enzyme resulting in prolonged active incretin levels. Incretin hormones (e.g., glucagon-like peptide-1 [GLP-1] and glucose-dependent insulinotropic polypeptide [GIP]) regulate glucose homeostasis by increasing insulin synthesis and release from pancreatic beta cells and decreasing glucagon secretion from pancreatic alpha cells	Linagliptin (Tradjenta) Saxagliptin (Onglyza) Sitagliptin (Januvia)	Infrequent: headache, diarrhea	Oral therapy for type 2 DM; does not cause hypoglycemia when used as monotherapy (i.e., the only agent used).
Incretin mimetic (GLP-1 analogs): An analog of the hormone incretin (glucagon-like peptide 1 or GLP-1) which increases insulin secretion, increases B-cell growth/replication, slows gastric emptying, and may decrease food intake	Exenatide (Byetta, Bydureon) Liraglutide (Victoza)	Hypoglycemia (when combined with sulfonylurea), nausea (45%); constipation, vomiting, diarrhea, nausea (less with Bydureon), headache	Administered subcutaneously with morning and evening meals to type 2 DM patients; can cause weight loss. Liraglutide is contraindicated in patients with a history of multiple endocrine neoplasia type 2 and medullary thyroid carcinoma. Bydureon is the long-acting form of exenatide and is only to be used once weekly.
Insulin: Insulin acts via specific membrane-bound receptors on target tissues to regulate metabolism of carbohydrate, protein, and fats. Normally secreted by the pancreas, insulin products are manufactured for pharmacologic use through recombinant DNA technology and are categorized based on promptness and duration of effect.	Ultra-rapid acting: Aspart (Novolin), glulisine (Apidra), insulin inhalation (Exubera), lispro (Humalog) Rapid acting: Regular (Humulin R, Novolin R) Intermediate: NPH (Humulin N, Novolin N) Intermediate to long-acting: detemir (Levemir) Long-acting: glargine (Lantus)	Atrophy or hypertrophy of subcutaneous fat tissue; hypoglycemia, weight gain; respiratory infection, cough, pharyngitis (with insulin inhalation; contraindicated in smokers and patients with respiratory disease)	Be aware of the time of onset and peak effect, and duration to peak effect, in order to determine when the hypoglycemia and hyperglycemia are most likely to occur. Rapid-acting insulins: onset within 30 minutes, peak 1-2 hours, duration 3-5 hours. Regular: onset 30 minutes, peak 2-4 hours, duration 6-8 hours. NPH: onset 1-2 hours, peak 6-12 hours, duration 18-24 hours. Detemir: onset 3-4 hours, duration (dose-dependent): 6-23 hours. Glargine: onset 3-4 hours, no peak, duration 24 hours

TABLE 19-39 Hypoglycemic Agents—cont'd

Mechanism of Action	Generic Name (Common Brand Name[s])	Adverse Effects	PT Considerations
Meglitinides (non-sulfonylurea secretagogues): Stimulates insulin release from the pancreatic beta cells	Nateglinide (Starlix), repaglinide (Prandin)	Hypoglycemia, weight gain	These agents are short-acting and are advantageous in controlling postprandial blood glucose. They should be taken with meals (skip a meal, skip the dose).
Sulfonylureas: Stimulates insulin release from the pancreatic beta cells; reduces glucose output from the liver; insulin sensitivity is increased at peripheral target sites	Glimepiride (Amaryl), glipizide (Glucotrol), glyburide (Micronase, Diabeta, Glynase)	Hypoglycemia, weight gain, photosensitivity	Monitor for hypoglycemia; design an exercise regimen to minimize weight gain; use caution when using ultraviolet light for therapy
Thiazolidinediones: Lower blood glucose by improving target cell response to insulin, without increasing pancreatic insulin secretion. It has a mechanism of action that is dependent on the presence of insulin for activity. Agonists for peroxisome proliferator-activated receptor-gamma (PPARgamma), which influences the production of a number of gene products involved in glucose and lipid metabolism	Pioglitazone (Actos), rosiglitazone (Avandia)	Edema, heart failure, weight gain; low risk of hepatotoxicity—requires periodic monitoring of LFTs; postmarketing data revealed increased risk of CVD with rosiglitazone	These drugs do not cause hypoglycemia when used as monotherapy; however, when added to existing insulin therapy, the risk of hypoglycemia is very high. These agents also have positive effects on lipid. Because of edema and heart failure risk, they should be avoided in patients with NYHA class III and IV heart failure. Postmarketing data revealed increased risk of CVD with rosiglitazone, which led to majority of prescribers switching their patients to pioglitazone.

Oral combinations: glimepiride + pioglitazone (Duetact), glimepiride + rosiglitazone (Avandaryl), glipizide + metformin (Metaglip), glyburide + metformin (Glucovance), metformin + rosiglitazone (Avandamet), metformin + saxagliptin (Kombiglyze XR), pioglitazone + sitagliptin (Janumet).

Combination insulin products are designed to decrease the number of injections and necessity to mix rapid-acting and long-acting insulins. The disadvantage of mixed insulin products is that it is more difficult to titrate the dose for tight glycemic control: insulin aspart suspension + insulin aspart (Novolog mix 70/30), regular + NPH (Novolin 70/30, Humulin 70/30), lispro suspension + lispro (Humalog mix 75/25 or 50/50).

BS, Blood sugar; *CVD,* cardiovascular disease; *DM,* diabetes mellitus; *DNA,* deoxyribonucleic acid; *GLP-1,* glucagon-like peptide 1; *LFTs,* liver function tests; *PT,* physical therapy.

TABLE 19-40 Treatment of Hyperparathyroidism

Indications: Decrease parathyroid hormone and prevent complications associated with hyperparathyroidism.

Mechanism of Action	Generic Name (Common Brand Name[s])	Adverse Effects	PT Considerations
Calcimimetic: Binds with the calcium-sensing receptor on the parathyroid gland and increases sensitivity of the receptor to extracellular calcium, thereby decreasing the stimulus for PTH secretion	Cinacalcet (Sensipar)	Hypocalcemia, nausea, vomiting, diarrhea, myalgias	Monitor calcium (will decrease); myalgias, GI side effects.
Vitamin D and analogs: Vitamin D promotes absorption of calcium in the intestines and retention at the kidneys, thereby increasing calcium levels in the serum; decreases excessive serum phosphatase levels, parathyroid hormone levels; decreases bone resorption; increases renal tubule phosphate resorption	Calcitriol (Calcijex, Rocatrol), doxercalciferol (Hectorol), ergocalciferol (Drisdol, Calciferol), paricalcitol (Zemplar)	Hypercalcemia, hyperphosphatemia, adynamic bone disease	Monitor calcium (will increase), phosphate (will increase), PTH (should decrease).

GI, Gastrointestinal; *PT,* physical therapy; *PTH,* parathyroid hormone.

TABLE 19-41 Treatment of Osteoporosis

Indications: Prevention and treatment of osteoporosis
In addition to medications described below, patients with osteopenia and osteoporosis should receive adequate calcium and vitamin D supplementation.

Mechanism of Action	Generic Name (Common Brand Name[s])	Adverse Effects	PT Considerations
Bisphosphonates: Inhibit osteoclast-mediated bone reabsorption and induces osteoclast apoptosis (zoledronic acid)	Alendronate (Fosamax or Fosamax plus D), ibandronate (Boniva), risedronate (Actonel or Actonel with Calcium), zoledronic acid (Reclast)	GI issues (mostly esophageal), fever (alendronate), nausea, visual disturbances Zoledronic acid: atrial fibrillation, bone metastasis	Zoledronic acid is given as an injection once yearly. The other agents are oral and must be taken on an empty stomach with a full glass of water; the patient then must wait 30-60 minutes upright before eating, drinking, or taking other medications.
Calcitonin: Reduces number of osteoclasts and prevents the resorptive activity, also increases osteoblast activity	Salmon calcitonin (Fortical and Miacalcin)	Mild: nausea	Available as an intranasal spray or injection.
Estrogen/hormone therapy: Bind to estrogen-responsive tissues and reduce the levels of gonadotropins, luteinizing hormone, and follicle-stimulating hormone in postmenopausal women	Conjugated estrogens (Premarin), conjugated estrogens/medroxyprogesterone acetate (Premphase and Prempro), ethinyl estradiol/norethindrone acetate (Femhrt), estradiol (Climara, Estrace, Vivelle dot), estradiol/norethindrone acetate (Activella), estropipate (Ogen, Ortho-Est)	Mild: headache, edema, nausea Serious: breast cancer, DVT, myocardial infarction, pulmonary emboli, stroke	Women who have not had a hysterectomy require one of the compounds containing medroxyprogesterone acetate or norethindrone acetate. Monitor for abnormal vaginal bleeding; estrogens can increase the risk of endometrial cancer. Activella, Climara, Estrace, and Premarin come in different formulations.
Estrogen agonists/antagonists: Reduce bone resorption and increases bone mineral density by selectively activating and blocking estrogenic pathways	Raloxifene (Evista)	Mild: hot flashes Serious: DVT	Avoid in women with a history of venous thromboembolism.
Parathyroid hormone: Reduces the number of osteoclasts and prevents resorptive activity of the bone	Teriparatide (Forteo)	Constipation, indigestion, leg cramps, nausea, spasms	Causes an increase in the incidence of osteosarcoma.
RANK inhibitor: Binds to the protein RANKL, inhibiting the formation, function, and survival of osteoclasts	Denosumab (Prolia)	Diarrhea, headache, fatigue, musculoskeletal pain, nausea, vomiting	

DVT, Deep vein thrombosis; *GI*, gastrointestinal; *PT*, physical therapy.

TABLE 19-42 Treatment of Thyroid Disorders

Indications: Treatment of hypothyroidism and hyperthyroidism.

Mechanism of Action	Generic Name (Common Brand Name[s])	Adverse Effects	PT Considerations
Hyperthyroidism Inhibit synthesis of thyroid hormones by preventing the incorporation of iodine into iodotyrosines and by inhibiting the coupling of monoiodotyrosine and diiodotyrosine to form thyroxine (T_4) and triiodothyronine (T_3); PTU also inhibits peripheral conversion of T_4 to T_3	Methimazole (Tapazole), propylthiouracil (commonly abbreviated as PTU)	Fever, headache, paresthesias, rash, arthralgia, urticaria, jaundice, hepatitis, agranulocytosis, leukopenia, bleeding	Monitor for improvement of signs and symptoms of hyperparathyroidism; monitor blood counts (will decrease, patient will complain of fever, malaise, sore throat).
Iodides: Block hormone release, inhibit thyroid hormone synthesis	Strong iodide solution (Lugol's solution), saturated solution of potassium iodide (SSKI)	Rash, swelling of salivary glands, metallic taste, burning of the mouth, GI distress, hypersensitivity, goiter	Monitor for improvement of signs and symptoms of hyperparathyroidism.
Hypothyroidism Thyroid hormones: Enhance oxygen consumption by most tissues and increase basal metabolic rate and metabolism of carbohydrates, lipids, and proteins	Desiccated thyroid (Armour Thyroid, Nature-Throid), levothyroxine (Levothroid, Levoxyl, Synthroid, Thyro-Tabs, Unithroid), liothyronine (Cytomel, Triostat), liotrix (Thyrolar)	Tachycardia, arrhythmia, angina, MI, tremor, headache, nervousness, insomnia, hyperactivity, diarrhea, nausea, vomiting, cramps, weight loss, fatigue, menstrual irregularities, excessive sweating, heat intolerance, fever, muscle weakness, decreased bone mineral density	Mostly well tolerated as long as patient maintains normal thyroid state. Dose that is too high will produce signs and symptoms of hyperthyroidism.

Organ Transplantation

TABLE 19-43 Immunosuppressants

Immunosuppressive therapy is essential to prevent organ rejection after transplantation. Immunosuppression protocols vary by transplant center and specific organ transplanted. The principles remain the same, however. Initially, immunosuppression is more aggressive, with the ultimate goal of reducing the doses and number of agents used to optimize graft and patient survival. To achieve this, several immunosuppressive agents must be monitored by serum concentration levels (these levels vary depending on time since transplant and other concomitant agents). Multidrug regimens are common to reduce doses of individual agents and, therefore, side effects, while maintaining the efficacy. Systemic corticosteroids (see Table 19-8) are often used immediately posttransplant, but can be used for maintenance immunosuppression at low doses. Patients on immunosuppressive therapy are at high risk for typical and atypical infections, and infection control measures must be used to reduce their exposure to bacteria and viruses. Most immunosuppressants have drug-drug interactions, so advise your patients to notify providers of any medication changes. Grapefruit and grapefruit juice have potential to interact with many immunosuppressive drugs, so avoid or check for drug interaction potential with a specific regimen.

Indications: For treatment and prevention of graft rejection in patients with solid organ transplants.

Mechanism of Action	Generic Name (Common Brand Name[s])	Adverse Effects	PT Considerations
Antimetabolites: azathioprine is a pro-drug of 6-MP; through the process of metabolism these agents are converted to active metabolites that, when incorporated into the nucleic acid, disrupt DNA, RNA, and protein synthesis decreasing proliferation of immune cells	Azathioprine (Azasan, Imuran), 6-mercaptopurine (6-MP, Purinethol)	Nausea, vomiting, thrombocytopenia, leukopenia, increased risk of melanoma	

Continued

TABLE 19-43 Immunosuppressants—cont'd

Mechanism of Action	Generic Name (Common Brand Name[s])	Adverse Effects	PT Considerations
Antimetabolites: Mycophenolate—inhibits inosine monophosphate dehydrogenase resulting in decreased nucleotide synthesis, ultimately reducing lymphocyte proliferation	Mycophenolate mofetil (CellCept), mycophenolic acid (Myfortic)	Diarrhea, nausea, vomiting, leukopenia	Strategies to reduce diarrhea include dose decrease, separating dose into 3-4 times a day administration, or taking it with food; assess patient side effects before scheduling PT.
Antithymocyte globulin: These are polyclonal antibodies that bind to a wide array of lymphocyte receptors that leads to cell lysis and subsequent lymphocyte depletion	ATG (Atgam), RATG (Thymoglobulin)	Dose-limiting myelosuppression; anaphylaxis, hypotension, hypertension, tachycardia, dyspnea, urticaria, rash	These are very potent immunosuppressants used short term as induction therapy or for treatment of acute rejection.
Calcineurin inhibitors: Block T-cell proliferation by inhibiting the production of IL-2 and other cytokines by T cells	Cyclosporin modified (Gengraf, Neoral), cyclosporin nonmodified (Sandimmune), tacrolimus (FK506, Prograf)	Both: nephrotoxicity, hypertension, hyperglycemia, tremor. Cyclosporin: hyperlipidemia, gingival hyperplasia, hirsutism. Tacrolimus: diarrhea, nausea, hepatotoxicity, headache, hyperkalemia, hypomagnesemia	Monitor blood pressure (cyclosporin causes more hypertension than tacrolimus). Hyperlipidemia is more common with cyclosporin, whereas hyperglycemia is more common with tacrolimus (monitor signs such as increase in thirst and urination). Monitor and report changes in urine output.
Interleukin-2 receptor antagonist: Binds to the alpha chain on the surface of activated T cells and to IL-2 receptors, preventing IL-2 mediated activation and proliferation of T cells	Basiliximab (Simulect)	Hypersensitivity reactions and increase in risk of infections	Exercise infection-control measures.
Mammalian target of rapamycin (mTOR) inhibitors: Bind to FKBP12, forming a complex that binds to mTOR, which inhibits the response to cytokines; ultimately this inhibits T-cell proliferation	Everolimus (Afinitor, Zortress), sirolimus (also called rapamycin, Rapamune)	Dose-related myelosuppression—thrombocytopenia, anemia, and neutropenia (all improve with continued treatment); hyperlipidemia	Monitor complete blood counts. Patients with low platelets are at an elevated risk of bleeding; low hemoglobin—will complain of fatigue; low WBC—puts patients at higher risk of infection
Muromonab-CD3: Murine monoclonal antibody that binds to the CD3 receptor of mature T cells leading to T-cell depletion and functional alteration	Muromonab-CD3 (Orthoclone OKT3)	Cytokine release syndrome is common with first dose: fever, chills, rigors, pruritis, changes in blood pressure.	This is a very potent immunosuppressants used short term as induction therapy or for treatment of acute rejection

PT, Physical therapy; *WBC,* white blood cell.

References

1. Ciccone CD: Chapters 6 through 37. In Pharmacology in rehabilitation, ed 4, Philadelphia, 2007, FA Davis.

2. Lacy CF: In Lexi-Comp's drug information handbook, ed 20, Hudson, OH, 2011, Lexi-Comp.

CHAPTER 20

Anesthesia: Perioperative Considerations for the Physical Therapist

Michele P. West

CHAPTER OBJECTIVES

The objectives of this chapter are the following:

1. Describe the types of anesthesia and the perioperative physiological effects of anesthesia on the body
2. List the potential complications that can occur with anesthesia by body system
3. Provide an introduction to the basic operative body positions and discuss the potential for complications related to OR positioning
4. Discuss the physical therapy considerations related to postoperative effects of anesthesia on the patient

PREFERRED PRACTICE PATTERNS

The acute care setting is multifactorial in nature and applies to many body systems. For this reason, specific practice patterns are not delineated in this chapter. Please refer to Appendix A for a complete list of the preferred practice patterns in order to best delineate the most applicable practice pattern for a given diagnosis.

The physical therapist should have a general understanding of the types of anesthesia and the physiological impact that anesthesia can have on a patient in the perioperative phase: that is, before (preoperative), during (intraoperative), and after (postoperative) surgery. This includes an understanding of the intraoperative effects, postoperative recovery phases, and potential complications of anesthesia. Insight into these factors allows the physical therapist to intervene as safely as possible, prioritize the plan of care, modify interventions and treatment parameters, and more accurately predict length of stay, discharge disposition, and physical therapy goals.

Surgery may be classified by urgency (elective, required, urgent, or emergent) and by purpose (diagnostic, explorative, reconstructive, transplant, curative, or palliative). The surgical classification determines the preoperative preparations, operative setting, and type of anesthesia.[1]

Types of Anesthesia

There are two types of anesthesia: general and regional. General anesthesia is a reversible state of unconsciousness consisting of four components (amnesia, analgesia, inhibition of noxious reflexes, and skeletal muscle relaxation) and is achieved by the use of intravenous and inhalation anesthetics, analgesics, and muscle relaxants.[2] Regional anesthesia is used for site-specific surgical procedures of the upper or lower extremity or lower abdomen and is achieved by spinal (subarachnoid), epidural (thoracic or lumbar), or peripheral nerve blocks.[2] Local anesthesia is considered a subset of regional anesthesia and involves the topical or direct application of an anesthetic to the skin or mucosa and the injection of a local anesthetic to a superficial site.[1]

The administration of anesthesia to a patient for a brief diagnostic or surgical procedure has transitioned from the operating room (OR) to other inpatient and outpatient settings.[3] Procedural sedation (formerly conscious sedation) is characterized by the patient's ability to maintain a patent airway without intervention, spontaneously ventilate, maintain cardiovascular function, and respond purposely to verbal or tactile stimulation.[2]

Intraoperative Effects of Anesthesia

The major intraoperative effects of general anesthesia include the following[4]:

A. Neurological effects. Decreased cortical and autonomic function.
B. Metabolic effects. Hypothermia or malignant hyperthermia (in patients with a genetic predisposition).
C. Cardiovascular effects. The potential for arrhythmia, hypotension, hypertension, decreased myocardial contractility, and decreased peripheral vascular resistance.[5]
D. Respiratory effects.[6]
   1. Anesthesia has multiple effects on the lung, including decreased or altered:
      a. Arterial oxygenation
      b. Response to hypercarbia or hypoxia
      c. Vasomotor tone and airway reflex
      d. Respiratory pattern
      e. Minute ventilation
      f. Functional residual capacity
   2. The shape and motion of the chest are altered because of decreased muscle tone, which causes the following:
      a. Decreased anteroposterior diameter
      b. Increased lateral diameter
      c. Increased cephalad position of the diaphragm
   3. Other factors that affect respiratory function and increase the risk of postoperative pulmonary complications (e.g., atelectasis, pneumonia, lung collapse) include the following[7]:
      a. Underlying pulmonary disease such as chronic obstructive pulmonary disease (COPD)
      b. Incisional pain, especially if there is a thoracic or upper abdominal incision
      c. Smoking history
      d. Obesity
      e. Obstructive sleep apnea
      f. Advanced age
      g. The need for large intravenous fluid administration intraoperatively
      h. Prolonged operative time (more than 180 minutes)
      i. Emergency surgery

Postoperative Effects of Anesthesia

Immediate Postoperative Phase

In the immediate postoperative phase, the patient is transported from the OR to a postanesthesia care unit (PACU) (after general anesthesia) or to an ambulatory surgery recovery room (after regional anesthesia); both are located near the OR for continuous nursing care. The recovery period after surgery is characterized as a time of physiological alteration as a result of the operative procedure and the effects of anesthesia.[3] During this initial postoperative phase, the priorities of care are to assess emergence from anesthesia and the status of the surgical site, to determine the patient's physiological status and vital sign trends, and to identify actual or potential postsurgical problems.[8]

Discharge from the PACU is often now dependent on clinical criteria rather than time-based criteria. Specific discharge criteria and/or the use of scoring systems varies among institutions; however, the general criteria for discharge from the PACU includes stable vital signs with normothermia, adequate respiratory function, return to baseline level of consciousness, return of motor function, satisfactory pain control, satisfactory management of nausea and vomiting, and control of surgical wound bleeding/drainage.[1]

The criteria for discharge from the ambulatory recovery room are similar to those for the PACU and include recovery from sedation or nerve block.

Postsurgical Complications

During the days to weeks of the postsurgical phase, the patient is monitored for the proper function and return of all of the major body systems. The prompt prevention and recognition of potential or actual postsurgical complications is the cornerstone of high-quality care by all health care providers, including physical therapists. The development of postsurgical complication(s) in the immediate or secondary phase may be expected or unexpected and determines further medical-surgical management and treatment parameters. The most common postoperative complications include the following[9]:

A. **Neurological complications**
   1. Delayed arousal, altered consciousness, agitation, or delirium
   2. Cerebral edema, seizure, or stroke
   3. Peripheral muscle weakness or altered sensation
B. **Cardiovascular and hematological complications**
   1. Hypotension, cardiogenic shock, or both
   2. Hypertension
   3. Dysrhythmia
   4. Myocardial ischemia and/or infarction
   5. Hemorrhage
   6. Deep vein thrombosis
   7. Pulmonary embolism
C. **Respiratory complications**
   1. Airway obstruction
   2. Hypoxemia or hypercapnia

3. Atelectasis, pneumonia, or both
4. Aspiration of gastric contents
5. Hypoventilation
6. Pulmonary edema, acute lung injury, acute respiratory distress syndrome (ARDS)

D. Renal complications
1. Acute renal failure/acute kidney injury (ARF/AKI)
2. Urine retention
3. Urinary infection

E. Gastrointestinal complications
1. Nausea and vomiting
2. Hiccups
3. Abdominal distention
4. Paralytic ileus or obstruction

F. Integumentary complications
1. Wound infection
2. Wound dehiscence, evisceration, or both
3. Hematoma or seroma

G. Other complications
1. Fever
2. Sepsis
3. Hyperglycemia
4. Fluid overload or deficit
5. Electrolyte imbalance
6. Acid-base disorders

Operative Positioning

Occasionally, a patient may experience postoperative pressure-induced nerve or skin damage as a result of operative positioning, especially during a lengthy procedure. The physiological effects of anesthesia such as hypothermia, hypotension, and pharmacologically blocked pain and pressure receptors make a patient vulnerable to pressure injuries.[10] When combined with risk factors such as advanced age; poor skin integrity; altered nutrition; diabetes; peripheral vascular disease; or the presence of cancer or neurological or cardiac disease, the incidence of pressure injury increases.[10] Judicious proper operative positioning with pads, limb holders, and drawsheets can prevent or minimize these injuries.

Standard operative positions include supine (dorsal decubitus), prone (ventral decubitus, low or full jackknife), side-lying (left or right lateral decubitus, jackknife, or flexed lateral), seated, and lithotomy (standard, low, or exaggerated) (Figure 20-1).[11]

The physical therapist may be consulted in the postoperative phase to evaluate for extremity weakness related to neuropathy from stretch, compression, ischemia, metabolic derangement, and/or surgical injury or for back or joint pain related to joint stiffness from immobility or connective tissue injury.

Physical Therapy Considerations

- Typically there is a brief written operative note and a more detailed operative report that is dictated by the attending surgeon in the chart. The brief note is similar to a procedure note and may be helpful to confirm the date and time of surgery as well as the name of surgery performed. The full operative report specifically states the patient position during surgery, the exact surgical technique used, specimens that were taken, estimated blood loss, unexpected findings, and/or complications.

- A review of the anesthesiologist's notes can provide information about the patient's surgical procedure(s) and type of anesthesia, intraoperative hemodynamic and vital sign status including electrocardiographic changes, unexpected anesthetic effects, operative time, and medications given intraoperatively.

- The physical therapist should monitor vital signs such as heart rate, blood pressure, oxygen saturation, and respiratory rate when intervening with the patient because of the altered or potentially altered physiology of multiple body systems after general anesthesia.

- Careful examination of sensation and motor control in the lower extremity after a local or regional anesthetic (e.g., after knee arthroplasty) is important to prevent falls, especially when the patient is not fully aware of the impairment.

- Nausea and vomiting are among the most common patient complaints after anesthesia and may continue for days after surgery. Nausea and vomiting may make the patient reluctant to mobilize out of bed. The physical therapist may need to consider the timing of the physical therapy session relative to these symptoms as well as antiemetic medication use, mealtimes, and rest between patient position changes or other activities in the day.

- Be aware that blood sugar levels may be elevated in the diabetic or nondiabetic patient postoperatively and that hyperglycemia can be caused by medications (e.g., corticosteroids), stress, acute pain, blood loss, and lengthy surgical procedures.[12] Check for the current blood glucose levels as you would other vital signs.

- Document the development and/or resolution of any postoperative complications or changes in the physical therapy evaluation and/or treatment notes. Discuss the relevance and impact of these changes on the patient's performance in the assessment of your note.

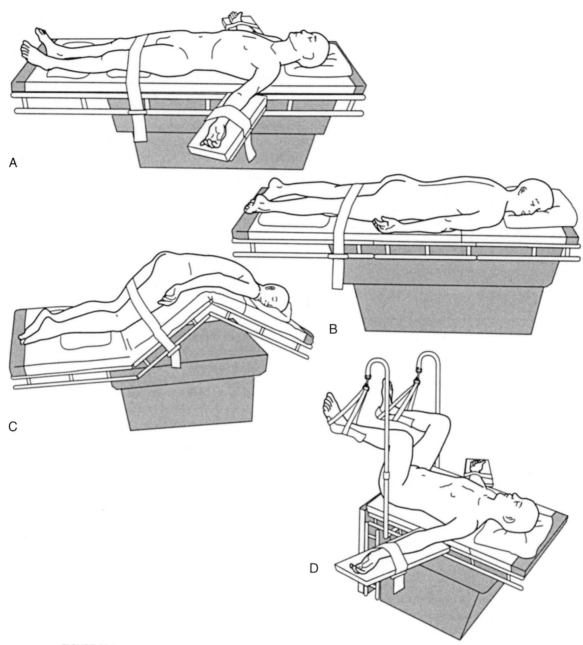

FIGURE 20-1

A, Supine position. Patient is placed on back with arms at sides or extended to 90 degrees and head in alignment with body. Legs are uncrossed, with a safety strap placed above knees. **B,** Prone position. Patient is usually anesthetized while supine, and then turned. Arms are placed at sides, with rolls beneath axillae to facilitate respiration. **C,** Jackknife position. Patient is usually anesthetized while supine, and then turned. Knees are flexed slightly to reduce lumbosacral stress. **D,** Lithotomy position. Patient is on back, and foot section of operating table is removed or lowered to 90-degree angle. Buttocks are moved to table's edge. Feet are suspended in straps to flex knees. Legs are placed into or removed from the stirrups simultaneously to avoid hip injuries.

References

1. Moe KL: Perioperative nursing. In Craven RF et al, editors: Fundamentals of nursing: human health and function, ed 7, Philadelphia, 2013, Wolters Kluwer Lippincott Williams & Wilkins, pp 534-563.

2. Sherwood E, Williams CG, Prough DS: Anesthesiology principles, pain management, and conscious sedation. In Townsend CM et al, editors: Sabiston textbook of surgery, ed 19, Philadelphia, 2012, Saunders, pp 389-417.

3. Neumeyer L, Vargo D: Principles of preoperative and operative surgery. In Townsend CM et al, editors: Sabiston textbook of surgery, ed 19, Philadelphia, 2012, Saunders, p 237.

4. Wadlund DL: Prevention, recognition, and management of nursing complications in the intraoperative and postoperative surgical patient, Nurs Clin North Am 41:151-171, 2006.

5. Wilson RS: Anesthesia for thoracic surgery. In Baue AE, Geha AS, Hammond GL et al, editors: Glenn's thoracic and cardiovascular surgery, ed 96, Stamford, CT, 1996, Appleton & Lange, p 23.

6. Hedenstierna G: Respiratory physiology. In Miller RD et al, editors: Miller's anesthesia, ed 7, Philadelphia, 2009, Churchill Livingstone, pp 361-391.

7. Lane JL: Postoperative respiratory insufficiency. In Atlee RL, editor: Complications of anesthesia, ed 2, Philadelphia, 2006, Saunders, pp 877-880.

8. Barnes D: Perianesthesia management. In Urden LD, Stacy KM, Lough ME, editors: Critical care nursing, ed 6, St Louis, 2010, Mosby, p 260.

9. Nicholau D: Postanesthesia recovery. In Miller RD, Pardo MC, editors: Basics of anesthesia, ed 6, Philadelphia, 2011, Saunders, pp 631-647.

10. Primiano M, Ffiend M, McClure C et al: Pressure ulcer prevalence and risk factors during prolonged surgical procedures, AORN J 94(6):555-566, 2011.

11. O'Connell MP: Positioning impact on the surgical patient, Nurs Clin North Am 41:173-192, 2006.

12. Rutan L, Sommers K: Hyperglycemia as a risk factor in the perioperative patient, AORN J 95(3):352-361, 2012.

CHAPTER 21

Acute Pain Management

Jaime C. Paz
Danika Quinlan

CHAPTER OBJECTIVES

The objectives of this chapter are to provide the following:

1. An overview of pain evaluation scales most applicable to the acute care setting
2. A description of physical therapy considerations when evaluating pain
3. An overview of commonly utilized management strategies for acute pain including pharmacologic agents
4. A brief description of physical therapy management strategies for acute pain

PREFERRED PRACTICE PATTERNS

Pain is multifactorial in nature and applies to many body systems. For this reason, specific practice patterns are not delineated in this chapter. Please refer to Appendix A for a complete list of the preferred practice patterns in order to best delineate the most applicable practice pattern for a given diagnosis.

This chapter provides information on the evaluation and management of acute pain with the goal of facilitating patient care. The characteristics of acute pain include less than 6 months in duration, often associated with tissue damage such as surgery or traumatic injury, the cause of pain is easily recognized, pain can be treated readily, and the duration of pain is predictable.[1] Acute pain in the medical patient may result from nonsurgical abdominal pain, renal or biliary stones, and phantom limb pain.[2]

Pain Evaluation

The subjective complaint of pain is often difficult to objectify in the inpatient setting. Patients may be mechanically ventilated, pharmacologically sedated, or in too much pain to articulate their discomfort.[3] Furthermore, patients who may be cognitively impaired are at higher risk for their pain to be undertreated with a resultant decreased quality of life.[4-6] Despite these difficulties, an effective pain treatment plan depends on an accurate evaluation of the patient's pain.[7,8]

Each evaluation requires a complete physical and diagnostic examination of the patient's pain. The criterion standard for pain assessment is through self-report by the patient because it is the most accurate indicator of the existence or intensity of his or her pain, or both.[4,5,9] The goal for evaluation should be directed toward individualization while maintaining consistency among patients. To assist with this process, various pain-rating tools have been developed to address both verbal and nonverbal (conscious or unconscious) patients.

Verbal pain scales (Table 21-1) include:
- Numeric rating scale (NRS)
- Visual analog scale (VAS)
- Verbal descriptor scale (VDS)
- Wong-Baker Faces Scale
- Functional pain scale
Nonverbal pain scales include:
- Adult Nonverbal Pain Scale (Table 21-2)
- Behavioral Pain Scale (Table 21-3)

TABLE 21-1 Verbal Pain Scales

Tool	Description
Verbal descriptor scales	The patient describes pain by choosing from a list of adjectives representing gradations of pain intensity.
Numeric Rating Scale (NRS)	The patient picks a number from 0 to 10 to rate his or her pain, with 0 indicating no pain, and 10 indicating the worst pain possible.
Visual Analog Scales (VAS)	
Line scale	The patient marks his or her pain intensity on a 10-cm line, with one end labeled "no pain," and the other end labeled "worst pain possible."
Wong-Baker Faces scale	The patient chooses one of six faces, portrayed on a scale that depicts graduated levels of distress, to represent his or her pain level.
Functional Pain Scale	A zero (0) to five (5) scale with corresponding pain descriptions 0 = No pain 1 = Tolerable (and does not prevent any activity) 2 = Tolerable (but does prevent some activities) 3 = Intolerable (but can use telephone, watch TV, or read) 4 = Intolerable (cannot use telephone, watch TV, or read) 5 = Intolerable (and unable to verbally communicate because of pain)

Data from Kittelberger KP, LeBel AA, Borsook D: Assessment of pain. In Borsook D, LeBel AA, McPeek B, editors: The Massachusetts General Hospital handbook of pain management, Boston, 1996, Little, Brown, p 27; Carey SJ, Turpin C, Smith J et al: Improving pain management in an acute care setting: the Crawford Long Hospital of Emory University experience, Orthop Nurs 16(4):29, 1997; Wong DL, Hockenberry-Eaton M, Wilson D et al: Wong's essentials of pediatric nursing, ed 6, St Louis, 2001, Mosby, p 1301; Puntillo K, Pasero C, Li D et al: Evaluation of pain in ICU patients, Chest 135:1069-1074, 2009; Gloth FM, Cheve AA, Stober CV et al: The functional pain scale: reliability, validity, and responsiveness in an elderly population, J Am Med Dir Assoc 2:110-114, 2001; Chanques G, Viel E, Constantin JM et al: The measurement of pain in intensive care unit: comparison of 5 self-report intensity scales, Pain 151:711-721, 2010.

TABLE 21-2 Adult Nonverbal Pain Scale

Categories	0	1	2
Face	No particular expression or smile	Occasional grimace, tearing, frowning, wrinkled forehead	Frequent grimace, tearing, frowning, wrinkled forehead
Activity (movement)	Lying quietly, normal position	Seeking attention through movement or slow, cautious movement	Restless, excessive activity and/or withdrawal reflexes
Guarding	Lying quietly, no positioning of hands over areas of body	Splinting areas of the body, tense	Rigid, stiff
Physiologic I (vital signs)	Stable vital signs (no change in past 4 hours)	Change over past 4 hours in any of the following: SBP > 20 mm Hg, HR > 20/min, RR > 10/min	Change over past 4 hours in any of the following: SBP > 30 mm Hg, HR > 25/min, RR > 20/min
Physiologic II	Warm, dry skin	Dilated pupils, perspiring, flushing	Diaphoretic, pallor

From Odhner M, Wegman D, Freeland N et al: Assessing pain control in nonverbal critically ill adults, Dimens Crit Care Nurs 22:260-267, 2003.
HR, Heart rate; *RR,* respiratory rate; *SBP,* systolic blood pressure.

Pain scales used for both verbal and nonverbal patients include:
- Face, Legs, Activity, Cry, Consolability (FLACC) scale (Table 21-4)
- Critical Care Pain Observational Tool (CPOT) (Table 21-5)

The validity of these scales may be improved by asking the patient about his or her current level of pain, rather than asking the patient to speculate about "usual" or "previous" levels of pain.[10]

✎ CLINICAL TIP

The therapist should be sensitive to, and respectful of, how different cultures perceive pain, as pain expression may vary among cultures.[5,11]

The therapist should be aware that some physiologic indicators exist normally in critically ill patients. One needs to analyze the behavioral trend and differentiate pain from physiologic changes.[12] The Adult Nonverbal Pain Scale is targeted toward adult patients who are intubated and sedated and is adapted from the FLACC Pain Assessment Tool.[12] The Behavioral Pain Scale (BPS) is used for mechanically ventilated, sedated patients in the intensive care unit (ICU).[4] Validity measured by BPS scores increase with painful stimuli.[13] Good construct validity (p < 0.001) has been reported for the FLACC as evidenced by decreased pain scores after administration of analgesics and from painful to nonpainful situations. The FLACC has also demonstrated good interrater reliability when assessing pain in critically ill patients.[14] This was consistent when compared among use with adults, children, and patients who are mechanically ventilated. However, there is some disagreement concerning the use of this scale with adults because of their inability to demonstrate some behaviors associated with the pediatric population. Those who disagree suggest utilizing the NVPS, as it has good interrater reliability and validity with critically ill, sedated, mechanically ventilated, and/or cognitively impaired adults.[12,14,15]

The CPOT was developed to assess pain in critically ill ICU patients and was mainly used with those recovering from cardiac surgery. It is reliable and valid in this population and further research is required for its use in other populations.[16] The CPOT can be used with both verbal and nonverbal patients.[4,16]

Physical Therapy Considerations for Pain Evaluation

- Observe pain-related behaviors to appropriately select an assessment tool. Use nonverbal assessment tools when self-report is unattainable.[5]
- Select the appropriate tool based on the clinical environment and relevance to the specific patient population.[5]

TABLE 21-3 Behavioral Pain Scale

Item	Description	Score
Facial expressions	Relaxed	1
	Partially tightened (e.g., brow lowering)	2
	Fully tightened (e.g., eyelid closing)	3
	Grimacing	4
Movements of upper limbs	No movement	1
	Partially bent	2
	Fully bent with finger flexion	3
	Permanently retracted	4
Compliance with ventilation	Tolerating movement	1
	Coughing but tolerating ventilation for most of the time	2
	Fighting ventilator	3
	Unable to control ventilation	4

From Payen JF, Bru O, Bosson JL et al: Assessing pain in critically ill sedated patients by using a behavioral pain scale, Crit Care Med 29(12):2258-2263, 2001.

- Table 21-6 provides a comparison of the various pain scales to aid in selecting an appropriate tool. The VAS and NRS tend to be used commonly in the clinical setting.[5,17]
- Patients report a preference for the NRS because of its ease of use and accuracy.
- In consideration of Joint Commission requirements, each patient interaction needs a pain rating, even if the patient reports 0/10 on the NRS.
- A pain grade is generally accompanied by location, description, and most importantly, an "intervention," especially if pain is graded greater than 4/10 on the NRS.
- The physical therapist should recognize when the patient is weaning from pain medication (e.g., transitioning from intravenous to oral administration), as the patient may complain of increased pain with a concurrent reduced activity tolerance during this time period.
- To optimize consistency in the health care team, the physical therapist should use the same pain rating tool as the medical-surgical team to determine adequacy of pain management.
- Often the best way to communicate the adequacy of a patient's pain management to the nurses or physicians is in terms of the patient's ability to complete a given task or activity (e.g., the patient is effectively coughing and clearing secretions). Therapists should communicate both verbally and in written form to the medical team if the pain management is insufficient to allow the patient to accomplish functional tasks.

Pain Management

The primary goal in acute pain management is to promote the resolution of the underlying causes of pain while providing effective analgesia.[18] Acute pain can be managed using both pharmacologic and nonpharmacologic techniques (including physical therapy) either in isolation or more often in combination.[19,20] This section focuses on pharmacologic management while the next section will describe physical therapy management considerations.

TABLE 21-4 FLACC Pain Assessment Tool

Categories	Score = 0	Score = 1	Score = 2
Face	No particular expression or smile	Occasional grimace or frown, withdrawn, disinterested	Frequent to constant frown, clenched jaw, quivering chin
Legs	Normal position or relaxed	Uneasy, restless, tense	Kicking, or legs drawn up
Activity	Lying quietly, normal position, moves easily	Squirming, shifting back/forth, tense	Arched, rigid, or jerking
Cry	No cry (awake or asleep)	Moans or whimpers, occasional complaint	Crying steadily, screams or sobs, frequent complaints
Consolability	Content, relaxed	Reassured by occasional touching, hugging, or "talking to," distractible	Difficult to console or comfort

Indication: For nonverbal patients, particularly the pediatric population.
From Merkel SI, Voepel-Lewis T, Shayevitz JR et al: The FLACC: a behavioral scale for scoring postoperative pain in young children, Pediatr Nurs 23(3):293-297, 1997.

TABLE 21-5 Critical-Care Pain Observation Tool (CPOT)

Indicator	Descriptor	Score
Facial expression	No muscular tension observed	0 = Relaxed, neutral
	Presence of frowning, brow lowering, orbit tightening and levator contraction	1 = Tense
	All of the above facial movements plus eyelid tightening	2 = Grimacing
Body movements	Does not move at all (does not necessarily mean absence of pain)	0 = Absence of movement
	Slow cautious movements, touching or rubbing the pain site, seeking attention through movements	1 = Protection
	Pulling tube, attempting to sit up, moving limbs/thrashing, not following commands, striking at staff, trying to climb out of bed	2 = Restlessness
Muscle tension (evaluation by passive flexion and extension of UEs)	No resistance to passive movements	0 = Relaxed
	Resistance to passive movements	1 = Tense, rigid
	Strong resistance to passive movements, inability to complete them	2 = Very tense, rigid
Compliance with mechanical ventilator (intubated patient)	Alarms not activated, easy ventilation	0 = Tolerating ventilator or movement
	Alarms stop spontaneously	1 = Coughing but tolerating machine
	Asynchrony: blocking ventilation, alarms frequently activated	2 = Fighting ventilator
Vocalization (extubated patient)	Talking in normal tone or no sound	0 = Talking in normal tone or no sound
	Sighing, moaning	1 = Sighing, moaning
	Crying out, sobbing	2 = Crying out, sobbing

Modified from Gélinas C: Nurses' evaluations of the feasibility and the clinical utility of the Critical-Care Pain Observation Tool, Pain Manag Nurs 11(2):115-125, 2010.

✎ **CLINICAL TIP**

Communication among therapists, nurses, physicians, and patients on the effectiveness of pain management is essential to maximize the patient's comfort. This includes a thorough review of the patient's medical history and the doctor's orders by the physical therapist before prescribing any modalities or therapeutic exercises.

Pharmacologic management of acute pain is based on the World Health Organizations (WHO) Analgesic Ladder[21,22] originally designed to promote ongoing assessment of pain management during the palliative care of patients with cancer.[20] The WHO ladder is a stepwise process in which step 1 is for patients with mild pain in whom the use of nonopioid analgesia is recommended, step 2 is for moderate pain and advocates the use of weak opioids with or without nonopioids, and step 3 is for patients with severe pain in whom strong opioids with or without nonopioids are recommended.[20] Table 21-7 provides an overview of commonly utilized opioid agents in the management of acute pain.

Nonopioid drugs typically comprise nonsteroidal antiinflammatory drugs (NSAIDs) (Table 21-8) and acetaminophen (paracetamol), which is a centrally acting analgesic that interacts with the cyclooxygenase system.[18,19] Acetaminophen also has antipyretic effects and is an effective analgesic when used alone or as an adjunct to opioid analgesia.[18]

As a group, NSAIDs are nonselective cyclooxygenase inhibitors. Cyclooxygenase (COX) is an enzyme that exists in two forms (COX-1 and COX-2).[23] The homeostatic pathways, which include production of prostaglandins and thromboxane, primarily involve the COX-1 enzyme, while COX-2 is involved with pathways that produce pain and inflammation. Prostaglandins have a protective role for the mucosal lining of the gastrointestinal tract; therefore nonselective inhibition of these substances can result in gastrointestinal (GI) dysfunction (see Chapter 8). Selective inhibition of COX-2 was found to decrease injury to the mucosal lining of the stomach, leading to the development of COX-2 selective agents, which were aimed at reducing inflammation without adverse GI effects. Unfortunately, these agents were also correlated with an increased risk of cardiovascular events in susceptible individuals, resulting in agents such as rofecoxib (Vioxx) and valdecoxib (Bextra) being taken off the market. Currently celecoxib (Celebrex) is the only COX-2 selective agent still available.[23,24] Careful patient selection regarding all NSAIDs and overall cardiovascular risk need to be considered.[23] Acetylsalicylic acid (aspirin) is the oldest form of NSAID prescribed for patients to help manage pain and inflammation, as well as providing antiplatelet effects for vascular conditions.[23]

Opioid agents and NSAIDs can be administered by oral, intravenous, or intramuscular routes. Alternative routes of administration for pain medications include local anesthetics (Tables 21-9A and 21-9B) and patient-controlled analgesia (PCA) (Table 21-10).

TABLE 21-6 Comparison of Pain Assessment Scales

Tool	Targeted Population	Benefits	Reliability	Validity	Verbal or Nonverbal
Numeric Rating Scale (NRS)	Adults	Easy to use	Interrater reliability coefficient = 0.54	$p < 0.001$ Compared to VDS and VAS	Verbal
Visual Analog Scale (VAS)	Adults	Visual face and number scale to rate pain	Reliability coefficient range = 0.95-0.98	$p < 0.001$ Compared to NRS and VDS	Verbal
Functional Pain Scale (FPS)	Geriatric	Relates pain to function	Reliability coefficient range = 0.95-0.98	$p < 0.0054$ Compared to VAS	Verbal
Verbal Descriptor Scale (VDS)	Adults, geriatrics	Descriptions aid patient to rate pain	Interrater reliability coefficient range = 0.77-0.89	$p \leq 0.002$ Compared to NRS and VAS	Verbal
Face, Legs, Activity, Cry, Consolability (FLACC)	Pediatrics mostly	Clinically useful and efficient in the ICU	Interrater reliability coefficient = 0.84	Criterion validity $p < 0.01$ Compared to Checklist of Nonverbal Pain Indicators (adults) and COMFORT scale for children	Both
Critical-Care Pain Observation Tool (CPOT)	Verbal and nonverbal Mechanically ventilated patients	Good reliability and validity when applied to cardiac surgical patients	Interrater reliability coefficient = 0.74	Criterion validity $p < 0.001$ Compared to NVPS and BPS	Both
Nonverbal Pain Scale (NVPS)	Sedated ICU patients Conscious adults	Assessment of burn and trauma patients	Interrater reliability coefficient = 0.78	Criterion validity $p < 0.005$ Compared to FLACC	Nonverbal
Behavioral Pain Scale (BPS)	Unconscious critically ill, mechanically ventilated, sedated ICU patients	Widely used for sedated patients	Interrater reliability Intraclass correlation coefficient = 0.95	Construct validity $p < 0.0.001$ when used for measuring pain in nonverbal ICU patients	Nonverbal

Data from Chanques G, Viel E, Constantin JM et al: The measurement of pain in intensive care unit: comparison of 5 self-report intensity scales, Pain 151:711-721, 2010; Gloth FM, Cheve AA, Stober CV et al: The functional pain scale: reliability, validity, and responsiveness in an elderly population, J Am Med Dir Assoc 2:110-114, 2001; Odhner M, Wegman D Freeland N et al: Assessing pain control in nonverbal critically ill adults, Dimens Crit Care Nurs 22:260-267, 2003; Cade CH: Clinical tools for the assessment of pain in sedated critically ill adults, Br Assoc Crit Care Nurse 13:288-297, 2008; Gelinas C, Fillion L, Puntillo K et al: Validation of the critical-care pain observation tool in adult patients, Am J Crit Care 15:420-427, 2006; Aissaoui Y, Zeggwagh AA, Zekraoui A et al: Validation of a behavioral pain scale in critically ill, sedated, and mechanically ventilated patients, Anesth Analg 101:1470-1476, 2005; Voepel-Lewis T, Zanotti J, Dammeyer JA et al: Reliability and validity of the face, legs, activity, cry, consolability behavioral tool in assessing acute pain in critically ill patients, Am J Crit Care 19:55-61, 2010.

ICU, Intensive care unit.

TABLE 21-7 Systemic Opioids

Indication	Moderate to severe postoperative pain; can also be used preoperatively
Mechanism of action	Blocks transmission of pain from the periphery to the cerebrum by interacting with opioid receptors Can be administered orally, intravenously, intramuscularly, subcutaneously, and intrathecally
General side effects	Decreased gastrointestinal motility, nausea, vomiting, and cramps Mood changes and sedation Pruritus (itching) Urinary retention Bradycardia, hypotension Respiratory and cough depression Pupillary constriction, blurred vision
Medications: Generic name (trade name)	Buprenorphine (Buprenex, Subutex) Butorphanol (Stadol) Codeine (Paveral) Fentanyl (Actiq, Sublimaze, Duragesic) Hydromorphone (Dilaudid, Hydrostat) Levorphanol (Levo-Dromoran) Meperidine (Demerol, Pethidine) Methadone (Dolophine, Methadose) Morphine (MS Contin, Kadian, Morphine sulfate) Nalbuphine (Nubain) Naloxone (Narcan)* Oxycodone (Oxycontin, Roxicodone, Percocet [oxycodone with acetaminophen], Percodan [oxycodone with aspirin]) Oxymorphone (Numorphan) Pentazocine (Talwin) Propoxyphene (Darvon, Dolene, Doloxene, Novopropoxyn) Remifentanil (Ultiva) Sufentanil (Sufenta) Tramadol (Ultram)

Data from Ciccone CD: Pharmacology in rehabilitation, ed 4, Philadelphia, 2007, FA Davis, pp 183-198; Opioid analgesics and antagonists. In Panus PC, Katzung B, Jobst EE et al: Pharmacology for the physical therapist, New York, 2009, McGraw-Hill, pp 278-279; Analgesics, sedatives and hypnotics. In Woodrow R, Colbert BJ, Smith D: Essentials of pharmacology for health occupations, ed 6, Clifton Park, NY, 2011, Delmar, pp 327-333.
*Opioid antagonist.

TABLE 21-8 Nonsteroidal Antiinflammatory Drugs (NSAIDs)

Indications	To decrease inflammation Sole therapy for mild to moderate pain Used in combination with opioids for moderate postoperative pain, especially when weaning from stronger medications Useful in children younger than 6 months of age Contraindicated in patients undergoing anticoagulation therapy, with peptic ulcer disease, or with gastritis, renal dysfunction, and NSAID-induced asthma
Mechanism of action	Accomplishes analgesia by inhibiting the enzyme cyclo-oxygenase (COX), which in turn stops the production of prostaglandins, resulting in antiinflammatory effects (prostaglandin is a potent pain-producing chemical) A useful alternative or adjunct to opioid therapy
General side effects	Platelet dysfunction and gastritis, nausea, abdominal pain, anorexia, dizziness, and drowsiness Severe reactions that include nephrotoxicity (dysuria, hematuria) and cholestatic hepatitis
Commonly prescribed medications: Generic name (trade name)	Aspirin/acetylsalicylic acid (Bayer) Celecoxib (Celebrex) Choline salicylate (Arthopan) Diclofenac (Cataflam, Voltaren) Etodolac (Lodine) Flurbiprofen (Ansaid) Ibuprofen (Motrin, Advil) Indomethacin (Indocin, Indocin SR, Indomethacin, Novomethacin, Nu-Indo) Ketoprofen (Orudis) Ketorolac (Toradol) Naproxen (Anaprox, Naprosyn, Aleve) Oxaprozin (Daypro) Sulindac (Clinoril) Tolmetin (Tolectin)

Data from Ciccone CD: Pharmacology in rehabilitation, ed 4, Philadelphia, 2007, FA Davis, pp 199-216; Frampton C, Quinlan J: Evidence for the use of non-steroidal anti-inflammatory drugs for the acute pain in the post anaesthesia care unit, J Perioper Pract 19(12):418-423, 2009; Cox F: Basic principles of pain management: assessment and intervention, Nurs Stand 25(1):36-39, 2010; Musculoskeletal and anti-inflammatory drugs. In Woodrow R, Colbert BJ, Smith D: Essentials of pharmacology for health occupations, ed 6, Clifton Park, NY, 2011, Delmar, p 389; Drugs affecting the musculoskeletal system. In Panus PC, Katzung B, Jobst EE et al: Pharmacology for the physical therapist, New York, 2009, McGraw-Hill, pp 522-523.

TABLE 21-9A Local Anesthetics

Type	Indication	Description
Topical administration	Minor injuries; surgical procedures; hypertonicity	Direct application to skin, mucous membrane, cornea, or other areas requiring anesthesia
Transdermal administration	Pain relief in subcutaneous structures such as tendons and bursae	Direct application to skin or other surfaces in concentrations to allow penetration to deeper tissues
Infiltration anesthesia	Suturing of skin lacerations	Injection directly into selected tissue in order to diffuse to sensory nerve endings
Peripheral nerve block	Minor surgical procedures; management for chronic pain; specific nerve pain	Injection close to nerve trunk to interrupt signal transmission
Central nerve blockade	Obstetric procedures; alternative anesthesia for orthopedic procedures such as lumbar surgery; acute or chronic pain management	Injection within the epidural or intrathecal spaces
Sympathetic block	Complex regional pain syndrome	Selective interruption of sympathetic efferent pathways
Intravenous regional anesthesia (Bier block)	Short surgical procedures	Injection into a peripheral distal limb vein with a proximally placed tourniquet to isolate limb circulation

Adapted from Local anesthetics. In Panus PC, Katzung B, Jobst EE et al: Pharmacology for the physical therapist, New York, 2009, McGraw-Hill, pp 218-225.

TABLE 21-9B Local Anesthetics

Mechanism of action	Blocks action potential propagation, thereby preventing transmission of sensation from the periphery to the central nervous system
General side effects	Somnolence, confusion, agitation, restlessness Hypotension, bradycardia, fatigue, dizziness
Medications: Generic (trade name)	Articaine (Septocaine) Benzocaine (Americaine) Bupivacaine (Marcaine, Sensorcaine) Butamben picrate (Butesin Picrate) Chloroprocaine (Nesacaine) Dibucaine (Nupercainal) Dyclonine (Dyclone) Levobupivacaine (Chirocaine) Lidocaine (Xylocaine) Mepivacaine (Carbocaine) Pramoxine (Tronothane) Prilocaine (Citanest) Procaine (Novocain) Proparacaine (Alcain) Ropivacaine (Naropin) Tetracaine (Pontocaine)

Data from Local anesthetics. In Panus PC, Katzung B, Jobst EE et al: Pharmacology for the physical therapist, New York, 2009, McGraw-Hill, pp 218-225; Ciccone CD: Pharmacology in rehabilitation, ed 4, Philadelphia, 2007, FA Davis, pp 149-160.

- Patients should be educated on the need to request pain medicine or push their PCA button when they need it, particularly when they are on an "as needed" (PRN) pain medication schedule.[25]
- Patients should be asked about the specific type of pain that the medication is intended for, such as postsurgical incisional pain. Pain medications, such as opioids, may mask the occurrence of a new type of pain, such as angina.[25]
- The physical therapist should also use a pillow, blanket, or his or her hands to splint or support a painful area, such as an abdominal or thoracic incision or rib fractures, when the patient coughs or performs functional mobility tasks, such as going from a sidelying position to sitting at the edge of the bed.[26]
- The physical therapist can also use a corset, binder, or brace to support a painful area during intervention sessions that focus on functional mobility.
- Patients may experience pain induced by exercise or mobilization (PIEM), which can be perceived by patients as a decreased quality of life and result in fears about participation in physical therapy and refusal of care. Enhanced communication among care providers and with the patient about expected pain responses during therapy may lessen the adverse results of PIEM.[27]

Physical Therapy Considerations for Pain Management

- The physical therapist should be aware of the patient's pain medication schedule and the duration of the effectiveness of different pain medications when scheduling treatment sessions, particularly if premedication is necessary to optimize intervention.

> ✎ **CLINICAL TIP**
>
> Patients, particularly those who are postsurgical, are often prescribed more than one type of pain medication in order to achieve "breakthrough" pain levels. In other words, they require additional medicine to break their pain.

TABLE 21-10 Patient-Controlled Analgesia

Indications	For patients with moderate to severe acute pain who are not cognitively impaired and are capable of properly using the pump
Considerations	Preoperative education of the patient on the use of patient-controlled analgesia Ensuring that only the patient doses himself or herself Dosage, dosage intervals, maximum dosage per set time, and background (basal) infusion rate can be programmed Pump apparatus, tubing and power lines could limit mobility
Side effects	Similar to those of opioids (see Table 21-7)
Medications	Morphine, meperidine, fentanyl, and hydromorphone

Types	Description
Intravenous patient-controlled analgesia (IV PCA)	An intravenous line to a peripheral vein is connected to a microprocessor pump, and a patient is provided a button to allow self-dosing.
Patient-controlled epidural analgesia (PCEA)	The tip of a small catheter is placed in either the epidural or the subarachnoid space and connected to a pump. For short-term use, the catheter exits through the back to connect to a pump. For long-term use, the catheter is tunneled through the subcutaneous tissue and exits through the front for patient control.
Patient-controlled regional analgesia (PCRA)	The catheter tip is inserted directly into a specific anatomic site such as a wound (incisional PCRA), near a peripheral nerve (perineural PCRA), or into a peripheral joint (intra-articular [IA] PCRA). The other end of the catheter is attached to a pump with a button for patient control. Ropivacaine and bupivacaine are also used in PCRA.
Patient-controlled intranasal analgesia (PCINA)	Intranasal opioids are delivered using a syringe, nasal spray or dropper, or nebulized inhaler either in dry powder or water or saline solution. A pump mechanism is adapted to provide PCINA.
Fentanyl iontophoretic transdermal system (ITS)	A needle-free, self-contained fentanyl delivery system that does not require venous access for administration. System adheres to outer arm or chest with an adhesive backing and, via iontophoresis, delivers fentanyl across intact skin. Patient has on-demand dosing up to 6 doses/hour.

Data from Ciccone CD: Pharmacology in rehabilitation, ed 4, Philadelphia, 2007, FA Davis, pp 237-249; Viscusi E: Patient-controlled drug delivery for acute post-operative pain management: a review of current and emerging technologies, Region Anesth Pain Med 33(2):146-158, 2008; Chumbley G, Mountford L: Patient-controlled analgesia infusion pumps for adults, Nurs Stand 25(8):35-40, 2010.

References

1. Mackintosh C: Assessment and management of patients with post-operative pain, Nurs Stand 22(5):49-55, 2007.
2. Helfand M, Freeman M: Assessment and management of acute pain in adult medical inpatients: a systematic review, Pain Med 10(7):1183-1199, 2009.
3. Young J, Siffleet J, Nikoletti S et al: Use of a behavioral pain scale to assess pain in ventilated, unconscious and/or sedated patients, Intensive Crit Care Nurs 22:32-39, 2006.
4. Cade CH: Clinical tools for the assessment of pain in sedated critically ill adults, Nurs Crit Care 13:288-297, 2008.
5. Puntillo K, Pasero C, Li D et al: Evaluation of pain in ICU patients, Chest 135:1069-1074, 2009.
6. Shega JW, Rudy T, Keefe FJ et al: Validity of pain behaviors in persons with mild to moderate cognitive impairment, J Am Geriatr Soc 56:1631-1637, 2008.
7. Kittelberger KP, LeBel AA, Borsook D: Assessment of pain. In Borsook D, LeBel AA, McPeek B, editors: The Massachusetts General Hospital handbook of pain management, Boston, 1996, Little, Brown, p 26.
8. Cristoph SD: Pain assessment: the problem of pain in the critically ill patient, Crit Care Nurs Clin North Am 3(1):11-16, 1991.
9. Acello B: Meeting JCAHO standards for pain control, Nursing 30(3):52-54, 2000.
10. Turk DC, Okifuji A: Assessment of patients' reporting of pain: an integrated perspective, Lancet 353(9166):1784, 1999.
11. American Physical Therapy Association: Cultural competence. http://www.apta.org/CulturalCompetence. Accessed March 16, 2012.
12. Odhner M, Wegman D, Freeland N et al: Assessing pain control in nonverbal critically ill adults, Dimens Crit Care Nurs 22:260-267, 2003.
13. Aissaoui Y, Zeggwagh AA, Zekraoui A et al: Validation of a behavioral pain scale in critically ill, sedated, and mechanically ventilated patients, Anesth Analg 101:1470-1476, 2005.
14. Voepel-Lewis T, Zanotti J, Dammeyer JA et al: Reliability and validity of the face, legs, activity, cry, consolability behavioral tool in assessing acute pain in critically ill patients, Am J Crit Care 19:55-61, 2010.
15. Kabes AM, Graves JK, Norris J: Further validation of the nonverbal pain scale in intensive care patients, Crit Care Nurse 29:59-66, 2009.
16. Gelinas C, Harel F, Fillion L et al: Sensitivity and specificity of the critical-care pain observation tool for the detection of pain in intubated adults after cardiac surgery, J Pain Symptom Manage 37:58-67, 2009.
17. Garra G, Singer AJ, Taira BR et al: Validation of the Wong-Baker FACES Pain Rating Scale in pediatric emergency department patients, Acad Emerg Med 17(1):50-54, 2010.
18. Keene DD, Rea WE, Aldington D: Acute pain management in trauma, Trauma 13(3):167-179, 2011.
19. Cox F: Basic principles of pain management: assessment and intervention, Nurs Stand 25(1):36-39, 2010.

20. McMain L: Principles of acute pain management, Pain Manage 18(11):472-478, 2008.

21. World Health Organization: WHO 1986 cancer pain relief, Geneva, World Health Organization.

22. World Health Organization: WHO 1996 cancer pain relief: with a guide to opioid availability, ed 2, Geneva, World Health Organization.

23. Ciccone CD: Pharmacology in rehabilitation, ed 4, Philadelphia, 2007, FA Davis, pp 183-249.

24. Chakraborti AK, Garg SK, Kumar R et al: Progress in COX-2 inhibitors: a journey so far, Curr Med Chem 17:1563-1593, 2010.

25. Chumbley G, Mountford L: Patient controlled analgesia infusion pumps for adults, Nurs Stand 25(8):35-40, 2010.

26. Cahalin L, Lapier T, Shaw D: Sternal precautions: is it time for change? Precautions versus restrictions—a review of literature and recommendations for revision, Cardiopulm Phys Ther J 22(1):5-15, 2011.

27. Alami S, Desjeux D, Lefèvre-Colau MM et al: Management of pain induced by exercise and mobilization during physical therapy programs: views of patients and care providers, BMC Musculoskelet Disord 12:172, 2011.

22 Postural Drainage

Michele P. West

CHAPTER OBJECTIVES

The objectives of this chapter are to provide the following:

1. A review of the relative and absolute contraindications for postural drainage positioning.
2. A review of the situations and conditions in which traditional postural drainage positions and/or chest wall manipulation may require modification.
3. A discussion of clinical considerations for postural drainage that maximize treatment effectiveness and patient comfort.

PREFERRED PRACTICE PATTERNS

The most relevant practice patterns for the diagnoses discussed in this chapter, based on the American Physical Therapy Association's *Guide to Physical Therapist Practice*, second edition, are as follows:

- Impaired Ventilation, Respiration/Gas Exchange, and Aerobic Capacity/Endurance Associated with Airway Clearance Dysfunction: 6C

Please refer to Appendix A for a complete list of the preferred practice patterns, as individual patient conditions are highly variable and other practice patterns may be applicable.

Postural drainage is the positioning of a patient with an involved lung segment such that gravity has a maximal effect of facilitating the drainage of bronchopulmonary secretions from the tracheobronchial tree.[1] The validity of postural drainage (with or without breathing exercises and chest wall manipulation) has been scrutinized in the literature over the past years, and the evidence is unequivocal. However, the use of postural drainage as an adjunct to other airway clearance techniques (ACTs) such as percussion, active cycle of breathing, autogenic drainage, oscillatory positive expiratory pressure (PEP), high-frequency chest compression, and exercise is recommended for patients with cystic fibrosis.[2]

Contraindications and Considerations

The physical therapist should note that there are many clinical contraindications and considerations for postural drainage.

The relative contraindications for the use of the Trendelenburg position (placing the head of the bed in a downward position) include the following[3]:

- Patient with an intracranial pressure (ICP) greater than 20 mm Hg or in whom increased intracranial pressure should be avoided
- Uncontrolled hypertension
- Uncontrolled or unprotected airway with a risk of aspiration
- Recent gross hemoptysis
- Recent esophageal surgery
- Significantly distended abdomen
- Orthopnea

The relative contraindications for the reverse Trendelenburg position (placing the head of the bed in an upward position) include the following[3]:

- Hypotension
- Use of vasoactive medications

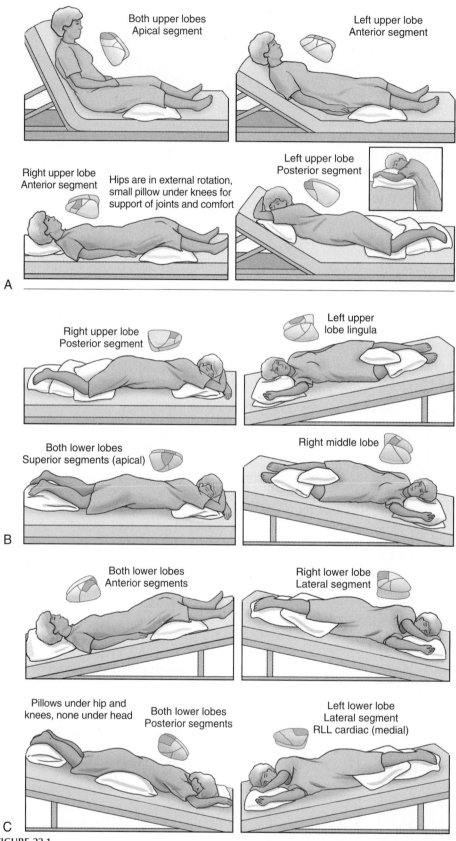

FIGURE 22-1

Postural drainage positions. **A,** Upper lobes. **B,** Upper, middle, and lower lobes. **C,** Lower lobes. (From Frown-felter D, Dean E, editors: Cardiovascular and pulmonary physical therapy: evidence to practice, ed 5, St Louis, 2012, Mosby.)

The following are absolute and relative contraindications for postural drainage[3]:

- Acute hemorrhage with hemodynamic instability (absolute contraindication)
- Unstabilized head or neck injury (absolute contraindication)
- ICP greater than 20 mm Hg
- Acute spinal injury or recent spinal surgery
- Rib fracture, with or without flail chest
- Bronchopleural fistula (BPF)
- Empyema
- Large pleural effusion(s)
- Unstable pneumothorax
- Pulmonary embolism
- Pulmonary edema or congestive heart failure
- Active hemoptysis
- Altered skin integrity of the chest wall

The use of postural drainage with or without other bronchopulmonary hygiene techniques should be considered on an individual patient basis if any of the aforementioned relative contraindications exist. This can include a discussion with the medical-surgical team and an analysis of the risk(s) versus benefit(s) for the patient, as well as any possible modifications of therapy.

Postural drainage positions with or without airway clearance techniques may require modification to maximize patient safety, comfort, and/or tolerance. In the acute care setting, there are many situations and conditions in which the patient cannot obtain or maintain traditional postural drainage positions or tolerate chest wall manipulation. These situations and conditions include the following[1,4]:

- The presence of multiple lines and tubes or mechanical ventilation
- Obesity
- Massive ascites
- Diaphragmatic hernia or reflux
- Chest wall abnormalities such as skin grafting, open wound, the presence of a vacuum-assisted wound closure dressing, rib fracture, flail chest, rib osteomyelitis, or rib metastasis
- Subcutaneous emphysema (air in the subcutaneous tissue)
- The elderly or long-term bedridden patient with cachexia or a spinal deformity
- Anxiety or confusion

- Inadequate pain control, especially in the postsurgical patient
- Recent pacemaker placement
- Uncontrolled dysrhythmia
- Platelet count less than 20,000 per mm[3]

Postural Drainage Positioning

Figure 22-1 demonstrates the 12 traditional postural drainage positions. Examples of postural drainage position modifications frequently used in the acute care setting are shown in Figure 22-2.

Physical Therapy Considerations

Therapists incorporating postural drainage in the plan of care should be mindful of all of the following:

- The timing of postural drainage after pain medication or bronchodilators can improve its effectiveness.
- Monitor vital signs with position changes to evaluate patient tolerance, especially for critically ill patients or those who have undergone cardiothoracic surgery and have a history of blood pressure and heart rate changes when turned to one side.
- Modify the position of the patient if anxiety, pain, skin breakdown, abnormal posture, decreased range of motion, or positioning restrictions exist.
- To improve patient tolerance of postural drainage, consider modifying the time spent in each position, the angle of the bed, or patient position.
- Provide time for the patient to rest or become acclimated to position changes if necessary.
- Use pillows, blankets, foam rolls, or wedges to maximize comfort or provide pressure relief.
- Bed mobility training can be incorporated during position changes with patients who have decreased independence with rolling or supine-to-sit transfers.
- Have a good working knowledge of the controls on the patient's bed that are needed to position the patient for postural drainage. Each bed model, especially pressure relief or rotating beds, has different controls, locks, and alarms.

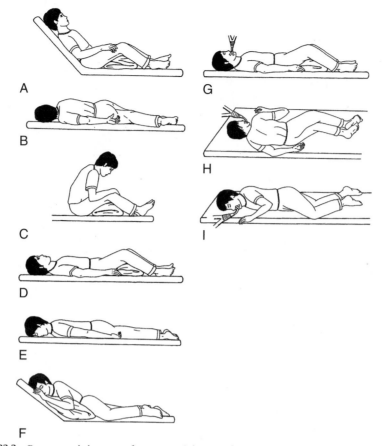

FIGURE 22-2 Recommended postures for segmental drainage from the upper lobe of the lung. **A** through **F,** Patient positions for postural drainage of S_1, S_2, S_{1-2}, S_3, and S_6 as recommended by Potter and Perry. **G** through **I,** Positions recommended for patients with tracheal intubation by Miyagawa. Potter and Perry described another 6 postures (i.e., 12 postures in all) to cover all lung segments, whereas Miyagawa included another 5 postures (8 postures total). **A,** Bending backward to drain S_1. When bending backward or forward (see **C**), the craniocaudal axis of the lung is tilted at 45 degrees from the horizontal. **B,** 45 degrees rotative prone with right-side-up position for draining the right S_2. In this position, the craniocaudal axis of the lung is the same as in the prone or supine positions, but the coronal plane of the lung is tilted at 45 degrees. **C,** Bending forward is recommended for drainage of the posterior portion of the left and right upper lobes. **D,** Supine position for draining S_3. **E,** Prone position for draining S_6 and S_{10}. **F,** 45 degrees relative prone with head-raised position, which is recommended for S_{1-2} drainage in the left lung. "Head raised" means that the craniocaudal axis of the lung is raised to 30 degrees. **G,** The supine position is also useful for S_3 drainage during tracheal intubation. It is also useful for S_1 drainage during tracheal intubation. **H** and **I,** 45 degrees rotative prone positions with right and left sides up, respectively. These positions are recommended for S_2 and S_{1-2} drainage during intubation. (From Takahashi N, Murakami G, Ishikawa A, et al: Anatomic evaluation of postural bronchial drainage of the lung with special reference to patients with tracheal intubation, Chest 125(3):935-944, 2004.)

References

1. Mejia-Downs A: Airway clearance techniques. In Frownfelter D, Dean E, editors: Cardiovascular and pulmonary physical therapy: evidence to practice, ed 5, St Louis, 2013, Mosby.
2. Flume PA, Robinson KA et al: Cystic fibrosis pulmonary guidelines: airway clearance therapies, Respir Care 54(4):522-537, 2009.
3. AARC clinical practice guideline: postural drainage therapy, Respir Care 36(12):1418-1426, 1991. http://www.rcjournal.com. Accessed July 7, 2012.
4. Sciaky A, Pawlik A: Interventions for acute cardiopulmonary conditions. In Hillegass EA, editor: Essentials of cardiopulmonary physical therapy, ed 3, St Louis, 2012, Saunders.

CHAPTER 23

Functional Tests

Paul E.H. Ricard

CHAPTER OUTLINE

CHAPTER OBJECTIVE

To provide a description of functional tests applicable to the inpatient acute care setting, including a description of how to perform each test, the applicable population, and how results may be interpreted.

PREFERRED PRACTICE PATTERNS

These functional tests and outcome measures apply to many body systems. For this reason, specific practice patterns are not delineated in this chapter. Please refer to Appendix A for a complete list of the preferred practice patterns in order to best delineate the most applicable practice pattern for a given patient.

Clinicians frequently look for the "best" test for particular functional activities (e.g., balance). To date, however, few if any "gold standard" functional tests have been identified in the literature. Several contributing factors are that functional activities have multisystem components and outcomes can vary based on environment, time of day, or prior patient practice. The purpose of this chapter is therefore to describe more common functional tests that can objectively measure the functional levels of various patient populations in the acute care setting, and not to compare one test to another.

Fortunately, the literature on functional tests and measures is consistently expanding. Although attention should be paid to the patient population used to validate each test described in this section, a particular functional test still may be useful in patient examination and evaluation in a population not yet specifically studied. A clinician should consider all factors when interpreting the outcomes of any clinical test and continue to read current literature to keep abreast with changes in test validation and interpretation.

✎ CLINICAL TIP

The American Physical Therapy Association (APTA) has online tools to assist with making evidence-based practice decisions, such as "Hooked on Evidence," and "Open Door."[1] Individual hospital facilities may also have online resources that are updated and reflect evidence-based practice for particular patient populations.[2]

The functional tests presented in this chapter were selected because of their ease of use, reliable and valid test results, and the appropriate population in the acute care setting. Where applicable, interrater (tested by different therapists) and intrarater (retested over time by a single therapist) reliability[3] and content,* construct,† and predictive‡ validity will be noted in the respective description of each test.[3]

Berg Balance Scale

The Berg Balance Scale (BBS) is a 56-point scale that evaluates 14 tasks. Katherine Berg developed this test to assess the level of function and balance in various patient

---

*Content validity: Degree to which a test actually measures what it was designed for.
†Construct validity: Degree to which a theoretical construct is measured against the test.
‡Predictive validity: Ability of a test to predict future performance.

TABLE 23-1 Overview of the Berg Balance Scale

Population	Equipment	Time	Reliability	Validity
Elderly patients who have sustained acute cerebrovascular accident and/or are in a rehabilitation setting	Ruler Stopwatch Chair Step stool Flat surface	10-20 minutes required to complete test	Interrater reliability: $ICC = 0.98$ $rs = 0.88$ Intrarater reliability: $ICC = 0.98$ Internal consistency: Cronbach's alpha $= 0.96$	Concurrent validity: Tinetti, $r = 0.91$ Get up and go, $r = -0.76$ Predictive validity: <45 score predicts falls (sensitivity 53%)

Data from Thorbahn L, Newton R: Use of the Berg Balance Test to predict falls in elderly persons, Phys Ther 76(6):576-583, 1996; Conradsson M, Lundin-Olsson L, Lindelof N et al: Berg Balance Scale: intrarater test-retest reliability among older people dependent in activities of daily living and living in residential care facilities, Phys Ther 87:1155-1163, 2007; Thompson M, Medley A: Performance of community dwelling elderly on the timed up and go test, Phys Occup Ther Geriatr 13(3):17-30, 1995; Whitney S, Poole J, Cass S: A review of balance instruments for older adults, Am J Occup Ther 52(8):666-671, 1998; Berg K, Wood-Dauphinee S, Williams JI, et al: Measuring balance in the elderly: preliminary development of an instrument, Physiother Can 41:304, 1989.

ICC, Intraclass correlation coefficient; r, correlation coefficient; rs, Spearman's rank correlation coefficient.

populations.[4] Table 23-1 describes the appropriate population, required equipment, completion time, reliability, and validity of the BBS.

> **✎ CLINICAL TIP**
>
> For patients with multiple sclerosis, the BBS is reported to be less efficient in discriminating between patients who tend to fall as compared to patients less likely to fall.[5]

Procedure

The patient is evaluated and graded on a sequence of balance activities, such as sitting unsupported with arms folded, rising, standing, transferring between one surface and another, reaching forward in standing, picking up objects off the floor, turning around in a full circle, and standing on one leg.[4] Scoring for each task ranges from 0 to 4. A score of 0 indicates that the patient is unable to complete a particular task. A score of 4 indicates that the patient can completely carry out the task.[4] The 14 tasks consist of[6]:

- Sitting to standing
- Standing unsupported
- Sitting unsupported
- Standing to sitting
- Transfers
- Standing with eyes closed
- Standing with feet together
- Reaching forward with an outstretched arm
- Retrieving object from floor
- Turning to look behind
- Turning 360 degrees
- Placing alternate foot on stool
- Standing with one foot in front of the other foot
- Standing on one foot

A short form of the BBS has been developed and demonstrates psychometric test properties similar to those of the original BBS. The short form of the BBS includes 7 activities rather than 14, and the scoring levels are reduced to three (0, 2, 4). This modified BBS has been shown to have good validity and reliability in patients who have had a cerebrovascular accident (CVA).[6] Box 23-1 outlines the seven items on this modified BBS.

> **BOX 23-1 Short Form of Berg Balance Scale**
>
> Items:
> - Reaching forward with outstretched arm
> - Standing with eyes closed
> - Standing with one foot in front
> - Turning to look behind
> - Retrieving object from floor
> - Standing on one foot
> - Sitting to standing

Data from Chou CY, Chien CW, Hsueh IP et al: Developing a short form of the Berg Balance Scale for people with stroke, Phys Ther 86:199, 2006.

> **✎ CLINICAL TIP**
>
> The modified BBS was developed with patients who have had a CVA. To date, the validity of this test has not been evaluated on any other patient populations.

Interpretation of Results

Higher scores on the BBS indicate greater independence and better ability to balance.[7] In contrast, lower scores indicate a greater fall risk. Prior evidence suggested that a total score of less than 45 predicted that the patient is at risk for falls.[8,9] However, more recent literature by Katherine Berg discourages the use the score as a dichotomous scale (i.e., determining fall risk based on values being greater than or less than 45 points).[10] Rather, the score should be used to represent a continuum of balance, through the use of likelihood ratios.[10]

> **✎ CLINICAL TIP**
>
> In patients who are over 65 years of age and are dependent in at least one personal activity of daily living, a change of 8 points on the BBS is necessary to demonstrate a genuine change in function.[11]

Timed "Up and Go" Test

The "up and go" test was originally developed in 1986 to serve as a clinical measure of balance in elderly people.[12] The original

TABLE 23-2 Overview of the Timed "Up and Go" Test

Population	Time	Equipment	Reliability	Validity
Geriatric population with various diagnoses	1 to 3 minutes to complete test	Armchair Stopwatch Assistive device*	Interrater reliability: $r = 0.99$ Intrarater reliability: $r = 0.99$ $ICC = 0.99$	Content validity: none reported Concurrent validity: Berg balance scale

Data from Whitney S, Poole J, Cass S: A review of balance instruments for older adults, Am J Occup Ther 52(8):666-671, 1998; Posiadlo D, Richardson S: The timed "up and go": a test of basic functional mobility for frail elderly persons, J Am Geriatr Soc 39:142-148, 1991; Berg KO, Wood-Dauphinee SL, Williams JI et al: Measuring balance in the elderly: validation of an instrument, Can J Public Health 83:S7-S11, 1992; Portney LG, Watkins MP, editors: Foundations of clinical research applications to practice, Norwalk, CT, 1993, Appleton & Lange.

ICC, Intraclass correlation coefficient; *r*, correlation coefficient.

*If necessary, an assistive device may be used while performing this test.

test used a numeric scoring system to determine a patient's level of balance but was later modified to a timed version by Posiadlo and Richardson in 1991.[13] The TUG test uses a time score to assess gait and balance in the elderly population and is summarized in Table 23-2.[14]

Procedure

The patient is timed during a five-part mobility task from start to finish. The task consists of the following[15]:

1. Rising from an armchair
2. Walking 3 meters
3. Turning around
4. Walking 3 meters back to the armchair
5. Sitting down

It is important to instruct the patient to walk at a comfortable and normal pace to maintain safety throughout the test. It is appropriate to provide assistance for the patient if it is needed. Documenting the level of assistance (i.e., assistive device, contact guard) is essential in demonstrating progress when performing the test over time.

Interpretation of Results

Test completion in fewer than 20 seconds indicates that the patient is independent with functional mobility.[15] The time needed to complete the test may improve for many reasons, including: (1) altering the use of an assistive device, (2) actual change in function, and (3) increased familiarity of the test, or a combination of these. Therefore it is important to periodically perform this test over the course of a patient's physical therapy intervention to allow for comparison to baseline results.

As described in Table 23-2, when compared to other functional tests (i.e., BBS), with regard to balance testing, the TUG test is a consistent test of the balance characteristics in this population. The ability or inability to complete the TUG test helps to stratify patients according to their fall risk. Patients who are unable to complete the TUG test for nonphysical reasons (including refusal or inability to follow instructions [e.g., dementia or delirium]) appear to have higher rates of falling as compared to patients who are unable to do the TUG test for physical reasons (inability to sit, stand, or walk independently, or with standby assistance).[16]

Additionally, patients who have undergone hip fracture surgery and are discharged from the acute care setting with a TUG score of 24 seconds or more are more likely to fall in the next 6 months than are patients with scores of less than 24 seconds.[17] When used in an acute care setting, this test can objectively demonstrate improvements in balance and ambulation. Over the course of therapy, it is expected that the time the patient takes to complete the TUG test will decrease as the patient improves.[14]

> ✎ **CLINICAL TIP**
>
> Caution should be exercised in interpreting the scores of the TUG test when administered to a frail elderly patient who has multisystem impairments. Patients with these characteristics may have TUG scores as low as 10 seconds but may still be at risk for falling.[18]

Functional Reach Test

The functional reach test was developed to assess the risk for falls in the elderly population and is a dynamic measure of stability during a self-initiated movement.[19] The functional reach test evaluates balance by measuring the maximum distance an elderly person can reach forward, backward, and out to the side while standing on the floor at a fixed position (Table 23-3).[7]

Procedure

The procedure involves a series of three trials of the distance a patient is willing to reach from a fixed surface.[7] After every reach, distance is measured with a yardstick attached to the wall at shoulder level. The difference in inches between a person's arm length and maximal forward, backward, and sideward reach with the shoulder flexed to 90 degrees while maintaining a fixed base of support in standing is then recorded.[12,20] The mean of three trials is the score.

Interpretation of Results

The functional reach in inches correlates with the patient's relative risk for falling (Table 23-4).[19]

When working with an elderly patient in an acute care setting, this test may be an objective way to quickly gauge balance abilities and determine the need for balance treatment,

TABLE 23-3 Overview of the Functional Reach Test

Population	Equipment	Time	Reliability	Validity

Elders who are community ambulators, patients who have undergone hip fracture surgery
 	
Population limitation excludes patients with dementia, extreme spinal deformities, severely restricted upper extremity function, frail elders, and nursing home residents
	Yardstick
	Level
	Assistive device*
		<5 minutes to complete test	Test-retest reliability:
			  $r = 0.89$
			Interrater reliability:
			  $ICC = 0.99$
				Concurrent validity:
				  Walking speed, $r = 0.71$
				  Tandem walk, $r = 0.71$
				  Center of pressure, $r = 0.71$
				Predictive validity:
				  >10 inches: not likely to fall
				  6-10 inches: two times more likely to fall
				  1-6 inches: four times more likely to fall
				  0 inches: 28 times more likely to fall

Data from Thapa PB, Gideon P, Fought RL et al: Comparison of clinical and biomechanical measures of balance and mobility in elderly nursing home residents, J Am Geriatr Soc 42:493-500, 1994; Portney LG, Watkins MP, editors: Foundations of clinical research applications to practice, Norwalk, CT, 1993, Appleton & Lange, p 689; Sherrington C, Lord SR: Reliability of simple portable tests of physical performance in older people after hip fracture, Clin Rehabil 19:496-504, 2005.

  ICC, Intraclass correlation coefficient; *r,* correlation coefficient.

  *An assistive device may be used while performing this test if it is necessary.

TABLE 23-4 Functional Reach Test Results

Reach	Likelihood of Falling
>10 inches	Not likely
6-10 inches	2 times more likely
1-6 inches	4 times more likely
Subject unwilling to reach	28 times more likely

Data from Duncan PW, Weiner DK, Chandler J, et al: Functional reach: a new clinical measure of balance, J Gerontol 45:M192-M197, 1990.

an assistive device, or both. It is important to remember that there are limitations to the population that can participate in this test. Elderly patients who are frail, demented, or both, are excluded, because participation in this test may lead to unnecessary injury or falls.

✎ CLINICAL TIP

If the procedure of the functional reach test is followed correctly, then scores of either the first or second trial or the mean of the first two trials will have no significant difference from that of the mean of all three trials.[21] This may be useful for clinicians who do not have time to perform three trials or if the patient does not have the endurance to perform three trials.

Tinetti Performance Oriented Mobility Assessment

The Tinetti Performance Oriented Mobility Assessment (POMA) is a performance test of balance and gait maneuvers used during normal daily activities.[22] This test has two subscales of balance and gait, as described in Table 23-5. There are 13 maneuvers in the balance portion and 9 maneuvers in the gait portion. The balance subscale, the performance oriented assessment of balance (POAB), can be used individually as a separate test of balance.

Procedure

The balance maneuvers are graded on an ordinal scale as normal (2 points), adaptive (1 point), or abnormal (0 points). The gait maneuvers are graded as normal or abnormal, with the exception of a few items. A combination of the total points for the balance and gait portions are summed together to determine the final score.[12,23] A summary of the Tinetti POMA can be found in Appendix 23A.

Interpretation of Results

A total combined score on the balance and gait subscales of the Tinetti POMA correlates with the patient's relative risk of falling (Table 23-6).[24] This functional test is an effective and objective measure to predict falls in elderly and adult population, as well as assist in determining progress over time in therapy.

Sit-to-Stand Tests

There are several sit-to-stand tests[25-35] currently being used in the clinical setting with some supporting evidence. These tests have been utilized for the assessment of balance or lower extremity strength and function, with validity not fully established for either use. Definitive agreement on the specific procedure for the sit-to-stand test has not been established.

    The procedures for sit-to-stand tests have included timing the patient's ability to complete 5 or 10 repetitions, counting the number of stands completed by the patient in 30 seconds, and varying the conditions such as the use of arms to stand up. A meta-analysis by Bohannon cautiously reports normative values for the 5-repetition sit-to-stand test in elders. In persons who are 60 to 69 years of age, mean times to complete this test

TABLE 23-5 Overview of the Tinetti Performance Oriented Mobility Assessment

Population	Equipment	Time	Reliability	Validity
Balance portion: adult or geriatric population with a wide variety of diagnoses	Chair Stopwatch	10-15 minutes to complete test	Interrater reliability: 85% ± 10% agreement balance portion	Concurrent validity: Berg, $r = 0.91$ Predictive validity: ≤18 total score predicts high fall risk

Data from King MB, Judge JO, Whipple L et al: Reliability and responsiveness of two physical performance measures examined of a functional training intervention, Phys Ther 80(1):8-16, 2000; Tinetti M: Performance oriented assessment of mobility problems in elderly patients, J Am Geriatr Soc 41:479, 1986; Nakamura DM, Holm MB, Wilson A: Measures of balance and fear of falling in the elderly: a review, Phys Occup Ther Geriatr 15(4):17-32, 1998; Wee JYM, Bagg SD, Palepu A: The Berg Balance Scale as a predictor of length of stay and discharge destination in an acute stroke rehabilitation setting, Arch Phys Med Rehabil 80(4):448-452, 1999; Anemaet W, Moffa-Trotter M: Functional tools for assessing balance and gait impairments, Top Geriatr Rehabil 15(1):66-83, 1999.

r, Correlation coefficient.

TABLE 23-6 Tinetti Results

Score	Risk
<18	High
19-23	Moderate
>24	Low

From Tinetti ME, Williams TF, Mayewski R: Fall index for elderly patients based on number of chronic disabilities, Am J Med 80:429-434, 1986.

TABLE 23-7 SPPB Score Classifications

Classification	Score
Severe limitations	0-3
Moderate limitations	4-6
Mild limitations	7-9
Minimal limitations	10-12

From Puthoff ML: Outcome measures in cardiopulmonary physical therapy: short physical performance battery, Phys Ther 19(1):17-22, 2008.

were 11.4 seconds, whereas persons who were 80 to 89 had mean times of 12.7 seconds.[35]

Despite some of the inconsistencies reported in the literature about this test, performing a suitable version of the sit-to-stand test during the examination of patients can still yield helpful information, as there is a relationship between the sit-to-stand test with instrumental activities of daily living and balance. In addition, a sit-to-stand test can be used to describe the limitations during a functional activity and measure improvement over time. Repeating the same procedure within the same clinical facility will help to improve reliability of these results.

> ✎ **CLINICAL TIP**
>
> When documenting a sit-to-stand test, make sure to describe the test characteristics such as seat height, use of arms or no arms, repetitions (5 or 10), and/or time to complete the test, as well as when to stop timing, either at the last stand or sit.

Short Physical Performance Battery

The Short Physical Performance Battery (SPPB) was initially developed in 1994 and involved a cohort of people aged 65 years or older living in the community.[36] It has since been validated for larger patient demographics.[37-40] The test consists of three subsections: balance, walking speed, and chair stand time (see Appendix 23A). Each section is scored on a 0- to 4-point scale. The total score is then compared to predictive values to describe the degree of limitation to mobility (Table 23-7).[37,41]

The reliability for the SPPB subsections varies, with the balance subscore having the weakest score.[37] The standard error

of measurement for the SPPB has been calculated to 1.42 points, whereas the minimal clinically important difference (MCID) has been reported to be from 0.54 to 1.34 points.[37,42] Although the original authors indicated that a 1-point score change was significant, score improvements closer to 2 would more greatly support actual change.[36,37]

Acute Care Index of Function

The Acute Care Index of Function (ACIF) was developed in 1988 to standardize the assessment of functional status in patients with acute neurologic deficits.[43,44] The test is based on patient performance measured in four domains: mental status, bed mobility, transfers, and mobility. Higher scores denote better patient performance.

For the functional aspects of the exam (bed mobility, transfers, and mobility) there are three possible choices for scoring performance: unable, dependent, or independent; point values are 0, 4, and 10, respectively.[43] For the mental status portion of the test, only the absence or presence of patient performance is issued point values. The sums of all the scores for each of the domains are then averaged.[43] Finally, each domain is independently weighted by a multiplier to help detect change in performance and to discriminate between discharge disposition.[44]

This test possesses good validity ($r_s = 0.81$, $p < 0.01$) and good interrater reliability (weighted kappa 0.88-0.98), except in the area of "impaired safety awareness" (weighted kappa 0.60), which was due to the more subjective nature of the question.[43,44] The test has subsequently been used to describe the functional status of patients with lower extremity orthopedic

TABLE 23-8 Overview of the Six-Minute Walk Test

Population	Equipment	Time	Reliability	Validity
Patients with cardiac and/or pulmonary disease and osteoarthritis of the knee	Chair Stopwatch Pulse oximeter Portable blood pressure cuff Rate of perceived exertion scale Visual pain analog scale Measuring wheel	10-15 minutes to complete test	Test-retest reliability: ICC = 0.93	Responsiveness index validity: 0.6

Data from King MB, Judge JO, Whipple L et al: Reliability and responsiveness of two physical performance measures examined of a functional training intervention, Phys Ther 80(1):8-16, 2000; Woo MA, Moser DK, Stevenson LW et al: Six-minute walk test and heart rate variability: lack of association in advanced stages of heart failure, Am J Crit Care 6(5):348-354, 1997; Kovar PA, Allegrante JP, MacKenzie CR et al: Supervised fitness walking in patients with osteoarthritis of the knee: a randomized controlled trial, Ann Intern Med 116:529-534, 1992; Guyatt GH, Sullivan MJ, Thompson PJ et al: The 6-minute walk: new measure of exercise capacity in patients with chronic heart failure, Can Med Assoc J 132:919-923, 1985; McGavin CR, Gupta SP, McHardy GJR: Twelve-minute walking test for assessing disability in chronic bronchitis, BMJ 1:822, 1976; Butland RJ, Pang J, Gross ER et al: Two-, six-, and twelve-minute walking tests in respiratory disease, BMJ 284:1607, 1982.

ICC, Intraclass correlation coefficient.

health conditions.[45] To date the minimal clinically detectable change score for this test has not yet been calculated.[44]

> ✎ **CLINICAL TIP**
>
> Clinicians may want to consider using the ACIF to help make appropriate discharge recommendations, thereby reducing readmissions and helping patients get to the appropriate level of care.

Exercise Testing

Although maximal exercise testing with evaluation of exhaled gases is considered the gold standard to evaluate a person's cardiopulmonary capacity, maximal testing is not commonly performed in the acute care setting. Submaximal tests, however, can be used safely to help a clinician with differential diagnosis of the etiology of a patient's fatigue or shortness or breath (SOB), describing a person's current aerobic capacity, estimating maximal capacity, or prescribing exercise, or as an outcome assessment.[46] Despite the submaximal design, these exercise tests may result in a symptom-limited test that, in some patient populations, approaches a maximal effort, particularly in a very deconditioned patient.

Although not within the scope of this test, exercise prescription based on actual effort during an exercise test can be more accurate than exercise prescribed on heart rate or perceived effort alone. The clinician is referred to the text *American College of Sports Medicine Guideline for Exercise Testing and Prescription*[47] for further details on exercise testing and prescription.

Six-Minute Walk Test

The 6-minute walk test (6MWT) is a time-limited measure of functional capacity in which a patient walks as far as possible on a course for 6 minutes.[48] This test evolved from the 12-minute walk test, originally designed to assess disability levels in patients with chronic bronchitis.[49] The 6MWT was found to provide similar measures of exercise tolerance and therefore was adopted by clinicians for its convenience (Table 23-8).[49,50]

Although this test is considered a time-limited, submaximal exercise test, it may cause patients with advanced heart disease and end-stage lung disease to approach their maximal work effort.[48,51] In patients with advanced heart disease, regression equations have been used to predict peak oxygen uptake values (peak $\dot{V}O_2$).[52]

> ✎ **CLINICAL TIP**
>
> There is also a 2-minute walk test that has been used for the functional capacity assessment of patients after cardiac surgery, those patients with chronic obstructive pulmonary disease, and for persons after amputation.[53-55] Although the 2-minute walk test may lack normative data, it may be considered in places with lack of space such as in the home setting.

Procedure

Premeasure the course in a flat, straight, enclosed corridor, approximately 30 meters (100 feet) in length to minimize turns.[56] Patients should use their usual walking aid and footwear and have rested in a chair for 10 minutes before the start of the test. For standardization of the test, patients are encouraged to carry their own oxygen source, are asked not to talk to anyone during the test, and are not followed by the clinician during the test. Standardized encouragement, or lack thereof, has been shown to influence the results of the walking test.[57] Standard encouragement, if used, should be said with a normal tone and identify only the time left (i.e., "You have 2 minutes left. You are doing a good job").[57] The standardized initial instructions to the patient, according to the American Thoracic Society (ATS), can be found in Box 23-2.

Although following ATS guidelines is preferred, it is recommended that the performance of the 6MWT in the acute setting be altered to maximize patient safety in recognition of the larger potential for medical or physical variability in this patient population. During the test, it is recommended that the

BOX 23-2 Standardized Instructions for the 6-Minute Walk Test

"The object of this test is to walk as far as possible for 6 minutes. You will walk back and forth in this hallway. Six minutes is a long time to walk, so you will be exerting yourself. You will probably get out of breath or become exhausted. You are permitted to slow down, to stop, and to rest as necessary. You may lean against the wall while resting, but resume walking as soon as you are able. You will be walking back and forth around the cones. You should pivot briskly around the cones and continue back the other way without hesitation. Now I'm going to show you. Please watch the way I turn without hesitation." Demonstrate by walking one lap yourself. Walk and pivot around a cone briskly. "Are you ready to do that? I am going to use this counter to keep track of the number of laps you complete. I will click it each time you turn around at this starting line. Remember that the object is to walk AS FAR AS POSSIBLE for 6 minutes, but don't run or jog. Start now or whenever you are ready."

From American Thoracic Society Board of Directors: ATS Statement: Guidelines for the six-minute walk test, Am J Resp Crit Care Med 166:111-117, 2002.

TABLE 23-9 Prediction Equations for 6-Minute Walk Test Distance

Author	Equation
Enright, 1998[63]	Healthy men between 40 and 80 years of age Expected 6 MWD = (7.57 × height in cm) − (5.02 × age) − (1.76 × weight in kg) − 309 meters Healthy women between 40 and 80 years of age Expected 6 MWD = (2.11 × height in cm) − (2.29 × weight in kg) − (5.78 × age) + 667 meters
Troosters, 1999[64]	Age range = 50 to 85 years of age Expected 6 MWD = 218 + (5.14 × height in cm − 5.32 × age) − (1.80 × weight in kg + (51.31 × gender*) *Male = 1, female = 0
Gibbons, 2001[65]	Age range = 22 to 79 years of age Expected 6 MWD = 868.8 − (2.99 × age) − (74.7 × gender*) *Male = 0, female = 1
Enright, 2003[66]	Age range greater than or equal to 65 years of age Healthy women: Expected 6 MWD = 493 + (2.2 × height in cm) − (0.93 × weight in kg) − (5.3 × age) Healthy men: Add 17 meters to results of above equation

6 MWD, 6-Minute walk distance.

therapist walk slightly behind the patient to allow close monitoring of heart rate (HR) and saturation of peripheral oxygen (SpO_2), but also to guard the patient if necessary. Because of the potential for variations in vital signs from baseline values, HR, SpO_2, respiratory rate (RR), rate of perceived exertion (RPE), and rate of perceived dyspnea (RPD) should be monitored every 2 minutes and for at least 2 minutes after the test has terminated to assess patient recovery. If the patient is unable to complete the full 6 minutes, then the distance covered on termination is measured along with establishing the reason for termination by the patient.

✎ CLINICAL TIP

Although the 6MWT was initially performed in a 30-meter hallway, studies have attempted to validate the test in other formats such as on a treadmill for space, safety, and monitoring issues frequently found in the acute care patient population. The conclusions reached in the literature thus far are currently mixed regarding a 6MWT performed on a treadmill.[58-61] It is important to consider the validity and patient safety when choosing how to perform the 6MWT.

Interpretation of Results

Many studies have examined the usefulness of the 6-minute walk test in specific populations and have found it to be effective in predicting oxygen consumption and determining the efficacy of surgical intervention on functional mobility.[49,50,52,62] A number of regression equations have been developed to predict 6-minute walk test distance in healthy adults (Table 23-9).[63-66] These prediction equations can be used by physical therapists as a means of determining the level of deficits in their patients and ultimately in prescribing exercise and measuring progress in patients' functional activity tolerance. A minimal change in walking distance of 54 to 70 meters has been shown to be clinically significant for improving functional status for patients with chronic obstructive pulmonary disease (COPD).[67] For frail, elderly patients with chronic heart failure the 6-minute walk test is a responsive measure of cardiac status.[68]

Incremental or Ramp Exercise Tests

In the case of persons who are not sufficiently challenged during time-based exercise testing, an incremental or ramp exercise test should be considered. Most incremental exercise test protocols described in the literature, such as the Bruce Protocol, may be too challenging even at the initial stage for the inpatient population. Modified incremental tests however, such as the Modified Balke-Ware, should be considered for special patient populations.

The Modified Balke-Ware consists of nine stages at a constant velocity of 5.6 kph (approximately 3.47 mph) while increasing the elevation from 6% to 22% in 2% increments each minute.[69] Modified tests, such as the Modified Balke-Ware, have lower initial workloads, thus reducing the floor effect while efficiently increasing the workload in a short period of time to both engage the aerobic pathways and reduce the impact of a ventilation impairment to performance. For example, most persons with cystic fibrosis admitted to the hospital for an exacerbation of their illness may not be challenged sufficiently by the 6MWT but are significantly challenged during the Modified Balke-Ware treadmill test.

Conclusion

Functional tests are quick and useful tools by which a clinician can objectively measure change in a patient's performance over time. The clinician is encouraged to review recent literature as the body of evidence for established functional tests grows and new tests are described. With the increasing push to provide efficient and effective care across health care, physical therapists need to continue to objectively document how we positively affect patient performance while reducing the overall cost of care.

References

1. American Physical Therapy Association: Evidence and research. http://www.apta.org/EvidenceResearch. Accessed February 16, 2012.
2. Brigham & Women's Hospital Department of Rehabilitation Services: Physical therapy standards. http://www.brighamandwomens.org/Patients_Visitors/pcs/rehabilitationservices/StandardsofCare.aspx?sub=1. Accessed February 16, 2012.
3. Portney LG, Watkins MP, editors: Foundations of clinical research applications to practice, Norwalk, CT, 1993, Appleton & Lange, pp 680, 689.
4. Wee JYM, Bagg SD, Palepu A: The Berg Balance Scale as a predictor of length of stay and discharge destination in an acute stroke rehabilitation setting, Arch Phys Med Rehabil 80(4):448-452, 1999.
5. Cattaneo D, Regola A, Meotti M: Validity of six balance disorders scales in persons with multiple sclerosis, Disabil Rehabil 28(12):789-795, 2006.
6. Chou CY, Chien CW, Hsueh IP et al: Developing a short form of the Berg Balance Scale for people with stroke, Phys Ther 86:195-204, 2006.
7. Nakamura DM, Holm MB, Wilson A: Measures of balance and fear of falling in the elderly: a review, Phys Occup Ther Geriatr 15(4):17-32, 1998.
8. Berg KO, Wood-Dauphinee SL, Williams JI et al: Measuring balance in the elderly: validation of an instrument, Can J Public Health 83:S7-S11, 1992.
9. Berg K, Wood-Dauphinee S, Williams JI et al: Measuring Balance in the elderly: preliminary development of an instrument, Physiother Can 41:304, 1989.
10. Muir SW, Berg K, Chesworth B et al: Use of the Berg Balance Score for predicting multiple falls in community-dwelling elderly people: a prospective study, Phys Ther 88(4);449-459, 2008.
11. Conradsson M, Lundin-Olsson L, Lindelof N et al: Berg Balance Scale: intrarater test-retest reliability among older people dependent in activities of daily living and living in residential care facilities, Phys Ther 87:1155-1163, 2007.
12. Whitney S, Poole J, Cass S: A review of balance instruments for older adults, Am J Occup Ther 52(8):666-671, 1998.
13. Posiadlo D, Richardson S: The timed "up and go": a test of basic functional mobility for frail elderly persons, J Am Geriatr Soc 39:142-148, 1991.
14. Thompson M, Medley A: performance of community dwelling elderly on the timed up and go test, Phys Occup Ther Geriatr 13(3):17-30, 1995.
15. White J: Functional assessment tools-use them! Phys Ther Case Rep 3(4):188-189, 2000.
16. Large J, Gan N, Basic D et al: Using the timed up and go test to stratify elderly inpatients at risk of falls, Clin Rehabil 20:421-428, 2006.
17. Kristensen MT, Foss NB, Kehlet H: Timed "up & go" test as a predictor of falls within 6 months after hip fracture surgery, Phys Ther 87:24-30, 2007.
18. Nordin E, Rosendahl E, Lundin-Olsson L: Timed "up & go" test: reliability in older people dependent in activities of daily living-focus on cognitive state, Phys Ther 86(5):646-655, 2006.
19. Duncan PW, Weiner DK, Chandler J et al: Functional reach: a new clinical measure of balance, J Gerontol 45:M192-M197, 1990.
20. Newton R: Reach in four directions as a measure of stability in older adults, Phys Ther 76:S23, 1996.
21. Billek-Sawbney B, Gay J: The functional reach test; are 3 trials necessary? Top Geriatr Rehabil 21(2):144-148, 2005.
22. Umphred DA, editor: Neurological rehabilitation, ed 3, St Louis, 1995, Mosby, pp 808-809, 812, 816-817, 822-823, 828-829.
23. Tinetti ME: Performance oriented assessment of mobility problems in elderly patients, J Am Geriatr Soc 41:479, 1986.
24. Tinetti ME, Williams TF, Mayewski R: Fall index for elderly patients based on number of chronic disabilities, Am J Med 80:429-434, 1986.
25. Csuka M, McCarty DJ: Simple method for measurement of lower extremity muscle strength, Am J Med 78:77-81, 1985.
26. Lord SR, Murray SM, Chapman K et al: Sit-to-stand performance depends on sensation, speed, balance, and psychological status in addition to strength in older people, J Am Geriatr Soc 57:M539-M543, 2002.
27. Bohannon RW: Alternatives for measuring knee extension strength of the elderly at home, Clin Rehabil 12:434-440, 1998.
28. Bohannon RW, Smith J, Hull D et al: Deficits in lower extremity muscle and gait performance among renal transplant candidates, Arch Phys Med Rehabil 76:547-551, 1995.
29. Cheng PT, Liaw MY, Wong MK et al: The sit-to-stand movement in stroke patients and its correlation with falling, Arch Phys Med Rehabil 79:1043-1046, 1998.
30. Hughes C, Osman C, Woods AK: Relationship among performance on stair ambulation, functional reach, and Timed Up and Go tests in older adults, Issues Aging 21:18-22, 1998.
31. Newcomer KL, Krug HE, Mahowald ML: Validity and reliability of the timed-stands test for patients with rheumatoid arthritis and other chronic diseases, J Rheumatol 20:21-27, 1993.
32. Bohannon RW, Shove ME, Barreca SR et al: Five-repetition sit-to-stand performance by community-dwelling adults: a preliminary investigation of times, determinants, and relationship with self-reported physical performance, Isokinet Exerc Sci 15(2):77-81, 2007.
33. Judge JO, Schechtman K, Cress E: The relationship between physical performance measures and independence in instrumental activities of daily living, J Am Geriatr Soc 44:1332-1341, 1996.
34. Whitney SL, Wristley DM, Marchietti GF et al: Clinical measurement of sit-to-stand performance in people with balance disorders: validity of data for the five-times-sit-to-stand test, Phys Ther 85(10):1034-1045, 2005.
35. Bohannon RW: Reference values for the five-repetition sit-to-stand test: a descriptive meta-analysis of data from elders, Percept Motor Skills 103:215-222, 2006.
36. Guralnik JM, Simonsick EM, Ferrucci L et al: A short physical performance batter assessing lower extremity function: associated with self-reported disability and prediction of mortality and nursing home admission, J Gerontol 49:M85-M94, 1994.

37. Puthoff ML: Research corner outcome measures in cardiopulmonary physical therapy: short physical performance battery, Phys Ther 19(1):17-22, 2008.

38. Ostir GV, Volpato S, Fried LP et al: Reliability and sensitivity to change assessed for a summary measure of lower body function: results from the Women's Health and Aging Study, Clin Epidemiol 55:916-921, 2002.

39. Wolinsky FD, Miller TR, Malmstrom TK et al: Four year lower extremity disability trajectories among African American men and women, J Gerontol A Biol Sci Med Sci 62:525-530, 2007.

40. Ostir CV, Markides KS, Black SA et al: Lower body functioning as a predictor of subsequent disability among older Mexican Americans, J Gerontol A Biol Sci Med Sci 53:M491-M495, 1998.

41. Guralnik JM, Ferrucci L, Simonsick EM et al: Lower-extremity function in persons over the age of 70 years as a predictor of subsequent disability, N Engl J Med 332:556-561, 1995.

42. Perera S, Mody SH, Woodman RC et al: Meaningful change and responsiveness in common physical performance measures in older adults, Am Geriatr Soc 54:743-749, 2006.

43. Roach KE, Van Dillen LR: Reliability and validity of the Acute Care Index of Function for patients with neurologic impairment, Phys Ther 68(7):1098-1101, 1988.

44. Scherer SA, Hammerick AS: Research corner outcomes in cardiopulmonary physical therapy: acute care index of function, Cardiopulm Phys Ther J 19(3):94-97, 2008.

45. Roach KE, Ally D, Finnerty B et al: The relationship between duration of physical therapy services in the acute care setting and change in functional status in patients with lower-extremity orthopedic problems, Phys Ther 78(1):19-24, 1998.

46. Balady GJ, Arena R, Sietsema K et al: Clinician's guide to cardiopulmonary exercise testing in adults: a scientific statement from the American Heart Association, Circulation 122:191-225, 2010.

47. American College of Sports Medicine: ACSM's guidelines for exercise testing and prescription, ed 8, Philadelphia, 2010, Lippincott Williams & Wilkins.

48. Guyatt GH, Sullivan MJ, Thompson PJ et al: The 6-minute walk: new measure of exercise capacity in patients with chronic heart failure, Can Med Assoc J 132:919-923, 1985.

49. McGavin CR, Gupta SP, McHardy GJR: Twelve-minute walking test for assessing disability in chronic bronchitis, BMJ 1:822, 1976.

50. Butland RJ, Pang J, Gross ER et al: Two-, six-, and twelve-minute walking tests in respiratory disease, BMJ 284:1607, 1982.

51. Olsson LG, Swedberg K, Clark AL et al: Six minute corridor walk test as an outcome measure for the assessment of treatment in randomized, blinded intervention trials of chronic heart failure: a systematic review, Eur Heart J 26(8):778-793, 2005.

52. Cahalin LP, Mathier MA, Semigran MJ et al: The six-minute walk test predicts peak oxygen uptake and survival in patients with advanced heart failure, Chest 110:310, 1996.

53. Leung ASY, Chan KK, Sykes K et al: Reliability, validity, and responsiveness of a 2-minute walk test to assess exercise capacity of COPD patients, Chest 130(1):119-125, 2006.

54. Brooks D, Parsons J, Tran D et al: The two-minute walk test as a measure of functional capacity in cardiac surgery patients, Arch Phys Med Rehabil 85(9):1525-1530, 2004.

55. Brooks D, Hunter JP, Parsons J et al: Reliability of the two-minute walk test in individuals with transtibial amputation, Arch Phys Med Rehabil 83(11):1562-1565, 2002.

56. American Thoracic Society Board of Directors: ATS statement: Guidelines for the six-minute walk test, Am J Respir Crit Care Med 166:111-117, 2002.

57. Guyatt GH, Pugsley SO, Sullivan MJ et al: Effect of encouragement on walking test performance, Thorax 39:818-822, 1994.

58. Stevens D, Elpern E, Sharma K et al: Comparison of hallway and treadmill six-minute walk tests, Am J Respir Crit Care Med 160(5 Pt 1):1540-1543, 1999.

59. Camargo VM, do Carmo dos Santos Martins B, Jardim C et al: Validation of a treadmill six-minute walk test protocol for the evaluation of patients with pulmonary arterial hypertension, J Bras Pneumol 35(5):423-430, 2009.

60. de Almeida FG, Victor EG, Rizzo JA: Hallway versus treadmill 6-minute-walk tests in patients with chronic obstructive pulmonary disease, Respir Care 54(12):1712-1716, 2009.

61. Olper L, Cervi P, De Santi F et al: Validation of the treadmill six-minute walk test in people following cardiac surgery, Phys Ther 91(4):566-576, 2011.

62. Laupacis A, Bourne R, Rorabeck C et al: The effect of elective total hip replacement on health-related quality of life, J Bone Joint Surg [Am] 75:1619, 1993.

63. Enright PL, Sherrill DL: Reference equations for the six minute walk in healthy adults, Am J Respir Crit Care Med 158:1384-1387, 1998.

64. Troosters T, Gosselink R, Decramer M: Six minute walking distance in healthy elderly subjects, Eur Respir J 14:270-274, 1999.

65. Gibbons WJ, Fruchter N, Sloan S et al: Reference values for a multiple repetition 6-minute walk test in healthy adults older than 20 years, J Cardiopulm Rehabil 21:87-93, 2001.

66. Enright PL, McBurnie MA, Bittner V et al: The 6 minute walk test: a quick measure of functional status in elderly adults, Chest 123:387-398, 2003.

67. Redelmeier DA, Bayoumi AM, Goldstein RS et al: Interpreting small differences in functional status: the six minute walk test in chronic lung patients, Am J Respir Crit Care Med 155:1278-1282, 1997.

68. O'Keefe ST, Lye M, Donnellan C et al: Reproducibility and responsiveness of quality of life assessment and six minute walk test in elderly heart failure patients, Heart 80:377-382, 1998.

69. Marinov B, Kostianev S, Turnovska T: Submaximal treadmill test for screening of physical capacity in pediatric age group, Pediatria 15(2):38-41, 2000.

APPENDIX 23A. FUNCTIONAL TESTS

A. Performance Oriented Mobility Assessment I

Element	Scoring
Balance	Instructions: Subject is seated in hard, armless chair. The following maneuvers are tested.
1. Sitting balance	2 = Steady, stable 1 = Holds onto chair to keep upright 0 = Leans, slides down in chair
2. Arising from chair	2 = Able to rise in a single movement without use of arms 1 = Uses arms (on chair or walking aid) to pull or push up; and/or moves forward in chair before attempting to arise 0 = Multiple attempts required or unable without human assistance
3. Immediate standing balance (first 5 seconds)	2 = Steady without holding onto walking aid or other object for support 1 = Steady, but uses walking aid or other object for support 0 = Any sign of unsteadiness
4. Standing balance	2 = Steady, able to stand with feet together without holding object for support 1 = Steady, but cannot put feet together 0 = Any sign of unsteadiness regardless of stance or holds onto object
5. Balance with eyes closed (with feet as close together as possible)	2 = Steady without holding onto any object with feet together 1 = Steady with feet apart 0 = Any sign of unsteadiness or needs to hold onto an object
6. Turning balance (360 degrees)	2 = No grabbing or staggering; no need to hold onto any objects; steps are continuous (turn is a flowing movement) 1 = Steps are discontinuous (patient puts one foot completely on floor before raising other foot) 0 = Any sign of unsteadiness or holds onto an object
7. Nudge on sternum (patient standing with feet as close together as possible, examiner pushes with light even pressure over sternum three times)	2 = Steady, able to withstand pressure 1 = Needs to move feet, but able to maintain balance 0 = Begins to fall, or examiner has to help maintain balance
8. Neck turning (patient asked to turn to side and look up while standing with feet as close together as possible)	2 = Able to turn head at least halfway side to side and able to bend head back to look at ceiling; no staggering, grabbing, or symptoms of lightheadedness, unsteadiness, or pain 1 = Decreased ability to turn side to side or to extend neck, but no staggering, grabbing, or symptoms of lightheadedness, unsteadiness, or pain 0 = Any sign of unsteadiness or symptoms when turning head or extending neck
9. One leg standing balance	2 = Able to stand on one leg for 5 seconds without holding object for support 1 = Some staggering, swaying, or moves foot slightly 0 = Unable
10. Back extension (ask patient to lean back as far as possible, without holding onto object)	2 = Good extension without holding object or staggering 1 = Tries to extend, but decreased range of motion (compared with other patients of same age) or needs to hold object to attempt extension 0 = Will not attempt or no extension seen or staggers
11. Reaching up (have patient attempt to remove an object from a shelf high enough to require stretching or standing on toes)	2 = Able to take down object without needing to hold onto other object for support and without becoming unsteady 1 = Able to get object but needs to steady self by holding onto something for support 0 = Unable or unsteady
12. Bending down (patient is asked to pick up small objects [e.g., a pen] from the floor)	2 = Able to bend down and pick up the object and able to get up easily in a single attempt without needing to pull self up with arms 1 = Able to get object and get upright in a single attempt but needs to pull self up with arms or hold onto something for support 0 = Unable to bend down or unable to get upright after bending down, or takes multiple attempts to become upright
13. Sitting down	2 = Able to sit down in one smooth movement 1 = Needs to use arms to guide self into chair, or movement is not smooth 0 = Falls into chair, misjudges distances (lands off center)

A. Performance Oriented Mobility Assessment I—cont'd

Element	Scoring
Gait	Instructions: Subject stands with examiner, then walks 15 ft down a premeasured hallway, turns, and walks back to starting point. Subject should use customary walking aid as necessary.
1. Initiation of gait (patient is asked to begin walking down hallway)	1 = Begins walking immediately without observable hesitation; initiation of gait is single, smooth motion 0 = Hesitates; multiple attempts; initiation of gait is not a smooth motion
2. Step height (begin observing after first few steps; observe one foot, then the other; observe from side)	1 = Swing foot completely clears floor but by no more than 1 to 2 inches 0 = Swing foot is not completely raised off floor (may hear scraping) or is raised too high (>2 inches)
3. Step length (observe distance between toe of stance foot and heel of swing foot; observe from side; do not judge first few or last few steps; observe one side at a time)	1 = At least the length of individual's foot between the stance toe and swing heel (step length usually longer, but foot length provides basis for observation) 0 = Step length less than the individual's foot
4. Step symmetry (observe the middle part of walking, not the first or last steps; observe from side; observe distance between heel of each swing foot and toe of each stance foot)	1 = Step length same or nearly same on both sides for most step cycles 0 = Step length varies between sides or patient advances with same foot with every step
5. Step continuity	1 = Begins raising heel of one foot (toe off) as heel of other foot touches the floor (heel strike); no breaks or stops in stride; step lengths equal over most cycles 0 = Places entire foot (heel and toe) on floor before beginning to raise other foot; or stops completely between steps; or step length varies over cycles
6. Path deviation (observe from behind; observe one foot over several strides; observe in relation to line on floor [e.g., tiles] if possible; difficult to assess if patient uses a walker)	2 = Foot follows close to straight line as patient advances 1 = Foot deviates from side to side or toward one direction, or patient uses a walking aid 0 = Marked deviation from straight line
7. Trunk stability (observe from behind; side to side motion of trunk may be a normal gait pattern, need to differentiate this from instability)	2 = Trunk does not sway; knees or back are not flexed; arms are not abducted in effort to maintain stability 1 = No sway but flexion of knees or back or spreads arms out while walking 0 = Any of the preceding features are present
8. Walk stance (observe from behind)	1 = Feet should almost touch as one passes the other 0 = Feet apart with stepping
9. Turning while walking	2 = No staggering or use of a walking aid; turning is continuous with walking; and steps are continuous while turning 1 = Steps are discontinuous but no staggering, or uses walking aid 0 = Staggers; unsteady; stops before initiating turn

Data from Tinetti ME: Performance-oriented assessment of mobility problems in elderly patients, J Am Geriatr Soc 34:119-126, 1986; Tinetti ME, Williams TF, Mayewski R: Fall index for elderly patients based on number of chronic disabilities, Am J Med 80:429-434, 1986.

B. Short Physical Performance Battery

Directions for the Short Physical Performance Battery

Balance Subscale

Side by side – Patient will stand with feet together, side by side for up to 10 seconds. Patient may use arms, bend knees or move body to maintain balance, but may not move feet. First demonstrate the position to the patient. Then stand next to the patient to help him or her into the side-by-side position. Supply just enough support to the patient's arm to prevent loss of balance. When the patient has his or her feet together and is ready, let go and begin timing as you say, "Ready, begin." Stop the stopwatch and say "stop" after 10 seconds or when the patient steps out of position or grabs your arm. If patient is unable to hold the position for 10 seconds, record results, and go to the next subscale. If patient can maintain for 10 seconds, go onto the next posture.

Semi-tandem – Patient will stand with feet together, the toes of one foot aligned with the midpoint of the other foot. Follow the same directions as in the side by side stand. If patient is unable to hold the position for 10 seconds, record results, and go to the next subscale. If patient can maintain for 10 seconds, go onto the next posture.

Tandem – Patient will stand with one foot in front of the other with the heel of the front foot in contact with the toes of the back foot. Follow the same directions as in the side by side stand. Record results, and go to the next subscale.

Four Meter Walk Subscale

Mark off a four meter (13.12 foot) course with two cones or pieces of tape. The patient will start at one end of the course. Instruct the patient to walk at their normal pace as if they are walking down the street or going to the store. The patient will begin walking on the command "begin." Patient should walk past the other end of the course and not slow down until outside the four meter marker. Start on "begin" and stop timing when one of the patient's feet is all the way across the four meter marker. Walk behind and to the side of the patient. Patients are allowed to use a cane or any other walking device they normally use. Patient should repeat this walk twice, with the best time used for scoring.

Sit to Stand Subscale

Single Chair Stand – The patient should be seated in a standard height chair. The patient should fold arms across chest and sit so feet are resting on the floor. Ask the patient to stand while keeping arms folded across the chest. If patient cannot stand without using arms, the test is over. Record results on the score sheet. If patient can complete the stand, go onto the five chair stands.

Five Chair Stands – Instruct patient that you will now time how long it takes to complete five chair stands. Patient starts with arms folded across chest and sits so feet are resting on the floor. On the command "begin," patient should stand up straight as quickly as possible, sit back down and repeat for a total of five times. Count out loud as the patient completes each stand. Start timing on "begin" and stop the stopwatch when the patient has straightened up completely for the fifth time. Stop the test if the patient becomes tired, short of breath, uses arms, or one minute has passed without all five stands completed.

Directions adapted from Guralnik JM, Ferrucci L, Pieper CF, et al: Lower extremity function and subsequent disability: consistency across studies, predictive models, and value of gait speed alone compared with the short physical performance battery, *J Gerontol A Biol Sci Med Sci* 55:M221-231, 2000.

B. Short Physical Performance Battery—cont'd

Score Sheet for the Short Physical Performance Battery

Patient Name: _____

Date: _____

Balance Score

Unable to hold side by side stance for > 9 seconds	0 points
Side by side stance for 10 sec, but unable to hold semitandem for 10 sec	1 point
Semitandem for 10 sec, unable to hold full tandem for > 2 sec	2 points
Full tandem for 3-9 sec	3 points
Full tandem for 10 sec	4 points

Walk Score (4 Meter or 13.12 feet)

Unable to walk		0 points
If time is more than 8.70 seconds		1 point
If time is 6.21 to 8.70 seconds	Time 1: _____	2 points
If time is 4.82 to 6.20 seconds		3 points
If time is less than 4.82 seconds	Time 2: _____	4 points

Chair Stand Score

If the participant was unable to complete the 5 chair stands		0 points
If chair stand time is 16.7 seconds or more		1 point
If chair stand time is 13.7 to 16.6 seconds		2 points
If chair stand time is 11.2 to 13.6 seconds		3 points
If chair stand time is 11.1 seconds or less	Time: _____	4 points

Total Score _____
Converted Gait Velocity (13.12/time in seconds)*0.68 = mph _____

Date: _____

Balance Score

Unable to hold side by side stance for > 9 seconds	0 points
Side by side stance for 10 sec, but unable to hold semitandem for 10 sec	1 point
Semitandem for 10 sec, unable to hold full tandem for > 2 sec	2 points
Full tandem for 3-9 sec	3 points
Full tandem for 10 sec	4 points

Walk Score (4 Meter or 13.12 feet)

Unable to walk		0 points
If time is more than 8.70 seconds		1 point
If time is 6.21 to 8.70 seconds	Time 1: _____	2 points
If time is 4.82 to 6.20 seconds		3 points
If time is less than 4.82 seconds	Time 2: _____	4 points

Chair Stand Score

If the participant was unable to complete the 5 chair stands		0 points
If chair stand time is 16.7 seconds or more		1 point
If chair stand time is 13.7 to 16.6 seconds		2 points
If chair stand time is 11.2 to 13.6 seconds		3 points
If chair stand time is 11.1 seconds or less	Time: _____	4 points

Total Score _____
Converted Gait Velocity (13.12/time in seconds)*0.68 = mph _____

From Puthoff ML: Outcome measures in cardiopulmonary physical therapy: short physical performance battery, Cardiopulm Phys Ther J 19(1):17-22, 2008.

APPENDIX A

Preferred Practice Patterns

Musculoskeletal

4A: Primary Prevention/Risk Reduction for Skeletal Demineralization

4B: Impaired Posture

4C: Impaired Muscle Performance

4D: Impaired Joint Mobility, Motor Function, Muscle Performance, and Range of Motion Associated with Connective Tissue Dysfunction

4E: Impaired Joint Mobility, Motor Function, Muscle Performance, and Range of Motion Associated with Localized Inflammation

4F: Impaired Joint Mobility, Motor Function, Muscle Performance, and Range of Motion and Reflex Integrity Associated with Spinal Disorders

4G: Impaired Joint Mobility, Muscle Performance, and Range of Motion Associated with Fracture

4H: Impaired Joint Mobility, Motor Function, Muscle Performance, and Range of Motion Associated with Joint Arthroplasty

4I: Impaired Joint Mobility, Motor Function, Muscle Performance, and Range of Motion Associated with Bony or Soft Tissue Surgery

4J: Impaired Motor Function, Muscle Performance, Range of Motion, Gait, Locomotion, and Balance Associated with Amputation

Neuromuscular

5A: Primary Prevention/Risk Reduction for Loss of Balance and Falling

5B: Impaired Neuromotor Development

5C: Impaired Motor Function and Sensory Integrity Associated with Nonprogressive Disorders of the Central Nervous System—Congenital Origin or Acquired in Infancy or Childhood

5D: Impaired Motor Function and Sensory Integrity Associated with Nonprogressive Disorders of the Central Nervous System—Acquired in Adolescence or Adulthood

5E: Impaired Motor Function and Sensory Integrity Associated with Progressive Disorders of the Central Nervous System

5F: Impaired Peripheral Nerve Integrity and Muscle Performance Associated with Peripheral Nerve Injury

5G: Impaired Motor Function and Sensory Integrity Associated with Acute or Chronic Polyneuropathies

5H: Impaired Motor Function, Peripheral Nerve Integrity and Sensory Integrity Associated with Non-progressive Disorders of the Spinal Cord

5I: Impaired Arousal, Range of Motion and Motor Control Associated with Coma, Near Coma, or Vegetative State

Cardiovascular/Pulmonary

6A: Primary Prevention/Risk Reduction for Cardiovascular/Pulmonary Disorders

6B: Impaired Aerobic Capacity/Endurance Associated with Deconditioning

6C: Impaired Ventilation, Respiration/Gas Exchange, and Aerobic Capacity/Endurance Associated with Airway Clearance Dysfunction

6D: Impaired Aerobic Capacity/Endurance Associated with Cardiovascular Pump Dysfunction or Failure

6E: Impaired Ventilation and Respiration/Gas Exchange Associated with Ventilatory Pump Dysfunction or Failure

6F: Impaired Ventilation and Respiration/Gas Exchange Associated with Respiratory Failure

6G: Impaired Ventilation, Respiration/Gas Exchange, and Aerobic Capacity/Endurance Associated with Respiratory Failure in the Neonate

6H: Impaired Circulation and Anthropometric Dimensions Associated with Lymphatic System Disorders

Integumentary

7A: Primary Prevention/Risk Reduction for Integumentary Disorders

7B: Impaired Integumentary Integrity Associated with Superficial Skin Involvement

7C: Impaired Integumentary Integrity Associated with Partial-Thickness Skin Involvement and Scar Formation

7D: Impaired Integumentary Integrity Associated with Full-Thickness Skin Involvement and Scar Formation

7E: Impaired Integumentary Integrity Associated with Skin Involvement Extending into Fascia, Muscle, or Bone and Scar Formation

From APTA: Guide to physical therapist practice, revised second edition, Alexandria, VA, 2003, American Physical Therapy Association.

Index

A

Abacavir (Ziagen, ABC), for HIV/AIDS, 441t-443t

Abarelix (Plenaxis), in chemotherapy, 430t-432t

Abatacept (Orencia), for rheumatoid arthritis, 421t-423t

Abbreviations, prohibitive, 12t

Abciximab (ReoPro), as antiplatelet agent, 417t

Abdomen, quadrants of, 204f

Abdominal aortic aneurysm, 174

Abdominal excursion measurement, 62

Abducens nerve (CN VI), 134t-135t

ABGs. *See* Arterial blood gas(es) (ABGs).

AbioCor Implantable Replacment Heart, 405-406

AbioNed AB 5000 ventricular assist device, 404t

Abiraterone (Zytiga), in chemotherapy, 430t-432t

Ablation procedures, for rhythm disturbances, 37

Acarbose (Precose), for hyperglycemia, 445t-447t

Acebutolol (Sectral), as antihypertensive, 413t-415t

Acetabulum fractures, 94-95, 95f

Acetaminophen (paracetamol), in pain management, 460

Acetazolamide (Diamox), as antihypertensive, 413t-415t

Acetylsalicylic acid (Bayer), in pain management, 462t

Achalasia, 209

Acid-base imbalances, causes of, 64t

Acidosis, causes of, 64t

Acquired immunodeficiency syndrome (AIDS)
complications from, 326t
drugs for, 441t-443t

Acromegaly, 247-248

ACTH. *See* Adrenocorticotropic hormone (ACTH).

Actinobacter baumannii, multidrug-resistant, 318-319

Activity
patient response to, evaluating, 40-41, 41f-42f
progression of, in respiratory dysfunction, 81

Activity tolerance, monitoring, 41-43

Acute care setting, 1-9
end-of-life issues in, 6-7
intensive care unit in, 5-6. *See also* Intensive care unit (ICU).
medical-surgical equipment in, 371-408. *See also* Medical-surgical equipment, in acute care setting.
pain management in, 459-463. *See also* Pain, management of.
safe caregiver and patient environment in, 1-5

Page numbers followed by f indicate figures; t, tables; b, boxes.

Acute care setting (*Continued*)
sleep pattern disturbance in, 6
substance abuse and withdrawal in, 6

Acute contagious osteomyelitis, 323

Acute coronary syndrome, 31-32, 31t, 32f

Acute graft rejection, 338-339

Acute hematogenous osteomyelitis, 323

Acute inflammatory demyelinating polyradiculopathy, 153

Acute interstitial nephritis, 232

Acute kidney injury (AKI), 229-230, 230t

Acute pyelonephritis, 231

Acute quadriplegic myopathy, 5-6

Acute vestibular neuronitis, 153

Acyclovir (Zovirax), for viral illnesses, 444t

Adalimumab (Humira), for rheumatoid arthritis, 421t-423t

Adaptive support ventilation, 394t

Addison's disease, 251

Adenoma, thyroid, hyperthyroidism from, 246t

Adenosine (Adenocard, Adenoscan), for arrhythmias, 411t

ADH. *See* Antidiuretic hormone (ADH).

Admission note format, 13

Adrenal cortical hormones, tests of, 249-250, 250t

Adrenal gland, 249-251
disorders of, 251-258
hormones of, target sites and actions of, 250t
structure and function of, 249, 250t

Adrenal hyperfunction, 250

Adrenal insufficiency, 251

Adrenal medulla
hormones of, tests of, 243-244, 250t
tumor of, pheochromocytoma from, 251

Adrenergic agonists, as antihypertensives, 413t-415t

Adrenergic antagonists, as antihypertensives, 413t-415t

Adrenocortical steroids, for respiratory disorders, 419t

Adrenocorticotropic hormone (ACTH)
overproduction of, 248
tests of, 248t

Adult respiratory distress syndrome (ARDS), 75t, 76

Adventitious breath sounds, 61

Afterload, cardiac output and, 18

Age, wound healing and, 299

Agonal rhythm, ECG characteristics and causes of, 47t

AIDS
complications from, 326t
drugs for, 441t-443t

Air entrainment mask, in oxygen delivery, 375t, 376f

Air trapping, in respiratory dysfunction, 68

Airway clearance techniques, 80

Airway injury, thermal, 291

Airway pressure release ventilation (APRV), 394t

Alanine aminotransferase (ALT), in hepatic testing, 207t-208t

Albumin, clinical indications and outcomes for, 191t

Albuterol (Proventil, Ventolin), as bronchodilator, 420t

Alcohol use disorders, in acute care setting, 6

Aldesleukin (Proleukin), in chemotherapy, 430t-432t

Aldosterone
cardiac effects of, 19t
target sites and actions of, 250t

Alemtuzumab (Campath), in chemotherapy, 430t-432t

Alendronate (Fosamax, Fosamax plus D), for osteoporosis, 448t

Alert state, 132t

Alfuzosin (Uroxatral), for benign prostatic hyperplasia, 436t

Aliskiren (Tekturna), as antihypertensive, 413t-415t

Alkaline phosphatase, in hepatic and biliary testing, 207t-208t

Alkaline phosphatase isoenzymes, in hepatic and biliary testing, 207t-208t

Alkalosis, causes of, 64t

Alkylating agents, in chemotherapy, 430t-432t

Allen's test, in vascular evaluation, 165t-166t

Allergic rhinitis, 319

Allergy, latex, 3

AlloDerm, in burn and wound treatment, 293t

Allogenic graft, for burns, 292t

Allograft, for burns, 292t

Alpha-1 blockers, for benign prostatic hyperplasia, 436t

Alpha fetoprotein, in hepatic and biliary testing, 207t-208t

Alpha-glucosidase inhibitors, for hyperglycemia, 445t-447t

5-Alpha-reductase inhibitors, for benign prostatic hyperplasia, 436t

Alprazolam (Xanax), as antianxiety medication, 424t

Alteplast (Activase, Cathflo), as thrombolytic, 419t

Aluminum carbonate (Badaljel), as antacid, 433t

Aluminum hydroxide (Amphojel, ALternaGEL), as antacid, 433t

Alveolar ventilation (VA), description and significance of, 70t-71t

Alveoli, description and function of, 54t

Alzheimer's disease (AD), 147-148

Amantadine (Symmetrel), for Parkinson's disease, 429t

Amebic meningoencephalitis, 323

American Spinal Injury Association (ASIA) Impairment Scale, 142, 144t

American Thoracic Society Dyspnea Scale, 58, 58t

Amikacin (Amikin), for infectious diseases, 437t-439t

Amiloride (Midamor), as antihypertensive, 413t-415t

Cefoperazone (Cefobid), for infectious diseases, 437t-439t

Cefotaxime (Claforan), for infectious diseases, 437t-439t

Cefotetan (Cefotan), for infectious diseases, 437t-439t

Cefoxitin (Mefoxin), for infectious diseases, 437t-439t

Cefpodoxime (Vantin), for infectious diseases, 437t-439t

Cefprozil (Cefzil), for infectious diseases, 437t-439t

Ceftaroline (Teflaro), for infectious diseases, 437t-439t

Ceftazidime (Fortaz), for infectious diseases, 437t-439t

Ceftibuten (Cedax), for infectious diseases, 437t-439t

Ceftizoxime (Cefizox), for infectious diseases, 437t-439t

Ceftriaxone (Rocephin), for infectious diseases, 437t-439t

Cefuroxime (Ceftin), for infectious diseases, 437t-439t

Celecoxib (Celebrex), in pain management, 462t

Cellulitis, 323

Central brain systems, 128

Central cord syndrome, 144t

Central nerve blockade, 463t

Central nervous system (CNS), 124-129
  amyotrophic lateral sclerosis and, 153
  antianxiety agents acting on, 424t
  anticonvulsants acting on, 425t
  antidepressants acting on, 426t
  antipsychotics acting on, 427t
  brain in, 124-128. *See also* Brain.
  cancers of, 277
  cerebrovascular disease/disorders and, 144-147. *See also* Cerebrovascular disease/disorders.
  degenerative diseases of, 153-154, 154b
  dementia and, 147-148
  drugs acting on, 424
  Guillain-Barré syndrome as, 153
  infections of, 322-323
  mood stabilizers acting on, 427t
  multiple sclerosis and, 154, 154b
    drugs for, 428t
  neuroinfectious diseases of, 150
  Parkinson's disease and, 154
    drugs for, 429t
  seizure and, 149, 149t
  spinal cord in, 128-129, 129f, 129t
    injury to, 142-143, 144t
  syncope and, 149-150
  traumatic brain injury and, 142, 143t
  ventricular dysfunction and, 148
  vestibular dysfunction and, 150-153, 150f, 151t-152t, 152f. *See also* Vestibular dysfunction.

Central venous catheter
  in hemodynamic monitoring, 378t-379t
  in medical-surgical management, 383t-388t
  tunneled, in medical-surgical management, 383t-388t

Cephalexin (Keflex), for infectious diseases, 437t-439t

Cephalosporins, for infectious diseases, 437t-439t

Cephapirin (Cefadyl), for infectious diseases, 437t-439t

Cephradine (Anspor), for infectious diseases, 437t-439t

Cerebellar arteries, 128t

Cerebellum, structure, function, and dysfunction of, 126t

Cerebral aneurysm, 147, 147t

Cerebral angiography, in neurologic examination, 140

Cerebral arteries, 128t

Cerebral blood flow (CBF), in brain monitoring, 382t

Cerebral hemispheres, structure, function, and dysfunction of, 125t

Cerebral microdialysis, in brain monitoring, 382t

Cerebral perfusion pressure (CPP), 155
  monitoring of, equipment for, 380-381, 381t

Cerebrospinal fluid (CSF)
  drainage of, to decrease ICP, 156t
  flow of, 125-128, 127f
  lead of, 148

Cerebrovascular accident (CVA), 144-146, 145f, 146t

Cerebrovascular disease/disorders, 144-147
  arteriovenous malformation as, 146-147
  cerebral aneurysm as, 147, 147t
  cerebrovascular accident as, 144-146, 145f, 146t
  subarachnoid hemorrhage as, 147, 147t
  transient ischemic attack as, 144

Certolizumab pegol (Cimzia), for rheumatoid arthritis, 421t-423t

Ceruloplasmin, in hepatic testing, 207t-208t

Cervical collar, 118t

Cervicothoracic orthoses, 118t

Cetirizine (Zyrtec), for respiratory disorders, 420t

Cetuximab (Erbitux), in chemotherapy, 430t-432t

CF (cystic fibrosis), 72-74, 73t

Chemical burns, 288

Chemoreceptors, 19
  in ventilatory control, 54-56

Chemotherapy, for cancer, 269-270
  drugs used in, 430t-432t
  physical therapy considerations on, 270

Chest, flail, 78

Chest pain
  angina-like, 209-210
  etiologies, patterns, and signs associated with, 368t
  incidence of, 367-368
  patients with, physical therapy considerations for, 367-369
  physiology of, 367
  preferred practice patterns for, 367
  presentation of, 368

Chest radiography. *See also* Chest X-rays (CXRs).
  in cardiac evaluation, 27

Chest tube, in medical-surgical management, 383t-388t, 389f

Chest wall excursion measurement, 62

Chest wall restrictions, 78

Chest X-rays (CXRs), in pulmonary evaluation, 66, 66f

Cheyne-Stokes respirations, description and conditions associated with, 59t

Chlordiazepoxide (Librium), as antianxiety medication, 424t

Chloroprocaine (Nesacaine), for local anesthesia, 463t

Chlorpheniramine maleate (Chlor-Trimeton), for respiratory disorders, 420t

Chlorpromazine (Thorazine), as antipsychotic, 427t

Chlorthalidone (Hygroton), as antihypertensive, 413t-415t

Chlorzoxazone (Parafon Forte), as muscle relaxant, 423t-424t

Cholangiopancreatography
  magnetic resonance, 208t
  retrograde, endoscopic, 208t

Cholecystectomy, 219

Cholecystitis, 216-217

Cholelithiasis, 216-217

Cholesterol, total, 26

Cholesterol absorption inhibitor, as lipid-lowering agent, 417t-418t

Cholestyramine (Questran), as lipid-lowering agent, 417t-418t

Choline salicylate (Arthopan), in pain management, 462t

Chordae tendineae, description and function of, 17t

Christmas disease, 187

Chromomycin, in chemotherapy, 430t-432t

Chronic graft rejection, 339

Chronic kidney disease (CKD), 230-231

Chronic osteomyelitis, 323

Chronic pyelonephritis, 231

Chronic venous insufficiency, 182-183, 182f

Cidofovir (Vistide), for viral illnesses, 444t

CIM (critical illness myopathy), 5-6

Cimetidine (Tagamet), in gastric acid suppression, 434t

Cinacalcet (Sensipar), for hyperparathyroidism, 447t

CIP (critical illness polyneuropathy), 5

Ciprofloxacin (Cipro), for infectious diseases, 437t-439t

Circle of Willis, 128, 128f

Circulation
  in brain, 128, 128f, 128t
  systemic, 19, 20f
  in wound assessment, 302

Circulatory assist devices, 397-408
  percutaneous, 398-402
    enhanced external counterpulsation as, 399, 399f
    intraaortic balloon pump as, 398-399, 398f
    percutaneous cardiopulmonary support as, 399-402. *See also* Cardiopulmonary support, percutaneous.
  surgical, 402-407
    total artificial heart as, 405-407, 406f
    ventricular assist devices as, 402-405, 403f, 404t

Circulatory complications, of musculoskeletal dysfunction, physical therapy interventions to prevent, 90

Cirrhosis, 216, 216f

Cisplatin (Platinol-AQ), in chemotherapy, 430t-432t

Citalopram (Celexa), as antidepressant, 426t

CK (creatine kinase), 26-27, 27t

Clarithromycin (Biaxin), for infectious diseases, 437t-439t

Claudication
  intermittent, in atherosclerosis, 172
  pseudoclaudication differentiated from, 173, 174t

Clavicle fractures, 85

Cleaning, wound, 304

Clemastine (Tavist), for respiratory disorders, 420t